Biological Foundations of Human Sexuality

Santa Ana
(714) 834-8187
Nat'l Aids Service
hotline
1800 342 AIDS

Aids Response program
O.C.
714 534 0961

Biological Foundations of Human Sexuality

William H. Masters

Virginia E. Johnson

Robert C. Kolodny

HarperCollinsCollegePublishers

Executive Editor: Glyn Davies
Sponsoring Editor: Susan Penney-McLaughlin
Project Editor: Cynthia Funkhouser
Design Superviser: Teri Delgado
Cover Design: Delgado Design, Inc.
Cover Photo: Takahisa Ide
Production Administrator: Linda Murray
Compositor: Ruttle, Shaw & Wetherill
Printer and Binder: R. R. Donnelley & Sons Company
Cover Printer: The Lehigh Press, Inc.

Library of Congress Cataloging-in-Publication Data

Masters, William H.
Biological foundations of human sexuality / William H. Masters, Virginia E. Johnson, Robert C. Kolodny.
p. cm.
Includes bibliographical references and index.
ISBN 0-06-501517-7
1. Human reproduction. 2. Sex. I. Johnson, Virginia E. II. Kolodny, Robert C. III. Title.
QP251.M349 1993 92-36367
612.6—dc20 CIP

93 94 95 96 9 8 7 6 5 4 3 2 1

Brief Contents

Detailed Contents

Preface

As the authors of a comprehensive college textbook of human sexuality that has gone through four editions in the past decade, we are especially aware of how the growing complexity of this broad field has resulted in a rapid expansion of material that is presented to college students studying the subject. Since much of this information is of direct relevance to virtually every reader's life—for example, learning about AIDS and other sexually transmitted diseases, as well as learning about conception and contraception—it is clear to us that a format providing core coverage of this subject that permits flexibility in use by college professors in presenting different types of courses is very much in order.

We have designed *Biological Foundations of Human Sexuality* with this in mind. As the title suggests, we have drawn a subset of material from our larger textbook that focuses primarily on biological aspects of sexual function, human reproduction, and sexual health. In doing so, we do not mean to suggest that biology has supremacy over psychological or social aspects of human sexuality, since sexuality is very clearly a multifactorial, multidimensional phenomenon. Instead, we offer a textbook that can be used in a number of different situations and a number of different ways: for example, as a core text to be supplemented by specifically selected readings from the psychosocial literature; as a primer for use in college courses that are shorter than one semester; as a textbook for students entering the allied health care professions; or as one of several sources of readings for college courses about AIDS.

Although the emphasis of our coverage in this book is squarely on the biological underpinnings of human sexuality, there is more than incidental discussion of psychosocial aspects of sexuality interwoven throughout. For example, in Chapter 1 (Perspectives on Sexuality), we examine historical themes showing how modern-day sexual attitudes have evolved from various historical, cultural, and religious influences. Chapters 2 and 3, dealing respectively with sexual anatomy and physiology, include consideration of many myths about the sex organs and sexual response, as well as a thorough discussion of PMS (premenstrual syndrome). Chapter 4 (Human Reproduction) presents a variety of topics of a psychosocial nature such as feelings about pregnancy, psychological aspects of childbirth, psychological reactions during the postpartum days, and the emotional impact of fertility. Similarly, Chapter 5 (Birth Control and Abortion) includes sections on psychological aspects of abortion and the psychology of contraceptive use. Chapter 6 is devoted to topics in developmental sexuality that, while primarily biological, bear on the issue of how sexual feelings evolve across the lifespan. Chapters 7 and 8, dealing respectively with sexually transmitted diseases and HIV infection and AIDS, include considerable attention to the psychosocial aspects of these broad topics. Of necessity, the major focus of Chapter 9 (Sexual Dysfunctions and Sex Therapy) is on psychological issues. And, while our concluding chapter (Sexual Disorders and Sexual Health) is mainly concerned with biomedical topics, it includes extensive discussion of the emotional reactions of people with health problems to their situations, including a detailed section on sexual aspects of psychiatric illnesses. In addition, many of the boxed items integrated within the text deal primarily with material that is psychosocially oriented.

This book is drawn entirely from our *Human Sexuality,* Fourth Edition. We believe that it is the most authoritative, practical, and engaging book of its type that you can find. This didn't just happen automatically, however; the success of *Human Sexuality* has been very much a result of the continuing input from a variety of colleagues and editors whose assistance we greatly appreciate (and acknowledge below), as well as the lessons we learn day in and day out from working with patients, people who volunteer for our research studies, and students we encounter in learning dialogues.

ACKNOWLEDGMENTS

We are grateful for the assistance of many people in the planning and production of *Human Sexuality,* Fourth Edition, from which this book is drawn. In addition to a general thank you to the staff at HarperCollins College Publishers, we should single out Melonie Parnes, our Project Editor, for diligent attention to detail in *Human Sexuality,* Fourth Edition, and patience whenever we missed a deadline. Dorothy Bungert, Assistant Art Director, should also be thanked for her creative, eye-pleasing design. We would also like to thank Cindy Funkhouser, Project Editor, and Heather Ziegler, Designer, for their attention to the production of the text and to the design of the cover for this shorter book.

Portions of the manuscript for *Human Sexuality,* Fourth Edition, were reviewed in draft form by:

C. L. M. Carnrike
Syracuse University

Ryda Rose
University of Pennsylvania

Jerome Cerney
Indiana State University

James Calhoun
University of Georgia

Myles Anderson
Walla Walla Community College

Grace Galliano
Kennesaw State College

Ann Auleb
San Francisco State University

Marlene Tufts
Clackamas Community College

The text drawn from *Human Sexuality,* Fourth Edition, to create this book was reviewed by:

M. Betsy Bergen
Kansas State University

Leslie McBride
Portland State University

Special mention is mandatory for two people who have made extraordinarily valuable comments and suggestions throughout the preparation of all four editions of *Human Sexuality.* Marlene Tufts, of Clackamas Community College, has given us detailed critical feedback as well as a large number of creative suggestions for improving earlier drafts of the book. She has also skillfully prepared the Thought Questions that appear in each chapter of the fourth edition and of this shorter version. Jane Tufts, the developmental editor who helped shape *Human Sexuality* in its first three editions—and who in many ways should share authorship credit with us—once again worked to help us attain the best book possible in the fourth edition.

In addition, we are grateful to the following professors who provided essential and helpful advice in setting the direction for *Human Sexuality,* Fourth Edition:

Marlene Tufts
Clackamas Community College

Jerome Cerny
Indiana State University

Clive Davis
Syracuse University

C. L. M. Carnike
Syracuse University

Ryda Rose
University of Pennsylvania

Carole Zawid
Atlantic Community College

James Johnson
Sam Houston State University

H. H. Milaelian
University of New Brunswick

We also want to extend our thanks to staff members at the following institutions who were helpful in the preparation of *Human Sexuality,* Fourth Edition: the Alan Guttmacher Institute, the Harvard Medical School Library, the SIECUS Library, the SUNY Purchase Library, the libraries of Columbia University, the New York Academy of Medicine Library, and the U.S. Centers for Disease Control.

In closing, we restate our final paragraph from the preface to the first edition of *Human Sexuality* because it makes a point we should all remember:

> Sexuality is an intensely personal subject, and we hope that this book reflects our view of each individual's potential to experience his or her sexuality in a unique way. We also hope that this book conveys our belief that today's knowledge may be short-lived when judged against the standards of time, so that we must all guard against assuming too certain a view of sexual matters.

William H. Masters
Virginia E. Johnson
Robert C. Kolodny

About the Authors

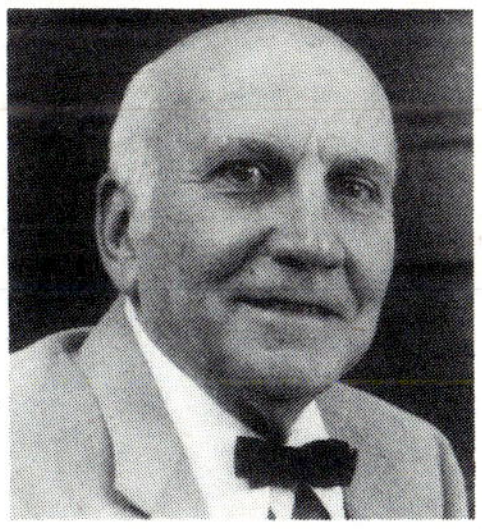

William H. Masters, M.D., is internationally acclaimed as one of the pioneer sex researchers and therapists of the twentieth century. Co-author of *Human Sexual Response* (1966), *Human Sexual Inadequacy* (1970), *The Pleasure Bond* (1975), and *Homosexuality in Perspective* (1979), among more than 200 publications, Dr. Masters has been instrumental in establishing the legitimacy of the scientific study of sex. Dr. Masters has been the recipient of more than a dozen awards from professional organizations in recognition of his outstanding career.

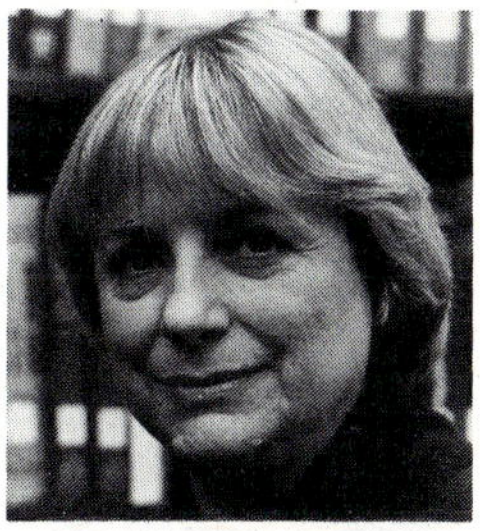

Virginia E. Johnson, D.Sc. (Hon.), is world-renowned for her innovative contributions to sex therapy and sex research. As Director of the Masters & Johnson Institute in St. Louis, she oversees clinical, research, and educational operations at this multidisciplinary organization, while continuing to maintain her own special interests in women's studies and the psychology of sexual behavior. Co-author of nine books and hundreds of journal articles, Dr. Johnson has been the recipient of more than a dozen awards from professional organizations during her remarkable career.

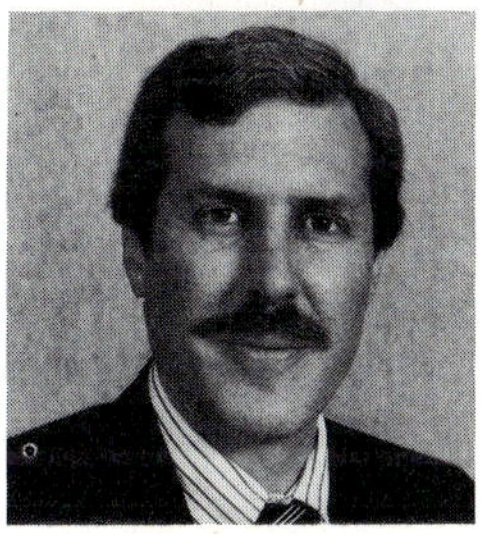

Robert C. Kolodny, M.D., is Medical Director of the Behavioral Medicine Institute in New Canaan, Connecticut. He was previously Associate Director and Director of Training at the Masters & Johnson Institute, where he continues to serve as a Consultant. In 1983, he received the National Award from the Society for the Scientific Study of Sex. A member of more than a dozen professional organizations, he currently serves on the Board of Advocates of Planned Parenthood Federation of America. Dr. Kolodny has co-authored a number of previous books with Masters and Johnson, including *Textbook of Sexual Medicine* (1979), *Ethical Issues in Sex Therapy and Research* (Volume 1, 1977; Volume 2, 1980), *On Sex and Human Loving* (1986), and *Crisis: Heterosexual Behavior in the Age of AIDS* (1988), and has also written two books with his wife on adolescence.

1

Perspectives on Sexuality

Every person has sexual feelings, attitudes, and beliefs, but everyone's experience of sexuality is unique because it is processed through an intensely personal perspective. This perspective comes from both private, personal experience and public, social sources. It is impossible to understand human sexuality without recognizing its multidimensional nature.

Sexuality has fascinated people in all walks of life from ancient times until the present. Sexual themes have been common in art and literature. Religions, philosophies, and legal systems—all concerned with shaping human behavior—have typically tried to establish sexual values and sexual taboos. At various times in history, illness, creativity, aggression, emotional disorders, and the rise and fall of cultures have all been "explained" as the result of too much or too little sexual activity or unusual sexual practices or thoughts.

While keeping in mind the private, public, and historical sources of our sexual heritage, we can broaden and deepen our understanding by studying sexuality from biological, psychosocial, behavioral, clinical, and cultural perspectives. In examining sexuality from these varied viewpoints, however, we must be careful not to forget that learning about sexuality, in all its forms, is really learning about people and the complexities of human nature.

WHY STUDY SEXUALITY?

While there are a number of different reasons for studying sexuality, many college students who enroll in sexuality courses do so for personal rather than academic reasons. This is because learning about sexuality—as contrasted to learning about physical chemistry or calculus—can provide people with knowledge that has a high potential for use in their everyday lives. This does not mean that there is no academic value to studying sexuality (since quite the opposite is true), but it does indicate that learning about sexuality has a number of practical applications that other subjects may not provide as easily.

Acquiring accurate information about sexuality can help prevent sexual problems, and it can enable us to educate our children better about sex. Becoming well informed about sex can also help us to deal more effectively with certain types of problems if they occur in our lives (e.g., infertility, sexual dysfunctions, sexually transmitted diseases, sexual harassment). Even more important, studying sexuality can help us become more sensitive and aware in our interpersonal relationships, thus contributing to the growth of intimacy and sexual satisfaction in our lives.

There is a particularly powerful reason to become knowledgeable about sexual matters today. In the age of the HIV epidemic (HIV is the abbreviation for the human immunodeficiency virus that causes AIDS), being knowledgeable can help you make sexual choices that are, quite literally, life-saving. In addition, since it is now apparent that unless a cure is found, in the decade of the 1990s virtually everyone's life will be touched in some way by the tragedies the HIV/AIDS epidemic engenders, acquiring accurate information about sexuality can increase your tolerance and understanding of the toll this takes on our society and its impact around the world.

Unfortunately, it is also true that these results do not happen automatically. There is no guarantee that careful study of this text will make finding (or keeping) sexual partners any easier, nor that it will lead to sexual bliss. Instead, we believe that learning about sexuality in an objective fashion will enable our readers to examine important sexual issues—some intensely personal, some social, some moral—and emerge with deeper insight into themselves and others. We also believe that sexual knowledge can lead to reasoned, responsible interpersonal sexual behavior and can help people make important personal decisions about sex. In short, learning about sexuality is an invaluable preparation for living.

DIMENSIONS OF SEXUALITY: SOME DEFINITIONS

> One would certainly think that there could be no doubt about what is to be understood by the term "sexual." First and foremost, of course, it means the "improper," that which must not be mentioned. (Freud, 1943, p. 266)

> Sex is not a mere physiological transaction to the primitive South Sea Islander any more than it is to us; it implies love and lovemaking; it becomes the nucleus of such venerable institutions as marriage and the family; it pervades art and it produces its spells and its magic. It dominates in fact almost every aspect of culture. *Sex*, in its widest meaning . . . is rather a sociological and cultural force than a mere bodily relation of two individuals. (Malinowski, 1929, p. xxiii)

> "Francie, you bloody fucker," I used to say, "you've got the morals of a clam." "But you like me, don't you?"

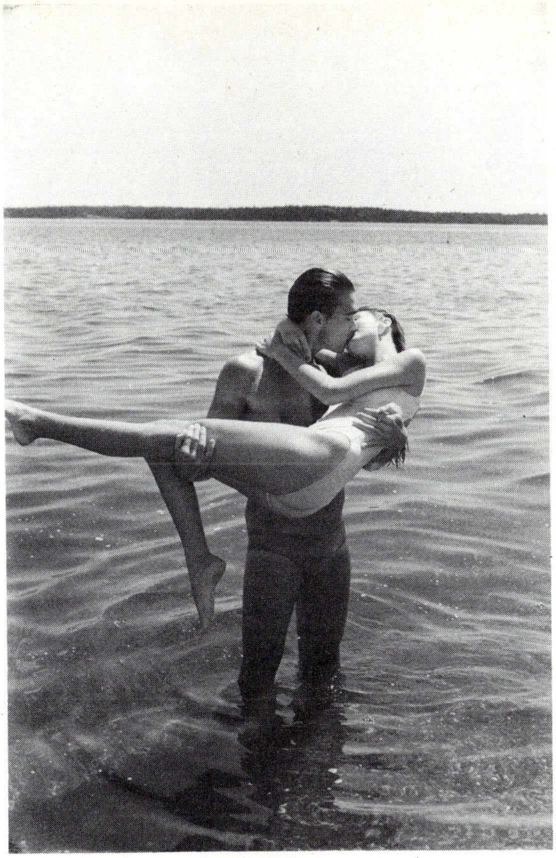

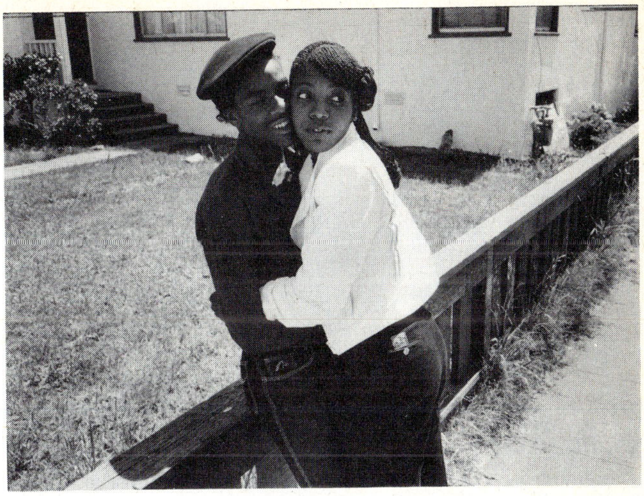

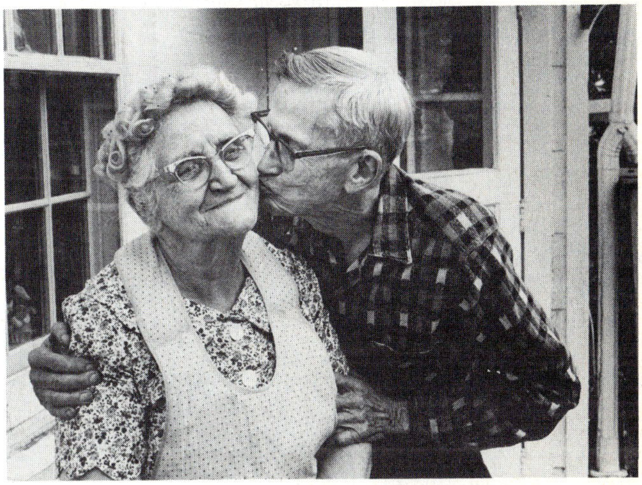

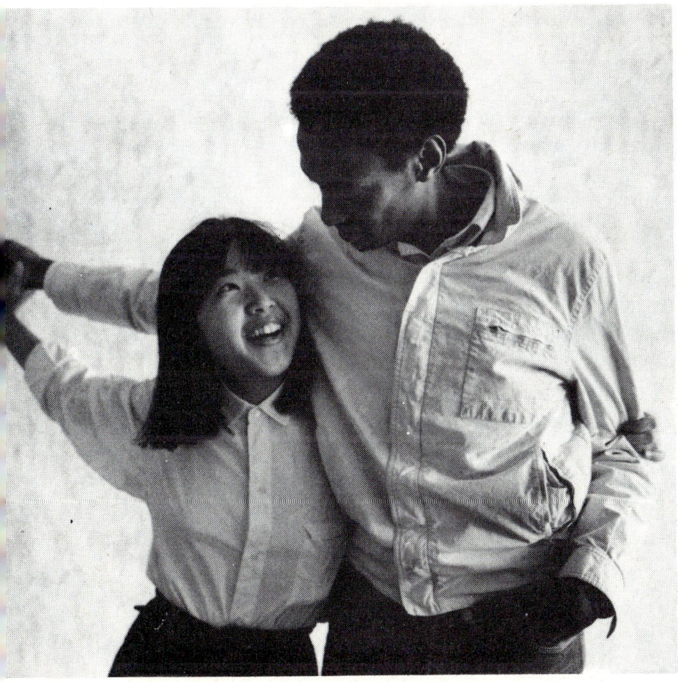

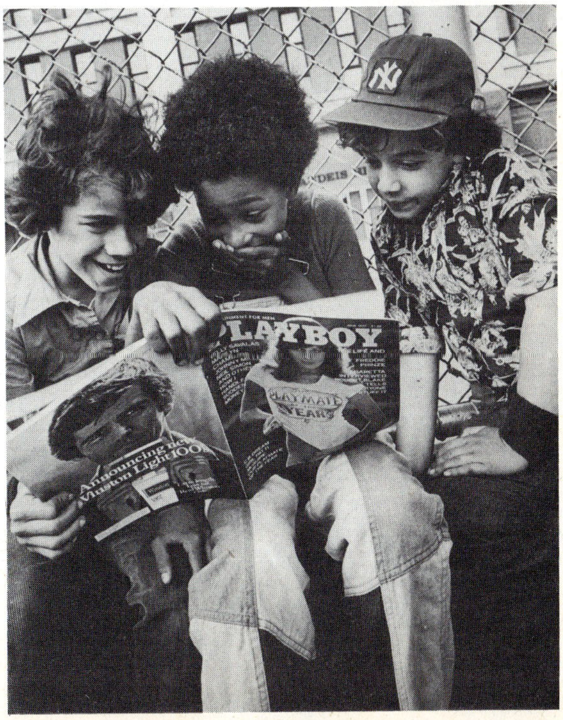

Sexuality is a part of everyone's life.

she'd answer. "Men like to fuck, and so do women. It doesn't harm anybody and it doesn't mean you have to love everyone you fuck, does it?" (Miller, 1961, p. 262)

What is sexuality? As shown by the preceding quotes, there is no simple answer to this question. Freud saw sex as a powerful psychological and biological force, while Malinowski emphasized its sociological and cultural dimensions. Henry Miller used frank portrayals of sex in his novels to make a philosophical statement about the human condition. In everyday life, the word *sex* is often used to mean male or female (biological gender) or to refer to physical activity involving the genitals ("having sex"). The word **sexuality** generally has a broader meaning since it refers to all aspects of being sexual. Sexuality means a dimension of personality instead of referring to a person's capacity for erotic response alone.

Unfortunately, our language for talking about sex and sexuality is very limited.[1] We may distinguish between sex acts (such as masturbation, kissing, and sexual intercourse) and sexual behavior (which includes not only specific sex acts but being flirtatious, dressing in certain ways, reading *Playboy*, and dating) without having yet scratched the surface of sexuality. We may describe different types of sex as **procreational** (for having children), **recreational** (for having fun, with no other goal), or **relational** (for sharing with a cared-for person) and find that our categories are still too few. While we cannot fully answer the question "What is sexuality?" in this chapter, we can briefly introduce the dimensions of sexuality that are the subject of this book.

A CASE PROFILE

David and Lynn sat anxiously in the waiting room at a sex therapy clinic. Although feeling embarrassed and unsure, they were determined to seek a solution to the sexual problems that had troubled their relationship for the past three months. Although they had been living together for almost two years and had planned to marry after their graduation from college, the dissatisfactions that now rocked their lives had thrown these future plans into doubt.

Once inside the clinic, they told their story in a straightforward fashion. They had met three years ago, at age 18, during their freshman year at school. Romance blossomed as they discovered many shared interests and easily developed an intimate sexual relationship. Neither David nor Lynn was a virgin when they met, and they felt a strong sexual attraction to each other. Their first shared lovemaking experience was passionate and sensuous. As their relationship matured, their sexual interaction continued to be a major source of pleasure. Living together was a natural outgrowth of these feelings, and it had been fun—until recently.

Trouble first appeared during Christmas vacation when they visited Lynn's parents in Boston. David was upset because he and Lynn were not allowed to share the same bedroom. Lynn was put off by her parents' apparent coolness toward David. Their only sexual opportunity (on a Sunday morning while Lynn's parents were at church) was hurried and felt mechanical. They were both relieved to return to school in time for a big New Year's Eve party with some friends.

The party lasted until 4:00 a.m. with great quantities of champagne consumed by all. Once back at their apartment, David and Lynn tried to make love but David was unable to get an erection. They laughed it off and fell asleep, happy to be "home."

The next morning David had a terrible hangover. He took some aspirin, ate a quick breakfast, and invited Lynn into their bedroom. She wasn't very enthusiastic, having a slight hangover herself, but didn't object. Once again David was unable to get an erection. Although Lynn was very understanding and supportive, David worried about his sexual performance (or lack of it) all day. He decided he needed some rest and relaxation before trying again, so he went to bed early that evening without any romantic overtures.

David awakened the next day feeling rested and refreshed and immediately turned to embrace Lynn.

Despite feeing good he found himself having only a partial erection, and even that disappeared when they tried to have intercourse. From that point on, David was plagued by difficulties getting or keeping an erection, and Lynn—despite initial attempts at helping him—was getting increasingly upset. Whereas their relationship *had* been relaxed and comfortable, now they were becoming short-tempered and abrupt. They talked about splitting up but believed they still loved each other and that they could—with some expert help—overcome this problem.

This real-life example, drawn from our files, allows us to introduce the various perspectives on sexuality that we examine in greater detail later in the book. By looking at David's and Lynn's situation, we can see the importance of the different dimensions of sexuality that interact in all of our lives.

The Biological Dimension

David's problem with erections first occurred after he had consumed a lot of champagne. This is not very surprising, since alcohol is a depressant to the nervous

[1] Wardell Pomeroy, a leading sexologist, likes to ask an audience for a four-letter word ending in the letter *k* that means "intercourse"—and then pauses knowingly before he says, "talk."

system. Because the nervous system normally transmits physical sensations to the brain and activates our sexual reflexes, too much alcohol can block *anyone's* sexual response.

The biological dimension of sexuality is far more inclusive than this, however. Biological factors largely control sexual development from conception until birth and our ability to reproduce after puberty. The biological side of sexuality also affects our sexual desire, our sexual functioning, and (indirectly) our sexual satisfaction. Biological forces are even thought to influence certain sex differences in behavior, such as the tendency of males to act more aggressively than females (Olweus et al., 1980; Reinisch, 1981). And sexual turn-ons, no matter what their source, produce specific biological events: the pulse quickens, the sexual organs respond, and sensations of warmth or tingling spread through our bodies.

The Psychosocial Dimension

David and Lynn reacted to their situation in different ways. David became anxious and goal-oriented and lost his self-confidence, while Lynn, who started out being supportive and understanding, became irritated and aloof. Clearly, the nature of their relationship changed in response to the stress of their sexual problem. David and Lynn even began to doubt whether they were in love and wanted to marry, although while visiting Lynn's parents they were convinced this plan was "right."

These responses illustrate the psychosocial dimension of sexuality, which includes psychological factors (emotions, thoughts, and personalities) in combination with social elements (how people interact). In this case, David's concern about his first sexual "failure" led him into further difficulties even when the original biological "cause"—too much alcohol—was removed from the situation. His anxieties led him into trying too hard to make sex work, with the result being exactly the opposite of what he and Lynn wanted.

The psychosocial side of sexuality is important because it sheds light not only on many sexual problems but also on how we develop as sexual beings. From infancy, a person's **gender identity** (the personal sense of being male or female) is primarily shaped by psychosocial forces. Our early sexual attitudes—which often stay with us into adulthood—are based largely on what parents, peers, and teachers tell us or show us about the meanings and purposes of sex. Our sexuality is also social in that it is regulated by society through laws, taboos, and family and peer group pressures that seek to persuade us to follow certain paths of sexual behavior.

The Behavioral Dimension

Talking with David and Lynn separately, we learned that the pattern of their sexual interaction changed considerably during the three months of their problem. The frequency of attempted lovemaking fell drastically, while in the past it had been four or five times per week. David masturbated several times a week (which he had not done for several years) after finding that he could easily get erections this way. On the other hand, Lynn masturbated only once, since she felt guilty about this activity. She also shied away from initiating sexual activity or even acting romantic with David because she thought this would put extra pressure on him.

These aspects of David's and Lynn's situation reflect the behavioral dimension of sexuality. Sexual behavior is a product of both biological and psychosocial forces, yet studying it in its own right can be enlightening. The behavioral perspective allows us to learn not only *what* people do but to understand more about *how* and *why* they do it. For example, David may have used masturbation to boost his self-confidence by "proving" to himself that he could still get erections. Lynn's withdrawal from initiating physical intimacy may have been well intended, but David may have interpreted it as rejection.

In discussing this topic, we should avoid judging other people's sexual behavior by our own values and experiences. Too often, people have a tendency to think about sexuality in terms of "normal" versus "abnormal." "Normal" is frequently defined as what we ourselves do and feel comfortable about, while the "abnormal" is what others do that seems different or odd to us. Trying to decide what is normal for others is not only a thankless task but one ordinarily doomed

sexuality a broadly encompassing term used to refer to all aspects of being and feeling sexual.

procreational sex (pro′ krē ā′ shun ul) sexual intercourse solely for reproduction. Sometimes advocated by some churches and groups as the only acceptable reason for sex.

recreational sex sexual activity primarily for pleasure. Emotional involvement and intimacy are purposefully limited.

relational sex sexual activity in the context of emotional involvement and intimacy in a relationship.

gender identity the inner sense a person has of being male or female.

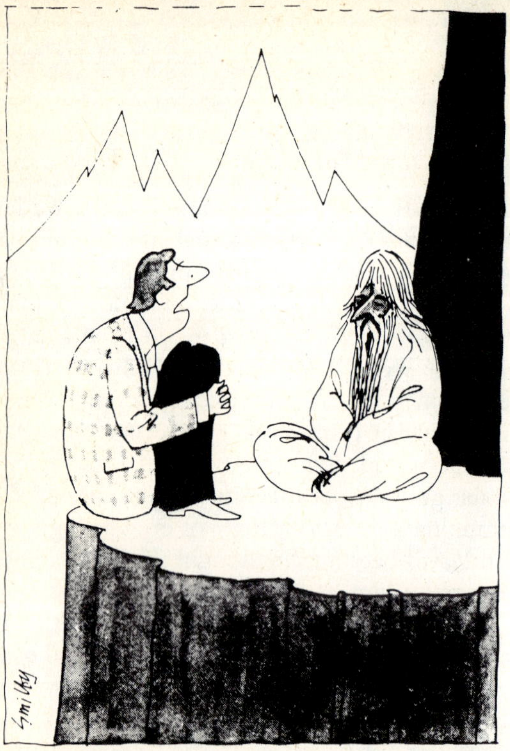

Smilby, copyright © Punch (Rothco).

"How often is normal?"

to failure because our objectivity is clouded by our values and experiences.

The Clinical Dimension

David and Lynn entered our sex therapy program and resolved their difficulties within two weeks. Not only did their sexual interaction return to its previously pleasurable state, but both felt that the therapy experience improved their relationship in other ways. As Lynn commented to us: "Overcoming the sexual problem was great, but we've also learned so much about ourselves. Our communication is about a thousand percent better now, and we really feel like we have a solid relationship that can cope with any kind of problem that comes up."

Although sex is a natural function, many types of obstacles can lessen the pleasure or spontaneity of our sexual encounters. Physical problems such as illness, injury, or drugs can alter our sexual response patterns or knock them out completely. Feelings such as anxiety, guilt, embarrassment, or depression and conflicts in our personal relationships can also hamper our sexuality. The clinical perspective of sexuality examines the solutions to these and other problems that prevent people from reaching a state of sexual health and happiness.

Greatly improved results have been obtained in the treatment of a wide variety of sexual difficulties in the last two decades. Two key changes have contributed to this success: a better understanding of the multidimensional nature of sexuality and the development of a new discipline, called sexology, devoted to the study of sex. Doctors, psychologists, nurses, counselors, and other professionals trained in sexology can integrate this knowledge with training in sex counseling or sex therapy to help a high percentage of their patients.

The Cultural Dimension

David's and Lynn's lives, like all of ours, reflect the input of the culture in which they live. For example, Lynn's parents refused to let them sleep in the same bedroom although they knew David and Lynn were living together. As another example, Lynn's sense of guilt toward masturbation stemmed largely from her religious upbringing. And David's anxiety over his sexual difficulties was partly a reaction to the prevailing American notion that men should be instantly erect at the first moment of a sexual encounter.

Our own cultural attitudes toward sexuality are far from universal. In some societies, a man's special obligations to a guest or a friend are discharged by an invitation to have sexual relations with his wife (Voger, 1961). Ford and Beach (1951, p. 49) listed eight cultural groups in which kissing was unknown, pointing out: "When the Thonga first saw Europeans kissing they laughed, expressing this sentiment: 'Look at them—they eat each other's saliva and dirt.' " While these cultural differences may shock or amuse us, they can also help us to understand that our viewpoint is not shared by all people in all places.

Sexual topics are often controversial and value-laden, but the controversy is often relative to time, place, and circumstance. What is labeled as "moral" or "right" varies from culture to culture, from century to century. Many of the moral issues pertaining to sex relate to certain religious traditions, but religion has no monopoly on morality. People who have no closely held religious creed are just as likely to be moral as those whose values are tied to a religious position. *There is no sexual value system that is right for everyone and no single moral code that is indisputably correct and universally applicable.*

In America, messages about sexual behavior that

CASE STUDY

Writer's Block

A 29-year-old woman who had won considerable acclaim for her deftly written first novel two years earlier entered psychotherapy because she had fallen far behind in work on her second novel, which was more than six months overdue. In fact, for nearly a year she had rarely been able to write more than a few paragraphs a day, often sitting and staring helplessly at the lines she jotted as though unable to focus her creative energies.

Shortly after her writer's block developed, she also began having difficulties in her sexual response with her husband, although she had previously been easily aroused and orgasmic with sexual activity. Gradually, she began to lose her sexual appetite, as well, which she thought was mainly a result of the tension caused by the writing difficulties she was having. She also began to have insomnia, which made her very tired all day long. Sometimes she was so frustrated by her problems that she found herself in tears.

When she had made no real progress in dealing with her writer's block after several months of psychotherapy, her therapist referred her and her husband to a sex therapy program in order to deal with the sexual problems in the hopes that improvement in that sphere would carry over to her writing.

In the initial intake interviews, the sex therapist suspected that the woman was clinically depressed. Further questioning revealed that she had thought about suicide from time to time and had lost more than ten pounds in the past six months. In addition, both her mother and a maternal aunt had been treated for depression.

Within weeks after being started on treatment with antidepressant medication, the woman began to notice that she was able to concentrate on her writing more effectively and that she was able to get a good night's sleep. Soon thereafter, she found that her interest in sex had returned, and she was once again able to have orgasms in her sexual relations.

Comment: Not all sexual problems require sex therapy, as this example shows. Here, the basic psychological problem was not the writer's block, although the writer's block was the presenting difficulty that masked the true diagnosis from the woman's first psychotherapist. Sexual symptoms are very common accompaniments to depression; fortunately, they usually are alleviated quickly when the underlying depression is properly treated.

Source: Authors' files.

prevailed in the first half of this century have changed considerably in the last 25 years. For example, while there used to be a high cultural premium placed on a woman being a virgin before marriage, today attitudes toward premarital sex have shifted in the opposite direction. Reflecting this change, the age of first sexual intercourse is now lower than it was 20 or 30 years ago, increasing numbers of adolescents are engaging in sexual intercourse, and substantial numbers of couples are living together before marriage. Another example that illustrates how times and attitudes have changed is the current degree of acceptance of masturbation as a harmless, pleasurable act, which is in sharp contrast to earlier views that regarded masturbation as a sign of moral weakness and a cause of physical and mental debility.

Three broad trends have played an important role in the evolution of cultural attitudes toward sex and sexuality in America in the last few decades. The first is a loosening of gender role stereotypes. **Gender role** is the public expression of gender identity—that is, how an individual asserts his or her maleness or femaleness in social settings (Money and Ehrhardt, 1972).[2] Traditionally, women and girls were cast as sexually passive and unresponsive creatures while men were seen as virile sexual aggressors. According to this view, the male was expected to be the sexual initiator and expert, and the female who was aggressive or enjoyed sex too much was frowned upon. This notion has now been replaced for many people by a concept of mutual participation and satisfaction. A second trend is the greater degree of openness about sexuality. All forms of the media from television to cinema to the printed word reflect this change, and, as a result, sex has become less shameful and mysterious. The third trend is the growing acceptance of relational and recreational sex as opposed to reproductive sex. This shift, which has been especially evident in the past 25 years, is due partly to improved contraceptive techniques and concern for overpopulation.

It is a mistake to think that cultural viewpoints are ever frozen in place. Currently, there is some evidence that alarm over increasing rates of sexually transmitted diseases coupled with a growing trend toward political and religious conservatism may cause a shift away from the sexual permissiveness that prevailed in the 1960s and 1970s. In fact, many observers now believe that the so-called sexual revolution is over, with a new era dawning that will emphasize commitment and fidelity in intimate relations instead of experimentation, instant gratification, and sexual variety. But cultural trends are notoriously changeable, so there is no certainty how this new direction will evolve.

HISTORICAL PERSPECTIVES ON SEXUALITY

> A major obstacle to understanding our own sexuality is realizing we are prisoners of past societal attitudes toward sex. *(Bullough, 1976, p. xi)*

To understand the present, it is helpful to begin by examining the past. In certain respects, we are bound by a sexual legacy passed on from generation to generation, but in other ways modern views of sex and sexuality differ drastically from past patterns.

Early Times

Although written history goes back almost 5000 years, only limited information is available describing sexual behavior and attitudes in various societies prior to 1000 B.C. Clearly, a prominent taboo against incest had already been established (Tannahill, 1980), and women were considered as property, with sexual and reproductive value (Bullough, 1976). Men were free to have many sexual partners, prostitution was widespread, and sex was accepted as a straightforward fact of life.

With the advent of Judaism, an interesting interplay of sexual attitudes began to emerge. In the first five books of the Old Testament, the primary source of Jewish laws, there are rules about sexual conduct: adultery is forbidden in the Ten Commandments (Exodus 20:13), for example, and homosexual acts are strongly condemned (Leviticus 18:22, Leviticus 21:13). At the same time, sex is recognized as a creative and pleasurable force, as depicted in the Song of Songs. Sex was neither considered inherently evil nor restricted to procreative purposes alone.

In ancient Greece, however, there was tolerance and even enthusiasm regarding male homosexuality in certain forms. Homosexual relations between an adult man and adolescent boy past the age of puberty were commonplace, usually occurring in an educational relationship where the man was responsible for the boy's moral and intellectual development (Bullough, 1976; Karlen, 1980; Tannahill, 1980). At the same time, exclusive homosexuality and homosexual acts between adults were frowned upon, and homosexual contact between adults and boys under the age of puberty was illegal. There was a strong emphasis on marriage and family, yet women were second-class citizens, if they could be considered citizens at all: "In Athens, women had no more political or legal rights than slaves; throughout their lives they were subject to the absolute authority of their male next-of-kin. . . . As everywhere else in the first millennium B.C., women were chattels, even if some of them were independent-minded ones. To the Greeks, a woman (regardless of age or marital status) was *gyne,* whose linguistic meaning is 'bearer of children' " (Tannahill, 1980, pp. 94–95).

As Christianity developed in its early forms, there was an intermingling of Greek and Jewish attitudes toward sexuality. In contrast to Judaism, which did

[2] Although the term "sex roles" is more widely used than "gender roles," we have chosen the second usage throughout this book to avoid the risk that "sex roles" implies an underlying biological mechanism (Unger, 1979).

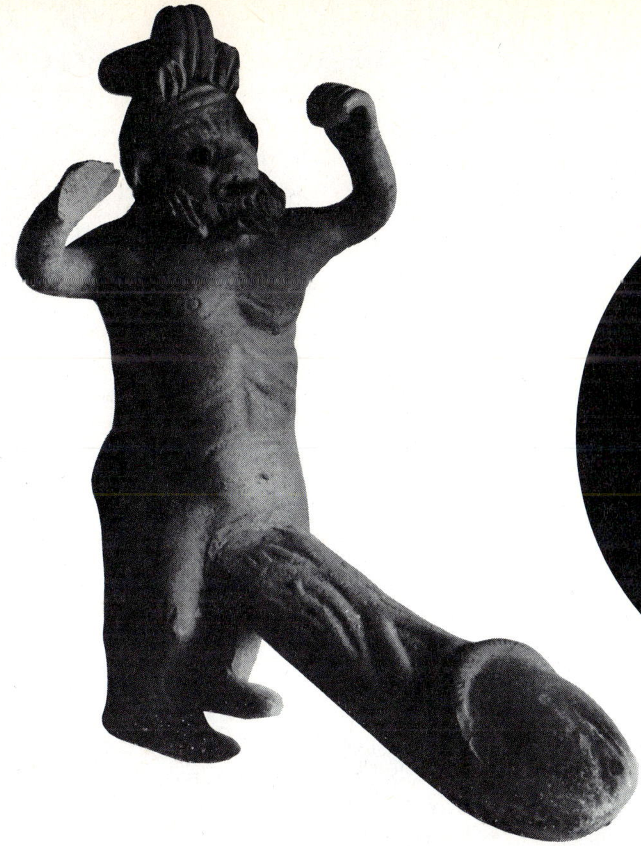

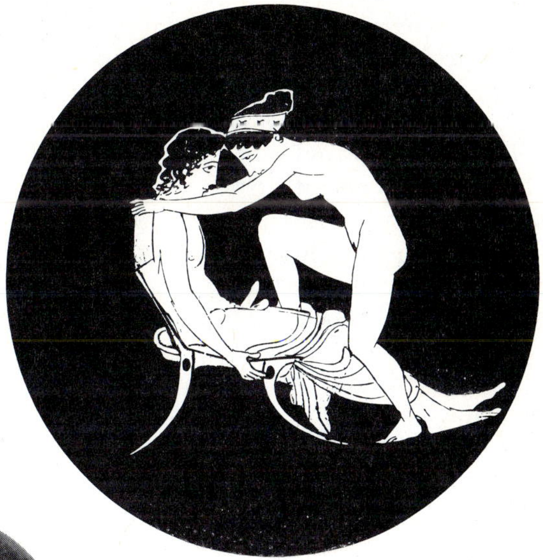

Sexual themes have been shown in art since ancient times. This Roman lamp, used to ward off evil spirits, and Greek dish, with its erotic scene, are two interesting examples.

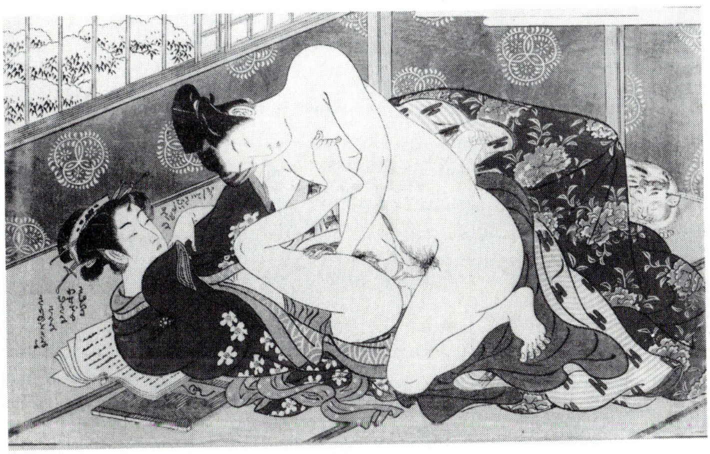

Oriental art has a long tradition of explicitly depicting erotic scenes, as this work from the eighteenth century shows.

not distinguish physical from spiritual love, Christian theology borrowed from the Greek and separated *eros*, or "carnal love," from *agape*, a "spiritual, nonphysical love" (Gordis, 1977). Bullough (1976) points out that the Hellenistic era in Greece (beginning in 323 B.C.) was marked by a denial of worldly pleasures in favor of developing the spiritual. Along with the New Testament portrayal of the imminent end of the world, this led to Christianity placing a high ideal on

gender role behavior that conveys to others that an individual is either male or female.

celibacy, although St. Paul allowed that while "it is good for a man not to touch a woman . . . it is better to marry than to burn" (1 Corinthians 7:1–12).

By the end of the fourth century A.D., despite small groups of Christians whose views of sexuality were less rigid and constrained, the church's negative attitudes toward sex were dramatically presented in the writings of St. Augustine, a religious leader whose background included a vivid and varied set of erotic experiences before he renounced worldly ways. Augustine confessed in stark terms, "I muddied the stream of friendship with the filth of lewdness and clouded its clear waters with hell's black river of lust" (*Confessions*, Book III:I). He believed that sexual lust came from the downfall of Adam and Eve in the Garden of Eden and that this sinfulness was transmitted to children by the inherent lust that separated humanity from God. Thus, sex was strongly condemned in all forms, although Augustine and his contemporaries apparently felt that marital procreative sex was less evil than other types.

Eastern Thought

Elsewhere in the world, sexual thinking varied remarkably from that just described. In particular, Islamic, Hindu, and ancient Oriental sexual attitudes were considerably more positive. Bullough states that "almost anything in the sexual field received approval from some segment of the Hindu society" and that in China "sex was not something to be feared, nor was it regarded as sinful, but rather, it was an act of worship" and even a path toward immortality (Bullough, 1976, pp. 275, 310). The *Kama Sutra*, compiled at about the same time Augustine was writing his *Confessions*, is a detailed Indian sex manual; in ancient China and Japan, similar manuals, which were abundant, glorified sexual pleasure and variety. These divergent patterns continued, although our focus for now will remain with the history of sex in the Western world.

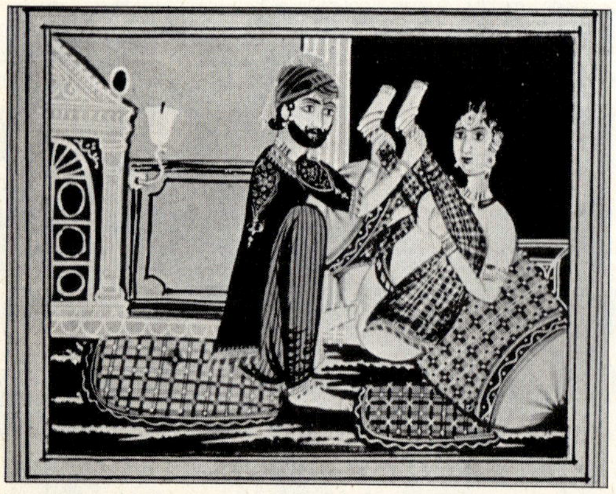

The ancient Kama Sutra *from India is one of the best-known sex manuals surviving from early times.*

Medieval and Renaissance Thought

The early Christian traditions regarding sexuality became more firmly entrenched in Europe during the twelfth and thirteenth centuries as the Church assumed greater power. Theology often became synonymous with common law, and there was a generally oppressive "official" attitude toward sex except for the purpose of procreation. There was, however, a certain hypocristy between professed Church policies and actual practices: "religious houses themselves were often hotbeds of sexuality" (Taylor, 1954, p. 19).

During this era, a new style of living emerged among the upper classes that brought about a drastic separation between actual practice and religious teachings. This style, called courtly love, introduced a new code of acceptable behavior in which women (at least high-ranking women) were elevated to an immaculate plane and romanticism, secrecy, and valor were celebrated in song, poetry, and literature (Tannahill, 1980). Pure love was seen as incompatible with the temptations of the flesh, and sometimes this concept was tested by lovers lying together in bed naked to see if they could prove the fullness of their love by refraining from sexual intercourse. Needless to say, it is unlikely that courtly love was always the unconsummated romantic ideal portrayed in story and verse.

Not too long after the era of courtly love began, chastity belts made their appearance. These devices allowed husbands to lock up their wives just as they would protect their money; while they may have been originally designed to prevent rape, they also served to guard "property":

> The belt of medieval times was usually constructed on a metal framework that stretched between the woman's legs from front to back. It had two small, rigid apertures that allowed for waste elimination but effectively prevented penetration, and once it was locked over the hips the jealous husband could take away the key. *(Tannahill, 1980, p. 276)*

The rebirth of humanism and the arts that subsequently engulfed Europe in the sixteenth and seventeenth centuries was accompanied by a loosening of sexual restrictions as well as less adherence to the formulas of courtly love. The Protestant Reformation, led by Martin Luther, John Calvin, and others, generally advocated less negative attitudes toward sexual matters than the Catholic church did. For example, although Luther was hardly liberal in his sexual attitudes, he thought that sex was not inherently sinful and that chastity and celibacy were not signs of virtue. At the same time, Europe was caught in a massive epidemic of syphilis—possibly imported from the Americas—that might have worked to limit sexual freedom.

The Eighteenth and Nineteenth Centuries

When we speak of the attitudes of a historical era, we must keep in mind that there was variance among different countries, levels of society, and religious groups. Although evidence can be cited to show a rather broad tolerance toward sexuality in England and France in the 1700s (Bullough, 1976), the Puritan ethic reigned in colonial America. Sex outside marriage was condemned, and family solidarity was exalted; those giving in to the passions of adultery or premarital sex, if discovered, were flogged, put in pillories or stocks, or forced to make public confessions. Some readers may be familiar with Nathaniel Hawthorne's *The Scarlet Letter*, which presents an account of sexual attitudes in colonial times.

In America, the Puritan ethic was carried over into the nineteenth century with a curious schism. As American frontiers expanded and as large cities took on a more cosmopolitan flair, there was a corresponding loosening of notions about sexual propriety, and prostitution became commonplace. This new development was met by the formation in the 1820s and 1830s of several groups whose primary mission was to combat the social evils of prostitution and rescue the "fallen women" who plied this trade (Pivar, 1973). Despite the organized resistance of such groups as the American Society for the Prevention of Licentiousness and Vice and the Promotion of Morality and the American Society for Promoting the Observance of the Seventh Commandment, prostitution flourished. During a three-year period in the 1840s, the government prosecuted 351 brothels in Massachusetts alone, and by the eve of the Civil War, a guidebook listing fashionable brothels in big cities described 106 establishments in New York, 57 in Philadelphia, and dozens of others in Baltimore, Boston, Chicago, and Washington, DC (Pivar, 1973).

By the mid-1800s, as the Victorian era began, reserve and prudery emerged once again in Europe, although this time less connected to religious edict. The spirit of Victorianism was sexual repression and a strong sense of modesty necessitated by the presumed purity and innocence of women and children. Taylor points out, "So delicate did the sensibilities of the Victorians become, so easily were their thoughts turned to sexual matters, that the most innocent actions were taboo in case they might lead to lurid imaginings. It became indelicate to offer a lady a *leg* of chicken." Clothing styles, showing not even a glimpse of ankle or bare neck, mirrored this conservatism (Taylor, 1954, pp. 214–215). The prudishness of this period is astonishing to us today: in some Victorian homes, piano legs were covered with crinolines, and books by authors of opposite sexes were not shelved side by side unless the authors were married to each other (Sussman, 1976).

In America, although the influence of Victorianism was strongly felt, crosscurrents sent the mainstream of moral thinking into a dizzying spin. For example, in 1870 the St. Louis City Council found a loophole in state law that allowed it to legalize prostitution, causing an uproar across the nation. Groups were again formed to combat sexual immorality and managed to find allies in other organizations dedicated to the cause of temperance (abolishing the sale of alcoholic beverages). This movement achieved several legislative successes. In 1886, for example, 25 states fixed the age of consent at 10 (thus permitting child prostitution to flourish), but by 1895, only 5 states retained this low age, and 8 states had raised the age of consent to 18.

Although the mainstream of Victorianism was antisexual—pornography was first banned by law in this era—there was another side to the times. A sexual "underground" of pornographic writings and pictures was widely read (Marcus, 1967). Prostitution was common in Europe, and in the 1860s it was legalized and regulated by an act of the British Parliament. Furthermore, Victorian prudery in sexual behavior and attitudes was not standard for all social classes (Gay, 1983). The middle and lower classes did not practice the sexual pretensions of the upper class. Indeed, it was the abject poverty of the lower classes that forced many young women into prostitution, and the middle classes—despite the ideal of the docile, sexless Victorian lady—not only had sexual feelings and desires but acted on them in much the same way women do today. Victorian women had (and enjoyed) marital sex and occasionally had torrid love affairs, as seen in a number of diaries which detailed the number and quality of their orgasms (Gay, 1983). In fact, a female sex survey conducted by a woman named Clelia Duel Mosher in 1892 has recently come to light, providing additional evidence that viewing the Victorian period as strictly antisexual is incorrect. In addition, an interesting viewpoint has been advanced about female sexuality in Victorian times:

> Although it is obvious that many Victorians suffered from sexual repression, it appears on closer observation that those women who contributed to the concept of prudishness were far closer to today's feminists than most are willing to admit. . . . The Victorian women sought to achieve a sort of sexual freedom by denying her sexuality . . . in an effort to keep from being considered or treated as a sex object. Her prudery was a mask that conveniently hid her more "radical" effort to achieve freedom of person. *(Haller and Haller, 1977, p. xii)*

Science and medicine reflected the antisexualism of the era thoroughly. Masturbation was variously branded as a source of damage to the brain and nervous system and a cause of insanity and a wide range of other illnesses (Bullough and Bullough, 1977; Haller and Haller, 1977; Tannahill, 1980). Women were thought to have little or no capacity for sexual response and were viewed as inferior to men both physically and intellectually. In 1878, the prestigious *British Medical Journal* printed a series of letters in which a number of physicians offered evidence supporting the idea that the touch of a menstruating woman would spoil hams. And even as eminent a scientist as Charles Darwin, the father of the theory of evolution, wrote in his *Descent of Man and Selection in Relation to Sex* (1871) that "man is more courageous, pugnacious, and energetic than woman, and has a more inventive genius" and that "the average of mental power in man must be above that of women."

In the latter part of the nineteenth century Richard von Krafft-Ebing, a German psychiatrist, undertook a detailed classification of sexual disorders. The impact of his *Psychopathia Sexualis* (1886), which went through 12 editions, was profound and influenced subsequent public attitudes and medical and legal practice for more than three-quarters of a century (Brecher, 1975). There were positive and negative aspects to this influence: on the one hand, Krafft-Ebing advocated sympathetic medical concern for the so-called sexual perversions and reform in laws dealing with sex criminals, while on the other hand his book seemed to lump sex, crime, and violence together. Much of his attention was devoted to aspects of sexuality he considered abnormal, such as sadomasochism (sexual arousal from inflicting or experiencing pain), homosexuality, fetishism (sexual arousal by an object rather than a person), and bestiality (sexual contact with animals). Because he frequently used lurid examples (sexual murders, cannibalism, and intercourse with the dead, to name just a few) which he presented in the same pages with less frightening sexual variations, many readers were left with a general loathing for almost all forms of sexual conduct. Nevertheless, Krafft-Ebing is often considered the founder of modern sexology.

The Twentieth Century

By the turn of the new century, sexuality began to be investigated in a more objective manner. Although Victorian attitudes still prevailed in many circles, the work of serious scientists such as Albert Moll, Magnus Hirshfeld, Iwan Bloch, and Havelock Ellis combined with the dynamic theories of Freud to initiate a striking reversal in thinking about sex.

FREUD

Sigmund Freud (1856–1939) was a Viennese physician who, more successfully than any figure before or since, demonstrated the central importance of sexuality to human existence. Today Freud's genius is recognized as partly a matter of original discovery and partly a reflection of his ability to synthesize emerging ideas into a cohesive and persuasive theoretical framework (Sulloway, 1979). Freud believed that sexuality was both the primary force in the motivation of all human behavior and the principal cause of all forms of **neurosis**, a mild form of mental disorder in which anxiety is prominent and coping skills are distorted although a sense of reality is maintained. He clearly described the existence of sexuality in infants and children, expanding views expressed by other sexologists between 1880 and 1905 (Kern, 1973; Sulloway, 1979), and formulated a detailed theory of psychosexual development.

Freud devised many innovative concepts related to sexuality. The best known, the **Oedipus complex**, refers to an inevitable sexual attraction of the young male child to his mother accompanied by an ambivalent mixture of love, hate, fear, and rivalry toward his father. Freud also believed that boys were concerned about the possible loss of their penis as a terrible form of punishment (**castration anxiety**) and that girls felt a sense of inadequacy and jealousy at not having a penis (**penis envy**). Freud saw these situations as operating primarily at the unconscious level—a level of the personality deeper than conscious awareness. From the rich theoretical tapestry of his thought, Freud wove a clinical method called psychoanalysis for assessing and treating the unconscious conflicts that lead to psychological problems. Although many modern sexologists disagree with Freud's formulations, psychoanalysis remains a widely used method of treatment today.

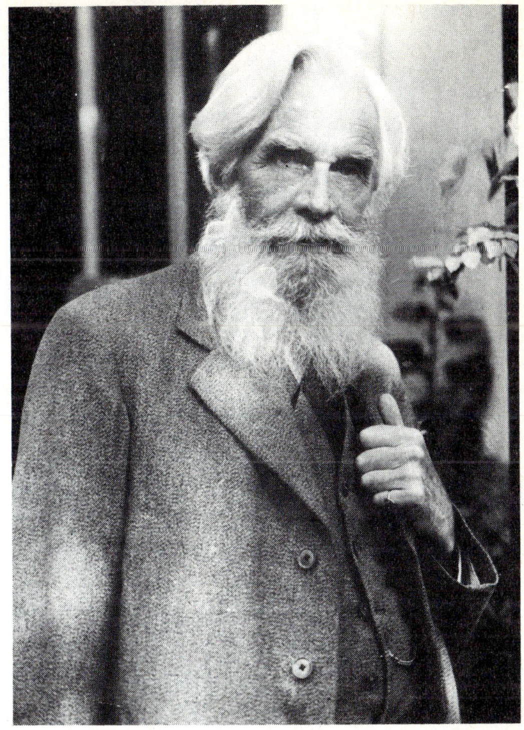

Havelock Ellis, through his prolific writings, became one of the most influential early sexologists.

ELLIS

At about this same time, an English physician named Havelock Ellis (1859–1939) was publishing a six-volume series called *Studies in the Psychology of Sex* (1897–1910). Ellis anticipated much that Freud later wrote about childhood sexuality and had remarkably modern views in certain areas. For example, he recognized the common occurrence of masturbation in both sexes at all ages, took exception to the Victorian idea that "good" women had no sexual desire, and emphasized the psychological rather than physical causes of many sexual problems. His writings also focused on the varied nature of human sexual behavior and provided an important balancing influence to Krafft-Ebing's view of sexual variations as diseases (Brecher, 1969, 1975).

1920–1950

By the end of World War I, massive social changes were emerging in both Europe and America that differed drastically from Victorian practices. Influenced by increasing social and economic freedom for women and the availability of the automobile, sexual attitudes became increasingly less inhibited in the Jazz Age and were accompanied by corresponding changes in fashion, dance, and literature. Women had become involved professionally in the sexual revolution that was brewing. Margaret Sanger was a leader of the birth control movement in America. Katherine Davis conducted a survey of the sex lives of 2200 women which was published initially as a series of scientific articles between 1922 and 1927 and then as a book (Davis, 1929). An Englishwoman, Marie Stopes, wrote an explicit marriage manual that sold well on both sides of the Atlantic.[3] By 1926, when a gynecologist named Theodore van de Velde published *Ideal Marriage*, providing specific details about a wide range of sexual techniques and endorsing such practices as oral–gen-

[3] It is interesting to note that Stopes, who had obtained a doctorate and was an accomplished scientific researcher, was very much a victim of Victorian prudishness about sex. Six months after her marriage to another scientist, Dr. Reginald Ruggles Gates, she "began to feel instinctively that something was lacking," and went to the British Museum to try to discover what it was. Finding out that her marriage had not been consummated, she successfully sued for divorce and later undertook the writing of her book to help others avoid such problems (Harrison, 1977).

neurosis a psychological disorder usually characterized by anxiety and/or tension. In contrast to more severe forms of psychological problems, called psychoses, with a neurosis a person's sense of reality is not greatly altered.

Oedipus complex (ed′ i pus) in Freudian theory, the sexual attraction of a young boy toward his mother, accompanied by a mixture of fear and rivalry toward his father.

castration anxiety (ka strā′ shun) according to Freud, the unconscious fear in boys about the possible loss of their penis as a terrible form of punishment.

penis envy in Freudian theory, the girl's unconscious sense of inadequacy and jealousy at not having a penis.

ital sex, his book became an instant international best-seller.

The Roaring Twenties came to a sudden end in 1929 with the stock market crash. In the Great Depression that followed, concern for sustenance, shelter, and survival seemed to take precedence over sex.

As Britain and America were drawn into World War II, the enormity of the conflict and its life-and-death drama provided a backdrop for wholesale changes in patterns of sexual behavior on both sides of the Atlantic. Women, who were enthusiastically enlisted in the workplace and in the armed forces, suddenly enjoyed a newfound economic freedom and personal independence but were also thrust into a confusing atmosphere of hasty marriages, anxious separation, loneliness, and fear. While their boyfriends or husbands were overseas, many turned to clandestine affairs, just as the male troops generally availed themselves of sexual opportunities near training camps, in overseas assignments, and on leave. As one social historian observed, "The lives and moral attitudes of many millions of people had undergone an extensive emotional trauma, and in the unsettled conditions of wartime many social inhibitions had lost their restraining force. Making the best of the present without thinking about the future had led to pleasure-seeking and increased promiscuity" (Costello, 1985, p. 258).

The postwar era, which was unsettled both for its burgeoning divorce rate and for the upheaval resulting from pushing women out of factories and offices back to their "rightful" place in the home, was also notable because it brought instant notoriety to another sexologist who was to leave an indelible mark on scientific history.

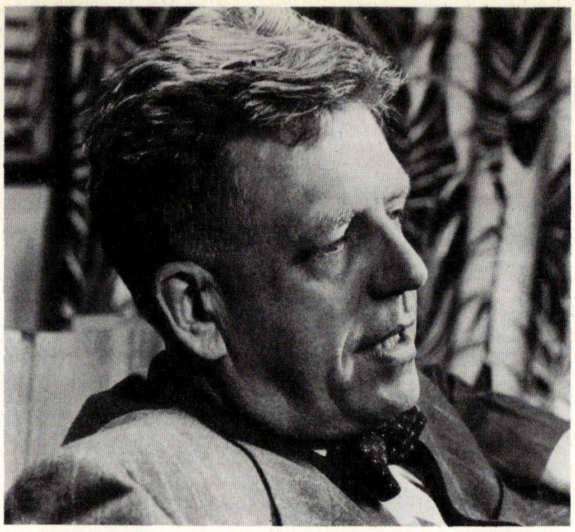

Alfred Kinsey brought boundless enthusiasm to his career in sex research despite the considerable controversies that his methods and findings provoked.

KINSEY

Alfred C. Kinsey (1894–1956), a zoologist at Indiana University, had been asked to participate in teaching a noncredit college course on marriage in the summer of 1938. Struck by the lack of scientific data about human sexual behavior, he used this opportunity to administer questionnaires to some of his students for the purpose of gathering information about their sexual histories. Soon thereafter, Kinsey decided that personal interviewing was a more promising technique for obtaining such case history material since it permitted greater flexibility and detail, and he embarked on a course of action that eventually led to interviews with thousands of men and women across the country. Joined by his coauthors and colleagues, Wardell Pomeroy and Clyde Martin, Kinsey published the monumental *Sexual Behavior in the Human Male* on January 5, 1948. Five years later, with Paul Gebhard, they published the companion volume, *Sexual Behavior in the Human Female* (Kinsey et al., 1953).

The Kinsey reports were based on extensive face-to-face interviews with 12,000 people from all segments of the population and the findings were often startling. For instance, 37 percent of American men were reported to have had at least one homosexual experience to the point of orgasm after the age of puberty; 40 percent of husbands had been unfaithful to their wives; and 62 percent of the women studied had tried masturbation.

The publication of *Sexual Behavior in the Human Male* instantly catapulted the Kinsey research into the public eye. By mid-March more than 100,000 copies had been sold, and the book remained on the best-seller list for 27 weeks.

Although Kinsey and his colleagues attempted to describe how people behave sexually without moral or medical value judgments, their work was severely criticized on methodological and moral grounds. Prestigious *Life* magazine called it "an assault on the family as a basic unit of society, a negation of moral law, and a celebration of licentiousness" (Wickware, 1948). Margaret Mead criticized Kinsey for dealing with sex "as an impersonal, meaningless act" (*The New York Times,* April 1, 1948), a charge that was echoed by many critics, including one professor from Columbia

University who stated that "there should be a law against doing research dealing exclusively with sex" (*The New York Times*, April 1, 1948). However, the Kinsey report was also praised as having "done for sex what Columbus did for geography" (Ernst and Loth, 1948).

All in all, the reception of Kinsey's first volume was fairly positive (Palmore, 1952), but the same cannot be said for his second book, *Sexual Behavior in the Human Female*. Many newspapers denounced this report in editorials and refused to give it coverage in their news columns. For example, the *Times* of New Philadelphia, Ohio, justified this decision by saying, "We believe it would be offensive to a large portion of our readers" (August 20, 1953). Church leaders and educators called Kinsey's findings amoral, antifamily, and even tainted with communism.

Kinsey died in 1956, embittered and disillusioned, but the impact of his energetic investigations was to be strongly apparent in the years ahead. In addition to the cultural and scientific legacy he left behind, he and his colleagues formed the Institute for Sex Research at Indiana University, which continues as a major center under the leadership of June Reinisch.

THE 1950s

In the aftermath of Kinsey's studies there was an era marked by quite a bit of sexual confusion in the United States. Premarital sex became more commonplace than it had been before, although it seems to have been restricted mainly to engaged couples. Popular descriptions of sex began to appear in books (such as the then-steamy *Peyton Place*) and movies (mostly imported from overseas), and even popular music began to present sexual themes. One observer, horrified by what he heard and saw, sourly noted that the "sexualization" of music made it "naked, seductive, . . . lusty and perverse," with performers whose "bleating is underscored by their gyrations, contortions, and bodily rhythms all too clear in sexual innuendo and undisguised meaning" (Sorokin, 1956).

At the same time, the 1950s were a time when females were expected to be glamorous but brainless creatures—something along the lines portrayed by Marilyn Monroe in her movies—whose primary ambitions should be directed toward marriage and motherhood. *Harper's Magazine* (January 1950) noted: "If an American girl wears plain, unadorned eyeglasses, instead of highly colored and fancifully shaped specs, she might just as well be dead, for all the dating it will get her." And *See* magazine (January 1950) solemnly advised readers: "It is quite legitimate for a girl to use falsies and not to tell her husband about them before marriage."

Albert Ellis (1959) succinctly summarized the prevailing mores of the times this way: "The fundamental law underlying all our sex, love, and marriage attitudes can be stated with absolute and appalling clarity in two simple statements: (a) if it's FUN you mustn't do it; (b) if it's DUTY you must" (p. 227).

THE 1960s

In the early 1960s, several factors influenced the start of a sexual revolution that was more visible than any America had previously seen. These included (1) the availability of birth control pills, (2) the protest movement among adolescents and young adults, (3) the reemergence of feminism in modern form, and (4) greater openness in discussions and displays of sex. While it isn't possible to render any final historical judgment on the relative importance of each of these factors in fueling the sexual revolution, it appears certain that each had a strong influence.

The pill made premarital sex considerably safer and permitted millions to think of sex as relational or recreational rather than procreative, as we have already noted. Indeed, the availability of the pill provided a sense of freedom for many women and probably contributed more to changing sexual behavior than has generally been imagined. The protest movement among the young, which began with the civil rights movement and expanded with the growing disillusionment with the Vietnam War, led teens and young adults to challenge their parents' generation ("the establishment") in every way imaginable. This challenge was expressed not only in the younger generation's clothing, long hair, and music but also in their recreational drug use and their support of sexual freedom ("Make love, not war").

With their consciousness raised at many levels to political and social injustices, young adults in the sixties also embraced the women's movement with enthusiasm. Since the pill had given women a new degree of control over their sexual destinies, it is not surprising that female sexuality was increasingly accepted as a natural fact of life.

In society at large, the initial reactions to the sexual revolution were mixed. While some sought to join the movement enthusiastically, many others seemed to regard it as a passing phase that would eventually fade away. And it's probably safe to say that a sizable segment of the population watched this upheaval with great distaste and alarm, concerned that the moral fabric of American society was disintegrating before their eyes. Nevertheless, sexuality became more talked about, shown, and studied, and the sixties saw the advent of "topless" bars, nudity in Broadway shows (first with *Hair*, later with *Oh! Calcutta!*), and the publication of a revolutionary study of human sexual function.

MASTERS AND JOHNSON

Kinsey and his collaborators had investigated the nature of human sexuality by interviews designed to find out how, when, and how often people behaved sexually. Since then, sex research has expanded in various directions in an attempt to answer questions that had not previously been resolved. Among the first and most significant departures from Kinsey's methods were those used by William H. Masters and Virginia E. Johnson, a physician and a behavioral scientist at Washington University Medical School in St. Louis.

Masters and Johnson believed that to understand the complexities of human sexuality, people must understand sexual anatomy and physiology as well as psychological and sociological data. Unsatisfied with the relevance to humans of information gathered by studies of sexual response in animals, Masters and Johnson decided that only a direct approach to the problem would be illuminating. They began a laboratory investigation in 1954 to observe and record the physical details of human sexual arousal. By 1965 more than 10,000 episodes of sexual activity by 382 women and 312 men had been observed, and the report that followed, *Human Sexual Response* (Masters and Johnson, 1966), drew rapid public attention. Although some health care professionals quickly grasped the importance of these findings, others were shocked by the methods employed. Amid the accusations of "too mechanistic an approach" and the cries of moral outrage, relatively few people recognized that the physiological information was not an endpoint but was instead a foundation on which a treatment method for people with sexual problems could be based.[4]

THE 1970s AND 1980s

In the 1970s and 1980s, the new openness about sexuality was readily apparent. In 1970, Masters and Johnson published *Human Sexual Inadequacy*, a landmark book that described a startlingly new approach to the treatment of sexual problems that had previously required lengthy treatments without very high rates of success. With a two-week treatment program and only a 20 percent failure rate, this work was soon to give rise to an entirely new profession—sex therapy—with the eventual proliferation of thousands of sex therapy clinics across the country before the end of the decade, and the development of other therapy approaches by doctors such as Helen Kaplan and Jack Anon.

[4] It is noteworthy that all of medical science is based on understanding normal anatomy and physiology before meaningful advances can be made in treating abnormalities. In 1966, when *Human Sexual Response* was published, many physicians seemed to forget this fact, which would have been unquestionable in the study of heart disease or skin disorders. Our files from that year contain many angry letters written by physicians criticizing the physiology work because of its impropriety and departure from traditional medical "respectability."

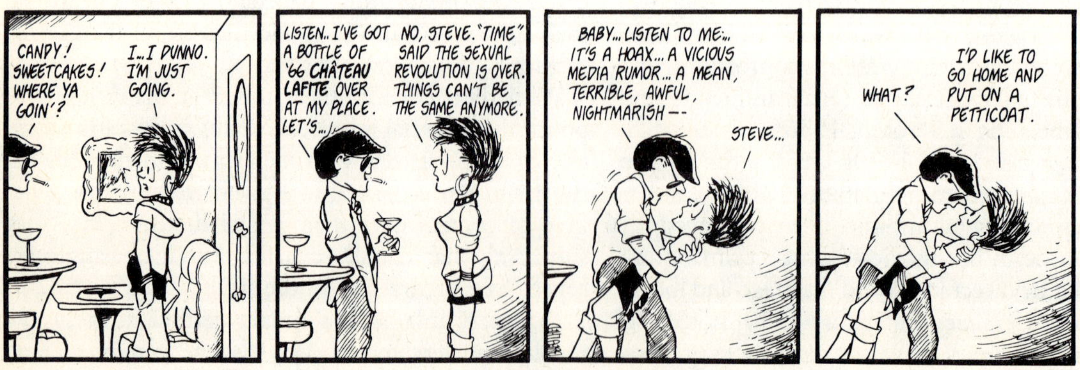
CANDY! SWEETCAKES! WHERE YA GOIN'?
I...I DUNNO. I'M JUST GOING.
LISTEN.. I'VE GOT A BOTTLE OF '66 CHÂTEAU LAFITE OVER AT MY PLACE. LET'S...
NO, STEVE. "TIME" SAID THE SEXUAL REVOLUTION IS OVER. THINGS CAN'T BE THE SAME ANYMORE.
BABY... LISTEN TO ME... IT'S A HOAX... A VICIOUS MEDIA RUMOR... A MEAN, TERRIBLE, AWFUL, NIGHTMARISH --
STEVE...
WHAT?
I'D LIKE TO GO HOME AND PUT ON A PETTICOAT.

Bloom County by Berke Breathed. © 1987 Washington Post Writers Group. Reprinted with permission.

Other, less technical books about sex were published by the dozens, with Alex Comfort's *The Joy of Sex* (1972) probably being the most accomplished and certainly the most successful (with sales of over nine million copies). Television became a notable force in the sexual revolution, too, as a number of programs tackled previously taboo sexual themes. Not to be outdone, movies became more sexually explicit, and, in the early days of the home video market, pornographic films were the single best-selling category.

A number of other trends occurred during this time that affected the ways Americans viewed sexuality: (1) the practice of nonmarital cohabitation—living together—began to assume increasing importance as a stage preceding marriage; (2) the legalization of abortion by the U.S. Supreme Court in 1973 made it possible to obtain safe abortions but also provoked considerable controversy about the morality of this practice; (3) the 1974 decision by the American Psychiatric Association to remove homosexuality from classification as a mental disorder set the stage for advances to be made in the gay rights movement; (4) a growing awareness of the significance of all forms of sexual victimization—in part an outgrowth of the women's movement and in part a result of the work of scientists and scholars who effectively showed that rape is a crime of violence rather than a crime of passion (e.g., Burgess and Holmstrom, 1974; Brownmiller, 1975; Metzger, 1976)—led to major legislative changes aimed at modernizing procedures for trying rape cases as well as the rapid growth in rape crisis centers across the country; (5) the appearance of new reproductive technologies encompassing the birth of the world's first "test-tube baby" in 1978 (with more than 15,000 babies conceived by similar means now alive) has proceeded to even more startling techniques, such as embryo transfer methods and the controversial surrogate mother practice.

The late 1970s and early 1980s were also a time for a backlash against what some perceived as overpermissive, even immoral sexual practices. The Moral Majority sought to block sex education in public schools and campaigned against "promiscuous" sexual behavior, which seemed to include anything other than marital sex. The right-to-life movement challenged the legality of abortion and unsuccessfully tried to pass a constitutional amendment that would have banned abortion under all circumstances. In 1983, the Reagan administration tried to implement a policy requiring notice to the parents of teenagers requesting contraceptives; this proposal, which became derisively known as the "squeal rule," fortunately never got off the ground.

Particularly alarming to some was the appearance in the late 1970s and early 1980s of seemingly new epidemics of sexually transmitted diseases: genital herpes, primarily among heterosexuals, and AIDS (acquired immune deficiency syndrome), which in America first affected homosexual and bisexual men but soon spread to involve heterosexuals as well. (AIDS results from infection with a virus that cripples the body's immune system, leading to a variety of severe infections, cancers, and neurologic disorders.) The AIDS epidemic—which has been likened by some to a modern-day plague—is particularly frightening because the disease now seems to be invariably fatal and because there are currently thought to be as many as two million Americans infected with the AIDS virus. Since cures were not available for either genital herpes or AIDS and since the two diseases seemed to be linked incontrovertibly to promiscuous sexual behavior, some observers suggested that they were a form of punishment from God for sexual transgressions.

With an avalanche of media publicity about AIDS and the realization that prevention cannot be guaranteed short of sexual abstinence or sexual monogamy with an uninfected partner, millions of people seem to have shifted their patterns of sexual behavior, with some choosing celibacy and others becoming more selective in their choice of sex partners (Kolodny and Kolodny, 1987; Stevens, 1987; Winkelstein et al., 1987). Others haven't changed their sexual practices at all or have simply added some cautionary steps to their sex lives (e.g., using condoms). While detailed research on the changes that AIDS awareness has brought about in different segments of the population remains to be done, it appears to us that the 1990s are a time in which growing numbers of people are rethinking their sexual behavior.

We cannot know, of course, if the changes and trends we see as significant today will have any lasting impact on our sexual behavior over time. Nor can we be certain that a century from now, historians won't label our era with a single word (like "Victorian") and reduce the many complexities of our sexual attitudes to a single notion. The only thing we can be sure of is that our attitudes and behaviors will continue to change—what directions those changes will take, however, is impossible to predict with any accuracy.

THE ABORTION ATTITUDE SCALE

One of the most controversial issues involving sexuality today is the abortion issue. If you are interested in seeing where you stand on this matter, complete the exercise below.

The self-administered, self-scored scale below is not a test. There are no right or wrong answers to any of the statements, so just answer as honestly as you can. The statements ask you to tell how you feel about legal abortion (the voluntary removal of a human embryo or fetus from a mother during the first three months of pregnancy by a qualified medical person). Tell how you feel about each statement by circling one of the choices beside each sentence. Here is a practice statement:

Abortion should be legalized. SA A SLA SLD D SD (SA = Strongly Agree; A = Agree; SLA = Slightly Agree; SLD = Slightly Disagree; D = Disagree; SD = Strongly Disagree)

Answer each statement and circle only one response.

1. The Supreme Court should strike down legal abortions in the United States.
   SA A SLA SLD D SD
2. Abortion is a good way of solving an unwanted pregnancy.
   SA A SLA SLD D SD
3. A mother should feel obligated to bear a child she has conceived.
   SA A SLA SLD D SD
4. Abortion is wrong no matter what the circumstances are.
   SA A SLA SLD D SD
5. A fetus is not a person until it can live outside its mother's body.
   SA A SLA SLD D SD
6. The decision to have an abortion should be made by the pregnant mother.
   SA A SLA SLD D SD
7. Every conceived child has the right to be born.
   SA A SLA SLD D SD
8. A pregnant female not wanting to have a child should be encouraged to have an abortion.
   SA A SLA SLD D SD
9. Abortion should be considered killing a person.

SUMMARY

1. Human sexuality is a multidimensional phenomenon having biological, psychosocial, behavioral, clinical, moral, and cultural aspects. No single dimension of sexuality is universally dominant.
2. History teaches us that sexual attitudes and practices vary considerably over time and place. For more than 2000 years, religion has been a principal force in shaping sexual thought. In the past century, the advent of sexology as a science—from the early approaches of Krafft-Ebing, Havelock Ellis, and Sigmund Freud to the dramatic research studies of Kinsey and Masters and Johnson—has greatly influenced contemporary attitudes toward sex and sexuality.
3. We must guard against interpreting sexual behavior too simplistically. For instance, although the Victorian era was certainly a time of sexual prudishness in many respects, it was clearly also a time when prostitution flourished, pornography was widely read, and the middle and lower

SA A SLA SLD D SD

10. People should not look down on those who choose to have abortions.

    SA A SLA SLD D SD

11. Abortion should be an available alternative for unmarried, pregnant teenagers.

    SA A SLA SLD D SD

12. Persons should not have the power over the life or death of a fetus.

    SA A SLA SLD D SD

13. Unwanted children should not be brought into the world.

    SA A SLA SLD D SD

14. A fetus should be considered a person at the moment of conception.

    SA A SLA SLD D SD

Score your answers in the following way:

Step One:

For items 2, 5, 6, 8, 10, 11, and 13:
SA = 6 points
A = 5 points
SLA = 4 points
SLD = 3 points
D = 2 points
SD = 1 point

For items 1, 3, 4, 7, 9, 12, and 14:
SA = 1 point
A = 2 points
SLA = 3 points
SLD = 4 points
D = 5 points
SD = 6 points

Step Two: Total your points for all 14 items.

Step Three: Use the following scoring scale to interpret your results.

0–15 Strong pro-life
16–26 Moderate pro-life
27–43 Unsure
44–55 Moderate pro-abortion
56–70 Strong pro-abortion

Source: "Abortion Attitude Scale," L. A. Sloan. This article is reprinted with permission from HEALTH EDUCATION, 1983, pp. 41–42. HEALTH EDUCATION is a publication of the American Alliance for Health, Physical Education, Recreation and Dance, 1900 Association Drive, Reston, VA, 22091.

classes paid scant attention to the sexual pretensions of the upper class.

4. In our recent past, many observers have pointed to the 1960s as a time when a sexual revolution began. Four factors contributed to this phenomenon: the availability of birth control pills, the protest movement among teenagers and young adults, a renewed interest in feminism, and a greater openness to discussion and displays of sex.
5. Alarm over new epidemics of sexually transmitted diseases—especially AIDS (acquired immune deficiency snydrome)—along with a growing trend toward conservatism seems to have brought the sexual revolution to a grinding halt. Millions of people are now adopting a more cautious attitude toward sexual behavior, with further changes likely to occur if the AIDS epidemic worsens.
6. Predicting the changes in sexual thinking and behavior that will occur in the future is difficult at best. All we can be sure of is that our attitudes and behaviors *will* change in one way or another.

Thought Questions

1. The authors state that "There is no sexual value system that is right for everyone and no single moral code that is indisputably correct and universally applicable." Do you agree with this assertion? Or are there some sexual values that are indisputably and universally right or wrong?
2. The text states that sexuality has biological, psychological, and social dimensions. However, many individuals and some religions take the position that only procreation justifies engaging in sexual activities. How would our attitudes toward proper sexual expression change if this were true? What kind of sex would be prescribed by society and what kind would be proscribed?
3. Some people regard Freud, Kinsey, and even Masters and Johnson as being "dirty old men" because of their interest in doing sexual research. How common is this perception and is it justified? What would motivate individuals to base a lifetime career on the study of sex?
4. "Make love, not war" was a slogan of the 1960s. Is there a relationship between these two activities? Is sexual repression somehow connected to war and sexual freedom to peace? Or is this slogan a catchy but meaningless piece of advice?
5. Has there been a true sexual revolution during the last few decades, or is this a myth? Does our society seem to be moving toward more or less diversity and freedom regarding sexual expression?
6. According to the text, prostitution and pornography flourished during Victorian times. Is there a cause and effect relationship here? Does sexual repression encourage an underground-type of sexual expression? Also, Victorian repression affected the sexes and the social classes differently. What might be the explanation for this?

Suggested Readings

Brecher, Edward. *The Sex Researchers*. Boston: Little, Brown, 1969. A collection of biographical sketches of the most influential sex researchers from Krafft-Ebing to Kinsey to Masters and Johnson.

Bullough, Vern, and Bullough, Bonnie. *Sin, Sickness and Sanity—A History of Sexual Attitudes*. New York: New American Library, 1977. A provocative study of how past attitudes to certain aspects of sexuality (e.g., masturbation, homosexuality, prostitution, pornography) have affected present sexual theorizing.

Costello, John. *Virtue Under Fire*. Boston: Little, Brown, 1985. A nicely done social history of the impact of World War II on sexual attitudes and behavior in America and Britain.

D'Emilio, J., and Freedman, E.B. *Intimate Matters: A History of Sexuality in America*. New York: Harper & Row, 1988. A lively historical survey of American sexual behavior, courtship etiquette, and public attitudes toward a broad spectrum of sexual matters.

Gay, Peter. *The Bourgeois Experience: Victoria to Freud*. Vol. 1, *Education of the Senses*. New York: Oxford University Press, 1983. An in-depth reassessment of sexuality during the Victorian era that shows why viewing this period as a strictly antisexual time is incorrect.

Tannahill, Reay. *Sex in History*. New York: Stein and Day, 1980. A lively, opinionated survey of sexual customs and attitudes from prehistoric to modern times.

2

Sexual Anatomy

Karen is a 20-year-old college junior who generally avoided dating because she felt her breasts were too small. She wrote: "I hate looking in a mirror or wearing a bathing suit because I see how flat I am. I would be *mortified* to let a guy touch or see my breasts." *(Authors' files)*

Brad is an athletic 17-year-old who quit his school's basketball team because his breasts were large. He told us that his teammates kidded him mercilessly in the locker room and showers about when he was going to get a bra. He was afraid he might "turn into a woman." *(Authors' files)*

A married couple in their mid-twenties who were sex therapy patients said they frequently used stimulation of the clitoris as part of making love. When asked to identify the clitoris during a physical exam, the husband pointed to a large freckle on the lower part of his wife's left labia majora. *(Authors' files)*

A class of 80 college sophomores was given a brief test on sexual anatomy the first day of their course on sexuality. The average student had more mistakes than right answers. *(Authors' files)*

As these examples show, many of us have inaccurate information or negative feelings about our sexual anatomy. This should not be surprising for a variety of reasons: we are taught to keep our sex organs covered by clothing; we are scolded or punished for touching our "private parts"; we are not likely to be told the correct terminology to describe our sexual anatomy; we are discouraged from conversations or questions about sex; and the sexual images we are exposed to in movies and magazines are likely to present almost unattainable standards to measure ourselves against. It is no wonder that our sexual anatomy can be a source of anxiety, shame, guilt, mystery, and curiosity, as well as a source of pleasure.

The mixed feelings we have about our sexual body parts are mirrored in the words we use to talk about them: some words are "clean" and "proper," while others are "dirty" or "impolite." These differences are a result of how we interpret words, not an innate property of the words themselves. Consider, for example:

> In Nigeria, the moral taboos of sex were taught by missionaries and administrators who used only clean words. These were the words that became taboo. The dirty words used as part of the vernacular of sailors, traders, and the like, became part of Nigerian vernacular English, with no taboo attached. In consequence, today it is as forbidden to say sexual intercourse, penis and vagina on Nigerian television as it is to say fuck, cock, and cunt on the national networks in the United States. In Nigeria, the latter terms are considered normal and respectable. *(Money, 1980, pp. 50–51)*

TABLE 2–1

Some Sexual Terminology: Science and Slang

Proper Name	Slang Terms
Vulva	Pussy, snatch, crotch
Pubic hair	Beaver, bush, pubes
Mons veneris	Love mound
Clitoris	Clit, button, joy button
Labia	—
Hymen	Cherry, maidenhead
Urethral meatus (urinary opening)	Peehole
Vagina	Cunt, box, pussy, hole, snatch, slit, twat, honeypot
Anus	Asshole
Breasts	Boobs, tits, knockers, bazooms
Buttocks	Ass, rear end, bottom, buns
Penis	Prick, cock, peter, tool, organ, meat (rod, boner, and hard-on usually refer to erect penis only)
Testes	Balls, nuts, jewels

In this book we do not use slang terms about sex because they convey a negative message to some people. As a matter of convenience, however, slang terms that describe sexual parts of the body are listed in Table 2–1. Sex organs in the pelvic region—in females the outer sexual structures and the vagina, in males the penis, scrotum, and testes—are customarily called the **genitals**.

People of all ages have common concerns about sexual anatomy: What is the normal size of the penis? Is something wrong if one breast is smaller than the other? Does circumcision lessen sexual pleasure? Do large breasts indicate a passionate woman? Is it abnormal if one testicle hangs lower than the other? Where and what is the clitoris? The answers to such questions begin with learning about sexual anatomy. The basis for understanding the way our bodies function sexually is discussed in the next chapter.

FEMALE SEXUAL ANATOMY

> We are encouraged to feel as if our bodies are not ours. Our "figure" is for a (potential) mate to admire. Our breasts are for "the man in our lives" to fondle during lovemaking, for our babies to suckle, for our doctors to examine. The same kind of "hands-off" message is even

stronger for our vagina. *(Boston Women's Health Book Collective, 1976, p. 24)*

Anyone who has been around young children knows that baby girls play with their genitals just as they touch and explore all parts of their body. Although this activity seems pleasurable and interesting, most girls are quickly taught that it's "not nice" or "dirty," a prohibition that is probably reinforced during toilet training when the two- or three-year-old girl is urged to "wipe carefully" and "be clean." The sex-negative tone of these early childhood messages is consistently reinforced for most girls as they grow up, commonly creating anxieties and inhibitions about sex in general and their sexual anatomy in particular (Hite, 1977; Long Laws, 1979; Barbach, 1980). These difficulties are compounded by many people's perception of the female sex organs as unattractive and unclean.

Menstruation is one source of such negative attitudes: menstrual periods are sometimes called "the curse," menstrual flow is contained by "sanitary" napkins (which suggests an underlying condition of uncleanliness), sex during menstruation is often avoided by men and women because it may be messy, and in some societies there are strong taboos surrounding menstruating women that isolate them so they will not contaminate food, plants, or people (Delaney, Lupton, and Toth, 1977). In our cosmetic-conscious society laden with perfumes, deodorants, and after-shave lotions, women have been told that their vaginal odors are unpleasant and should be hidden. As a result, "feminine hygiene deodorant sprays" were widely used until it became apparent that they frequently caused vaginal irritation and itching.

Many women have not taken a direct look at their own genitals or cannot accurately name and identify the parts of their sexual anatomy. While we cannot imagine a person unable to distinguish between eyes, nose, mouth, and chin, many men and women have no idea of the locations of the female urethra, clitoris, or hymen.

The Vulva

The external sex organs of the female, called the **vulva** (meaning "covering"), consist of the mons, the labia, the clitoris, and the perineum (Figure 2–1). Although the vagina has an external opening (the **introitus,** or entrance), it is principally an internal organ and discussed separately.

THE MONS

The **mons veneris** (Latin for mound of Venus; Venus was the Roman goddess of love) is the area over the pubic bone which consists of a cushion of fatty tissue covered by skin and pubic hair. Since this region has numerous nerve endings, touch and/or pressure here may lead to sexual arousal. Many women find that stimulation of the mons area can be as pleasurable as direct clitoral touch.

THE LABIA

The outer lips (**labia majora**) are folds of skin covering a large amount of fat tissue and a thin layer of smooth muscle. Pubic hair grows on the sides of the outer lips, and sweat glands, oil glands, and nerve endings are liberally distributed in them. In the sexually unstimulated state, the outer lips usually are folded together in the midline, providing mechanical protection for the urethral (urinary) opening and the vaginal entrance.

The inner lips (**labia minora**) are like curving petals. They have a core of spongy tissue rich in small blood vessels and without fat cells. The skin covering the inner lips is hairless but has many sensory nerve endings. The inner lips meet just above the clitoris, forming a fold of skin called the **clitoral hood** (see Figure 2–1). This portion of the inner lips is sometimes referred to as the female foreskin.

The labia are an important source of sexual sensations for most women since their many nerve endings serve as sensory receptors. When the skin of the labia is infected, sexual intercourse may be painful, and itching or burning may occur.

Women's external genitals may vary greatly in ap-

genitals (jen′ i tulz) sex organs in the pelvic region. Customarily refers to the penis, the testes, and scrotum in the male and the vulva and vagina in the female.

vulva (vul′ vuh) the external sex organs of the female: the mons, labia, clitoris, and vaginal orifice.

introitus the opening of the vagina.

mons veneris (mōnz ven′ e ris) the area over the pubic bone of the female which consists of a cushion of fatty tissue covered by skin and pubic hair. Also called mons pubis or mound of Venus.

labia majora (la′ bē uh muh jor′ uh) the two outer folds of skin on either side of the inner lips, the clitoris, and the urethral and vaginal openings.

labia minora (la′ bē uh mi nor′ uh) the two inner folds of skin enclosing the urethral and vaginal openings.

clitoral hood the fold of skin covering the clitoral shaft. Sometimes referred to as the female foreskin.

FIGURE 2–1

The Vulva

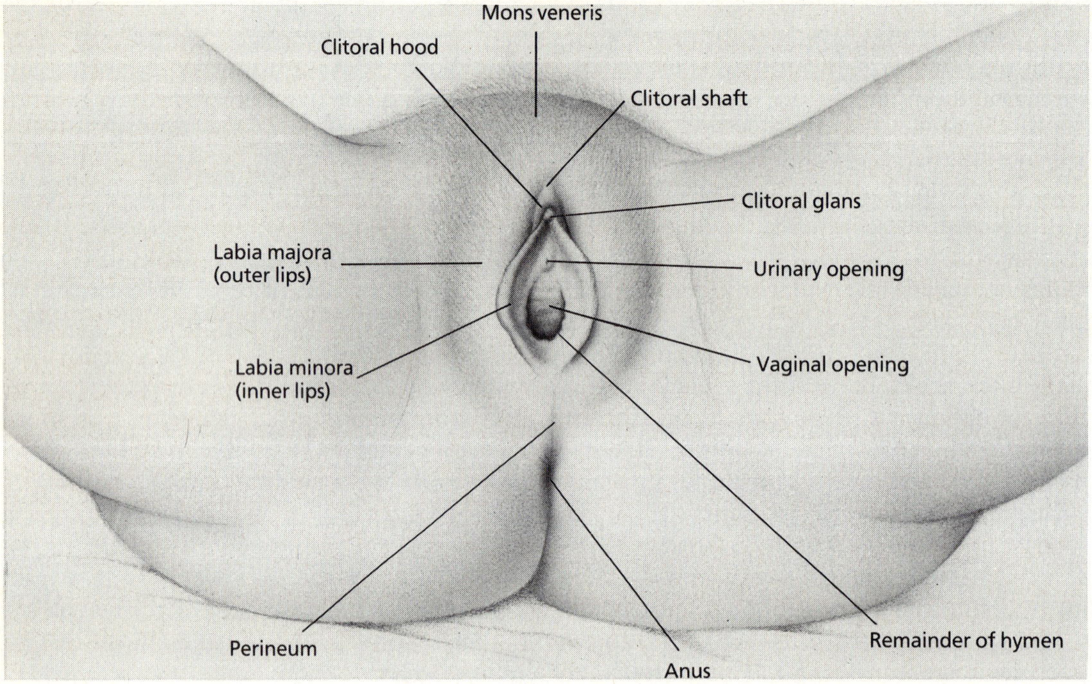

pearance. There are differences in the size, shape, and color of the labia (a few examples are shown in Figure 2–2), in the color, texture, amount, and distribution of pubic hair, and in the appearance of the clitoris, vaginal opening, and hymen. Sexual anatomy varies just as much as facial anatomy differs from one person to another.

Bartholin's glands lie within the labia minora and are connected to small ducts that open on the inner surface of the labia next to the vaginal opening (see Figure 2–3). Although they were once thought to play a major role in the production of vaginal lubrication, it is now clear that the few drops of secretion usually produced by these glands during sexual arousal are not important contributors to vaginal lubrication, although they may slightly moisten the labia.

THE CLITORIS

The **clitoris**, one of the most sensitive areas of a female's genitals, is located just beneath the point where the top of the inner lips meet. The only directly visible part of the clitoris is the head or **clitoral glans**, which looks like a small, shiny button. This head can be seen by gently pushing up the skin or clitoral hood that covers it. The clitoral hood also hides the **clitoral shaft**, the spongy tissue that branches internally like an inverted V into two longer parts or **crura**. The crura lead to the bony pelvis. The clitoris is richly endowed with nerve endings that make it highly sensitive to touch, pressure, and temperature. It is unique because it is the only organ in either sex whose only known function is to focus and accumulate sexual sensations and erotic pleasure (Masters and Johnson, 1970).

The clitoris is often regarded as a miniature penis, but this notion is sexist and incorrect. The clitoris has no reproductive or urinary function and does not usually lengthen like the penis when stimulated, although it does become engorged. The clitoris and the penis, however, are derived embryologically from the same tissue.

The size and appearance of the clitoris vary considerably among women, but there is no evidence that a

FIGURE 2–2

Some Variations in the Appearance of the Female Genitals

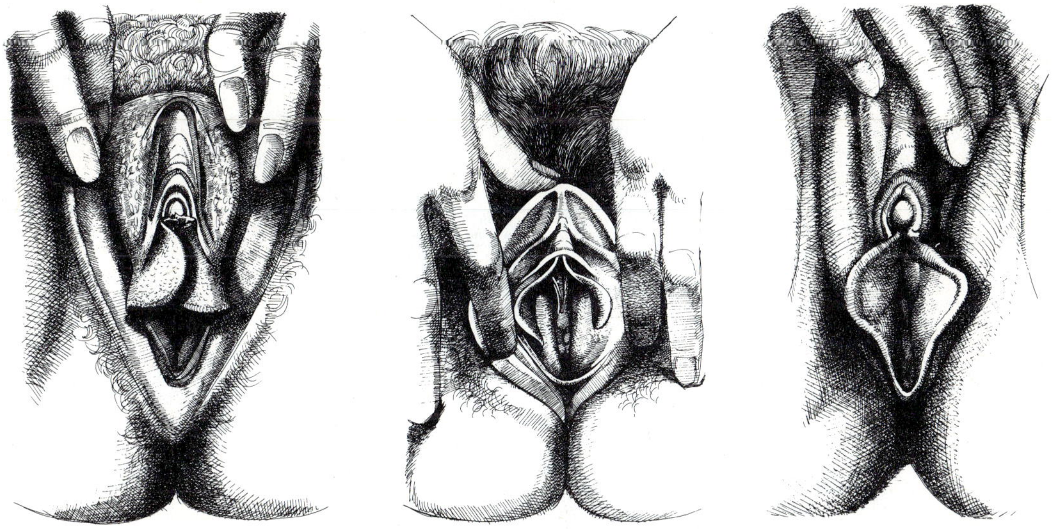

Betty Dodson's drawings of the female genitals reflect not only her artistic perspective but also the feminist view of the importance of women accepting their sexual anatomy as a positive attibute and a source of pleasure rather than shame.

Source: Betty Dodson, *Selflove & Orgasm* (1983), Box 1933 Murray Hill Station, New York, N.Y. 10156, $5.50 pp.

larger clitoris provides more intense sexual arousal. Contrary to the opinion of some physicians, masturbation rarely causes enlargement of this organ.

Clitoral circumcision—surgical removal of the clitoral hood—has been said to improve female sexual responsivity by exposing the clitoral glans to more direct stimulation.[1] We believe, however, that this procedure is rarely useful since it has two major drawbacks: (1) the clitoral glans is often exquisitely sensitive to direct touch, to the point of pain or irritation (in this sense, the clitoral hood serves a protective function),[2] and (2) during intercourse the thrusting of the penis indirectly stimulates the clitoris by mov-

[1] Some tribes in Africa and South America practice surgical removal of the clitoris (clitoridectomy) as a ritual rite of puberty. And, according to one Egyptian physician, more than one-half of all young girls in Egypt are still undergoing this painful procedure today (*Sexuality Today*, Vol. 6, No. 3, June 6, 1983). Although this practice is sometimes called "clitoral circumcision," it is not at all the same. Clitoridectomy does not destroy the capacity for sexual arousal or orgasm, but it certainly does not help it at all.

[2] In masturbation most women stroke areas around the clitoral glans but avoid its direct stimulation for this very reason. Apparently, the advocates of clitoral circumcision (usually men, oddly enough) have overlooked this finding.

Bartholin's glands (bahr′ tō linz) small glands adjacent to the vaginal opening. Although they produce minimal amounts of lubrication, their function is unknown.

clitoris (klit′ o ris) part of the external genitals of the female, situated at the anterior meeting of the labia minora and made up of two small erectile bodies, a glans and a hood. Its only known function is to focus and accumulate sexual sensations and erotic pleasure.

clitoral glans (klit′ o rul) the tip or head and the only visible part of the clitoris, resembling a small button.

clitoral shaft part of the external female genitals; two small erectile bodies enclosed in a fibrous membrane and ending in a glans. Corresponds to the **corpus cavernosa** in the penis.

crura (kroo′ ruh) the internal branches of the clitoral shaft and the corpus cavernosa attached to the bony pelvis.

FIGURE 2–3

Anatomy of the Clitoris

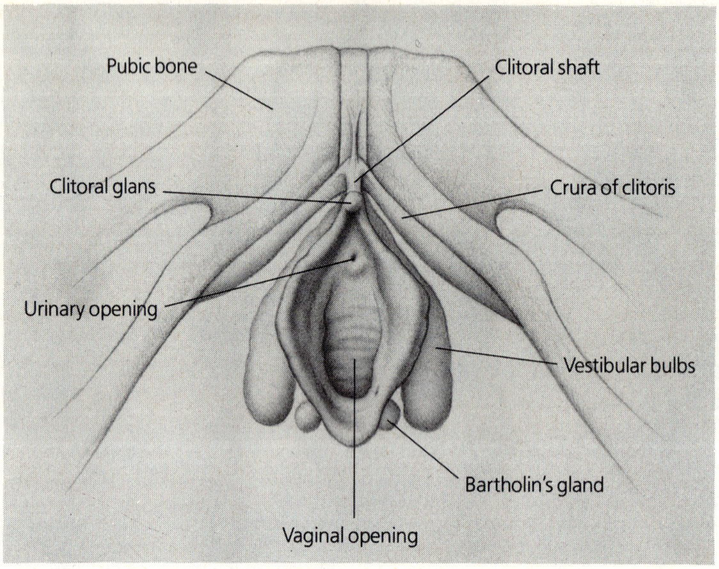

ing the inner lips of the vagina, causing the clitoral hood to rub back and forth across the clitoral glans (Masters and Johnson, 1966). A less drastic procedure than circumcision is advocated by several sexologists to improve some women's sexual responsiveness. A probe is used to loosen adhesions or thickened secretions (**smegma**) between the clitoral hood and clitoral glans (Graber and Kline-Graber, 1979). We have seen very few cases that required such an approach and remain skeptical about the use of this procedure on a routine basis.

THE PERINEUM

The **perineum** is the hairless area of skin between the bottom of the labia and the anus (the opening for evacuation of the bowels). This region is often sensitive to touch, pressure, and temperature and may be a source of sexual arousal.

The Hymen

The opening of the vagina is covered by a thin tissue membrane called the **hymen.** The hymen, which has no known function, typically has perforations in it that allow menstrual flow to pass from the body at puberty. The hymen usually stretches across some but not all of the vaginal opening and may vary in shape, size, and thickness, as Figure 2–4 reveals.

Historically, it has been important for a woman to have an intact hymen at the time of marriage as proof of her virginity. In some societies, a bride who does not have an intact hymen is returned to her parents, subjected to public ridicule, physically punished, or even put to death (Ford and Beach, 1951). Even in modern Japan and Italy, plastic surgeons are kept busy reconstructing the hymens of many engaged women to create "neovirginity" for those who wish to conceal their sexual histories from future husbands.

Contrary to the fears of some females, a doctor cannot usually tell if they are virgins by conducting a pelvic examination. The presence or absence of an intact hymen is not an accurate indication of prior sexual behavior. The hymen may be broken or stretched at an early age by various exercises or by inserting fingers or objects in the vagina. Some females are born with only a partial hymen or none at all. In addition, intercourse does not always tear the hymen; instead, it may simply stretch it. Under most circumstances, the first intercourse experience for a girl or woman is not painful or marked by a great deal of bleeding. The excitement of the moment is usually enough so that the pressure on the hymen is barely noticed.

FIGURE 2–4

Variations in the Hymen

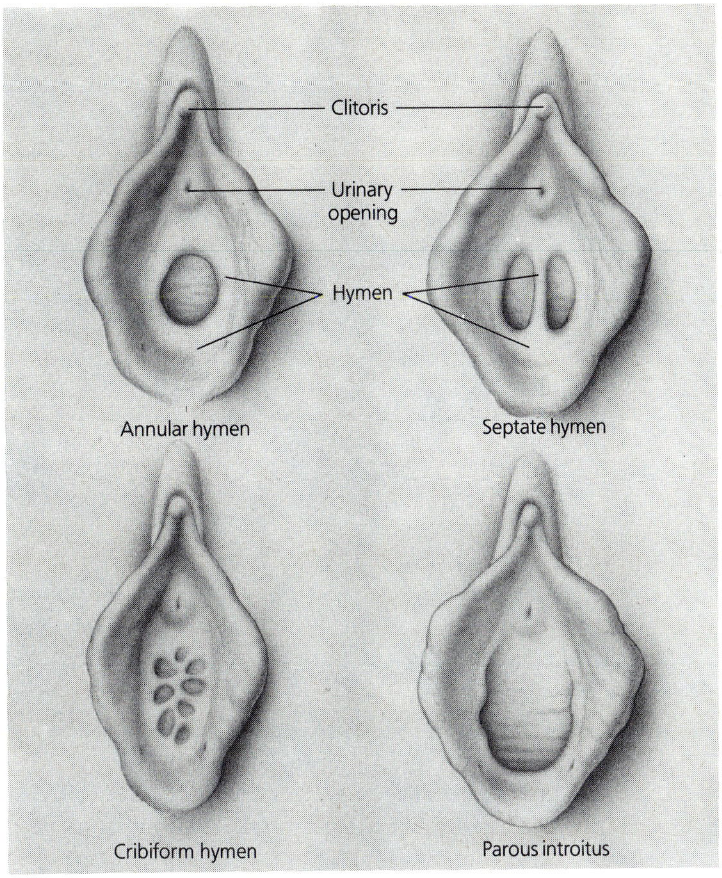

The annular *hymen forms a ring around the vaginal opening; the* septate *hymen has one or more bands of tissue that cross the diameter of the vaginal opening; and the* cribiform *hymen stretches completely across the vaginal opening but has many small perforations. The* parous introitus *is the opening of the vagina in a woman who has previously given birth to a child by vaginal delivery; only small remnants of the tissue of the hymen are visible.*

The Vagina

The **vagina** is a muscular internal organ that tilts upward at a 45° angle diagonally pointed toward the small of the back (Figure 2–5). In the sexually unstimulated state, the vagina's walls are collapsed. In a woman who has never had a child, the back wall of the vagina averages 8 centimeters (about 3 inches) in length, while the front wall is approximately 6 centimeters (2½ inches) long.

The vagina functions as a potential space that, like

smegma (smeg' muh) glandular secretions, dead cells, dirt particles, and bacteria that accumulate under the foreskin of the penis or the hood of the clitoris.

perineum (per i nē' um) the hairless area of skin between the vagina and anus in the female and between the scrotum and anus in the male.

hymen (hī' mun) a thin tissue membrane covering the opening of the vagina.

vagina (va jī' nuh) the canal in the female that receives the penis in copulation, existing as a potential space capable of contraction and expansion. The opening is called the vaginal introitus.

FIGURE 2–5

Internal Side View of the Female Reproductive System

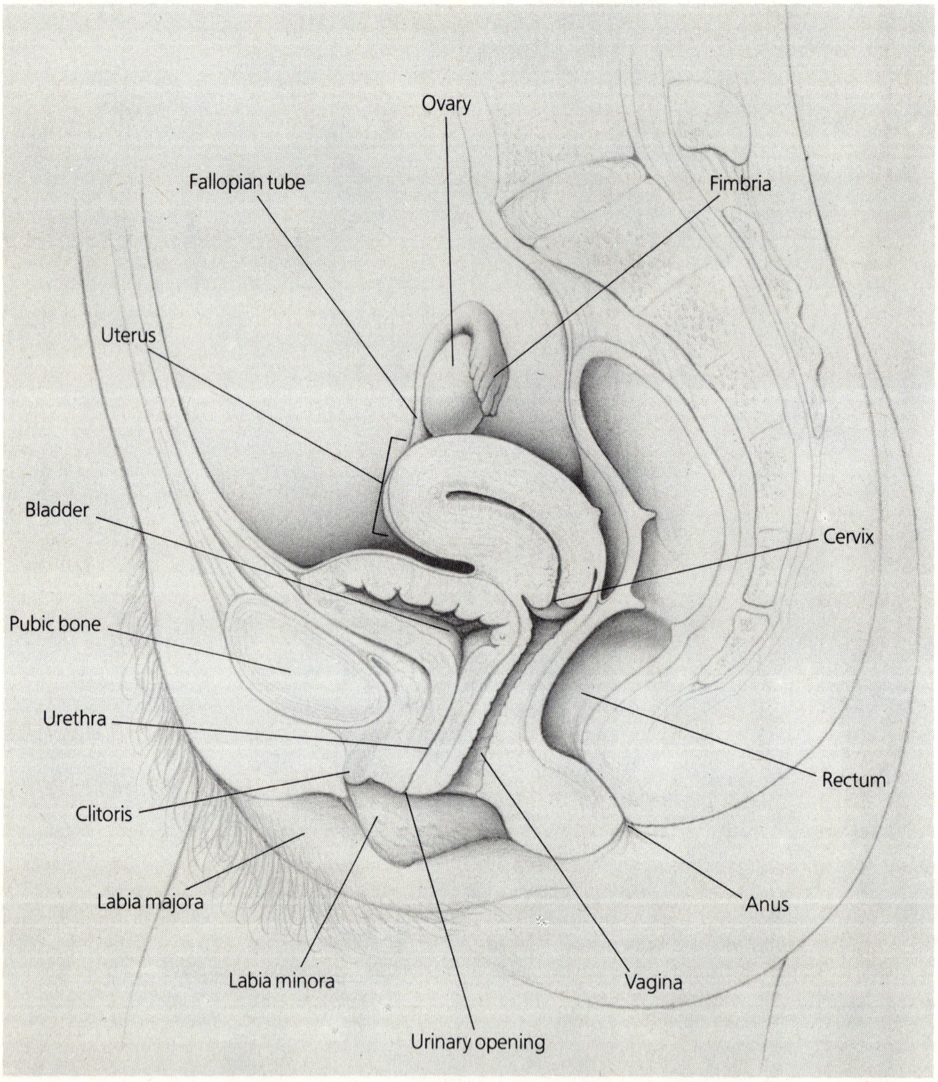

a balloon, can change shape and size. It can contract and expand, accommodate the passage of a baby during childbirth, or adjust in size to fit snugly around a finger.[3]

Many people wonder about the relationship between vaginal size and sexual gratification. Since the vagina adjusts equally well to a large or small penis, it is unusual for size differences between male and female sex organs to lead to sexual difficulties. Following childbirth, the vagina usually enlarges moderately and loses some degree of elasticity. Exercises to strengthen the muscles supporting the vagina are thought by some authorities to improve this condition

[3] Despite its ability to contract, the human vagina cannot "clamp down" on the penis during intercourse and make physical separation impossible. In dogs, there is a type of intravaginal "locking," but it occurs primarily because of expansion of the bulbar portion of the shaft of the penis.

and foster sexual responsiveness (Kegel, 1952; Kline-Graber and Graber, 1978).[4]

The inside of the vagina is lined with a surface similar to the lining inside the mouth. This **mucosa** is the source of vaginal lubrication. There are no secretory glands in the vagina, but there is a rich supply of blood vessels. The vagina has relatively few sensory nerve endings except near its opening. As a result, the inner two-thirds of the vagina are relatively insensitive to touch or pain.

In the last decade, there have been claims that a region in the front wall of the vagina midway between the pubic bone and the cervix has a special sensitivity to erotic stimulation. Called the **G spot** (or **Gräfenberg spot,** for the German physician who first suggested its presence in 1950), it has been described as a mass of tissue about the size of a small bean in the unstimulated state. When stimulated, the tissue swells to the size of a dime or larger (Ladas, Whipple, and Perry, 1982).

Ladas, Whipple, and Perry (1982) state that examinations of more than 400 women identified the "G spot" in each one; they explain that it has generally been overlooked in the past because "in its unstimulated state, it is relatively small and difficult to locate, especially since you can't see it." This explanation does not fit a research project in which Whipple herself participated in which the "G spot" could be found in only 4 out of 11 women (Goldberg et al., 1983), nor does it coincide with our studies at the Masters & Johnson Institute, where less than 10 percent of a sample of over 100 women who were carefully examined had an area of heightened sensitivity in the

[4] The "Kegel exercises" are done by contracting the pelvic muscles that support the vagina (most notably, the **pubococcygeus** and **bulbocavernosus** muscles). These same muscles are used when a woman stops the flow of urine or tightens the vagina against an inserted object such as a tampon, a finger, or an erect penis. The muscles are contracted firmly for one or two seconds and then released; this is repeated in a series of ten contractions several times a day for maximum results. In addition to strengthening muscular contractions, these exercises can improve a woman's sense of self-awareness. Whether they really improve sexual responsivity is less certain at present.

FOCUS IN BRIEF

Douching

Concerns about vaginal cleanliness have led many women to practice **douching** (using a liquid to flush out the vagina) on a regular basis as part of their personal hygiene, and commercial preparations of douching solutions are now even advertised on television. However, there is mounting evidence of negative health effects from douching.

- Frequent douching can destroy beneficial bacteria in the vagina, which sometimes leads to an overgrowth of pathological microorganisms that produce symptomatic vaginal infections.
- Frequent douching also reduces the acidity of the vagina, which can make a woman more susceptible to vaginal infections.
- Frequent douching is a risk factor for pelvic inflammatory disease (Forrest et al., 1989; Wolner-Hanssen et al., 1990), a serious infection involving the inner reproductive organs in females (see Chapter 7).
- Self-diagnosing and self-treating vaginal burning, itching, discharge, or odor by douching is ill-advised, since douching may mask the presence of a serious infection such as gonorrhea and thus delay the start of appropriate medical therapy (Covington and McClendon, 1987).

In short, while there is probably no major health risk associated with infrequent douching (once or twice a month or less), we consider it wisest to avoid this practice unless it has been medically recommended to a woman. ■

mucosa (mew kō′ suh) mucous membrane. The membrane lining of the body openings, especially of the vagina, kept moist by the secretions of various types of glands.

G spot (Gräfenberg spot) a proposed region of the front wall of the vagina claimed by some researchers to have a high degree of erotic sensitivity.

pubococcygeus (pew′ bō kock sij′ ē us) a muscle encircling and supporting the vagina.

bulbocavernosus (bul′ bō kav ur nō′ sus) a muscle encircling and supporting the entrance to the vagina.

douching (dūsh′ ing) using a liquid to flush the vagina.

front wall of the vagina or a tissue mass that fit the various descriptions of this area. Another study also was unable to find evidence supporting the existence of the "G spot" (Alzate and Londono, 1984), although many of the women studied showed signs of erotic sensitivity in the front wall of the vagina. A more recent report concluded that "evidence for the existence of the G spot . . . in an appreciable minority of women, let alone the majority of them, is so far inconclusive" (Alzate and Hoch, 1986). Thus, at the present time it seems that additional research is needed to establish whether the "G spot" exists as a distinct anatomic structure or whether, as Helen Kaplan (1983) says, "the knowledge that many women have erotically sensitive areas in their vaginas which contribute to pleasure and orgasm is not new or controversial." As one recent report noted, the greater sensitivity of the anterior vaginal wall does not seem to be restricted to one specific spot, so that it may be "part and parcel of the female's clitoral/vaginal sensory arm of the orgasmic reflex" (Schultz et al., 1989).

The Uterus

The **cervix** is the bottom part of the uterus that protrudes into the vagina. Through the vagina, the cervix of a woman who has never been pregnant looks like a smooth pink button with a rounded face and a small central hole. At the mouth of the cervix (the **cervical os**), sperm cells enter the uterus and menstrual flow passes into the vagina. The **endocervical canal** (a thin tubelike communication between the mouth of the cervix and the cavity of the uterus) contains many secretory glands that produce mucus. The consistency of cervical mucus varies during different phases of the menstrual cycle in response to changing hormonal stimulation: just before or at the time of ovulation (when the egg is released from the ovary), cervical secretions become thin and watery; at other times, these secretions are thick and form a mucous plug that blocks the entrance to the cervix.

The cervix has no surface nerve endings, so it experiences little in the way of sexual feelings. If the cervix is removed surgically, there is no loss of sexual responsivity.

The **uterus** (womb) is a hollow muscular organ shaped like an inverted pear somewhat flattened from front to back. It is about 7.5 centimeters (3 inches) long and 5 centimeters (2 inches) wide. Anatomically, the uterus consists of several parts (Figure 2–6). The inside lining of the uterus (the **endometrium**) and the muscular component of the uterus (the **myometrium**) have separate and distinct functions. The inner lining changes during the menstrual cycle and is where a fertilized egg implants at the beginning of a pregnancy. The muscular wall facilitates labor and delivery. Both aspects of uterine function are regulated by chemicals called **hormones**, which also play a part in the growth of the uterus during pregnancy.

The uterus is held loosely in place in the pelvic cavity by six ligaments. The angle of the uterus in relation to the vagina varies from woman to woman. Ordinarily, it is relatively perpendicular to the axis of the vaginal canal, but in about 25 percent of women, the uterus is tipped backward, and in approximately 10 percent, it is tilted farther forward. If the uterus is rigidly fixed in position by scar tissue or inflammation, it may be a source of pain during sexual activity, requiring surgical correction.

The Fallopian Tubes

The **Fallopian tubes**, or oviducts, begin at the uterus and extend about 10 centimeters (4 inches) laterally (Figure 2–6). The far ends of the Fallopian tubes are funnel-shaped and terminate in long fingerlike extensions called **fimbria**, which hover near the ovaries. The inside lining of the Fallopian tubes consists of long, thin folds of tissue covered by hairlike **cilia**. The Fallopian tubes pick up eggs produced and released

cervix (ser′ viks) the cylindrical part of the uterus that protrudes into the vagina. The point where sperm cells enter the uterus and menstrual flow exits is called the **cervical os.**

cervical os (ser′ vi kul oss′) the mouth or opening of the cervix.

endocervical canal (en′ dō ser′ vi kul) the tubelike connection between the mouth of the cervix and the uterine cavity containing numerous secretory glands that produce mucus.

uterus (ū′ tur us) a hollow, pear-shaped muscular organ, part of the female internal genitals, in which the fertilized egg becomes embedded and the embryo and the fetus are nourished. Sometimes called the womb.

endometrium (en′ dō mē′ trē um) the inner lining of the uterus in which the egg implants and which is partially shed during menstruation.

myometrium (mī′ ō mē trē um) the muscular component of the uterus, important in labor and delivery.

hormone chemical substance secreted by the endocrine system into the bloodstream to be carried directly to the tissue on which it acts.

Fallopian tubes (fuh lō′ pē un) the tubes that transport eggs from the ovaries to the uterus. Also called oviducts.

FIGURE 2–6

Front View of the Internal Female Reproductive System

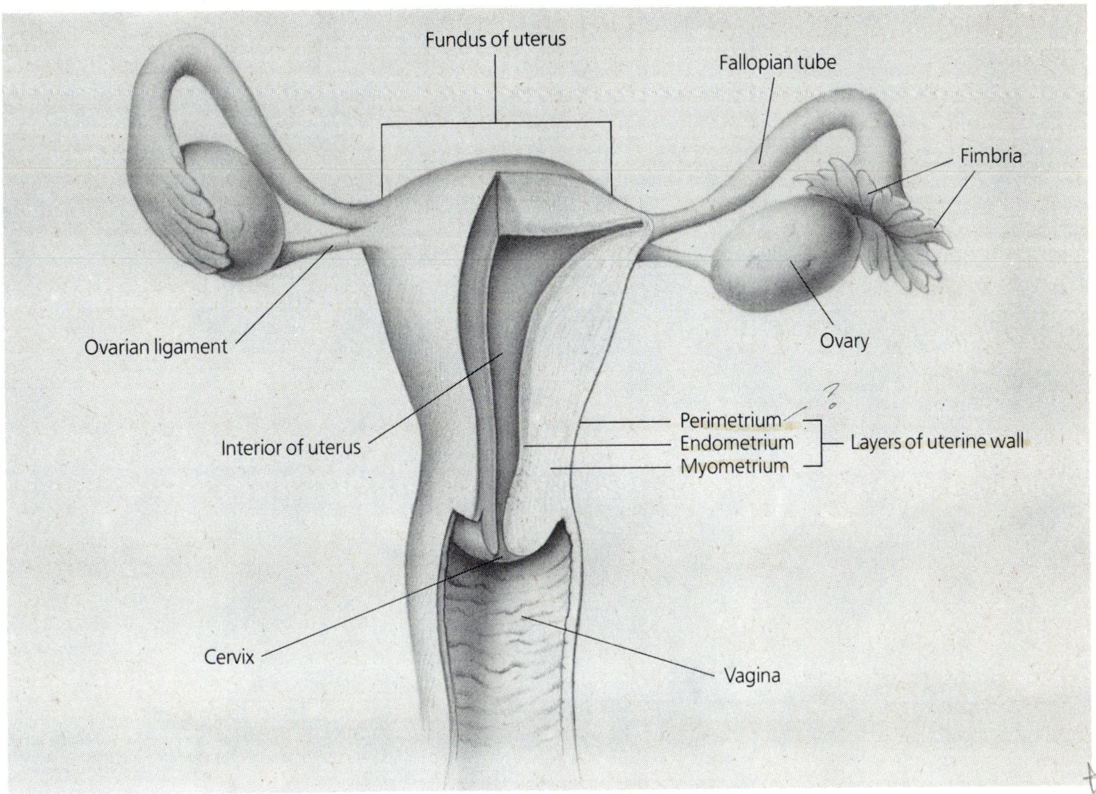

The uterus and vagina in this figure are shown partially cut away.

by the nearby ovary and then serve as the meeting ground for egg and sperm.

The Ovaries

The **ovaries**, or female gonads, are paired structures located on each side of the uterus. About the size of unshelled almonds (about 3 × 2 × 1.5 centimeters or 1.2 × 0.8 × 0.6 inches), they are held in place by connective tissue that attaches to the broad ligament of the uterus. The ovaries have two separate functions: manufacturing hormones (most notably, estrogen and progesterone) and producing and releasing eggs.

Before a baby girl is born, development of future eggs begins in her just-forming ovaries. About halfway through her mother's pregnancy, the girl's ovaries contain 6 or 7 million future eggs, most of which degenerate before birth. About 400,000 immature eggs are present in the newborn girl, and no new eggs are formed after this time. During childhood, continued degeneration reduces the number of eggs still further. The immature eggs are surrounded by a thin capsule of tissue forming a **follicle.**

When puberty arrives and girls begin to have menstrual cycles (see Chapter 6), each cycle is marked by a process of maturation in which some immature eggs divide twice, splitting their genetic material in half.

fimbria (fim′ brē uh) long, fingerlike extensions at the entrance to the Fallopian tubes.

cilia (sil′ ē uh) the hairlike filaments in the inside of the fallopian tubes that propel the egg along to the uterus.

ovaries (ō′ vur ēz) paired structures located on each side of the uterus that contain and release eggs and secrete hormones such as estrogen and progesterone. The female gonads.

follicle (fol′ i kul) a thin capsule of tissue surrounding immature eggs.

FIGURE 2–7

Photomicrograph of a Human Egg in a Secondary Follicle

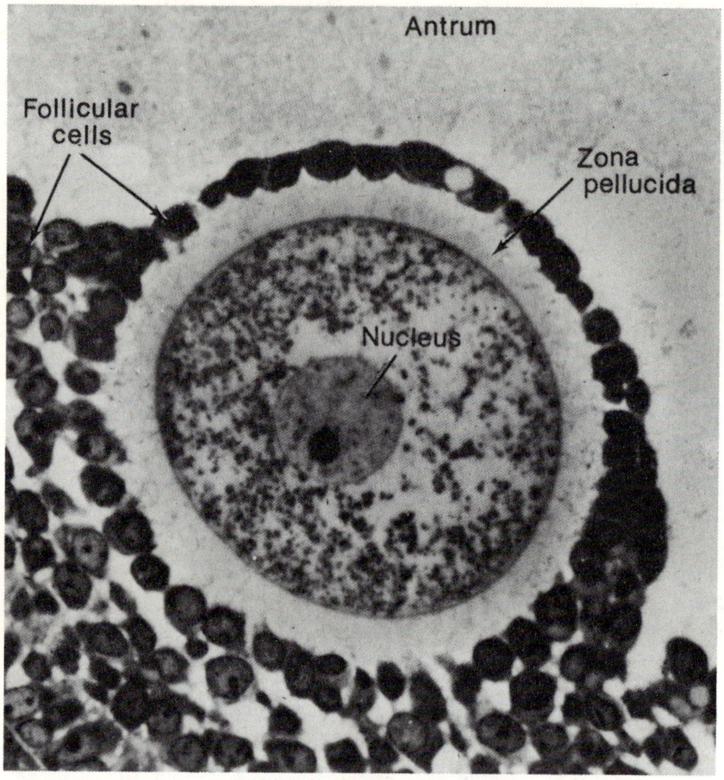

Through this process, called **meiosis**, each young egg divides into four cells, only one of which is a mature egg (**ovum**). A mature egg is about 0.135 millimeter (1/175 of an inch) in diameter and is surrounded by a zone of jellylike material called the **zona pellucida** (Figure 2–7). A human egg is just barely visible, appearing as a speck smaller than the period at the end of this sentence. The other three cells, called **polar bodies** (Figure 2–8), have no known function and eventually degenerate.

Although a number of different follicles begin growing in each cycle, usually only one develops to the point where it moves to the surface of the ovary and ruptures, releasing the egg in a process called **ovulation**. For every follicle that ovulates, about a thousand undergo various degrees of growth and then degenerate. Fewer than 400 follicles are usually involved in ovulation during the female's reproductive years.

After the release of the egg, the **granulosa cells** that made up the capsule of the follicle begin to enlarge, forming a structure called the **corpus luteum.** The corpus luteum produces hormones and is des-

meiosis (mī ō′ sis) the process by which each immature egg divides into four cells, only one of which is a mature egg.

ovum (ō′ vum) a mature egg cell that can, after maturation and fertilization, become another member of the same species.

zona pellucida (zō′ nuh pe lew′ sē duh) the jellylike material surrounding the mature egg.

polar bodies cells that arise in the development of the ovum during meiosis.

ovulation (ōv you lā′ shun) the second phase of the menstrual cycle; the release of the egg from the ovary.

granulosa cells (gran′ ū lō′ suh) the cells lining the ovarian follicle that enlarge and form the corpus luteum.

corpus luteum (kor′ pus lew′ tē um) part of the capsule of the ovarian follicle left in an ovary after an egg is expelled. It secretes hormones and, if pregnancy does not occur, degenerates.

FIGURE 2–8

Development of Sperm Cells (upper diagram) and Ovum (lower diagram)

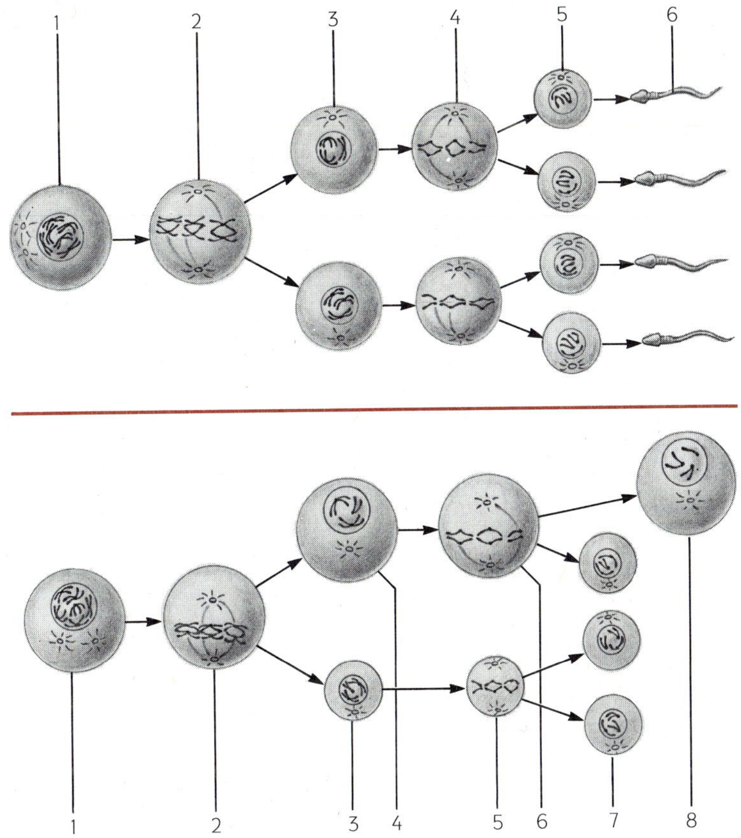

Development of sperm cells (upper diagram)
Stages 1 and 2: Primitive germ cell no. 1, the primary spermatocyte. At stage 1, the chromosomes in the nucleus double lengthwise. At stage 2, the chromosomal pairs are arranged in a plane for meiotic division. This will give rise to two new cells, each with half the normal complement of chromosomes.
Stages 3 and 4: Primitive germ cell no. 2, the secondary spermatocyte. At stage 3, the chromosomes in the nucleus again double longitudinally. At stage 4, the chromosomes are aligned in a plane for ordinary cell division, not meiosis.
Stage 5: Four sperm cell precursors, or spermatids, are produced from the original spermatocyte.
Stage 6: Mature sperm cells.

Development of an ovum (lower diagram)
Stages 1 and 2: The primitive germ cell, or the primary oocyte. At stage 1, the chromosomes in the nucleus double lengthwise. At stage 2, the chromosomes are aligned in a plane for meiotic division. This gives rise to a secondary oocyte and the first polar body, each with half the number of chromosomes.
Stages 3 and 5: First polar bodies. At stage 5, the chromosomes of the first polar body are arranged for ordinary cell division.
Stages 4 and 6: The second primitive germ cell, or the secondary oocyte. At stage 4, the chromosomes in the nucleus double longitudinally. At stage 6, the chromosomes are aligned in a plane for ordinary cell division, not meiosis.
Stage 7: Three secondary polar bodies are produced.
Stage 8: Mature ovum.

Source: "Development of Sperm Cells and Ovum" from BEHOLD MAN by Lennart Nilsson with Jon Lindberg. Copyright © 1973 by Albert Bonniers Forlag. English translation copyright © 1984 by Albert Bonniers Forlag. Reprinted by permission.

FIGURE 2–9

External and Internal Anatomy of the Female Breast

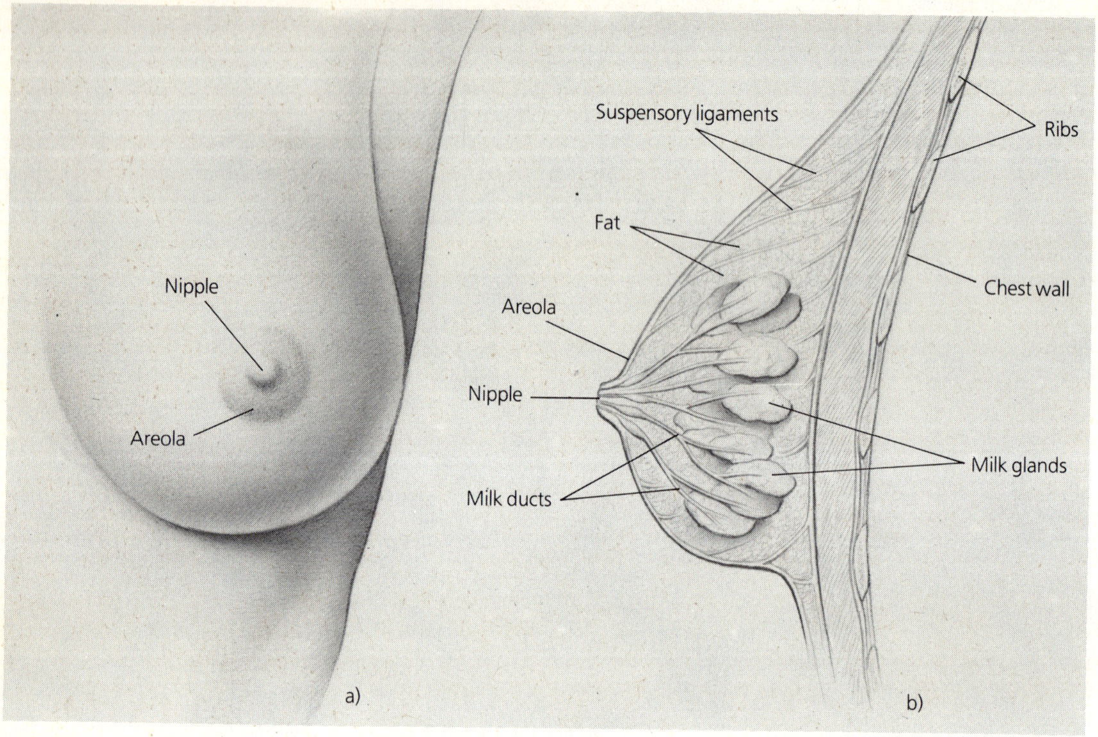

tined to degenerate within two weeks if pregnancy does not occur; with conception, the corpus luteum continues to develop and provides important hormonal support during early stages of pregnancy.

The Breasts

Although the breasts are not reproductive organs, they are clearly part of the sexual anatomy. In American society, the female breasts have a special erotic allure and symbolize sexuality, femininity, and attractiveness. Prominent attention is devoted to the breasts in clothing styles, men's magazines, advertising, television, and cinema. This attitude is not universal by any means, and in some cultures little or no erotic importance is attached to the breasts. For example, in Japan women traditionally bound their breasts to make them inconspicuous. Today, however, the westernization process has brought about changes in Japan and the breasts have become rather fully eroticized.

As the big-breasted female has become an almost universal sex symbol—the image used to promote everything from car sales to X-rated films—men and women have been bombarded daily with the not very subtle suggestion that a woman with large breasts has a definite sexual advantage. This has led to a number of harmful misconceptions. For example, men and women alike have come to believe that the larger a woman's breasts are, the more sexually excitable she is or can become. Another fallacy, still firmly subscribed to by many men, holds that the relatively flat-chested woman is less able to respond sexually and actually has little, if any, interest in sex.

There is absolutely no evidence to suggest that breast size bears any relation to a woman's level of sexual interest, to her capacity for sexual response, or to the ease with which she attains orgasm. Actually, many women experience very little sexual sensation when their breasts are fondled or caressed, and this is as true of those with large breasts as it is of those with small ones. Furthermore, the woman who does become sexually excited when her breasts are stimulated does so regardless of their size.

For all their erotic significance, breasts are actually just modified sweat glands. The female breasts undergo changes in size and shape during puberty, grad-

FIGURE 2–10

Variations in Appearance of the Female Breast

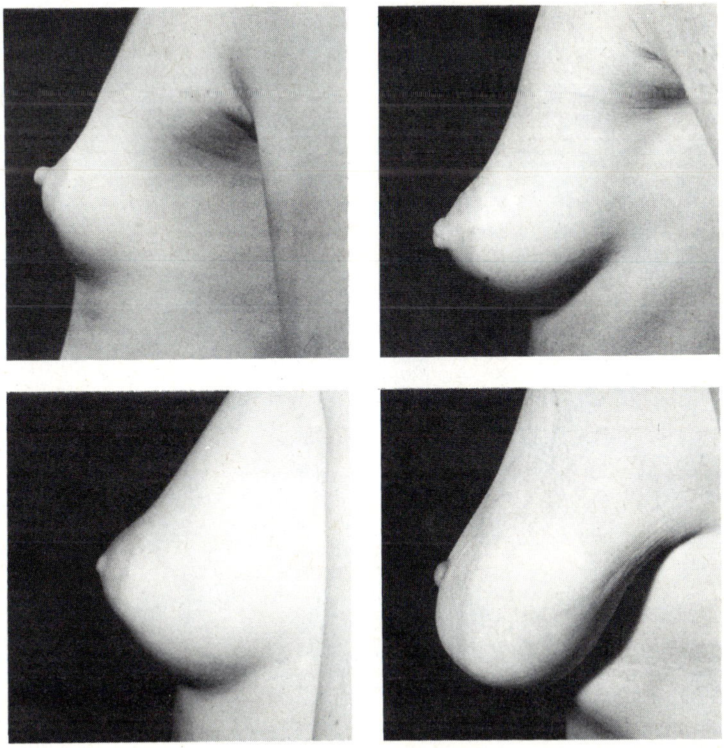

ually becoming conical or hemispherical, with the left breast usually slightly larger than the right (DeGowin and DeGowin, 1976). Each breast contains 15 to 20 subdivided lobes of glandular tissue arranged in a grapelike cluster, with each lobe drained by a duct opening on the surface of the nipple (Figure 2–9). The glandular lobes are surrounded by fatty and fibrous tissue, giving a soft consistency to the breast.

The **nipple** is located at the tip of the breast and mostly consists of smooth muscle fibers and a network of nerve endings that make it highly sensitive to touch and temperature. The dark wrinkled skin of the nipple extends 1 or 2 centimeters onto the surface of the breast to form the **areola**, a circular area of dark skin with many nerve fibers and with muscle fibers that cause the nipple to stiffen and become erect.

The sexual sensitivity of the breast, areola, and nipple do not depend on breast size or shape (Figure 2–10). Personal preference, learned habit, and biology all contribute to their responsiveness. Nevertheless, the American male's fascination with female breasts leads many women who consider themselves "flat-chested" or "underdeveloped" to seek to improve their sexual attractiveness and self-esteem by the use of exercises, lotions, or mechanical devices such as suction machines to enlarge their breasts. These methods, though widely advertised, do not work. For this reason, so-called breast augmentation surgery has become popular. In the past, liquid silicone was injected directly into the breasts to increase their size, but this technique proved to be highly unsatisfactory as it led to many medical complications. Today, soft thin plastic pouches filled with silicone gel are implanted through a simple breast incision to increase size while retaining a natural appearing and soft feeling breast.

Conversely, some women are troubled by breasts

nipple protuberance located at the tip of the breast consisting principally of smooth muscle fibers and a network of nerve endings and containing in the female the outlets of the milk ducts.

areola (a rē′ o luh) the circular area of dark skin around the nipple.

SELF-EXAMINATION OF THE BREASTS

It is important for women to examine their own breasts regularly because most breast lumps are self-discovered rather than found by a doctor or nurse. Although some people feel uncomfortable about this type of self-exam, two specific facts should be noted: (1) about nine out of ten breast lumps are *not* cancer and (2) women who examine their own breasts monthly have significantly higher survival rates after breast cancer than women who do not (Foster et al., 1978). The best time for a breast self-exam is right after your period ends because estrogen levels are low. Women who do not have periods should still examine their breasts once a month. The following technique should be used.

1. *Stand in front of a mirror with good lighting*. Inspect your breasts visually in the mirror, with your arms relaxed at your sides. Then raise your hands above your head. Finally, put your hands on your hips and push down. Look for flattening or bulging in one breast but not the other, puckering of the skin, dimpling or redness, or one nipple being unusually drawn up into the breast. Squeeze each nipple gently to see if there is any discharge.
2. *Lie flat on your back, with a pillow or folded towel underneath your left shoulder, and your left arm behind your head.* Imagine that your breast is divided into four quarters, as shown in the diagram.
3. *With the fingers of your right hand held together, press firmly but gently (using the flat part of your fingertips) to feel the inner, upper quadrant of your left breast.* Move your hand in small circles so the breast tissue slides underneath the skin. Start at the breastbone and work towards the nipple.
4. *Repeat step 3 for each of the remaining quadrants of your left breast.* Cover the entire area and also feel over the ribs to the side of the breast.
5. *Bring your left arm down to your side and feel under your left armpit for swellings.*
6. *Repeat steps 2 to 5 using your left hand to examine your right breast.*
7. *Repeat steps 2 to 6 in the sitting or standing position.* The position change redistributes the breast tissue and may allow you to feel a lump that was hidden when you were lying down. You may want to do this in the bath or shower, since hands glide more easily over wet skin.

Sources: Boston Women's Health Book Collective, 1976; Stewart et al., 1979, American Cancer Society, 1980.

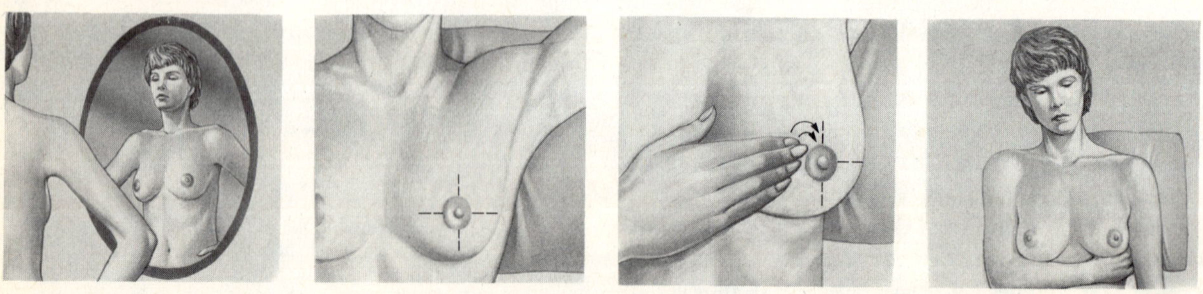

that are too large. This condition, called **mammary hyperplasia** or **macromastia**, can be treated by reduction mammaplasty, a fairly simple operation to reduce breast size and weight. Other common breast problems include **inverted nipples** (the nipples are pushed inward), a harmless anatomical variation that usually does not interfere with nursing, and **extra nipples**, which are minor errors of development that have no adverse health consequences but may be a source of embarrassment. Breast self-examination is discussed on page 36.

MALE SEXUAL ANATOMY

> It is not much of an exaggeration to say that penises in fantasyland come in only three sizes—large, gigantic, and so big you can barely get them through the doorway. . . .
>
> Accepting your own merely human penis can be difficult. You know it is somewhat unpredictable and, even when functioning at its best, looks and feels more like a human penis than a battering ram or a mountain of stone. But you do have one small advantage. You are alive and can enjoy yourself whereas the supermen of the model with the gigantic erections are unreal and feel nothing. *(Zilbergeld, 1978, pp. 23, 26)*

The male sex organs are more visible and accessible than the female sex organs. Unlike the clitoris or vagina, the penis is involved directly in the process of urination so that boys become accustomed to touching and handling their penises at a relatively early age. The sexual aspects of the male organ are hard for a boy to miss. He learns about them by watching, touching, and playing with his penis as it becomes erect (a pleasurable experience) or by hearing stories and jokes that graphically portray the sexual and reproductive purposes of the penis. Despite such exposure, many males are not fully informed about the details of the anatomy and function of the sex organs.

The Penis

The penis is an external organ that consists primarily of three parallel cylinders of spongy tissue bound in thick membrane sheaths (Figure 2–11). The cylindrical body on the underside of the penis is called the **spongy body** (**corpus spongiosum**). The **urethra** (a tube that carries urine or semen) runs through the middle of the spongy body and exits at the tip of the penis via the **urinary opening** (**urethral meatus**). When the penis is erect, the spongy body on the underside looks and feels like a straight ridge. The other two cylinders, called the **cavernous bodies** (**corpora cavernosa**), are positioned side by side above the spongy body. All three consist of irregular sponge-like tissue dotted with small blood vessels. The tissue swells with blood during sexual arousal causing the penis to become erect.

Internally, beyond the point where the penis attaches to the body, the cavernous bodies branch apart to form tips (**crura**) that are firmly attached to the pelvic bones. The penis has numerous blood vessels, both inside and apart from the cylindrical bodies; a pattern of veins is often visible on the outer skin of the erect penis. The penis also has many nerves, making it highly sensitive to touch, pressure, and temperature.

The tip of the penis, the **glans** or head, consists entirely of corpus spongiosum. This region has a higher concentration of sensory nerve endings than the shaft of the penis and is thus particularly sensitive to physical stimulation. Two other areas particularly sensitive to touch are the rim of tissue that separates the glans from the shaft of the penis (the **coronal ridge**) and the small triangular region on the underside of the penis where a thin strip of skin (the **frenulum**) attaches to the glans (Figure 2–11). Many males find that direct stimulation of the glans may become painful or irritating and prefer to masturbate by rubbing or stroking the penile shaft.

The skin that covers the penis is freely movable and

mammary hyperplasia or **macromastia** abnormally large breasts.

inverted nipples congenital condition in which the nipples are not protuberant.

extra nipples more than two paired nipples; about one person in 1000 has this condition.

corpus spongiosum (kor′ pus spon′ jē ō′ sum) the cylinder of erectile tissue along the underside of the penis containing the urethra. The distal portion expands to form the **glans.** Also called spongy body.

urethra (u rē′ thruh) a tube beginning at the bladder and ending at the urethral meatus, carrying urine in the female and urine or semen in the male.

urethral meatus (u re′ thral mē a′ tus) the urinary opening.

corpora cavernosa (kor′ po rhu kav ur nō′ suh) the two parallel cylindrical bodies of erectile tissue that make up the larger part of the shaft of the penis and the clitoris. Also called cavernous bodies.

glans (glanz) the tip or head of the penis or clitoris.

coronal ridge (kor′ ō nul) the rim of tissue that separates the glans from the shaft of the penis.

frenulum (fren′ ū lum) a small, triangular fold of skin on the underside of the penis connecting the glans with the foreskin.

FIGURE 2–11

Anatomy of the Penis

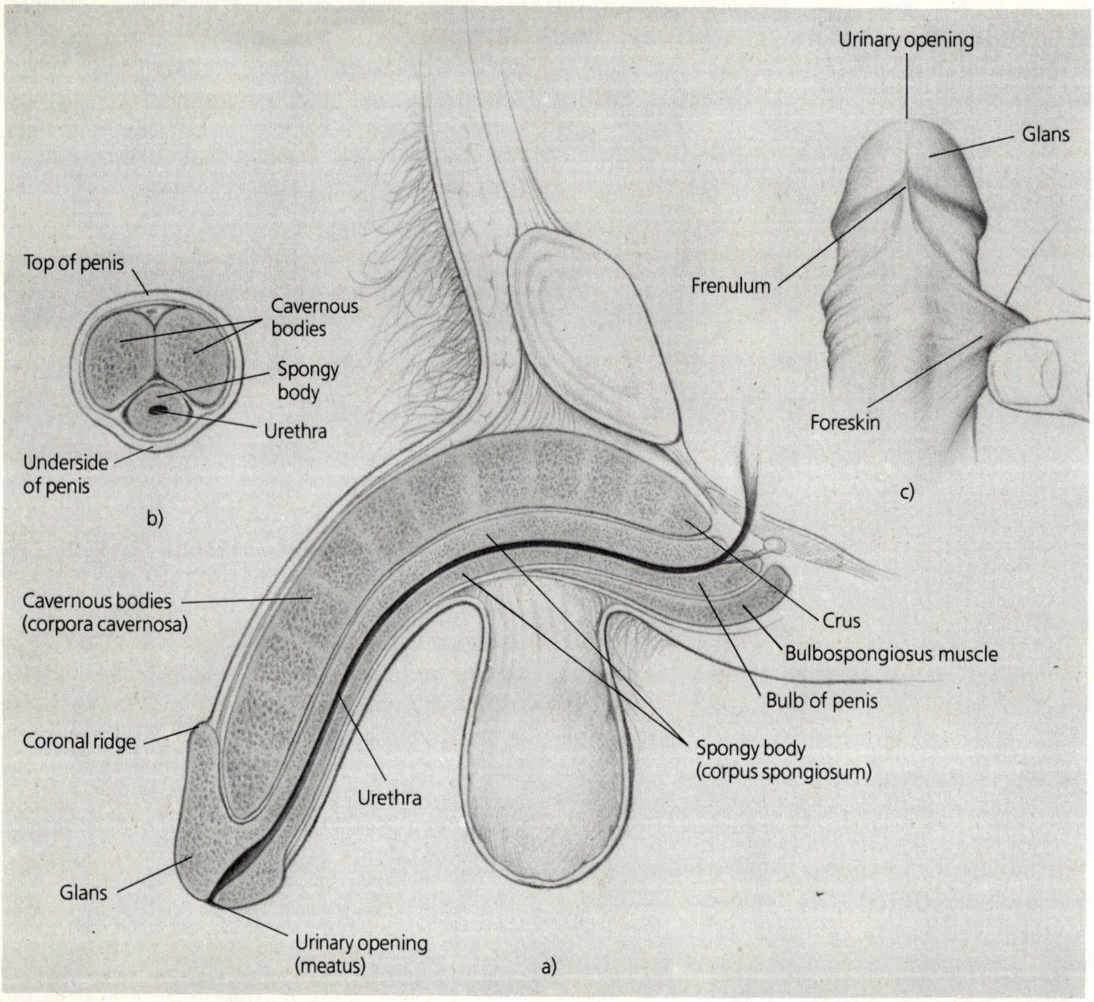

(a) Internal side view of the penis. (b) A cross section of the penis. (c) A view of the underside of the penis showing the location of the frenulum.

forms the **foreskin** or prepuce at the glans. Inflammation or infection of the foreskin or glans may cause pain during sexual activity. Sometimes the foreskin sticks to the underlying glans when smegma, a naturally occurring substance of cheesy consistency made up of oily secretions, dead skin cells, dirt particles, sweat, and bacteria, is not regularly washed away from underneath the foreskin. This type of problem occurs only in uncircumcised men and is one argument in favor of routine circumcision.

Circumcision is the surgical removal of the foreskin. As a result of this minor operation, usually done shortly after birth, the glans of the penis is fully exposed. Circumcision is sometimes a religious practice, as in Islam or in Judaism, where it symbolizes the covenant with God made by Abraham. In the United States, it is often done routinely for nonreligious reasons, whereas it is less common in Canada and Europe.

The advantages of circumcision are primarily related to hygiene and health: smegma does not collect, the glans of the penis is easier to clean, conditions of

FIGURE 2–12

Some Variations in the Appearance of the Male Genitals

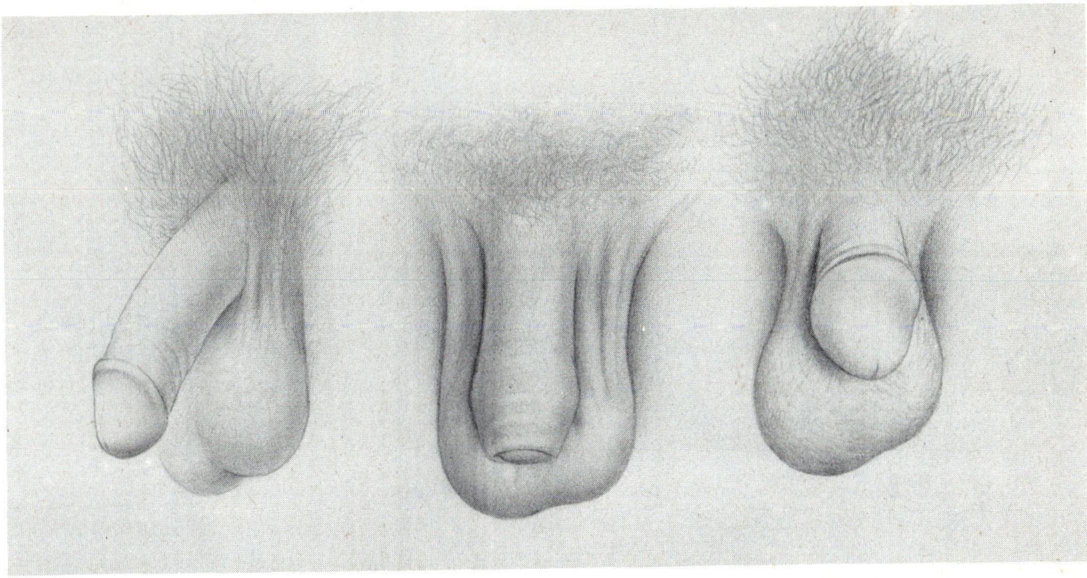

The middle drawing shows an uncircumcised penis.

inflammation or infection are less likely to occur, and cancer of the penis is far less frequent. Although the rate of cancer of the cervix is considerably lower in the spouses of circumcised men (Green, 1977, p. 403), it is not certain that this is a cause–effect relationship (Poland, 1990). In addition, urinary tract infections are many times higher in uncircumcised male infants than in those who are circumcised (Wissell et al., 1987; Herzog, 1989; Schoen, 1990). Potentially of even more importance, recent research suggests that circumcision provides some protection against infection with HIV (the AIDS virus) (Quinn et al., 1988; Marx, 1989; Schoen, 1990).

Opponents of routine circumcision see no clear reason for this operation and suggest that removing the skin protecting the glans weakens the region's sexual sensitivity since it constantly rubs directly against clothing. Others believe that circumcision increases the risk of premature ejaculation (this is probably not true, since the foreskin of the erect uncircumcised penis retracts, exposing the glans, and researchers have not found a difference in the rates of premature ejaculation in circumcised versus uncircumcised men). We are not aware of any believable evidence demonstrating that circumcision affects male sexual function one way or the other. On the other hand, uncircumcised men who practice routine hygienic care are unlikely to be at any major health disadvantage simply because their foreskin is intact.

Although it might sound surprising, a small number of men who were so dissatisfied with having been circumcised as infants have undergone a complicated series of operations to reconstruct the foreskin. While the results were reported as uniformly pleasing to these men (Greer et al., 1982), it was also noted that the reconstructed foreskin (which was taken from the scrotum) has a noticeable difference in skin texture, color, and contour from the skin on the shaft of the penis. The series of operations takes up to a year to complete.

The appearance of the penis varies considerably from one male to another. These variations are due to differences in color, size, shape, and the status of the foreskin (circumcised or uncircumcised). Some examples of different male genitals are shown in Figure 2–12.

Concerns about penile size are common in males of all ages. Although the size of the nonerect penis

foreskin (for′ skin) the freely movable skin that covers the penis. Also the hood of the clitoris.

circumcision (sur′ kum sizh′ un) surgical removal of the foreskin of the penis.

PENIS SIZE

We have already mentioned that many males are somewhat anxious about the size of their penis. More specifically, this concern is a comparative one: "How does *my* penis stack up against what others have?" This interest in penis size has several different components. First, it shows a concern for being "normal"—the same as everyone else. Second, it is related to a wish to be sexually adequate. Our society generally believes that "biggest is best," and the notion that a "big" penis will provide more sexual satisfaction to a woman is widespread. Actually, penile size has little physiological effect for the woman (although it may have positive or negative psychological significance) since the vagina accommodates its size equally well to an erect penis that is relatively smaller or larger in circumference. The length of the penis, which determines the depth of vaginal penetration, is also relatively unimportant, since the inner portion of the vagina and the cervix have few sensory nerve endings. Third, there is often an element of status-seeking in wishing to have a large penis. Finally, some males feel that a larger penis would make them more sexually attractive. Most of these points apply to both heterosexual and homosexual males.

In art and in the media (particularly erotic books, male magazines, and movies) there is a tendency to portray male genital size in "bigger than life" dimensions. This distortion reflects the triumph of anxious perception versus reality, literary and cinematic license (e.g., the use of particular camera angles or close-up shots), and the deliberate selection of male subjects whose genital proportions are decidedly larger than average. Male readers should remember, too, that there is a visual difference between the view you get of your own genitals (they appear shortened because of your viewing angle) and the view you get of someone else's penis size in the locker room or on the movie screen.

Recently a team of Canadian researchers studied the psychological impact of penis size

---

differs widely from one male to another (the average length is approximately 9.5 centimeters, or just under 4 inches), in adulthood this variation is less apparent in the erect state. Erection can be thought of as "the great equalizer" since men with a penis that is smaller when flaccid (nonerect) usually have a larger percentage volume increase during erection than men who have a larger flaccid penis (Masters and Johnson, 1966; Jamison and Gebhard, 1988).

The Scrotum

The **scrotum** is a thin loose sac of skin underneath the penis that is sparsely covered with pubic hair and contains the testicles (testes). The scrotum has a layer of muscle fibers that contract involuntarily as a result of sexual stimulation, exercise, or exposure to cold, causing the testes to be drawn up against the body. In hot weather, the scrotum relaxes and allows the testes to hang more freely away from the body. These reflexes of the scrotum help to maintain a stable temperature in the testes, an important function because sperm production (occurring in the testes) is impaired by heat or cold. In response to cold, the scrotum lifts the testes closer to the body to provide a warmer environment. In hotter conditions, the scrotum loosens, thereby moving the testes away from the body and providing a larger skin surface for the dissipation of heat. Tightening of the scrotum with sexual arousal on sexual arousal. They found that reading erotic passages that differed only in the description of the size of the penis produced no differences in the levels of arousal of male or female undergraduates (Fisher, Branscombe, and Lemery, 1983). Thus, they concluded that "penis size may be as unimportant on a psychological level as it appears to be on a physical level."

There *is* a rare medical condition called *micropenis* in which the penis is formed properly but is miniature in size. This condition is marked by a penis length of less than 2 centimeters (approximately ¾ inch) and sometimes is due to a treatable deficiency of testosterone. In other circumstances, there is no means of increasing penis size by drugs, creams, gadgets, hypnosis, or hormones although there are advertisements for such "treatments" which exploit the myth that bigger is necessarily better.

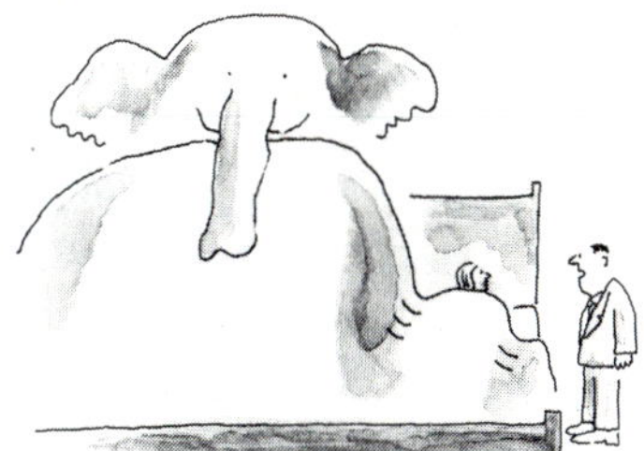

"Doris, I thought you told me size wasn't important!"

Playboy, April 1983, p. 182. Reproduced by special permission of *Playboy* Magazine; Copyright © 1983 by *Playboy*.

Men who are preoccupied or extremely anxious about the size of their penis appear to be more likely to develop sexual difficulties than other men. These difficulties range from the avoidance of potentially sexual relationships because of embarrassment or worry to difficulty in obtaining or maintaining an erection due to poor self-confidence, tension, and anxiety. Fortunately, this type of problem can usually be overcome by brief sex counseling or therapy (see Chapter 9).

or physical exercise may be a protective reflex that lessens the risk of injury to the testes.

The Testes

The **testes** (the male gonads) are paired structures usually contained in the scrotum (Figure 2–13). The two testes are about equal in size, averaging 5 × 2 × 3 centimeters (2 × 0.8 × 1.2 inches) in adults, although one testicle generally hangs lower than the other. Most often, the left testis is lower than the right one, but in left-handed men the reverse is usually true. There is no significance attached to the relative height of the testes within the scrotal sac, but if one testis is considerably larger or smaller than the other there could be a medical problem and a doctor should be seen.

The testes are highly sensitive to pressure or touch. Some men find that light caressing or stroking of the scrotum or gentle squeezing of the testes during sexual activity is arousing, but many others are uncomfortable with touching in this region.

The testes have two separate functions: hormone and sperm production. The cells that manufacture

scrotum (skrō′ tum) the thin, loose sac of skin that contains the testes and has a layer of muscle fibers that contract involuntarily.

testes (tes′ tēz) the paired male reproductive glands contained in the scrotum. The male gonads.

FIGURE 2–13

Internal Side View of the Male Reproductive System

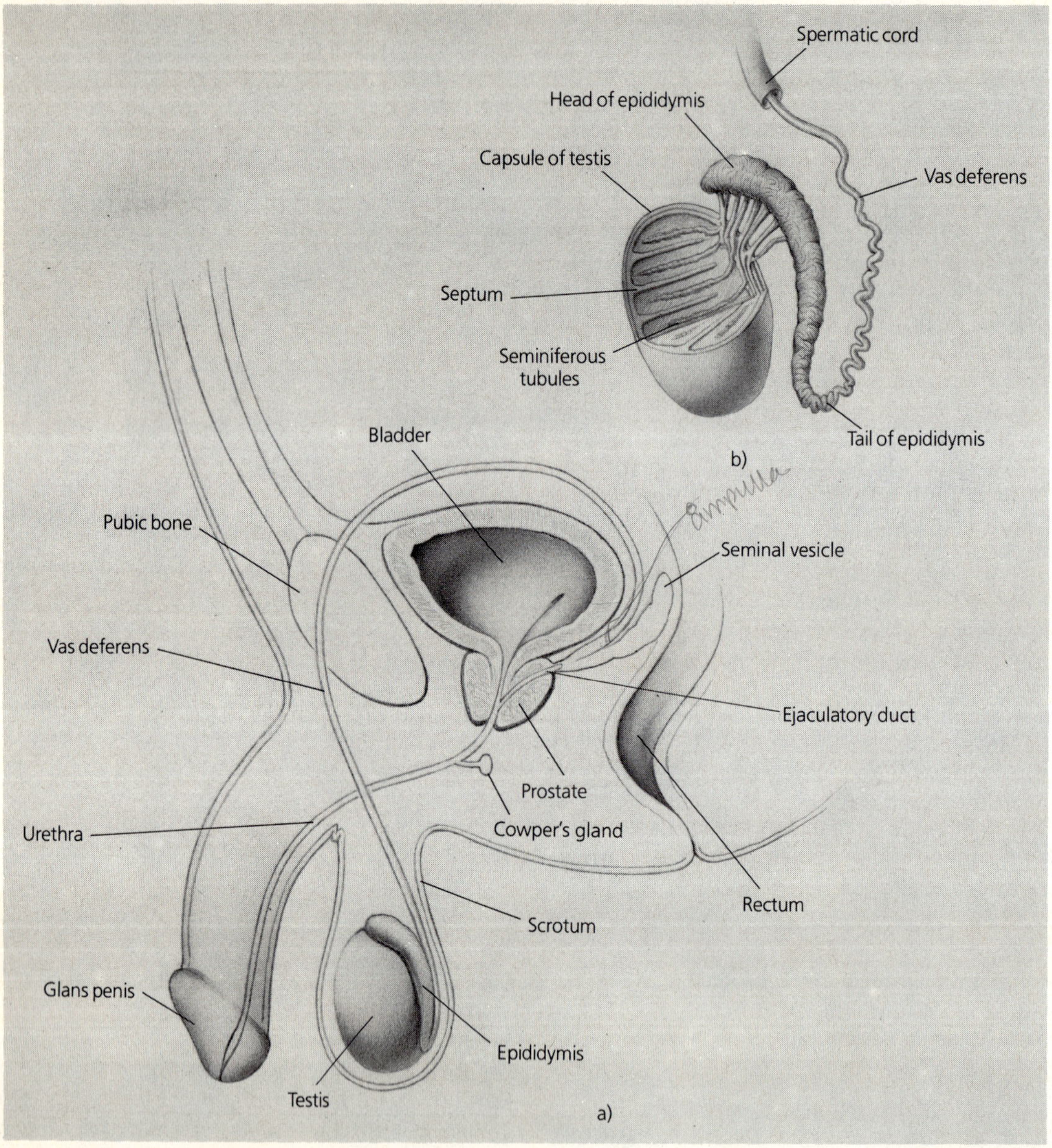

hormones—most importantly, **testosterone,** which controls male sexual development and plays an important part in sexual interest and function—are called **Leydig cells.** Sperm production occurs in the **seminiferous tubules,** tightly coiled tubes of microscopic size that collectively measure almost 500 meters (more than a quarter mile) in length. The entire process of sperm production takes 70 days. Unlike the female who creates no new eggs after birth, the male produces sperm from puberty on, manufacturing billions of sperm annually.

A mature spermatozoon is considerably smaller than the size of a human egg, being about 0.06 millimeter (1/500 of an inch) in length and thousands of

FIGURE 2–14

The Human Sperm

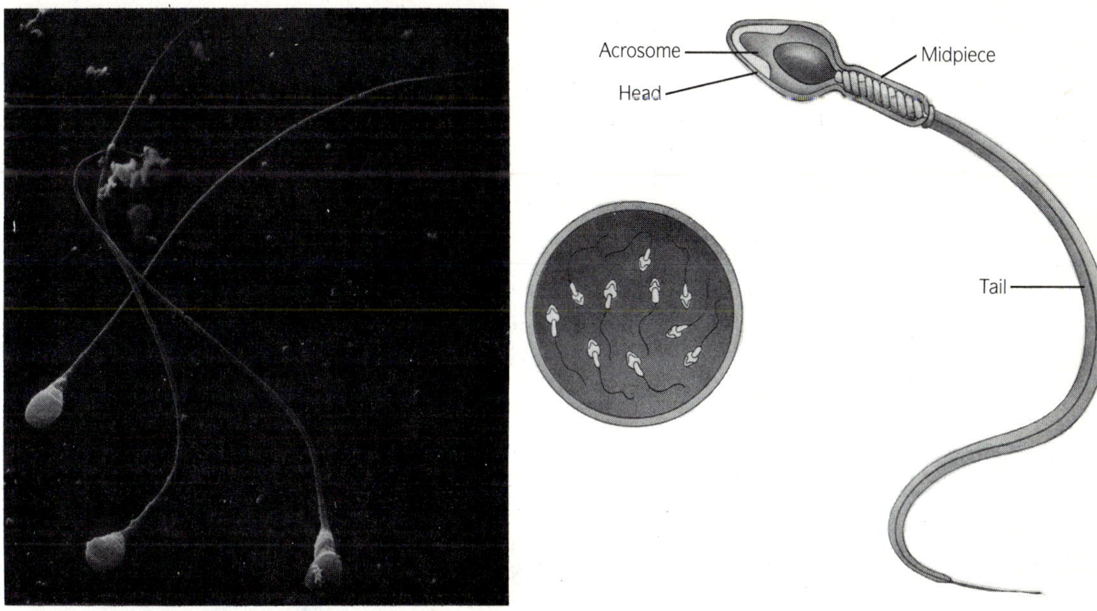

The insert shows live sperm as seen under a microscope, where their active swimming motion is apparent. The photograph of human sperm is taken with a scanning electron microscope.

times smaller than the egg in volume. Sperm are visible only with the aid of a microscope, which shows that they consist of three pieces: a head, a midpiece, and a tail (Figure 2–14). The head of the spermatozoon contains genetic material (**chromosomes**) and a chemical reservoir (the **acrosome**). The midpiece contains an energy system that allows the spermatozoon to swim by lashing its long tail back and forth.

The Epididymis and Vas Deferens

The seminiferous tubules (the tubes where sperm are produced) empty into the **epididymis,** a highly coiled tubing network folded against the back surface of each testis (Figure 2–13). Sperm cells generally spend several weeks traveling slowly through the epididymis as they reach full maturation. From here, sperm are carried into the **vas deferens,** long tubes (approximately 40 centimeters, or 16 inches) that leave the scrotum and curve alongside and behind the bladder. Both the right and left vas deferens are cut when a vasectomy is done (see Chapter 5).

The Prostate and Accessory Organs

The **prostate gland,** normally about the size of a chestnut, consists of a muscular and a glandular por-

testosterone (tes tos′ tur ōn) the most important hormone in sexual function, present in both sexes. Often called the male hormone, it is secreted by the testes and adrenals in the male and the ovaries and adrenals in the female.

Leydig cells (lī′ dig) the cells in the testes where hormone production occurs.

seminiferous tubules (sem′ i nif′ ur us tū′ bewls) microscopic tube-shaped structures in the testes where sperm is produced.

chromosomes (krō′ muh sōmz) the genetic material in the nucleus of every cell in the body. Sperm and eggs each have 23 chromosomes; all other cells normally have 46.

acrosome (ak′ ro som) chemical reservoir in the head of the spermatozoon.

epididymis (ep′ i did′ i mis) the tightly coiled tubing network folded against the back surface of each testis in which sperm cells spend several weeks maturing.

vas deferens (vas def′ ur enz) one of two long, tubelike structures that convey spermatozoa from the testes.

prostate gland (pros′ tāt) gland located directly below the bladder, surrounding the urethra as it exits the bladder. It secretes part of the seminal fluid.

EXAMINATION OF TESTICLES

After a 29-year-old film projectionist showed a movie about testicular self-examination to a group of doctors, he decided to take the film's recommendations and found a bean-sized lump in his right testicle. This simple act probably saved his life because he had a fast-growing cancer that required immediate surgery (P.C. Smith, 1980).

Men are not usually told about the importance of self-examination of the testes even though women are advised about checking their own breasts. This may partly reflect that cancer of the testis is statistically infrequent, with fewer than 5000 cases annually (Silverberg, 1981). It is the most common cancer in men between the ages of 20 and 34, however, and in many cases it does not produce pain or other symptoms.

The self-examination procedure is a simple one. After a warm bath or shower, when the scrotum is relaxed and loose, each testis should be felt individually. The surface of each testis should be covered, using the fingertips and thumb to feel for lumps, irregularities, hardening, or enlargement. If any suspicious areas are found, see your physician *immediately*.

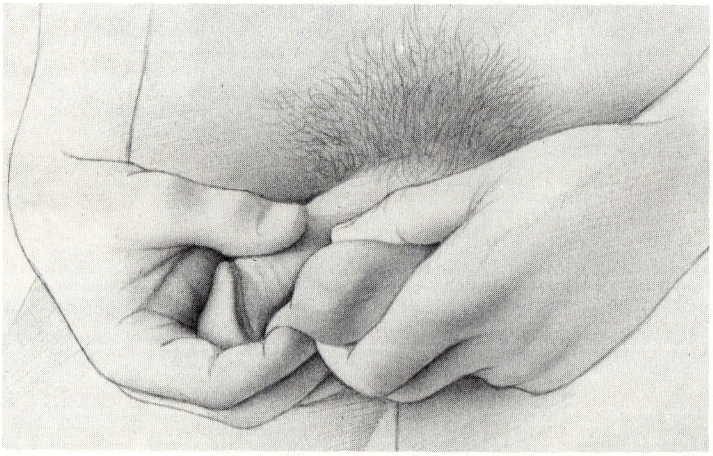

tion. The prostate is located directly below the bladder and surrounds the urethra (the tube through which urine passes) as it exits from the bladder. The relationship of the prostate to the urethra is like a large bead (the prostate) on a string (the urethra). Because the **rectum** (the lowest part of the bowels) is directly behind the prostate, the prostate can be examined by a physician during a rectal examination. This is important because the prostate can become infected or cancerous (Chapter 10).

The prostate produces clear fluid that makes up about 30 percent of **seminal fluid,** the liquid that is expelled from the penis during ejaculation. The other 70 percent of seminal fluid comes from the **seminal vesicles** (Eliasson and Lindholmer, 1976; Spring-Mills and Hafez, 1980). These two small structures lie against the back portion of the base of the bladder and join with the ends of the vas deferens to form the **ejaculatory ducts.** These ducts in turn join the urethra, thereby creating a continuous tubing system that leads to the end of the penis.

On the average, there are 3 to 5 milliliters (5 milliliters equal about 1 teaspoonful) of semen (seminal fluid plus sperm) per ejaculate. Although the concentration of sperm is highly variable, depending in part on the frequency of ejaculation, a count of 40 to 120 million per milliliter is considered normal. This means that there may be 120 to 600 million sperm in a single ejaculate.[5]

Seminal fluid ranges in color from whitish to tones of yellow or gray and has a creamy, sticky texture. Right after ejaculation, seminal fluid is rather thick but then liquefies quickly. It consists of water, mucus, and a large number of chemical substances that include sugar (providing an energy source for sperm), bases (for neutralizing the acidity of the male urethra and the female vagina), and prostaglandins (hormones that cause contractions in the uterus and Fallopian tubes, possibly aiding upward transit of sperm).

Cowper's glands are two pea-sized structures connected to the urethra just below the prostate gland. They produce a few drops of fluid which sometimes appear at the tip of the penis during sexual arousal but before ejaculation. Some men never notice this pre-ejaculatory fluid, while others may produce a teaspoonful or more of this slippery secretion. Although this pre-ejaculatory fluid may buffer the acidity of the urethra, there is no certainty about its function. Occasionally, the pre-ejaculatory fluid contains a small number of live sperm cells, accounting for at least some of the "failures" of withdrawal of the penis before ejaculation as a method of birth control.

The Breasts

The male breasts have a nipple and areola but have little underlying glandular tissue or fatty padding. The male nipple and areola seem to be less sensitive to touch and pressure than the same structures in adult females (Robinson and Short, 1977). Nevertheless, some males find that having their breasts or nipples stroked or licked is sexually arousing. Others do not notice any erotic pleasure from such practices.

Sometimes one or both of a male's breasts become enlarged. This condition, called **gynecomastia,** occurs in 40 to 60 percent of boys during puberty but usually disappears within a year or two (Lee, 1975; Kolodny, Masters, and Johnson, 1979). In adulthood, it may be caused by alcoholism, liver disease, thyroid disease, drug ingestion, or certain forms of cancer. When gynecomastia is so severe that it creates major psychological problems, it can be corrected by relatively simply surgery.

The male breasts can also become enlarged if a man takes estrogen over a period of time. Most male-to-female transsexuals undergo such treatment. We have also seen a case in which a man unwittingly took birth control pills for several months, causing the same result.

OTHER EROGENOUS ANATOMY

Many parts of the body besides those involved in reproduction are potential sources of sexual arousal in both sexes. Surprisingly, the largest sensory organ for both females and males is the skin itself. The insides of the thighs, the neck, and the perineum are often sources of sexual pleasure. In our genitally oriented society, where sex is often thought of as synonymous with intercourse, it is easy to overlook the importance of touching and body-to-body contact as a form of intimacy and gratification. Stroking, caressing, and massage can be forms of nonverbal communication, sensual pleasure, or invitations to further sexual activity.

Some people are well aware of the erotic sensations they can experience from touch, while others pay little attention to this component of their sexual arousal. However, there are wide differences from person to person in such matters: for some, the skin outside the genital region has relatively little sexual input or may actually dampen sexual feelings (what would happen to your level of arousal if a touch felt persistently ticklish or irritating?); at the other extreme, we have seen one woman who could be aroused to the point of orgasm by having the small of her back rubbed without any other stimulus (Masters and Johnson, 1966). (However, the likelihood of being or encoun-

rectum (rek′ tum) the lower part of the large intestine.

seminal fluid (sem′ uh nul) the thick white, yellow, or gray liquid portion of the male ejaculate.

seminal vesicles (sem′ uh nul ves′ e kulz) in the male, paired pouchlike bodies that empty into the ejaculatory ducts and provide the major part of fluid in the ejaculate.

ejaculatory ducts (ē jak′ you luh tō′ rē) paired tube-like structures that carry sperm from the vas deferens and fluid from the seminal vesicles into the prostatic urethra.

Cowper's glands (kow′ perz) two pea-sized structures connected to the urethra just below the prostate gland. They produce fluid before ejaculation but otherwise have no known function.

gynecomastia (jīn′ e kō mas′ tē uh) enlargement of one or both male breasts.

[5] After a vasectomy, although there are no longer sperm in the ejaculate, the amount of fluid in the ejaculate remains the same.

tering a female capable of reaching orgasm by back rubbing alone is probably less than one in a million.)

The mouth, including the lips and tongue, is an area of high erotic potential. Kissing is one practice that uses the sensitivity of this region in a sexually stimulating fashion. In addition to the sensory signals activated by kissing, it is also an act of intimacy that can symbolize passion and penetration (think of the form of kissing called "French kissing" or "soul kissing" in which one partner's tongue enters the other's mouth). Oral–genital contact—stimulation of one person's genitals in a licking or sucking fashion by the partner's lips or tongue—is another common form of sexual stimulation.

The anus, rectum, and buttocks are also potentially erogenous areas. The anus is highly sensitive to touch and the insertion of a finger, object, or penis in the anus and rectum is part of some people's sexual activity. Anal intercourse is often thought to be primarily an act of male homosexuals. However, numerically, far more heterosexual couples engage in this activity than homosexuals and many homosexual men have not had experience with this type of sexual behavior.

The buttocks are regarded in some cultures as symbolic of female sexuality in much the sense that our society regards the female breasts. The buttocks are bulky groups of muscles covered by fat and skin, with a relatively sparse distribution of nerves sensitive to touch. The underlying muscles are important in the mechanical process of pelvic thrusting during sexual intercourse. As a target for spanking, the buttocks are sometimes provocative for those of both sexes who find this activity erotically arousing. As a visible part of the anatomy, the buttocks (especially when displayed in tight jeans, swim trunks, bikinis, or similar apparel) commonly serve as a form of sexual enticement.

Many other parts of the body can also have erotic allure. For instance, hair can be sensual or sexual: some women are turned on by their partner's hairy chest and some lovers like to stroke each other's hair. Well-developed muscles make males more attractive to some females, whereas others are less impressed or actually turned off by this "he-man" appearance. Nibbling an earlobe, caressing the face, and touching fingertips can all be part of a sexual encounter and all may be a source of excitation. Our attempt here is not to provide an exhaustive catalogue but to demonstrate the wide range of what can be sexual.

We each have a unique appearance to our sexual anatomy and an even more individual experience of sexual feelings and interactions. As we have repeatedly stressed, the variations—even anatomically—from one person to another are considerable. Unfortunately, some people are preoccupied with the notion that "biggest is best" and others believe that sexual satisfaction is mainly a matter of "pushing the right buttons." Instead, we believe that a mechanical view of sex often leads to a mechanical experience, whereas a view of sex as a matter of comfort, mood, and feelings combined with physical sensations and response is more likely to be fulfilling and fun.

SUMMARY

1. Sexual anatomy includes the organs of reproduction and the parts of the body that are potential sources of sexual pleasure. Accurate knowledge about sexual anatomy can help people distinguish between fact and myth and can lead to a better understanding of one's self and one's partner.
2. The female vulva consists of the mons, the inner and outer labia, the clitoris, and the perineum. The clitoris is not a miniature penis. It is a unique organ, richly endowed with sensory nerves, that serves solely as a receptor and transformer of sexual sensations.
3. The opening of the vagina is partially covered by a membrane called the hymen, which is sometimes mistakenly thought to be a foolproof indication of female virginity. The vagina itself is an internal organ, capable of expanding and contracting, with relatively few sensory nerve endings except near its opening. The vaginal lining is similar to that found inside the mouth, and vaginal lubrication originates from this surface. There is currently considerable controversy over the possible existence of the "G spot," which is claimed by some to be an anatomic area in the front wall of the vagina that has a high degree of erotic sensitivity.
4. The uterus is a hollow muscular organ, part of which (the cervix) protrudes into the vagina.
5. The male sex organs include the penis, scrotum, testes, and various internal structures. The penis is made up of three cylinders of spongy tissue with a rich network of blood vessels. There is great variation from male to male in the size of the nonerect penis; but with erection, size differences tend to diminish.
6. The glans, or head, of the penis is covered by foreskin in the uncircumcised male but is ex-

posed in a male who has been circumcised. Circumcision has not been proved to have any effect, positive or negative, on sexual feeling or responsivity.

7. The scrotum is a sac of skin underneath the penis that contains the testes. Muscle fibers in the scrotum move the testes closer to or farther away from the body in response to temperature changes or exercise in order to facilitate sperm production.
8. Sperm made in the testes are carried by a long tubing system (the epididymis and vas deferens) inside the body. Sperm are mixed with seminal fluid from the prostate gland and seminal vesicles to make up semen.
9. The breasts are basically modified sweat glands, but in our society the female breasts have assumed major sexual importance. Not all women find that breast stimulation is a sexual turn-on, and many women are concerned about the size (or lack of size) of their breasts.
10. The mouth, tongue, lips, thighs, buttocks, anus, and skin are other parts of the body often involved in sexual activity and can be a source of erotic arousal.

Thought Questions

1. How do you think children should be taught about sexual anatomy? When should this teaching begin? Should children be encouraged to use the correct terms, or are slang words good enough? If slang words are used, are some more appropriate than others?
2. In what ways are females in our society often given negative messages about their anatomies? Are males also given such messages?
3. Compare the clitoris and the penis in terms of function, value, implications, and so on. The penis has at times been given a prominent role in myth, art, literature, and even scientific ideas (such as Freud's). Why not the clitoris?
4. Operations for breast enlargement or reduction are common in our society. Are these medically justifiable (and thus properly paid for by Medicaid and insurance), or are they primarily done for purposes of vanity?
5. Is the uncircumcised male at a disadvantage in our culture? Why or why not? Apart from religion, what other factors might contribute to parents deciding whether or not to have a baby boy circumcised?
6. The text states that "Under most circumstances, the first intercourse experience for a girl or woman is not painful or marked by a great deal of bleeding." What is your experience in this respect? What is it like "the first time" for both sexes?

Suggested Readings

Ayalah, D., and Weinstock, I. J. *Breasts*. New York: Summit Books, 1979. An informal and informative look at how women of all ages react to their breasts.

Boston Women's Health Book Collective. *The New Our Bodies, Ourselves*. New York: Simon & Schuster, 1984. A readable and practical collection of facts and insights into female sexuality and reproduction, updated extensively from an earlier edition.

Diagram Group. *Man's Body: An Owner's Manual*. New York: Paddington Press/Two Continents Publishing Group, 1976. Although there are no really good books on the subject of male sexual anatomy, this straightforward book includes some interesting material and diagrams.

Federation of Feminist Women's Health Centers. *A New View of a Woman's Body*. New York: Simon & Schuster, 1981. A profusely illustrated guide to female anatomy and health care. Excellent color photos of the cervix and vulva.

3

Sexual Physiology

> An orgasm is like a rocket ride. First the ascent, then the blackout, and after that the burst of light as the golden apple turns into the golden sun and azure skies with a slow parachute until the earth appears below, streams and meadows or a city street. You slowly touch and bounce up again. . . . Then you slowly touch once more, and then the afterglow and the deep refreshing sleep. *(Berne, 1971, p. 233)*

> Orgasm can be a very mild experience, like a ripple or peaceful sigh; it can be a very sensuous experience where our body glows with warmth; it can be an intense experience with crying out and thrashing movements; it can be an ecstatic experience with momentary loss of awareness. *(Boston Women's Health Book Collective, 1976, p. 45)*

> Sometimes I think orgasms are overrated. Getting there is more than half the fun. *(Comment by a 23-year-old woman, Authors' files)*

People interpret their sexual responses in various ways, as these quotations show. But the basic details of how the body responds to sexual arousal are identical whether the stimulation comes from touching, kissing, intercourse, masturbation, fantasy, watching a movie, or reading a book. This statement does not imply that sex is just a mechanical process, any more than dancing or playing the violin are "only" mechanical because certain parts of the body are involved in these activities. Human sexual response is multidimensional, with input from feelings and thoughts, learning and language, personal and cultural values, and many other sources combining with our biological reflexes to create a total experience.

To understand the complexities of human sexuality, it is helpful to become familiar with the details of sexual physiology (the functions of our sexual anatomy). Learning about the various responses of the body during sexual arousal and about the forces that regulate them will increase your awareness of your own and your partner's responses and may clarify many misconceptions, myths, and questions about sex. It is also important to understand sexual physiology to comprehend many sexual disorders discussed later in the book.

SOURCES OF SEXUAL AROUSAL

When people talk about sexual arousal, they frequently say they are "turned on," "revved up," or "hot." Each phrase likens sexual arousal to an energy system, and, as a starting point, this comparison is useful. From a scientific perspective, sexual arousal can be defined as a state of activation of a complex system of reflexes involving the sexual organs and the nervous system. The brain itself, the controlling part of the nervous system, operates with electrical and chemical impulses "wired" to the rest of the body through the spinal cord and peripheral nerves. Signals from other parts of the body (like the skin, genitals, breasts) are integrated and focused in the brain, for without sexual thoughts, feelings, or images, sexual response is fragmentary and incomplete. At times, sexual arousal may be largely a cerebral event: that is, a person may be aroused while no visible physical changes are occurring elsewhere in the body. On other occasions, genital sensations can be so intense that they block out awareness of almost everything else.

Sexual arousal can occur under a wide variety of circumstances. It may be the result of voluntary actions such as kissing, hugging, reading a sexy book, or going to an erotic movie. Sexual arousal can also be unexpected, unwanted, or even alarming. Consider, for instance, the following situations: (1) a 12-year-old boy gets an erection while taking a shower in a crowded all-male locker room at school; (2) a female college student who is an ardent feminist becomes sexually aroused while watching a rape scene in a movie; (3) a female medical student is sexually excited when she examines an elderly male patient; (4) a male lawyer is sexually aroused by discussions with a female client who hires him to help her obtain a divorce. These people may be embarrassed or uncomfortable temporarily, but unexpected sexual arousal is normal and happens to most of us occasionally.

The sources of sexual arousal are also varied. The process of getting "turned on" may be triggered by direct physical contact such as a touch or a kiss or may be activated by a verbal invitation ("let's make love"), a nonverbal message (body language), or a visual cue (such as nudity or a particular clothing style). It may also spring from fantasies or the most everyday occurrences—clothing rubbing against the genitals, the rhythm of a moving vehicle, or taking a bath or shower. Sexual arousal occurs in all age groups, from infants to the elderly, and it occurs when we are asleep as well as when we are awake. Men have about a half dozen erections during a night's sleep (the erections usually last five to ten minutes), and women have similar episodes of vaginal lubrication during sleep (Masters and Johnson, 1966; Abel et al., 1979). These reflex responses occur automatically and are not controlled by the specific content of dreams.

FIGURE 3–1

The Sexual Response Cycle

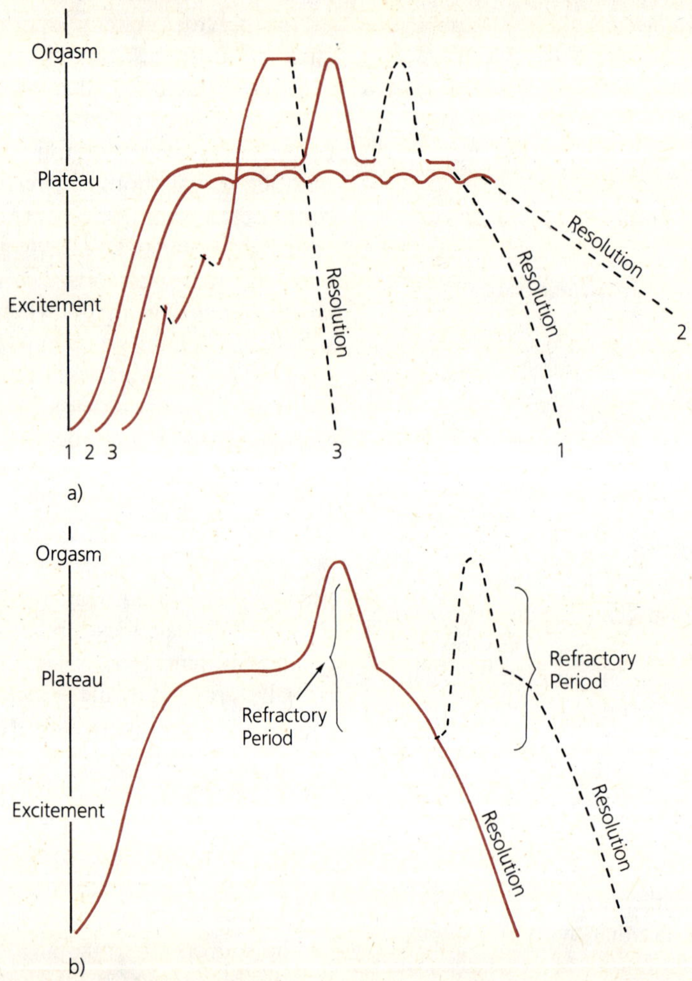

(a) Three representative variations of female sexual response. Pattern 1 shows multiple orgasm; pattern 2 shows arousal that reaches the plateau level without going on to orgasm (note that resolution occurs very slowly); and pattern 3 shows several brief drops in the excitement phase followed by an even more rapid resolution phase.
(b) The most typical pattern of male sexual response. The dotted line shows one possible variation: a second orgasm and ejaculation occurring after the refractory period is over. Numerous other variations are possible, including patterns that would match 2 and 3 of the female response cycle.

Source: From William H. Masters and Virginia E. Johnson, *Human Sexual Response*. © 1966 by William H. Masters and Virginia E. Johnson. Reprinted by permission of Little, Brown and Company.

THE SEXUAL RESPONSE CYCLE

Before the 1960s, relatively little was known about the way the body responds during sexual arousal. Scientists were not convinced by Kinsey's claims that some women had more than one orgasm at a time (Pomeroy, 1966), and it was thought that vaginal lubrication was produced by glands in the cervix and Bartholin's glands. The mechanisms controlling erection and ejaculation in the male were incompletely understood. As a matter of propriety, sexual response was studied in animals, not people. In this climate, the results of an investigation of sexual physiology based on direct laboratory observation of more than 10,000 episodes of sexual activity in 382 women and 312 men first appeared (Masters and Johnson, 1966).

The findings of this study indicated that human sexual response could be described as a cycle with four stages: **excitement, plateau, orgasm,** and **resolution**. These stages correspond to varying levels of sexual arousal and describe the typical responses people have during sexual function. Although it is convenient to use the cycle as a model for descriptive purposes, remember that the stages are arbitrarily defined. They are not always clearly separated from one another and may vary considerably both in one person at different times and between people. Bear in mind also that the physiological processes of sexual response are not simply mechanical movements detached from thoughts or feelings but are part of the sexual involvement and identity of the whole person.

Although the sexual response cycle usually follows a consistent pattern of progression, the simplified schematic patterns of sexual response may vary widely, as Figure 3–1 reveals. Sometimes excitation is rapid and leads quickly to orgasm. On other occasions, excitement mounts slowly over a period of hours—while having a romantic, intimate meal, for example—and the rest of the cycle may seem brief in comparison. The plateau stage may not always lead to orgasm as the high levels of arousal that characterize this phase may dissipate; and a person may slip back to the excitement phase. If sexual stimulation stops, a person may also drift back into an unaroused state.

There are two basic physiologic reactions during human sexual response. The first is **vasocongestion**, an increased amount of blood concentrated in body tissues in the genitals and female breasts. The second is increased **neuromuscular tension** or **myotonia**. Here, tension does not refer to a negative physical state ("feeling tense") but to a buildup of energy in the nerves and muscles. Myotonia occurs throughout the body in response to sexual arousal, not simply in the genital region.

Although there are some differences in male and female sexual response, many details are similar. The physiology of sexual response is also the same for heterosexuals and homosexuals (Masters and Johnson, 1979).

Before we discuss the specific details of sexual response, a note of caution is in order. It is often tempting to equate the speed, size, and strength of sexual responses (such as erection, vaginal lubrication, or muscular contractions during orgasm) with the gratification a person experiences or with his or her proficiency as a lover. This is like saying that a bowl of chili is "better" than sirloin steak simply because chili causes a faster and larger secretion of digestive juices than steak. In both cases ("better" digestive response, "better" sexual response), the degree to which one experience is "better" than the other depends on your perspective *and* on your personal satisfaction.

Excitement

Excitation results from sexual stimulation, which may be physical, psychological, or a combination of the two. Sexual responses are like other physiological processes that may be triggered not only by direct contact but by vision, smell, thought, or emotion. For example, thinking about food, smelling fresh baked goods, or watching a television commercial may prompt salivation and gastric acid production; and

excitement phase first phase of the human sexual response cycle caused by physical and/or psychological stimulation. It is characterized by increasing levels of myotonia and by vasocongestion.

plateau phase the phase of human sexual response following excitement, in which a leveling off of sexual tensions occurs. This phase can be short or long prior to reaching levels required to trigger orgasm.

orgasm (or′ gas um) the third and shortest phase of the human sexual response cycle. A total body response involving the sudden discharge of accumulated sexual tension.

resolution phase last phase of human sexual response following orgasm or maximum excitement in which the body returns to an unaroused state.

vasocongestion (vas′ o kun jes′ chun) an increased amount of blood concentrated in body tissues, especially in the genitals and female breasts during sexual arousal. In the male it causes erection and in the female an increase in the size of the clitoris and transudation of fluid in the vagina.

neuromuscular tension (new′ rō mus′ kew lur) buildup of energy in the nerves and muscles sometimes caused by sexual arousal.

myotonia (mī′ ō tō nē uh) involuntary contraction of muscle.

FIGURE 3–2

Internal Changes in the Female Sexual Response Cycle

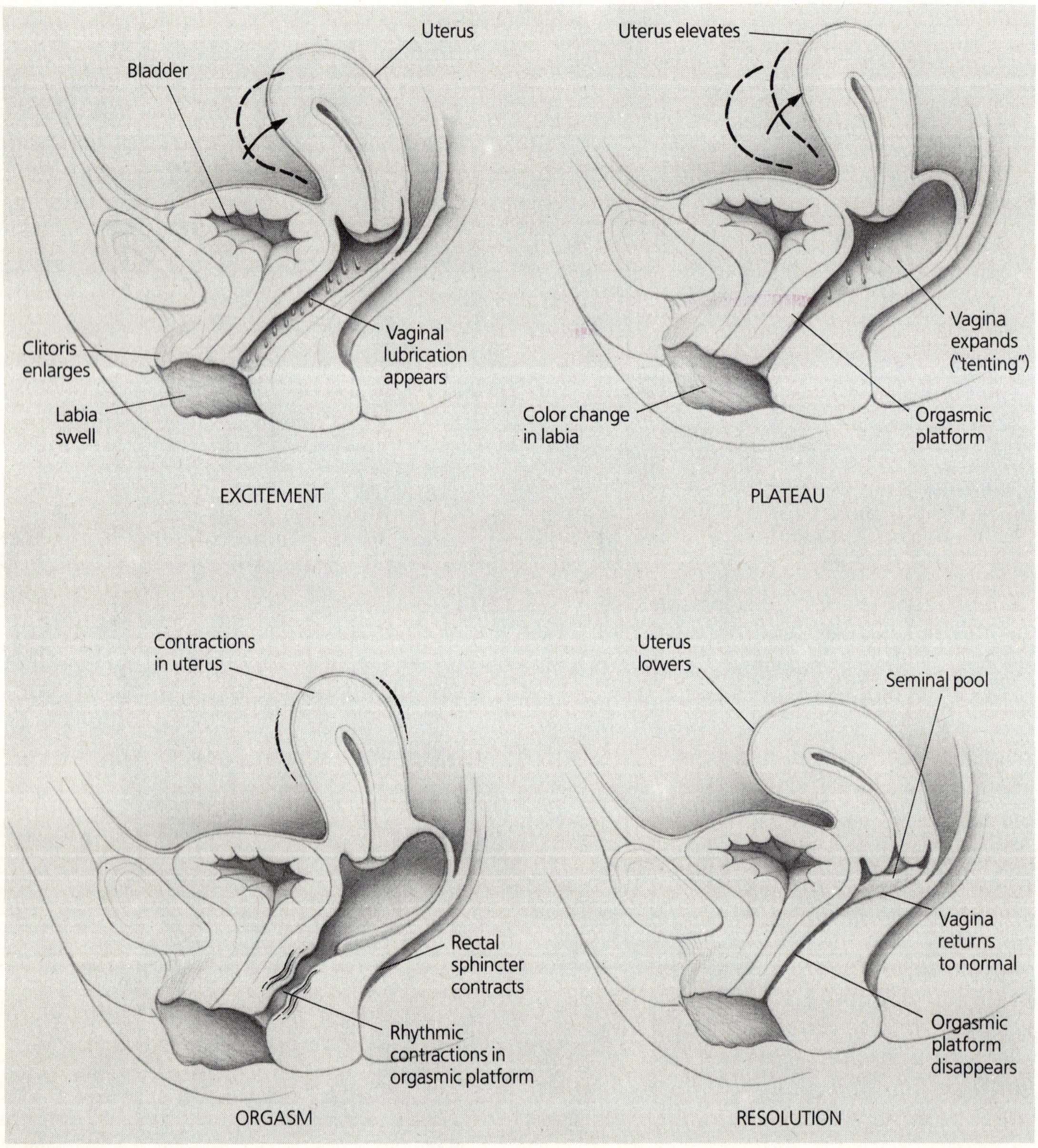

fear may activate a complex set of reflexes including sweating, a faster pulse rate, and increased blood pressure.

FEMALE

The first sign of sexual excitation in the female is the appearance of vaginal lubrication, which starts 10 to 30 seconds after the onset of sexual stimulation. Vaginal lubrication occurs because vasocongestion in the walls of the vagina leads to moisture seeping across the vaginal lining in a process called **transudation**. Beads of vaginal secretion first appear as isolated droplets which flow together and eventually moisten the entire inner surface of the vagina. Early in the excitement stage the quantities of fluid may be so small that neither the woman nor her partner notices it. As vaginal lubrication increases, it sometimes flows out of the vagina, moistening the labia and the vaginal opening, but this depends on the woman's position and the type of sexual play going on.

The consistency, quantity, and odor of vaginal lubrication varies considerably from one woman to another and also varies in the same woman from time to time. Contrary to commonly held beliefs, the amount of vaginal lubrication is *not* necessarily indicative of the woman's level of sexual arousal, and the presence of vaginal lubrication does not mean the woman is "ready" for intercourse. Vaginal lubrication makes insertion of the penis into the vagina easier and smoother and prevents discomfort during intravaginal thrusting.

Other changes also occur in women during the excitement phase. The inner two-thirds of the vagina expand, the cervix and uterus are pulled upward, and the outer lips of the vagina flatten and move apart (see Figure 3–2). In addition, the inner lips of the vagina enlarge in diameter, and the clitoris increases in size as a result of vasocongestion. A woman's nipples typically become erect during the excitement phase as a result of contractions of small muscle fibers. Late in the excitement phase (again as a result of vasocongestion), the veins on the breasts become more visible and there also may be a small increase in breast size.

MALE

The most prominent physical sign of sexual excitation in men is erection of the penis, which usually occurs within a few seconds after sexual stimulation starts (Figure 3–3). Although this response may seem very different from vaginal lubrication, they are parallel events that both occur because of vasocongestion. Erection results from the spongy tissues of the penis rapidly filling with blood. It is not certain at present whether engorgement occurs because the veins that drain the penis cannot keep up with this rapid filling or if special structures called "polsters" in the blood vessels of the penis limit outflow (Weiss, 1972; Krane and Siroky, 1981). Whatever the exact mechanism, the increased size and firmness of the erect penis are due to increased fluid pressure: erection can thus be viewed in simplest terms as a hydraulic event. Despite this seeming mechanical simplicity, a man may be physically and/or psychologically aroused and not have a firm erection, particularly under conditions of anxiety or fatigue. Contrary to some common misconceptions, there is neither a bone in the human penis (although erections are sometimes called "boners") nor a penis muscle that controls the process of erection.[1]

In addition to erection, the skin ridges of the scrotum begin to smooth out and the testes are partially drawn toward the body. Late in the excitement phase, the testes increase slightly in size. Nipple erection occurs during excitation for some men but not others.

Although many people think of male sexual response as nearly instantaneous and constant, in real life it does not always happen this way. Literary descriptions of a "pulsating," "throbbing," or "steel-hard" penis are common but often fictional. As Zilbergeld (1978) observes, in our unrealistic expectations, "the mere sight or touch of a woman is sufficient to set the penis jumping, and whenever a man's fly is unzipped, his penis leaps out. . . . Nowhere does a penis merely mosey out for a look at what's happening" (p. 24). In other words, a man is expected to be instantly erect at the drop of a bra, which of

[1] Many animals have a penis bone (**os penis**). The late Dr. Francis Ryan, a zoologist who taught a popular course on comparative anatomy at Columbia University, delighted in waving a large, baseball bat–sized bone in the air and asking, "Does anyone know what this is?" After no response from his all-male class, he would declare, "This, gentlemen, is the *os penis* of the Arctic Whale." He would pause then for effect before saying, "Life in the Arctic is a stiff proposition."

transudation (trans′ ū dā′ shun) the passing of a fluid through a membrane, especially the lubrication in the vagina during sexual arousal.

os penis penis bone present in some animal species but not in humans or other primates.

FIGURE 3–3

External and Internal Changes in the Male Sexual Response Cycle

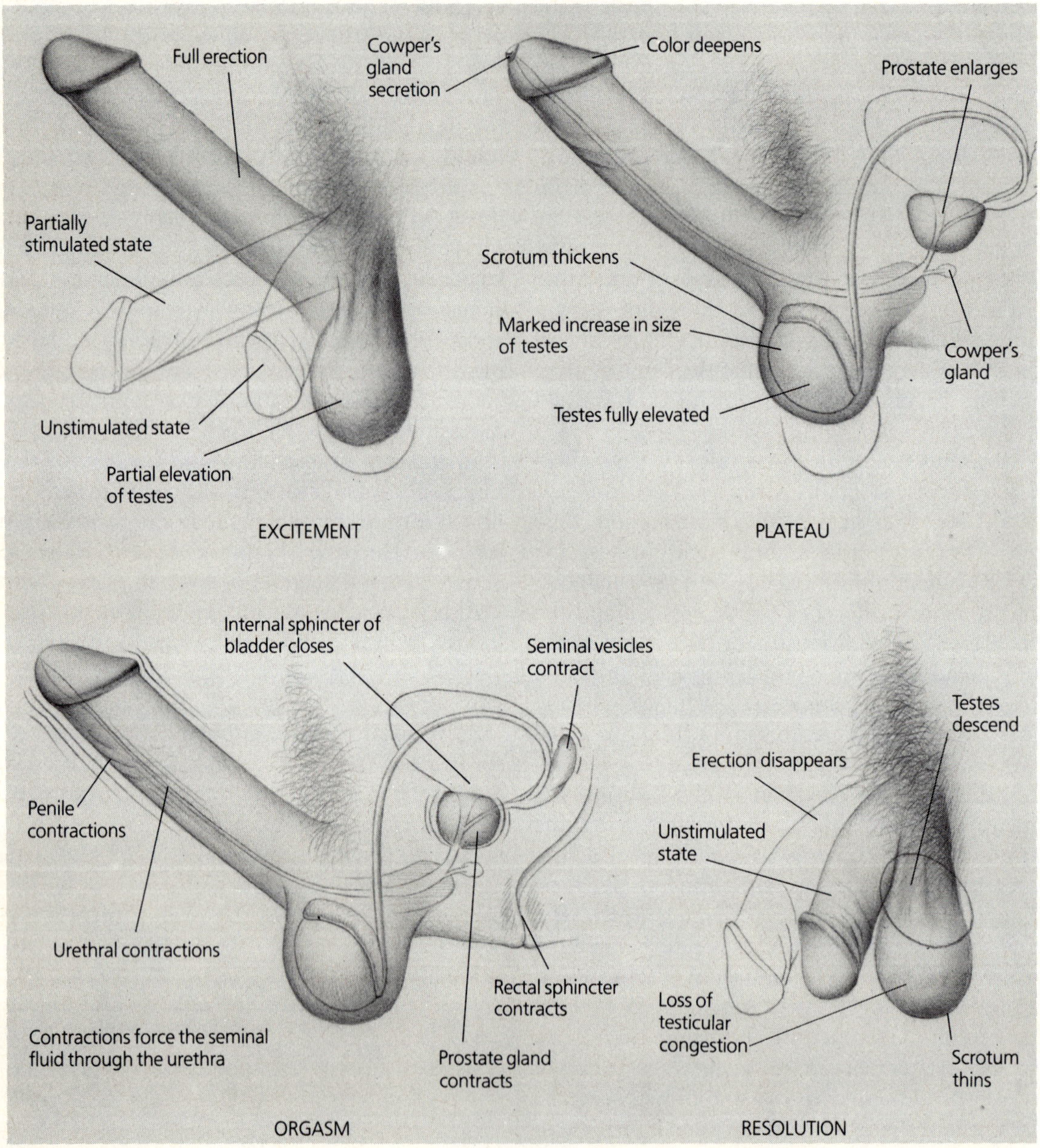

course creates a dilemma for anyone who finds that his arousal is not so dramatic or visible.

VARIATIONS IN EXCITEMENT

As we have seen, the physical changes of the excitement phase are neither constant nor always increasing for men and women. Mental or physical distractions can and often do decrease the buildup of sexual tension that is the hallmark of excitation. A honking horn, a knock on the door, an inopportune telephone ring, a shift in position, a muscle cramp, or a growling stomach are among the innumerable possible distractions. In addition, changes of tempo or manner of direct sexual stimulation can also temporarily disrupt sexual arousal, just as too much of a particular caress may temporarily cause a dulling of sensations.

Some people become upset or worried if their initial sexual arousal does not build steadily to a shattering peak. If a man's erection recedes even briefly, he may think, "I'm losing it" or his partner may wonder, "What am I doing wrong?" If a woman's vagina seems to get dry or her nipples lose their erection, she (or her partner) may have the same concerns. As a result, sexual spontaneity is likely to be lessened and awareness of body sensations is reduced. In such situations, the initial worry often becomes a self-fulfilling prophecy.

Vasocongestive mechanisms of sexual arousal wax and wane in everyone, just as most biological processes fluctuate a bit. An erection may be diminishing in firmness or size, or vaginal lubrication may seem to cease, although physical sensations and neuromuscular tension indicate that the man and woman are clearly nearing the plateau phase of the sexual response cycle. In this example, if the partners become alarmed or give up because they "see" that their physical response is less than what they want or expect it to be, they are not really giving themselves a chance.

Plateau

In the excitement phase, there is a marked increase in sexual tension above baseline (unaroused) levels. As Figure 3–1 shows, in the plateau phase, high levels of sexual arousal are maintained and intensified, potentially setting the stage for orgasm. The duration of the plateau phase varies widely. For men who have difficulty controlling ejaculation, this phase may be exceptionally brief. In some women, a short plateau phase may precede a particularly intense orgasm. For other people, a long, leisurely time at the plateau level is an intimate and erotic "high" that may be a satisfying end in its own right.

FEMALE

During the plateau phase in women prominent vasocongestion in the outer third of the vagina causes the tissues to swell. This reaction, called the **orgasmic platform**, narrows the opening of the vagina by 30 percent or more (Figure 3–2). One reason penis size is not so important to a woman's physical stimulation during intercourse is that her outer vagina or orgasmic platform "grips" the penis if plateau levels of arousal are reached.[2] During the plateau phase, the inner two-thirds of the vagina expand slightly more in size as the uterus becomes more elevated in a process known as "tenting." The production of vaginal lubrication often slows during this phase compared with excitation, especially if the plateau phase is prolonged.

The clitoris pulls back against the pubic bone during the plateau phase. This change, coupled with the vasocongestion occurring in the vaginal lips, hides the clitoris (Figure 3–4) and partially protects its head from direct touch. No loss of clitoral sensation occurs during these changes, however, and stimulation of the mons or the labia will result in clitoral sensations.[3]

The inner lips enlarge dramatically as a result of engorgement with blood, doubling or even tripling in thickness. As this happens, the inner lips push the outer lips apart, providing more immediate access to the opening of the vagina. Once this reaction has occurred, vivid color changes develop in the inner lips. The inner lips of women who have never been pregnant range from pink to bright red, while those in women who have been pregnant range from bright red to a deep wine color because of greater vascular supply delivering more blood flow to this area. Masters and Johnson (1966) noted that if effective sexual

---

[2] As we mentioned in Chapter 2, some women may find a large penis to be important for *psychological* stimulation, and some women claim to receive more physical stimulation from a large penis. As someone once said, "Different strokes for different folks."

[3] Marriage manuals in the 1950s all seemed to instruct the male that finding and stimulating the clitoris was the key to female sexual responsiveness. We wonder how many men panicked when this phase of clitoral retraction made the clitoris seem to disappear.

orgasmic platform the narrowing of the vagina during sexual excitement due to vasocongestion.

FIGURE 3–4

The Clitoris and Labia in the Female Sexual Response Cycle

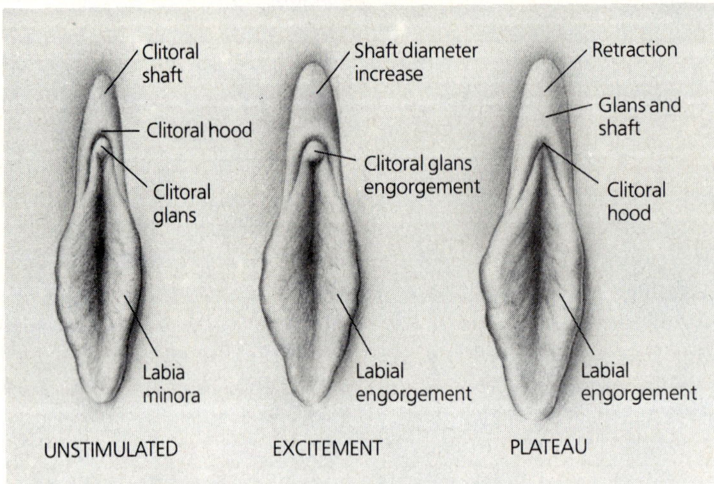

In the plateau phase, the clitoris seems to disappear beneath its hood, but it is actually quite engorged. The orgasmic phase is omitted because of lack of information.

stimulation continues once this "sex skin" color change appears, orgasm invariably follows. In more than 7500 cycles of female sexual response, an orgasm never occurred without the preceding color change of the inner lips.

Late in the excitement phase, the areola of the female breast begins to swell. During the plateau phase, swelling continues to the point that the earlier nipple erection usually becomes obscured (Figure 3–5). Increases in breast size during the plateau phase are striking in women who have not breast-fed a child, averaging 20 to 25 percent above baseline levels. For women who have previously nursed a child, this increase is much less pronounced or nonexistent because of their more developed venous drainage. However, this does not reduce erotic sensations in the breasts.

Late in the excitement phase or early in the plateau phase, a reddish, spotty skin color change resembling measles develops in 50 to 75 percent of women and about one-fourth of men. This **sex flush** generally begins just below the breastbone in the upper region of the abdomen and then spreads rapidly over the breasts and front of the chest. It may also appear on other parts of the body, including the neck, buttocks, back, arms, legs, and face. The sex flush results from changes in the pattern of blood flow just below the surface of the skin.

MALE

During the male's plateau phase (Figure 3–3), the diameter of the head of the penis near the coronal ridge increases slightly. This area often deepens in color due to pooling of blood. Vasocongestion also causes the testes to swell, and they become 25 to 50 percent larger than in the unstimulated state.

As sexual tension mounts toward orgasm, the testes not only continue to elevate but also begin to rotate forward so that their back surfaces rest in firm contact with the perineum (the area between the scrotum and the anus). Full elevation of the testes indicates that orgasm is imminent. In some men, particularly over age 50, the testes elevate only partially. Incomplete elevation of the testes during the plateau phase is frequently associated with reduction of ejaculatory pressure during the male's orgasmic experience (Masters and Johnson, 1966).

Small amounts of clear fluid may sometimes appear

FIGURE 3–5

Breast Changes During the Female Sexual Response Cycle

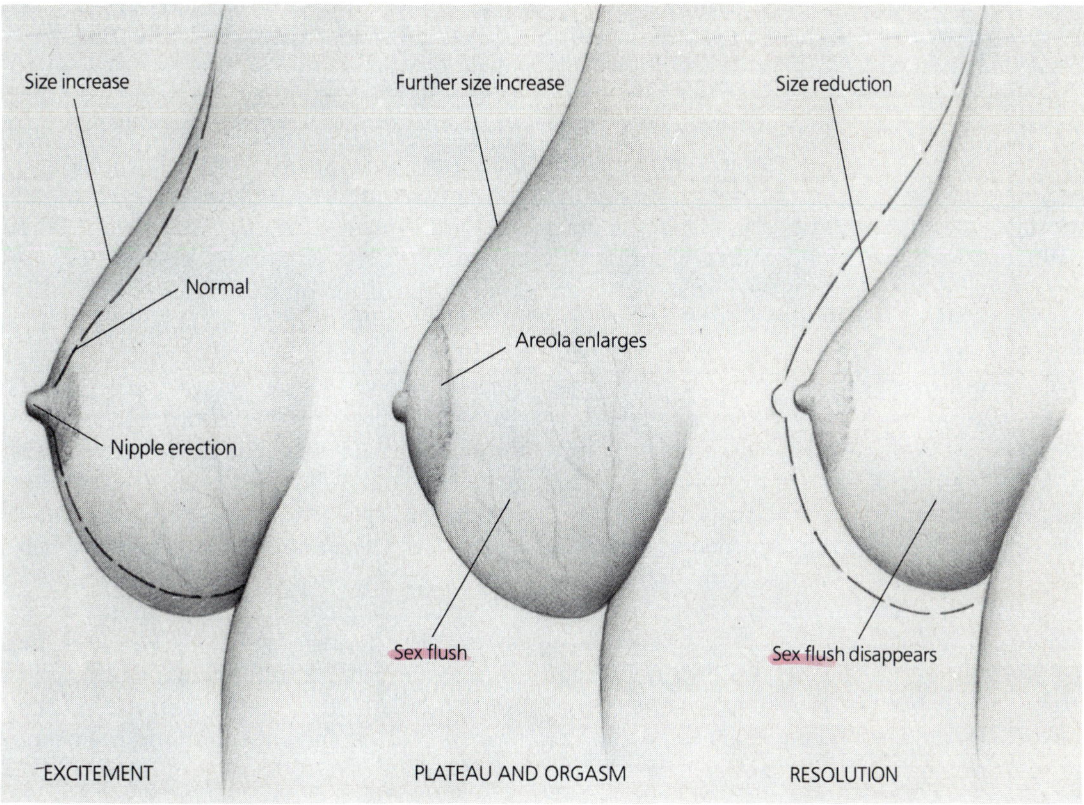

After orgasm, the rapid reduction in swelling of the areola often makes it appear as though the nipple has again become erect.

from the male urethra during the plateau phase. This fluid is thought to come from Cowper's glands and, as mentioned in the previous chapter, occasionally carries live sperm. Many men experience a sensation of internal pressure or warmth during the plateau phase that corresponds to vasocongestion in the region of the prostate gland and seminal vesicles.

In addition to the sensations and changes just described, men and women experience several changes throughout their bodies during the plateau phase. A generalized increase in neuromuscular tension is particularly apparent in the buttocks and thighs. The heart rate increases, sometimes leading to a prominent awareness of heart thumping inside the chest. Breathing also becomes faster and there is a small increase in blood pressure, too.

Orgasm

If effective sexual stimulation continues late in the plateau phase, a point may be reached where the body suddenly discharges its accumulated sexual tension in a peak of sexual arousal called **orgasm**. Orgasm is sometimes called climax or coming. Eric Berne (1971) observed, "Climax started off as a decent enough word, but it has been so overworked on the news-

sex flush a temporary reddish, spotty, rashlike color change sometimes developing during sexual excitement. Usually on the abdomen and breasts, it can spread to any areas of the body.

orgasm the third and shortest phase of the human sexual response cycle. A total body response involving the sudden discharge of accumulated sexual tension.

stands that it now sounds like the moment when two toasted marshmallows finally get stuck to each other" (p. 3). We also prefer the word *orgasm*. Biologically, orgasm is the shortest phase of the sexual response cycle, usually lasting for only a few seconds during which .rhythmic muscular contractions produce intense physical sensations followed by rapid relaxation. Psychologically, orgasm is usually a time of pleasure and suspended thought—the mind turns inward to enjoy the personal experience.

Orgasms vary not only for one person at different times but also for each individual. Sometimes orgasm is an explosive, ecstatic avalanche of sensations, while at other times it is milder, less intense, and less dramatic. While "an orgasm is an orgasm is an orgasm," one orgasm may differ from another just as a glass of ice water tastes better and is more satisfying if you are hot and thirsty than if you are cool and not thirsty at all. Different intensities of orgasms arise from physical factors such as fatigue and the time since the last orgasm as well as from a wide range of psychosocial factors, including mood, relation to partner, activity, expectations, and feelings about the experience.

For all these reasons, trying to define or describe orgasm is a difficult task because each individual's subjective experience includes a psychosocial as well as physiological dimension. Measuring intense muscular contractions during one orgasm does not mean that it is necessarily perceived as "better than" another orgasm with less intense bodily changes. A milder physiological orgasm may be *experienced* as bigger, better, or more satisfying than a physiologically more intense one.

FEMALE

Until the mid-twentieth century, many people (including some medical authorities) believed that women were not capable of orgasm. This belief undoubtedly reflected a cultural bias: sex was seen as something the man did *to* the woman for his own gratification. Women were told for centuries to "do their wifely duties" by making themselves available to their husbands for sex yet were also cautioned that "proper" women did not enjoy sex. Since a sign of physical pleasure or orgasm was thought to be "unladylike," it followed that women were not able to have orgasms. In other words, females were told, "You can't have any physical sexual release, and even if you can, you shouldn't." It is now clear, however, that orgasm occurs in both sexes.

Orgasm in the female is marked by simultaneous rhythmic muscular contractions of the uterus, the outer third of the vagina (the orgasmic platform), and the anal sphincter (Figure 3–2). The first few contractions are intense and close together (at 0.8-second intervals). As orgasm continues, the contractions diminish in force and duration and occur at less regular intervals. A mild orgasm may have only 3 to 5 contractions, while an intense orgasm may have 10 to 15.

Orgasm is a total body response, not just a pelvic event. Brain wave patterns show distinctive changes during orgasm (Cohen, Rosen, and Goldstein, 1976), and muscles in many different body regions contract during this phase of sexual response. In addition, the sex flush achieves its greatest intensity and its widest distribution at the time of orgasm.

Women often describe the sensations of an orgasm as beginning with a momentary sense of suspension, quickly followed by an intensely pleasurable feeling that usually begins at the clitoris and rapidly spreads throughout the pelvis. The physical sensations of the genitals are often described as warm, electric, or tingly, and these usually spread throughout the body. Finally, most women feel muscle contractions in their vagina or lower pelvis, often described as "pelvic throbbing."

Despite a popular misconception, most women do not ejaculate during orgasm. The erroneous belief that women ejaculate probably stems from descriptions in erotic novels of fluid gushing from the vagina as a woman writhes and moans at the peak moment of sexual passion. Such descriptions may sell books but are not particularly accurate.

There is conflicting opinion about whether a different form of female ejaculation occurs. Various workers have claimed that some women expel semen-like fluid from the urethra at the time of orgasm (Grafenberg, 1950; Sevely and Bennett, 1978; Belzer, 1981; Perry and Whipple, 1981). It has been theorized that this fluid may come from a "female prostate," rudimentary glands (Skene's glands) around the urethra near the neck of the bladder that derive embryologically from the same tissues that develop into the prostate gland in males. In fact, some suggest that this "female prostate" is the anatomical site of the "G spot," but this idea—although stirring considerable controversy and conjecture—has not yet been proved scientifically (Bohlen, 1982; Kaplan, 1983). And, while a report on one woman with this ejaculation-like phenomenon indicated that the fluid was not urine (Addiego et al., 1981), a more detailed study of six other women who "ejaculated" showed that the fluid they expelled was indistinguishable from urine (Goldberg et al., 1983).

Further confusion in this area is caused by uncertainty over the number of women who have this ejaculation-like response. Perry and Whipple (1981) initially claimed that "perhaps 10 percent of females" had this response but later reported that they were finding "closer to 40 percent" of women "had ever experienced" female ejaculation (Ladas, Whipple, and Perry, 1982, p. 60). A more recent questionnaire survey also found that 40 percent of the women queried reported having experienced ejaculation at the moment of orgasm (Darling, Davidson, and Conway-Welch, 1990). In our own studies, a survey of approximately 300 women aged 18 to 40 revealed only 14 who claimed to note any gushing or expulsion of fluid at orgasm. However, we *have* observed several cases of women who expelled a type of fluid that was not urine (Masters, 1982).

Although it is clear that at least *some* women experience this ejaculation-like response, it should be realized that a number of these cases represent a condition called **urinary stress incontinence** in which urine is expelled from the urethra due to physical straining such as occurs with coughing, sneezing, or sexual arousal. Since this condition is usually correctable either by the use of Kegel exercises or minor surgery, medical evaluation is warranted if a woman is bothered by such a response.

MALE

Orgasms in men, unlike those in women, occur in two distinct stages. In the first stage of orgasm, the vas deferens (the two tubes that carry sperm) and the prostate and seminal vesicles begin a series of rhythmic contractions that force semen into the bulb of the urethra (Figure 3–3). The man experiences a sensation of **ejaculatory inevitability**—that is, the feeling of having reached the brink of control—as these contractions begin. This sense of inevitability is quite accurate because at this point the ejaculatory process cannot be stopped.[4] In the second stage of the male orgasm, contractions of the urethra and penis combine with contractions in the prostate gland to cause ejaculation, the spurting of semen out of the tip of the penis.

During ejaculation, the neck of the urinary bladder is tightly shut to ensure that semen moves forward and to avoid any mixing of urine and semen. The rhythmic contractions of the prostate, perineal muscles, and shaft of the penis (creating the physical force that propels semen on its journey) occur initially at 0.8-second intervals, just as in women, and account for the spurting of the semen during ejaculation, After the first three or four contractions of the penis, the intervals between contractions become longer and the intensity of the contractions tapers off.

Male orgasm and ejaculation are not one and the same process, although in most men and under most circumstances the two occur simultaneously. Orgasm refers specifically to the sudden rhythmic muscular contractions in the pelvic region and elsewhere in the body that effectively release accumulated sexual tension and the mental sensations accompanying this experience. Ejaculation refers to the release of semen, which sometimes can occur without the presence of orgasm. Orgasm without ejaculation is common in boys before puberty (Kinsey, Pomeroy, and Martin, 1948) and can also occur if the prostate is diseased or with the use of some drugs. Ejaculation without orgasm is less common but can occur in certain cases of neurological illness.

In **retrograde ejaculation,** the bladder neck does not close off properly during orgasm so that semen spurts backward into the bladder. This condition occurs in some men with multiple sclerosis, diabetes, or certain types of prostate surgery. There are no harmful effects, but infertility results and the man may have a different sensation during ejaculation.

The subjective experience of orgasm in men starts quite consistently with the sensation of deep warmth or pressure (sometimes accompanied by throbbing) that corresponds to ejaculatory inevitability. Orgasm

[4] Women do not have a consistently identifiable point of orgasmic inevitability that corresponds to the stage of ejaculatory inevitability in the male response cycle. Distractions can interrupt women's orgasms, whereas if the male has reached "inevitability," orgasm occurs no matter what.

urinary stress incontinence a condition in which urine leaks from the urethra during coughing, laughing, and/or sexual arousal.

ejaculatory inevitability the first stage of orgasm in men, a feeling of having passed the point where ejaculation can be controlled as the vas deferens, seminal vesicles, and prostate start contracting.

retrograde ejaculation condition in which the semen spurts backward into the bladder during orgasm because the bladder neck does not close off properly. It occurs in men with multiple sclerosis and diabetes and following some types of prostate surgery.

is then felt as sharp, intensely pleasurable contractions involving the anal sphincter, rectum, perineum, and genitals, which some men describe as a sensation of pumping. A different feeling, sometimes called a warm rush of fluid or a shooting sensation, describes the actual process of semen traveling through the urethra. In general, men's orgasms tend to be more uniform than women's, although all male orgasms are certainly not identical.

During the orgasmic phase in both sexes, there are high levels of myotonia evident throughout the body. Late in the plateau phase or during orgasm, the myotonia is often visible in facial muscles, where a grimace or frown may be seen. While this expression is sometimes viewed by a partner as an indication of displeasure or discomfort, it is actually an involuntary response that indicates high levels of sexual arousal. Muscle spasms or cramps in the hands or feet may also occur late in the plateau phase or during orgasm, and at the peak of orgasm the whole body may seem to become rigid for a moment.

CONTROVERSIES ABOUT FEMALE ORGASM

While many controversies about the nature of female orgasms exist, several deserve special mention. The first controversy originated with Freud, who believed that there were two types of female orgasm, a clitoral and a vaginal orgasm. Freud stated that clitoral orgasms (those originating from masturbation or other noncoital acts) were evidence of psychological immaturity, since the clitoris was the center of infantile sexuality in the female. Vaginal orgasms (those deriving from coitus) were "authentic" and "mature" since they demonstrated that normal psychosexual development was complete. In his essay "Some Psychological Consequences of the Anatomical Distinction Between the Sexes," Freud wrote that "the elimination of clitoral sexuality is a necessary precondition for the development of femininity." Many women were considered neurotic or were pushed into psychoanalysis because of this view (Schulman, 1971; Sherfey, 1972; LoPiccolo and Heiman, 1978).

Physiologically, all female orgasms follow the same reflex response patterns, no matter what the source of sexual stimulation. An orgasm that comes from rubbing the clitoris cannot be distinguished physiologically from one that comes from intercourse or breast stimulation alone (Masters and Johnson, 1966). This does not mean that all female orgasms feel the same, have the same intensity, or are identically satisfying. As discussed earlier, feeling and intensity are matters of perceptions, and satisfaction is influenced by many factors.

Some women prefer orgasms that occur as a result of intercourse, while others prefer masturbatory orgasms. Those who prefer coital orgasms often say that the overall experience is more satisfying, but the actual orgasm is less direct and intense. One study notes that many women find masturbatory orgasms to be more satisfying than coital ones, perhaps because the woman is not affected by her partner's style, needs, or tempo (Hite, 1977). In other reports, attempts have been made to differentiate between "vulval orgasm," "uterine orgasm," and "blended orgasm" (Singer and Singer, 1972), or other classifications of orgasmic types (Fox and Fox, 1969; Clark, 1970; Fisher, 1973; Bohlen et al., 1982). Ladas, Whipple, and Perry (1982) have claimed that stimulation of the "G spot" produces a completely different type of orgasm than does stimulation of the clitoris: one in which no orgasmic platform forms, and in which the uterus, instead of elevating and expanding the inner portion of the vagina, "seems to be pushed down and the upper portion of the vagina compresses." However, data to support these claims have not yet been published. Despite the continued controversy about "types" of female orgasms, the idea that one type is immature or less good than another has generally been discarded (Masters and Johnson, 1966; Sherfey, 1972; Hite, 1977; Barbach, 1982).

A second controversy about female orgasm is the question of whether or not all women in good health are able to experience a coital orgasm without any other type of simultaneous stimulation. While Masters and Johnson (1966) and others (Sherfey, 1972; Barbach, 1980) believe all women have this ability, some sexologists believe that there may be a group of women who do not. Helen Kaplan (1974) seems to favor the latter view when she says "this pattern may represent a normal variant of female sexuality, at least for some women" (p. 374). And various studies show that the number of women who experience orgasm regularly during intercourse is about 40 to 50 percent (Kinsey et al., 1953; Fisher, 1973; Hite, 1977; Wilcox and Hager, 1980). Many authorities believe that lack of coital orgasm is usually caused by factors such as anxiety, poor communication between partners, hostility, distrust, or low self-esteem. However, if certain females are incapable of experiencing a sexual reflex due to physiological factors (Brindley and Gillan, 1982), it would have implications in diagnosing

PERSONAL PERSPECTIVES

Describing Orgasm

Previous research has shown that expert judges were unable to reliably distinguish between written reports of male and female orgasms (Proctor, Wagner, and Butler, 1974). The sex of the person describing orgasm in the following examples from our files may surprise you.

1. Like a mild explosion, it left me warm and relaxed after a searing heat that started in my genitals and raced to my toes and head.
2. Suddenly, after the tension built and built, I was soaring in the sky, going up, up, up, feeling the cool air rushing by. My insides were tingling and my skin was cool. My heart was racing in a good way, and breathing was a job.
3. Throbbing is the best word to say what it is like. The throbbing starts as a faint vibration, then builds up in wave after wave where time seems to stand still.
4. When I come it's either like an avalanche of pleasure, tumbling through me, or like a refreshing snack—momentarily satisfying, but then I'm ready for more.

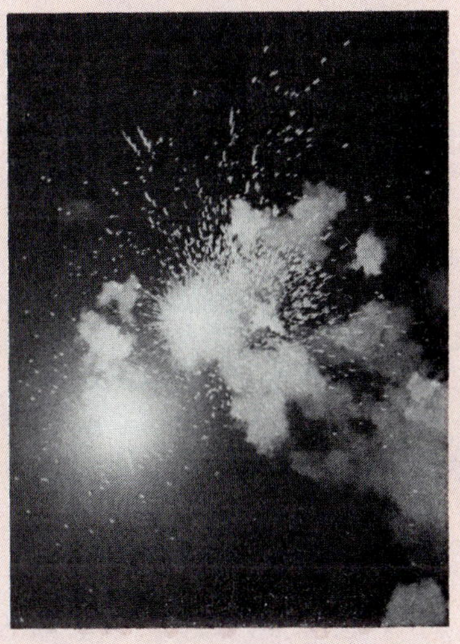

5. My orgasms feel like pulsating bursts of energy starting in my pelvic area and then engulfing my whole body. Sometimes I feel like I'm in freefall, and sometimes I feel like my body's an entire orchestra playing a grand crescendo.
6. An orgasm feels like a dive, magnified many times over. First I feel my muscles tensing, then there's a leap into a cool lake, a sense of suspension and holding my breath, and then my whole body feels relaxed and tingling.
7. Exhilaration is the best word I can find. I feel all pumped up and then, instead of exploding, I am one big wave of happiness and whooshing feelings.
8. Some orgasms feel incredibly intense and earth-shattering, but other times orgasms feel like small, compact, self-contained moments.
9. I feel like a cork popping out of a champagne bottle.
10. There is a warm rush from my toes to my head, with a strong, pulsing rhythm. Then everything settles down like a pink sunset.

1. M 2. F 3. M 4. F 5. F 6. M 7. F 8. M 9. F 10. M

and treating some women's sexual problems, as discussed in Chapter 9.

Another controversial area has to do with the role of the muscles surrounding the vagina in orgasm. Both Arnold Kegel (a surgeon who was the inventor of the "Kegel exercises") and other workers (Perry and Whipple, 1981; Ladas, Whipple, and Perry, 1982; Graber, 1982) claim the condition of the pubococcygeus muscle (PC muscle) is an important determinant of the occurrence of orgasms in women. However, other studies fail to document any correlation between PC muscle strength and female orgasmic responsiveness (Sultan and Chambles, 1982) and have also found that using the Kegel exercises did not improve orgasmic responsivity in nonorgasmic women (Trudel and Saint Laurent, 1983).

Finally, although many observers believe that most women don't feel that orgasm is a necessity for sexual satisfaction, a study by Waterman and Chiauzzi (1982) found that "orgasm consistency was significantly related to sexual satisfaction in females but not in males." While this doesn't mean that women who have the most frequent orgasms are happiest sexually, it does imply that not having orgasms (or not having them very often) may correlate with sexual dissatisfaction.

Resolution Phase

There is a major difference between male and female sexual response immediately following orgasm. Generally, females have the physical capability of being **multiorgasmic**: that is, they can have one or more additional orgasms within a short time without dropping below the plateau level of sexual arousal (Figure 3–1a, pattern 1). Being multiorgasmic depends on both continued effective sexual stimulation and sexual interest, neither of which is consistently present for most women. For this reason, some women never experience multiple orgasms, and others are multiorgasmic in only a small fraction of their sexual experiences. It is unusual for a woman to have multiple orgasms during most of her sexual activity.

Interestingly, multiple orgasm in females seems to occur more frequently during masturbation than intercourse. This may reflect several factors: (1) the relative ease of continuing sexual stimulation, (2) the lack of distraction by concerns about one's partner, and (3) the more frequent use of sexual fantasy by women during masturbation than during intercourse.

Men, on the other hand, are not able to have multiple orgasm if it is defined in the same way. Immediately after ejaculation, the male enters a **refractory period** (Figure 3–1b), a recovery time during which further orgasm or ejaculation is physiologically impossible. A partial or full erection may be maintained during the refractory period, but usually the erection subsides quickly. There is great variability in the length of the refractory period both within and between individual males, and it may last anywhere from a few minutes to many hours. For most males, this interval usually gets longer with each repeated ejaculation within a time span of several hours. In addition, as a man gets older, the refractory period gets longer. In 1978, Robbins and Jensen reported on 13 men who said they had multiple orgasms by withholding ejaculation (only one of whom they studied in the laboratory), but their claims have not yet been fully substantiated. However, it does appear that at least a few men have the capacity to have multiple orgasms before a true refractory period sets in, although it should be stressed that this usually does not happen once ejaculation has occurred. However, Dunn and Trost (1989) have reported that in a small number of men, multiple nonejaculatory orgasms sometimes occur following an initial orgasm with ejaculation.

The period of return to the unaroused state is called the resolution phase. In this phase, which includes the refractory period in men, the anatomic and physiologic changes that occurred during the excitement and plateau phase reverse. In females, the orgasmic platform disappears as the muscular contractions of orgasm pump blood away from these tissues. The uterus moves back into its resting position, the color changes of the labia disappear, the vagina begins to shorten in both width and length, and the clitoris returns to its usual size and position (Figure 3–2). If the breasts enlarged earlier in the response cycle, they decrease in size at this time, and their areolar tissue flattens out faster than the nipples themselves, giving the impression that the nipples are again erect (Figure 3–5). Stimulation of the clitoris, the nipples, or the vagina may be unpleasant or irritating during the postorgasmic phase.

In males, erection diminishes in two stages. First, as a result of orgasmic contractions that pump blood out of the penis, there is a partial loss of erection. In the slower, second stage of this process, genital blood flow returns to baseline (unaroused) patterns. The testes decrease in size and descend into the scrotum, moving away from the body, unless sexual stimulation is continued (Figure 3–3).

As both men and women return to their unaroused state, the "sex flush" disappears and prominent sweating is sometimes noticeable. A fast, heavy breathing pattern may be present just after orgasm, accompanied by a fast heartbeat, but both recede gradually as the entire body relaxes.

If there has been considerable excitement but orgasm has not occurred, resolution takes a longer time. Although certain changes occur quickly (such as disappearance of the orgasmic platform in women and the erection in men), there is sometimes a lingering sensation of pelvic heaviness or aching that is due to continued vasocongestion. This may create a condition of some discomfort, particularly if high levels of arousal were prolonged. Testicular aching ("blue balls") in men and pelvic congestion in women may be relieved by orgasms that occur during sleep or by masturbation. Although **nocturnal emissions** ("wet dreams") in young males are well known, females also can experience orgasm during sleep (Kinsey et al., 1953).

COMMON MYTHS ABOUT SEXUAL RESPONSE

In the preceding chapter, we discussed a number of misconceptions related to sexual anatomy and sexual satisfaction (e.g., a bigger penis always provides more stimulation to the female during intercourse). In light of the physiologic responses just considered, we can now debunk some other common myths about sex.

One commonly held belief is that males have a greater sexual capacity than females. The reverse is actually true. From the viewpoint of physical capability, females have an almost unlimited orgasmic potential, while men, because of the refractory period, are unable to have a rapid series of ejaculations. (While women do not have a true refractory period, orgasmic potential is undoubtedly restricted by fatigue. There may be other physiologic limitations not known at present.) Many males also find it difficult to obtain another erection shortly after ejaculation. From a mechanical perspective then, their capacity to participate in repeated intercourse usually does not match that of the opposite sex.

Another misconception about sexual response is that the male can *always* tell if his female partner had an orgasm. At times, the male may be unaware of his partner's orgasm because he is caught up in his own feelings of arousal or because he doesn't recognize the physical signs of female orgasm. This may occur either because his expectations are inaccurate, because he doesn't know what to expect, or because the accuracy of his sense of vision is lessened during high levels of sexual excitation. Some males are fooled by a partner who "fakes" orgasm by means of loud moans and groans, intense pelvic thrusting, heavy breathing, and voluntary contractions of the outer portion of the vagina.[5]

The notion that all orgasms are intense, earth-shattering, explosive events is another widespread sexual misconception that can probably be traced to the literary imagination. Although the reflex mechanisms of orgasmic response are fairly uniform, some orgasms are mild, fluttery, or warm, while others are blockbusters. These differences arise from variations in a person's physical state such as being tired, tense, having a sore throat or headache, or from variations in the emotions that accompany the sexual experience. The sensations of any physiologic process—drinking a glass of water, eating a meal, breathing, urinating, or sex—vary in different times and circumstances.

In the 1950s, the idea that "mutual orgasm" (both partners experiencing orgasm at the same time) was the ultimate peak in sexual pleasure became popular and was advocated enthusiastically in numerous marriage manuals. Many people tried to "fine-tune" the timing of their responses, but working at sex usually resulted in a loss of spontaneity and fun. While mutual orgasm can be exhilarating, each person can be so wrapped up in his or her own response that the experience of the partner's orgasm cannot be fully appreciated or can even be missed completely.

HORMONAL REGULATION OF SEXUAL FUNCTION AND BEHAVIOR

The physiologic processes of sex are not only vascular and neuromuscular. An important part of sexual physiology is under the control of the endocrine system, which consists of ductless glands that produce chemical substances called hormones. Hormones are secreted directly into the bloodstream where they are carried to tissues on which they act. Some hormones, such as cortisol (made in the adrenal glands, which lie just above the kidneys), are necessary for life itself and influence a wide range of body functions. Other hormones are required for reproduction or sexual de-

multiorgasmic (mul′ tē or gaz′ mik) the potential ability of women to have a series of identifiable orgasmic responses without dropping below the plateau level of arousal. Men do not share this capacity.

refractory period in the male, the period immediately following ejaculation during which further orgasm is physiologically impossible. This period is not present in the female response cycle.

nocturnal emissions involuntary male orgasm and ejaculation during sleep (sometimes called wet dreams).

[5] Men also sometimes resort to sexual fakery. For both women and men, this may be motivated by the wish to please their partner. For a fuller discussion, see Chapter 9.

velopment. Here, we consider the hormones that influence our sexual function.

The Sex Hormones

The most important hormone in sexual function is testosterone. This hormone, sometimes called the male sex hormone, is actually present in both sexes. In a normal man, 6 to 8 mg of testosterone are produced per day, with more than 95 percent manufactured in the testes and the remainder in the adrenal glands. In a woman, approximately 0.5 mg of testosterone is made daily in the ovaries and the adrenals.

Testosterone is the principal biologic determinant of the sex drive in both men and women. Deficiencies of testosterone may cause a drop in sexual desire (Bancroft, 1978; Kolodny, Masters, and Johnson, 1979), and excessive testosterone may heighten sexual interest. In men, too little testosterone may cause difficulty obtaining or maintaining erections, but it is not certain whether testosterone deficiencies interfere with female sexual functioning apart from reducing sexual desire. However, there is no evidence whatsoever to suggest that because women have less testosterone than men, they have lower sexual interest. Instead, it seems that men and women have different levels of behavioral sensitivity to the effects of this hormone, with women actually being more sensitive to small quantities in their circulation (Persky et al., 1978; Kolodny, Masters, and Johnson, 1979; Bancroft, 1984).

Estrogens, sometimes called female hormones, are also present in both sexes and are made primarily in the ovaries in women and in the testes in men. In women, they are important from a sexual viewpoint in maintaining the condition of the vaginal lining and in producing vaginal lubrication. Estrogens also help to preserve the texture and function of the female breasts and elasticity of the vagina. In men, estrogens have no known function. It does not seem that estrogens are important determinants of female sexual interest or capacity, since surgical removal of the ovaries does not reduce the sex drive in women or lessen sexual responsivity. Too much estrogen in males, however, dramatically reduces the sexual appetite and can cause difficulties with erection and enlargement of the breasts.

Progesterone, a hormone structurally related to both the estrogens and testosterone, is also present in both sexes. The effects of progesterone on sexual behavior and function have been studied primarily in animals, where it appears that large amounts suppress sexual interest. Some authorities speculate that it may also act as a sexual inhibitor in humans (Bancroft, 1984).

Regulatory Mechanisms

Two decades ago, it was thought that the "master gland" of endocrine function was the **pituitary,** an acorn-sized structure lying beneath the brain. It is now clear that the regulatory role of the pituitary is more like a relay station and that a portion of the brain itself—the **hypothalamus**—has primary control over most endocrine pathways.

The hypothalamus produces a substance called **gonadotropin releasing hormone** (**GnRH**) that controls the secretion of two hormones made in the pituitary gland which act on the gonads (ovaries and testes). **Luteinizing hormone** (**LH**) stimulates the Leydig cells in the testes to manufacture testosterone; in the female, LH serves as the trigger for ovulation (release of an egg from the ovary). **Follicle stimulating hormone** (**FSH**) stimulates the production of sperm cells in the testes; in the female, FSH prepares the ovary for ovulation.

The hypothalamus acts much like a thermostat in regulating hormonal function (Figure 3–6). Instead of reacting to temperature, as a thermostat does, the hypothalamus reacts to the concentrations of hormones in its own blood supply. For example, in adult males the amount of testosterone "registers" in the hypothalamus. If the amount is high, production of GnRH is turned off, leading to a drop in LH secretion by the pituitary. The decrease in LH in the bloodstream quickly results in reduced production of testosterone in the testes, and therefore lower amounts of testosterone are secreted into the blood. When the amount of testosterone reaching the hypothalamus drops below a certain level, it triggers the secretion of GnRH into the pituitary. The pituitary responds to this signal by sending more LH into the circulation, where it will soon reach the testes and cause an increased rate of testosterone production.

Hormones and Sexual Behavior

It is tempting to try to understand sexual behavior in terms of hormones. In many animal species, patterns of sexual interaction are tightly regulated by hormonal events that control both the sexual receptivity of the female (her willingness to mate) and sexual interest

FIGURE 3–6

Endocrine Regulation in the Adult Male (a) and Female (b)

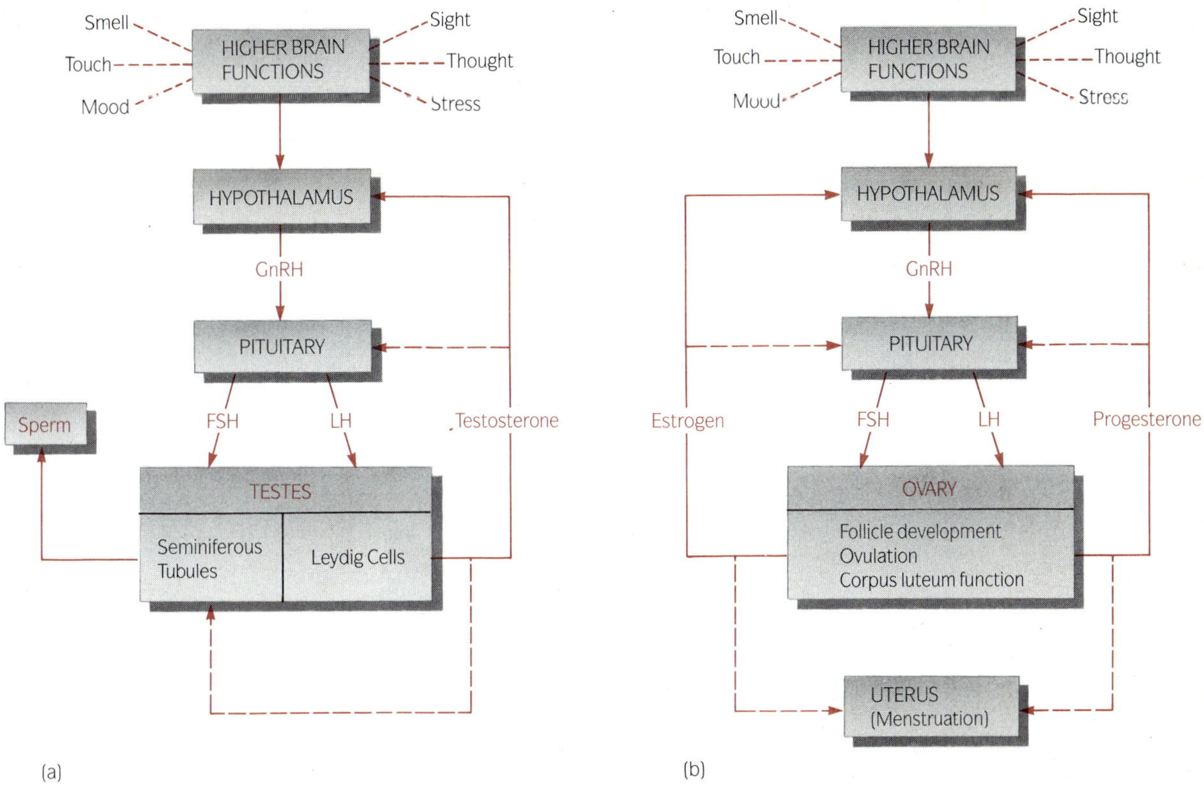

(courtship behavior) of the male, as well as male mounting and penile thrusting (Hutchison, 1978). Testosterone and estrogen have been found in mammals, birds, reptiles, amphibians, and fish: in all these groups, actions of sex hormones on the brain appear to be important determinants of sexual behavior (Kelley and Pfaff, 1978).

In humans, however, there is a more complicated relationship between hormones and sexual behavior. Although a marked testosterone deficiency usually reduces sexual interest in men or women, there are cases where this effect is not seen. Similarly, although many men with subnormal testosterone levels have difficulty with erection, others continue to have completely normal sexual function. Women who have low amounts of estrogen in their bodies do not usually lose their ability to be sexually aroused or to have orgasms. People's sex hormone levels do not "predict" their sexual behavior or interest.

Although there is no simple one-to-one relationship between sex hormones and human sexual behavior,

estrogens (es' tro jinz) hormones present in both sexes, but primarily considered female. Produced in the ovaries and adrenal glands in the female, they maintain the lining of the vagina and produce breast growth. Also important in controlling the menstrual cycle.

progesterone (prō jes' tur ōn) a hormone present in both sexes, but primarily known as a female hormone. Present in high levels during pregnancy.

pituitary (pi tew' i ter' ē) an acorn-sized gland at the base of the brain which, at the direction of the hypothalamus, secretes several hormones important to sexual development and function. Once believed to control most of the endocrine system, it is now known to act only as a relay station.

hypothalamus (hī' pō thal' uh mus) the portion of the brain that has primary control over most endocrine pathways. It reacts to the level of hormones in the blood supply which regulate many sexual responses and direct their production.

gonadotropin releasing hormone (GnRH) (gō nad' ō trō' pin) a substance produced by the hypothalamus that controls the production and release of LH and FSH by the pituitary.

luteinizing hormone (LH) (lū' tē in īz' ing) produced by the pituitary gland, LH triggers ovulation and stimulates the Leydig cells to manufacture testosterone.

follicle stimulating hormone (FSH) a substance produced in the pituitary gland that prepares the ovary for ovulation and stimulates the production of sperm cells in the testes.

fascinating questions about the role of hormones in sexuality abound. Later chapters will address such questions as: How do hormones influence sexual development (Chapter 6)? What kinds of sexual disorders are caused by hormone imbalance (Chapter 10)? How do hormone changes caused by aging affect sexual response (Chapter 6)? We now consider the hormonal patterns of the menstrual cycle and see whether they influence sexual behavior in women.

MENSTRUATION

Menstruation is a flow of blood that occurs about once a month in most women from approximately age 12 to 48. Although menstruation is a normal part of the female reproductive cycle, it is a subject of considerable misunderstanding and taboo. In ancient times, a menstruating woman was regarded as unclean and liable to pollute foods she handled or as contagious and liable to cause illness or even death in others (Delaney, Lupton, and Toth, 1977). In the modern era, menstruation is sometimes seen as a physical and emotional handicap that makes women "inferior" to men (Koeske, 1976; Frieze et al., 1978; Sherif, 1980). Whether menstruation is called the "curse," "the monthlies," or "being on the rag," it is often referred to in negative terms. In this section, we discuss the physiology of the menstrual cycle and consider the effects of menstruation on emotions and physical well-being.

Physiology of the Menstrual Cycle

The menstrual cycle is traditionally described as starting with the first day of menstrual flow (cycle day 1) and ending the day before the next menstruation begins. The length of the cycle varies, normally ranging from 21 to 40 days and averaging about 28 days (Vollman, 1977). Very few women are so regular that they can accurately and consistently predict the length of each cycle on the basis of their past pattern of cycle lengths.

The menstrual cycle consists of three phases, which we describe in terms of an "average" 28-day cycle (Figure 3–7). The **follicular phase** is the first portion of the menstrual cycle. Ovarian follicles, oval arrangements of cells around a young egg, begin to mature as FSH stimulates them. At the start of this phase, estrogen and progesterone levels are quite low and the uterus sheds its lining, resulting in three to six days of menstrual flow. Menstrual flow consists of a small amount of blood combined with tiny bits of tissue from the lining of the uterus, and the entire amount is usually only 2 or 3 ounces (4 to 6 tablespoons).

Midway in the follicular phase (around cycle days 7 to 10), estrogen output from the ovaries increases, which acts with FSH to prepare the developing follicle for ovulation. Estrogen also causes the lining of the uterus to thicken, or proliferate, due to growth of glands, connective tissue, and blood vessels. Just before ovulation, estrogen levels reach a broad peak, which acts on the hypothalamus to trigger the surge of LH and FSH released from the pituitary a day or two afterwards.

Ovulation, release of the egg from the ovary, typically occurs at about the fourteenth cycle day in most 28-day cycles. However, we have studied cycles in which ovulation ranged from the ninth day to the nineteenth day of a cycle of this length, and in some menstrual cycles ovulation does not occur at all (see Chapter 4). Ovulation usually follows the LH peak by 12 to 24 hours. The ovulatory phase is the shortest phase of the menstrual cycle.

The third portion of the menstrual cycle is the **luteal phase,** which encompasses the time from immediately after ovulation until the start of the next cycle. This phase is named for the corpus luteum, the mass of cells left in the ovary after the follicle ruptures during ovulation. The corpus luteum produces huge amounts of progesterone and estrogen, leading to increased levels of these hormones in this portion of the menstrual cycle (Figure 3–7). The progesterone causes the small blood vessels in the thickened endometrium to develop and produces coiling in the endometrial glands, changes that prepare the uterus to receive a fertilized egg if pregnancy occurs. The progesterone also registers in the hypothalamus, where it shuts off output of GnRH, resulting in a rapid decline in LH and FSH from the pituitary. Unless the egg is fertilized, the corpus luteum degenerates 10 to 12 days after ovulation, and its hormone production drops drastically. The next menstrual flow occurs as the lining of the uterus sheds in preparation for regrowth in the next cycle. Menstruation is thus the result of abrupt withdrawal of hormone stimulation.

Menstrual Cycle Effects

Brief comments from three women who participated in studies of the menstrual cycle at the Masters &

Johnson Institute show the great diversity in how women feel about menstruation:

> I have a tough time with my periods. First, I get irritable and depressed a day or two before my period starts—nothing seems to go right. Then, I have real bad cramps for two days. I have to stay in bed; it's sheer agony.
>
> A few days before my period, my breasts get swollen and tender, and I usually get a headache. Once my period starts, everything is back to normal.
>
> Menstruation is no big deal. One time when I was 13 or so I had some cramping, but I really don't have any problems at all.

Mirroring this diversity, there is also considerable scientific controversy about the physiological and psychological effects of the menstrual cycle. In 1931 an American physician reported that estrogen causes "varying degrees of discomfort preceding the onset of menstruation," including "increased fatigability, irritability, lack of concentration, and attacks of pain" (Frank, 1931). High doses of x-rays were sometimes prescribed to knock out the ovaries in severe cases of the condition, which Frank called *premenstrual tension*.

More recently, Dr. Katharina Dalton conducted an extensive series of studies on the subject, reporting that female criminal acts, accidents, hospital visits, poor judgments, and suicides are more common in the premenstrual and menstrual phases than at other times (Dalton, 1959, 1960, 1964, 1966, 1968, 1970, 1980). Numerous reports also indicate that the menstrual and premenstrual phases are associated with negative moods (Moos, 1969; Golub, 1976; May, 1976; Rossi and Rossi, 1977).

These findings, however, are not universal or interpreted in the same way by all scientists. For example, Persky (1974) found that mood was fairly consistent in college-aged women at three different points in the menstrual cycle. Dan (1976) noted that mood changes were very similar in women and their husbands over time regardless of the menstrual cycle. Webster, Bauman, and Kolodny (1978) noted that "menstrual or premenstrual symptoms" were unrelated to hormone levels and occurred with some frequency throughout the cycle, even around the time of ovulation. More recently, another research group found no evidence of menstrual cycle effects on academic performance as shown by examination grades (Walsh et al., 1981). Many investigators have suggested that social expectations and stereotypes seem to influence the occurrences of menstrual or premenstrual distress (e.g., Paige, 1973; Parlee, 1973; Koeske and Koeske, 1975; Brooks-Gunn and Ruble, 1980; Sherif, 1980). For example, some observers note that the title of one of the questionnaires most frequently used in menstrual cycle research, the Menstrual Distress Questionnaire, is inherently biased, as are the preponderance of questions asked.

> If the questionnaire were called the *Menstrual Joy Questionnaire*, if the majority of items asked for responses such as "happiness" or "feeling great" or "able to plot effective strategy" or "increased creativity," the end results would inevitably be different. *(Delaney, Lupton, and Toth, 1977, p. 84)*

Others in the field point out the problems associated with a person's attempts at remembering past events (including the exact timing of the onset of menstruation) months after they have happened, although this type of retrospective self-reporting has been a mainstay of much of Dalton's research (Sherif, 1980). And, as Ruble, Brooks-Gunn, and Clarke (1980) have noted, cultural factors influence both the anxiety about or acceptance of a biological event like menstruation. "If a woman believes that women normally experience a variety of premenstrual symptoms, she may report such symptoms in part to make herself appear normal" (p. 234).

While it is clear that women are not ruled by their monthly hormone cycles, two kinds of menstrual problems are very common: **dysmenorrhea** (painful menstruation) and the **premenstrual syndrome (PMS).**

DYSMENORRHEA

Dysmenorrhea, or painful menstruation, is usually marked by pelvic or lower abdominal cramping, back-

menstruation (men stroo′ ā′ shun) a flow of blood from the lining of the uterus occurring about once a month in females from puberty until the late forties or early fifties.

follicular phase (fol ik′ ū lar) the first phase of the menstrual cycle, in which ovarian follicles begin to mature as a result of stimulation by FSH.

ovulation (ōv you lā′ shun) the second phase of the menstrual cycle; the release of the egg from the ovary.

luteal phase (lū′ tē ul) the third phase of the menstrual cycle, after ovulation. The corpus luteum produces large amounts of progesterone and estrogen, which prepare the uterus to receive the fertilized egg.

dysmenorrhea (dis men′ or ē′ uh) painful menstruation, usually including backache, headache, cramps, and a bloated feeling.

premenstrual syndrome (PMS) fatigue, irritability, depression, and bloated feeling some women experience a few days before menstruation. Physical, psychological, and social causes are debated.

FIGURE 3–7

Hormone Changes During a Typical Menstrual Cycle

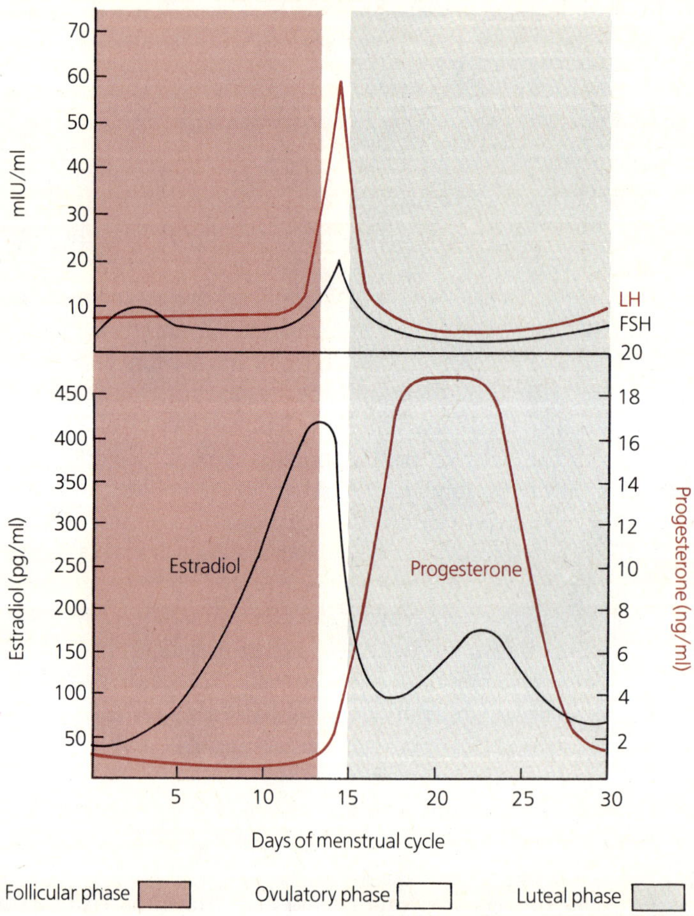

Source: Reproduced, with permission, from Benson, R. C. (editor), *Current Obstetric and Gynecologic Diagnosis and Treatment*, 3rd ed. Copyright 1980 by Lange Medical Publications, Los Altos, California.

ache, headache, and a feeling of being bloated, sometimes accompanied by diarrhea, nausea, or vomiting. These symptoms generally start in the 24 hours before menstrual flow begins and disappear spontaneously within 48 to 72 hours after menstruation starts.

There are two types of dysmenorrhea. Primary dysmenorrhea is defined as the group of symptoms mentioned above without the presence of any pelvic abnormalities. Secondary dysmenorrhea is diagnosed when a specific pelvic abnormality is found in the presence of the same symptoms. Common causes of secondary dysmenorrhea include endometriosis (the occurrence of the type of tissue lining the uterus in locations outside the uterus), pelvic inflammatory disease (scarring of Fallopian tubes, usually resulting from a sexually transmitted disease), ovarian cysts, and tumors of the uterus. Primary dysmenorrhea usually begins in adolescence and reaches its peak incidence and severity around age 25, whereas secondary dysmenorrhea tends to occur in women in their thirties and forties.

Although primary dysmenorrhea was once thought to be a psychosomatic condition, it is now clear that it has a biochemical basis. The trigger mechanism is an excess release of prostaglandins from the uterus. Various drugs, such as aspirin, naproxen (trade name Naprosyn), naproxen sodium (trade name Anaprox), ibuprofen (trade name Motrin), and mefenamic acid (trade name Ponstel), are highly effective in inhibiting prostaglandin production, so that they effectively prevent or relieve the discomfort associated with dysmenorrhea. If these drugs do not work, birth control pills can be used as an alternative, since they relieve dysmenorrhea in more than 90 percent of cases (presumably by indirectly affecting prostaglandin production). In addition, some women find that being orgasmic relieves the discomfort of dysmenorrhea by reducing pelvic heaviness (Masters and Johnson, 1966).

PMS: THE PREMENSTRUAL SYNDROME

The premenstrual syndrome is usually defined as occurring in the two to three days before menstrual flow begins and is marked by feelings of tension and irritability (Delaney, Lupton, and Toth, 1977; Frieze et al., 1978; Money, 1980). Other variable findings include feeling sluggish, impatient, dizzy, nervous, depressed, and indecisive, as well as having physical symptoms such as breast tenderness, constipation, headache, bloating, and alcohol intolerance. It is uncertain how many women have such premenstrual difficulties (estimates range from 20 to 75 percent). There do not appear to be any major differences in the premenstrual symptoms experienced by blacks and whites (see Table 3–1), although most women seeking help at PMS centes are white (Stout et al., 1986). Researchers are also trying to determine whether a woman's attitudes toward menstruation or her physiological events, such as shifting hormones or fluid retention, induce these mood changes and discomfort (González, 1981). The specific cause of the premenstrual syndrome is unclear, although some researchers think it might relate to the estrogen:progesterone ratio, the adrenal hormones controlling water retention, or the chemical substances in the brain influencing mood (see Table 3–2). Whatever the resolution of these interesting controversies, premenstrual symptoms are usually transient, do not always occur, and are often unobservable (Delaney, Lupton, and Toth, 1977). Moreover, most researchers agree that only 5 to 10 percent of women have premenstrual distress that is serious enough to interfere with their functioning (Keye, 1983). The severity of this problem may be as much a reflection of negative societal attitudes about menstruation as an indicator of physiological processes.

The numerous controversies over PMS present a particularly complex issue, with biomedical, social, political, legal, and economic ramifications. Most researchers feel that Dalton's studies are not credible (Koeske, 1983; Fausto-Sterling, 1985), yet her findings have been used in various court cases: for instance, in Brooklyn, New York, attorney Stephanie Benson decided to defend a client who was accused of beating her four-year-old daughter by claiming that the woman was a victim of hormonal imbalances associated with her menstrual cycle. Although the idea of using PMS as a legal defense was eventually dropped in this case as part of a plea-bargaining agree-

TABLE 3–1

Premenstrual Symptoms in Black and White Women from a Community, Nonpatient Sample

	Black Women (N = 321)	*White Women (N = 462)*
Feeling depressed, sad, or blue	29%	27%
Having wide mood swings	26%	21%
Feeling under stress	16%	18%
Having cravings for certain foods	25%	17%
Having decreased energy	29%	23%
Being irritable	28%	31%
Feeling unable to cope	10%	10%

Source: From Stout, A. L., et al. "Premenstrual Symptoms in Black and White Community Samples," *American Journal of Psychiatry* 143: 1436–1439, 1986. Copyright 1986, the American Psychiatric Association. Reprinted by permission.

TABLE 3–2

Proposed Causes and Treatments of PMS

Causes
Psychosomatic
Abnormality of brain neurotransmitters
Hormonal
  Estrogen excess
  Progesterone deficiency
  Antidiuretic hormone excess
  Aldosterone abnormality
  Hormone allergy
Vitamin A deficiency
Vitamin B deficiency
Low blood sugar (hypoglycemia)
Fluid retention

Treatments[a]
Exercise
Diet changes (especially restricting sugar and salt)
Birth control pills
Progesterone
Vitamin supplements
Diuretics
Dietary supplements (minerals, herbs, etc.)
Tranquilizers
Counseling

[a] There is no current evidence that suggests that any of these treatments is superior to a placebo in producing improvement in women with PMS.

ment, in at least two murders in England the so-called PMS defense was used successfully to claim mitigating circumstances (*American Medical News,* Nov. 26, 1982, p. 14).

While some lawyers appear interested in pursuing this line of legal ground-breaking, many feminists feel they are uncomfortably caught in a paradoxical situation. On the one hand, as Susan Edmiston (1982) points out, "Throughout the 1970s, the feminist attitude toward menstruation was to deny that it made a difference and to minimize any effects women feel . . . . The reasoning was that to admit that menstruation mattered was to open the door to charges of biological inferiority." Now, however, increasing numbers of women (including many feminists) have become concerned about the realities of PMS, which they realize can be addressed only by open and intensive study. To pretend that PMS doesn't exist or that it affects only a tiny fraction of women, they believe, is going to slow much-needed research and make women who suffer from PMS feel lonely and abnormal. But, as well-known politician–lawyer–feminist Elizabeth Holtzman has pointed out, the PMS defense could backfire to harm women in divorce proceedings and custody battles and might even be used to justify violence against women (Allen, 1982).

The problem is an especially complicated one since researchers seem surrounded on all sides by disagreement, methodological difficulties, and uncertainty over what their findings mean. According to a news report in the *Journal of the American Medical Association* (June 3, 1983), scientists attending a PMS workshop sponsored by the National Institute of Mental Health agreed that PMS existed but "were hard-pressed to define the disorder precisely." Instead, noting that PMS doesn't seem to have a single pattern, they suggested using the plural term "premenstrual syndromes" rather than the singular form.

Disagreement in PMS research seems to apply up and down the line. While some workers such as England's Dr. Katharina Dalton champion the notion that progresterone deficiency causes PMS, no studies have actually measured this deficiency in a way that

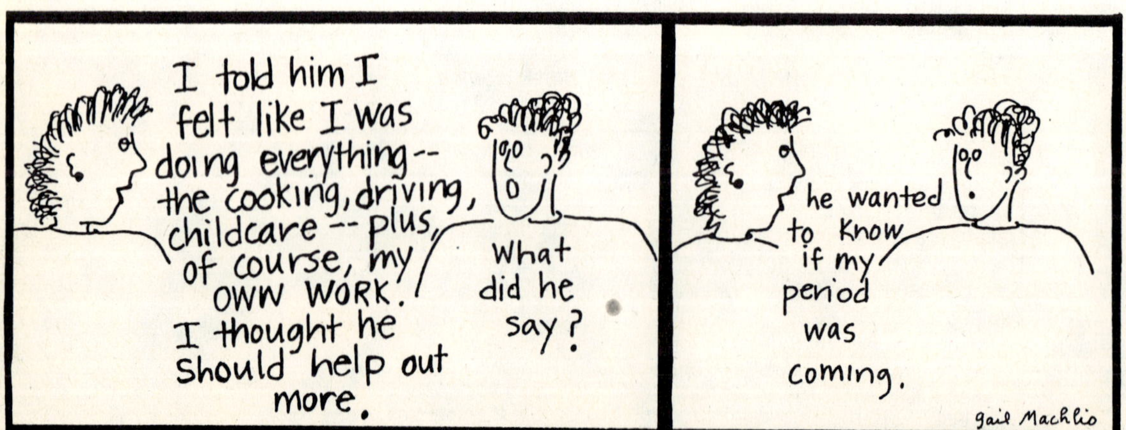
I told him I felt like I was doing everything-- the cooking, driving, childcare -- plus, of course, my OWN WORK. I thought he should help out more.
What did he say?
he wanted to know if my period was coming.
gail Machlis

shows a cause-and-effect relationship. Although one research team claims that even in its severest forms, PMS is *not* a form of depression (Haskett et al., 1980), others say that exactly the opposite is true (Shuckit et al., 1975; Halbreich, Endicott, and Nee, 1983). Worst of all, research on the treatment of PMS—which now includes literally hundreds of studies on dozens of different approaches—is often surprisingly slipshod, poorly designed, and difficult to interpret. As researcher Judith Green says, "No one approach has yielded consistent results, and no single agent has stood out as consistently useful."

Uncertainty among researchers is magnified, in a sense, by the large numbers of women who have read or heard about PMS and are now demanding treatment. Since progesterone use is not approved for treatment of PMS in the United States, many physicians are unwilling to prescribe it, particularly since it has been reported to cause cancer in animals. In addition, many of the most knowledgeable physicians in this field are aware that controlled, double-blind studies (in which neither the test subjects nor the investigators know whether a subject is taking progesterone or an inert look-alike pill called a placebo) have not been able to show that progesterone works better than a placebo in reducing premenstrual symptoms (Blume, 1983).

Despite this uncertainty, scores of PMS clinics have sprouted all over the country, with most of them offering progesterone therapy. Predictably, perhaps, they've been greeted by an avalanche of patients, partly because they've done a good job of selling American women on the idea that almost *any* symptom during the premenstrual week is a sign of PMS (Allen, 1982). In addition to offering the experimental hormone treatments, most of these clinics also prescribe dietary changes (e.g., avoiding salty foods, refined sugar, chocolate, and caffeine; eating six small meals a day), and they perform blood tests of dubious value. Not surprisingly, many of these centers charge high fees. The bottom line here seems to be "Let the buyer beware"—at least until the research community can provide better documentation for the causes and cures of this elusive but troublesome disorder.

Sex and the Menstrual Cycle

As part of our evolutionary heritage, there is some basis for assuming that women should be most interested in sex around the time of ovulation, when pregnancy can occur. In most animal species, the female follows this pattern of behavior rather exclusively, avoiding sexual contact at all other times. Some studies document a pattern of increased sexual activity around the presumed time of ovulation and do not find such a "peak" in women using birth control pills, which block ovulation (Udry and Morris, 1968, 1970; Adams, Gold, and Burt, 1978), but these findings appear to have been a result of imprecise determination of when ovulation occurred (James, 1971; Kolodny and Bauman, 1979). Other reports find no evidence of heightened female sexual interest during ovulation (James, 1971; Persky et al., 1978; Bancroft, 1984).

A well-designed study by Schreiner-Engel and coworkers (1981) found objective laboratory evidence of higher levels of vaginal vasocongestion during the follicular and luteal phases of the menstrual cycle. Subjective reports of sexual arousal were also higher at these times than during the ovulatory phase, providing further confirmation that an ovulatory peak in female sexual responsivity is unlikely. Another recent study confirmed that female sexual activity and sexual interest peak in the follicular phase well before ovulation (Bancroft et al., 1983). Nevertheless, individuals differ in unique ways, so that some women may well find themselves feeling sexier at midcycle while others are most interested in sex earlier or later in their cycles.

Taboos about sexual intercourse during menstruation are still a part of everyday life for many people. In some cases, avoiding sexual contact is a matter of religious practice. For example, Orthodox Jews are supposed to abstain from sex for seven days after the end of menstrual flow, and sex is resumed only after the woman has immersed herself in a ritual bath, called the *mikvah*. In other cases, abstinence seems to stem from cultural and psychological sources: "A man is as likely to be sexually aroused by a woman when she is menstruating as he is at any other time. But the blood of the menstruating woman is somehow dangerous, magical, and apparently not something he wants to get on his penis" (Delaney, Lupton, and Toth, 1977). The following comments illustrate the broad range of feelings people have about sexual activity during menstruation:

> I often find that I feel sexiest when I'm having my period, so making love is particularly enjoyable then. *(Authors' files)*

> I somehow feel like it's not right to have sex when my girlfriend is menstruating. I don't know why, but I just feel funny about it. *(Authors' files)*

Jill and I love to have sex during her periods. It's a particularly passionate time because we don't need to use any birth control then. *(Authors' files)*

In a word, I'm embarrassed about it. I feel like I'm not completely clean when I'm flowing, and tampons make me dry inside, so I really prefer waiting until my period is done. *(Authors' files)*

The notion that sexual activity, including intercourse, is "dangerous" to either partner during menstruation has no basis in fact (Masters and Johnson, 1966). Yet some people feel that intercourse is messy during menstruation and restrict their sexual experiences to noncoital options. It appears as though attitudes toward sex during menstruation are beginning to change, however, since younger people seem to be less affected by the negative attitudes concerning such activity than their parents' generation (Paige, 1978).

SUMMARY

1. Sexual physiology describes the functions and reflexes of sexual response. Sexual arousal is the activation of a complex network of reflexes that involves the sex organs and sensory, cognitive, and hormonal pathways in the brain.
2. The sexual response cycle of both sexes consists of four basic stages: excitement, plateau, orgasm, and resolution. The primary physical changes that occur during the cycle are a result of vasocongestion and the accumulation of neuromuscular tension.
3. Vaginal lubrication in the female and penile erection in the male are the most prominent signs of the excitement phase. This phase is also marked by internal vaginal expansion and nipple erection.
4. In the plateau phase of high sexual arousal, the outer portion of the vagina swells, forming the orgasmic platform, and the labia thicken and undergo a prominent color change. In the male, the testes increase in size and are pulled tightly against the body, and a preejaculatory fluid may appear. A measles-like rash called the "sex flush" is seen in the majority of women and in about 25 percent of men.
5. Orgasm is a highly pleasurable reflex discharging neuromuscular tension via a total body response. In both sexes, a series of muscular contractions occur initially at 0.8-second intervals and then diminish in intensity and rapidity. In females, orgasm includes contractions of the outer portion of the vagina, the uterus, and the anal sphincter. In males, orgasm begins with contractions in the prostate and seminal vesicles, which initiates the process of ejaculation.
6. The resolution phase is a period in which the foregoing changes reverse, with a return to the unaroused state.
7. The male is limited in terms of physiologic response capacity by a refractory period immediately after ejaculation during which he cannot ejaculate again. Females do not have a refractory period. While women have the capacity to be multiorgasmic, this pattern of response has been noted in only a small number of men.
8. The old notion that there are two types of female orgasm—vaginal and clitoral—has been disproved. The physiologic patterns of female orgasm are identical no matter what the source of sexual stimulation.
9. The sex hormones—principally testosterone, estrogens, and progresterone—are present in both sexes and are controlled by the hypothalamus and pituitary gland. Testosterone is an important influence on sexual drive in males and females, but sexual behavior in humans cannot be thought of as tightly controlled by the sex hormones.
10. The menstrual cycle consists of three phases: the follicular phase, ovulation, and the luteal phase. The length of the entire cycle and its effects on mood and physical symptoms vary considerably.
11. Dysmenorrhea (painful menstruation), which is marked by cramping, backache, and feeling bloated, is now thought to be due to excessive release of chemicals called prostaglandins; it can usually be controlled by drugs that inhibit these substances.
12. PMS (premenstrual syndrome) affects a substantial number of women, typically causing irritability and tensions in the few days before the period begins. Many theories abound about the causes of PMS, but there is little agreement on this or on the proper treatment.

Thought Questions

1. Which stage of the human sexual response cycle allows for the greatest experience of intimacy between the two partners? Which allows for the least? Do you have a favorite part of the cycle? Which part, or when?
2. The text indicates that excitement, plateau, and orgasm are brought on by "effective sexual

stimulation." What does "effective sexual stimulation" mean to you?

3. Researchers believe that only 40 to 50 percent of women regularly experience orgasm during intercourse. How do women who don't have orgasms during intercourse feel about it? How would men feel if they didn't regularly have orgasms during intercourse? Are the sexes different in how necessary they think it is to have an orgasm?
4. The text states that in ancient times a menstruating woman was regarded as unclean and dangerous and that, even today, many couples avoid having intercourse while the woman is menstruating. What are the reasons for these negative values? How do you feel about having sex during menstruation?
5. Do you think that men typically prefer to have intercourse during certain phases of a woman's cycle, rather than other phases?

Suggested Readings

Brecher, R., and Brecher, E. *An Analysis of Human Sexual Response*. New York: New American Library, 1966. A readable and accurate examination of Masters' and Johnson's physiology studies, with additional social and historical perspectives.

Delaney, J., Lupton, M. J., and Toth, E. *The Curse: A Cultural History of Menstruation*. New York: New American Library, 1977. A lively and authoritative account of taboos, myths, rituals, and contemporary research about menstruation and the menstrual cycle.

Hite, S. *The Hite Report*. New York: Dell, 1977. A detailed analysis of women's views of their own sexual responsivity, lacking in scientific precision but useful for women's descriptions of their sexual feelings.

Hite, S. *The Hite Report on Male Sexuality*. New York: Alfred A. Knopf, 1981. The male companion piece to the original *Hite Report;* unscientific but clearly showing the great diversity of male sexual feelings and fears.

Norris, R. V., and Sullivan, C. *PMS: Premenstrual Syndrome*. New York: Rawson Wade, 1983. An opinionated and not too scientific approach, but with some useful pointers.

Sherfey, M. J. *The Nature and Evolution of Female Sexuality*. New York: Random House, 1972. A detailed discussion integrating sexual physiology with female psychology. Heavy reading in parts, but a classic.

Zilbergeld, B. *Male Sexuality: A Guide to Sexual Fulfillment*. Boston: Little, Brown, 1978. An insightful, well-written view of male sexuality, with a nice touch of humor.

4

Human Reproduction

This chapter continues our look at sexuality in a biological perspective by focusing on one special aspect: how life begins. We start our discussion of reproduction by examining the process of conception (the union of egg and sperm) and then explore what happens during pregnancy, childbirth, and the first days of infancy. We conclude with a look at problem pregnancies and difficulties that prevent conception.

THE DYNAMICS OF CONCEPTION

In humans, pregnancy can result only when sperm meets egg. For this to happen, sperm must be deposited in the vagina close to the time of ovulation. In general, sperm retain their capability to penetrate the egg for 24 to 72 hours.

Although it may seem as though pregnancy happens almost instantaneously, fertile couples who are trying to have a baby or who have intercourse regularly without contraception take an average of 5.3 months for pregnancy to occur (Shane, Schiff, and Wilson, 1976). Only 25 percent of women conceive after one month of unprotected intercourse. Sixty-three percent conceive by the end of six months, and by the end of one year, 80 percent become pregnant. Clearly, even when intercourse in fertile couples is timed to be near ovulation, there is an element of luck in whether a pregnancy occurs.

The Union of Sperm and Egg

After ovulation, the egg is gently drawn from the surface of the ovary into the Fallopian tube, where it is propelled toward the uterus by movement of cilia (tiny hairlike outgrowths). If fertilization occurs, it is usually in the upper portion of the Fallopian tube, not in the uterus.

After ejaculation in the vagina, healthy sperm swim rapidly into the female reproductive system in an arduous race that has few survivors. Although 200 million or more sperm are in the vagina, only a few thousand get to the Fallopian tubes and only about 200 actually get near the egg. Most sperm never reach the cervix because they spill out of the vagina or are immobilized by clumping together. Other sperm are damaged along the way, and about half the sperm that swim into the uterus take a wrong turn and enter the eggless Fallopian tube (except in rare circumstances, ovulation occurs on only *one* side each month). The difficult journey is nature's way of making sure that only the healthiest sperm have a chance to fertilize the egg.

Fertilization

Sperm spend several hours in the female reproductive tract undergoing a poorly understood process called **capacitation,** which enables them to penetrate the egg. Some sperm can reach the egg in an hour, but they must still wait to undergo this process. The race to penetrate the egg then is not always won by the swiftest; in fact, usually there are about 40 sperm clustered about the egg at fertilization. After capacitation, sperm secrete a chemical that dissolves the **zona pellucida,** the jellylike coating around the egg.

The egg is not just a passive participant in this process. The egg actually embraces the sperm by extending tiny outgrowths called microvilli up from its surface. Then, to avoid penetration by more than one sperm, the egg first produces a brief electrical block on its surface (lasting only about 30 seconds), followed by a hard outer protein coat. Schatten and Schatten (1983, p. 32) describe it this way: "The successful sperm is held down on the egg membrane in the tight grip of microvilli, while the coat rises above it, pushing all other sperm away. It is rather as if the egg had opened an umbrella, holding the crowd of spermatozoa at a distance." Next, the egg pulls the sperm inside itself and moves its nucleus to meet that of the sperm. Once a sperm cell enters the egg, the zona becomes impenetrable (Figure 4–1).

Fertilization is a complex process that typically lasts for 24 hours or longer, so it is not biologically correct to speak of "the moment of fertilization" (Jones and Schrader, 1989). The process of fertilization begins with the first contact of the sperm with the zona pellucida of the egg and is generally considered to be completed when genetic material from sperm and egg combine.

This marks the start of the **pre-embryo stage,** which lasts until biologic individuation occurs—the establishment beyond any doubt of one and only one biologically unique individual from the developing fertilized egg. The pre-embryo stage lasts for 14 days,

capacitation (kuh pas′ i tā′ shun) the process by which sperm become capable of penetrating an egg.

zona pellucida (zō′ nuh pe lew′ sē duh) the jellylike material surrounding the mature egg.

pre-embryo stage the interval from the completion of fertilization until the appearance of a single primitive streak.

FIGURE 4–1

Human Egg Being Fertilized

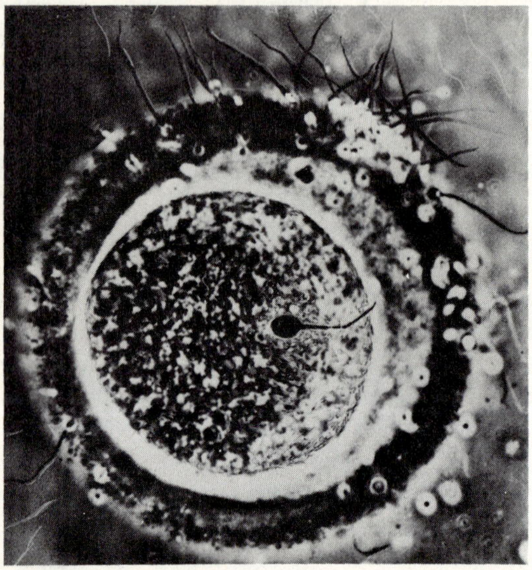

Note that only one sperm has penetrated the egg; the tails of many other sperm are visible at the border of the egg, where they have been blocked.

Source: Dr. Landrum B. Shettles

when the start of the **embryo stage** coincides with the appearance of the **primitive streak** (a thickened linear band that will ultimately develop into various types of tissue, including portions of the spinal cord and part of the heart) (Jones and Schrader, 1989).

Fertilization produces a single cell called the **zygote** (Figure 4–2). This cell contains 23 **chromosomes** (strands of genetic material) contributed by the sperm and 23 chromosomes from the egg. These 46 chromosomes provide programming for inherited characteristics such as blood type, height, skin color, and so forth. Two of the chromosomes, called the sex chromosomes, combine to determine the sex of the developing zygote. All eggs and half of the sperm cells contain an X sex chromosome, while the remaining sperm have Y sex chromosomes only. A zygote with two X chromosomes will become a female, and a zygote with one X and one Y will become a male.[1]

[1] Some exceptions and complications of this process of sex determination are discussed in Chapter 6.

Since eggs always have X chromosomes, the sex of the baby is determined by the contribution of the father, whether it be an X or a Y chromosome.

Despite this biological reality, some men mistakenly believe that the woman is responsible for determining the baby's sex, and in some cultures divorces have occurred when a wife "couldn't" produce a male heir for her husband.

Sex Preselection

The desire to choose the sex of a baby before conception is probably as old as written history. In some cultures, folklore provides advice about various ways of selecting a child's sex: for instance, wearing boots to bed will produce boys, or eating sweet foods improves the chances of having a girl. In an age of greater scientific sophistication, most Americans are unlikely to believe these sorts of notions, yet interest in predetermining the sex of a child is so high that numerous other methods have been advanced with a more "plausible" scientific ring to them but without much more value than the boots or sweets theories.

One popular set of ideas proposed by Shettles and Rorvik (1970) suggested that having intercourse as close as possible to the time of ovulation, increasing the alkalinity of vaginal secretions by douching with a baking soda solution, using deep penetration during intercourse, and having the woman be orgasmic before the male ejaculates all favor conceiving boys. These suggestions—which were each rationalized on detailed scientific grounds—have not yet been supported by any secure research data; in fact, one well-designed study of 3658 births actually found that the proportion of male births was higher when intercourse occurred two days or more after ovulation than when it occurred at or near ovulation (Harlap, 1979). The absence of supporting data after two decades has led several recent reviewers to conclude that Shettles' and Rorvik's methods are not only unproven but should be regarded with skepticism (Carson, 1988; Zarutskie et al., 1989)

A more promising but still unproven method of sex preselection involves separating X and Y sperm in test tubes by passing them through liquid albumin, a protein found in blood that is similar to the thick material of an egg white. The faster-swimming Y sperm migrate to the bottom of the tube in higher numbers than the somewhat slower X sperm, permitting their ultimate recovery and use via artificial insemination to increase the chances of conceiving a male (Glass and

FIGURE 4–2

Early Development After Fertilization

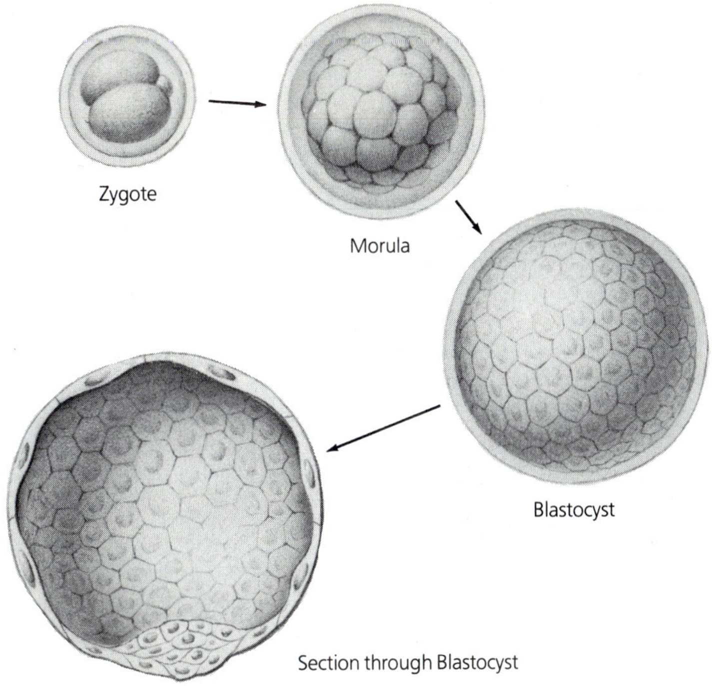

The blastocyst implants in the lining of the uterus.

Ericsson, 1982). However, sperm separation has not yet been shown to work, despite the fact that it is no longer a new technology. The current scientific consensus is that "albumin separation cannot be proved to separate X- from Y-bearing sperm" (Carson, 1988, p. 18).

If a sex preselection method is eventually found to work reliably, experts predict that it will lead to a substantially higher percentage of male births and possibly an overall decline in family size. One recent study of college students in Texas showed that 62 percent wanted their firstborn to be a boy, while only 6 percent wanted a firstborn daughter; furthermore, American couples often continue having children after giving birth to a girl, but stop after having a baby boy, both of which suggest a clear preference for male children in our society (Konner, 1987). In other countries, especially Japan, China, India, and elsewhere in the Orient and Africa, there is even a stronger bias toward having male children, which undoubtedly reflects socioeconomic factors (e.g., males earn more than females, and in some countries families must provide a dowry in order for their daughters to marry) and other cultural differences (Carson, 1988).

Some people are concerned about the ethics of us-

embryo stage (em′ brē ō) the unborn child during the first eight weeks after fertilization.

primitive streak an embryonic structure that appears on about the fourteenth day of development, eventually degenerating and disappearing.

zygote (zī′ gōt) the single cell created by the penetration of an egg by the sperm. An organism produced by the union of two gametes.

chromosomes (krō′ muh sōmz) the genetic material in the nucleus of every cell in the body. Sperm and eggs each have 23 chromosomes; all other cells normally have 46.

ing sex preselection techniques, which have been termed "one of the most stupendously sexist acts in which it is possible to engage" (Powledge, 1981). While many would disagree with this statement—including, for instance, couples who have several sons and would like to have a daughter, as well as couples trying to avoid the transmission of sex-linked genetic disorders—there is little question that past history strongly suggests that this practice might just become another form of discrimination against women.

Transport and Implantation

The single-celled zygote starts to divide about 30 hours after the process of fertilization begins. It splits initially into two cells, then these two cells split into four cells, eight cells, and so on. As this division occurs, the size of each cell becomes progressively smaller. This collection of cells, resembling a mulberry, is called a **morula** (Figure 4–2). During the three or four days after fertilization, the morula travels down the Fallopian tube and enters the cavity of the uterus. The morula now has a hollow inner portion containing fluid and is called a **blastocyst** (Figure 4–2).

The blastocyst undergoes further growth inside the uterus, receiving oxygen and nourishment from secretions of the lining of the uterus (the **endometrium**). After a few days, the blastocyst begins to attach itself to the lining of the uterus in a process called **implantation.** The endometrium of the uterus thickens and becomes richly endowed with blood vessels as a result of hormone secretions in the second half of the menstrual cycle. If fertilization does not occur, this hormonal stimulation ceases abruptly and the thickened tissue is shed during menstruation. However, if fertilization does occur, the thickened, spongy endometrium becomes a "bed" for the blastocyst, which usually attaches to the upper portion of the back wall of the uterus. If implantation occurs outside the uterus (e.g., in the tubes or in the abdomen), an **ectopic** (misplaced) **pregnancy** results.

Implantation is completed about 10 to 12 days after fertilization. There are no physical sensations that accompany implantation, so it is impossible to know just when it has occurred. In some women, implantation is accompanied by bleeding that may be confused with a menstrual period. As a result, women sometimes miscalculate when pregnancy began, leading to a wrong estimation of the expected date of delivery.

PREGNANCY

The average pregnancy lasts for 266 days. As a matter of convenience, the events of pregnancy are usually described in terms of three-month periods or **trimesters.** The first trimester includes the first three months after conception, the second trimester spans the fourth to the sixth month, and the third trimester ranges from the seventh month to delivery. As we have already noted, the first 14 days after fertilization is the pre-embryo stage; by definition, the embryonic stage lasts from this point until the end of eight weeks after fertilization. After that comes the period of fetal development.

First Trimester

EMBRYONIC AND FETAL DEVELOPMENT

Parts of the tiny, spherical blastocyst that implants in the lining of the uterus develop into the **placenta** and the **fetal membranes**. The placenta is the organ through which the embryo and fetus receive nourishment and oxygen from the mother's circulating blood. Waste products from the fetus are also passed through the placenta. The fetal membranes, an inner **amnion** and outer **chorion,** are thin sacs of tissue that enclose the developing fetus. The fetus is suspended in a liquid called **amniotic fluid** that keeps the temperature constant and serves as a shock absorber to protect the fetus against physical injury.

At the time of implantation, the blastocyst/pre-embryo is less than 1 millimeter (0.04 inch) in diameter. By the end of the first trimester, the fetus will be 9 centimeters (3.5 inches) long. This phenomenal rate of growth is accompanied by intricate patterns of organ formation that transform a small, undifferentiated mass of cells into an unmistakably human appearance.

By the end of the first month, the embryo has a primitive heart and digestive system, and the beginnings of the brain, spinal cord, and nervous system have been established. The outlines of eyes can be seen on the large head, but distinct facial features have not appeared. In the fifth week, arm and leg buds become visible, the jaws begin to form, and indentations are seen in the region where the ears will develop. The **umbilical cord,** which contains two arteries and a vein connecting the embryo to the placenta, becomes a distinct structure.

FIGURE 4–3

A Human Embryo Inside the Amniotic Sac Late in the Sixth Week of Development

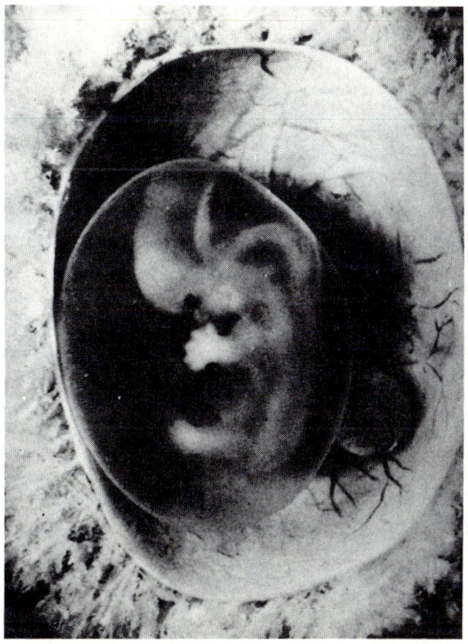

In the sixth and seventh weeks (Figure 4–3), the eyes and ears develop more fully, and teeth and facial muscles begin to form. A distinct neck becomes visible, and bone formation begins as well. Testicular tissue appears in male embryos at this point, but in a female embryo formation of the ovaries has not yet begun. Before this time, male and female embryos are anatomically indistinguishable (see Chapter 6). By eight weeks, the embryo has distinct hands and feet, and all major blood vessels are forming. At this point, the embryo weighs about 1 gram (0.04 ounce) and is 3 centimeters (1.2 inches) in length (Figure 4–4).

In the third month, fetal development proceeds with the appearance of fingernails, toenails, hair follicles, and eyelids. The limbs become more properly proportioned in relation to the rest of the body, and recognizable male and female genital organs are seen. By the end of the twelfth week, all the major organs are differentiated, although they are not all completely formed.

THE MOTHER

Early pregnancy is experienced in different ways by different women. Some have a strong sense of energy, radiance, and well-being even before they know they are pregnant. Others find that the first months of pregnancy are marked by fatigue, loss of appetite, or humdrum emotions.

Being tired is such a typical feature of the first trimester that it is considered a symptom of pregnancy. Another frequent symptom is nausea or vomiting, which usually begins around the end of the first month. This "morning sickness" can occur at any time of day and usually disappears spontaneously a month or two after it begins. Frequent urination, irregular bowel movements, breast swelling and tenderness, and an increased amount of vaginal secretion are among the other physical changes that may be noticed by the pregnant woman in the first trimester. However, the woman cannot feel the changes going on inside her uterus during this time.

Missing a period is not a sure sign of pregnancy (periods can be skipped because of stress or illness, among other reasons), but it raises a question in most

morula (more′ u lah) a spherical mass of cells resulting from cleavage of the fertilized egg.

blastocyst (blas′ tō sist) a spherical mass of cells with a hollow inner portion containing fluid produced by the cleavage of the fertilized egg.

endometrium (en′ dō mē′ trē um) the inner lining of the uterus in which the egg implants and which is partially shed during menstruation.

implantation the attachment of the blastocyst to the lining of the uterus.

ectopic pregnancy (ek top′ ik) a misplaced pregnancy. The implantation of the blastocyst occurs outside the uterus, for example in the tubes or abdomen.

trimester a three-month period; generally used to describe the progression of pregnancy in three such periods.

placenta (pluh sen′ tuh) the organ attached to the wall of the uterus that performs the functions of nutrition, respiration, and excretion for the unborn child. It is also an endocrine organ secreting large amounts of several hormones.

fetal membranes two thin sacs of tissue, the inner amnion and the outer chorion, that enclose the developing baby.

amnion (am′ nē on) the inner of the thin sacs of tissue (fetal membranes) that enclose the developing fetus.

chorion (kor ee on′) the outer sac of tissue that encloses the developing fetus inside the uterus.

amniotic fluid (am′ nē ot′ ik) the liquid in which the developing fetus is suspended. It keeps the temperature constant and cushions shock.

umbilical cord the cylindrical structure connecting the fetus to the placenta. It contains two arteries and a vein.

women's minds. To find the answer, a woman can purchase a kit for a self-administered home pregnancy test and then have the results confirmed by a physician, at a medical laboratory, or at a clinic.

In the past, biological tests using laboratory animals such as frogs, rabbits, or mice were employed to check for pregnancy, but these were cumbersome, time-consuming, expensive, and relatively inaccurate. Now there are many immunological tests that allow a diagnosis to be made in as short a time as 2 minutes. They work by detecting the presence of HCG (human chorionic gonadotropin), a hormone secreted by the placenta. A drop of urine is placed on a glass slide (or in a tube) and is mixed with several chemicals. If HCG is present, the mixture does not coagulate and the test is said to be positive, indicating pregnancy. These tests offer 99 percent accuracy as early as one week after conception when performed properly.

At-home pregnancy tests that do not require a prescription and are simple to perform are also available. Based on a technology using monoclonal antibodies—made-to-order proteins that latch onto HCG in urine in very small amounts—these tests give results within 5 to 10 minutes with a high degree of accuracy. The First Response Pregnancy Test Kit, which can be used as early as the first day after a missed period, gives its results—a simple color change from clear to pink—in only 5 minutes. Other monoclonal antibody pregnancy test kits currently being sold are called Advance, Daisy 2, Fact Plus, Q Test, and Answer Plus. Each kit typically costs $10 to $15. Recent research shows that home pregnancy tests, when performed and interpreted by laypersons, are almost 10 percent less accurate than testing done by qualified laboratory personnel (Hicks and Iosefsohn, 1989), so it is important for a woman to have a home test result confirmed before concluding whether or not she is pregnant.

FIGURE 4–4

A Human Fetus Early in the Ninth Week of Development

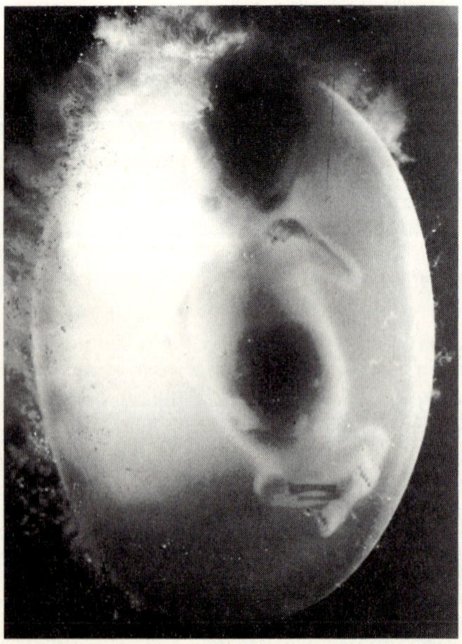

A negative pregnancy test, no matter what method is used, is *not* foolproof, and a repeat test done a week or two later may be in order. Women need to have an early knowledge of their pregnancy to begin proper health care (such as good nutrition and avoidance of cigarettes, alcohol, and drugs of all kinds—prescription, nonprescription, and illegal). Early diagnosis is also important so that those who want to terminate pregnancy can have an abortion in the first trimester, when this procedure is safest and simplest.

Pregnancy can also be detected in other ways. During a pelvic examination, a physician can note (1) a softening of the cervix, (2) a bluish color of the vagina and cervix, (3) a softening of the uterus just above the cervix, or (4) an irregular increase in the size of the uterus. These signs of pregnancy may be present at about the sixth week but are quite variable. The most conclusive physical signs of pregnancy—finding a fetal heartbeat, feeling the fetus move, and identifying the fetus by sound-wave tests—usually cannot be done before the second trimester.

One interesting fact to keep in mind is that many pregnancies end naturally before they reach the point where they are detected clinically. In one recent study which used highly sensitive testing for HCG, 22 percent of all pregnancies detected just after implantation (before the first missed period was noticed by the woman) failed to survive to the point at which they would be recognized clinically (Wilcox et al., 1988). (Overall, the total rate of pregnancy loss was 31 percent.) While the causes of early pregnancy loss are not well understood at present, some experts believe that it may be nature's way of eliminating pre-embryos that are defective in one way or another.

Once a woman knows that she is pregnant, she may be happy, proud, ambivalent, fearful, angry, depressed, or any combination thereof. Her reaction reflects many things—her age, marital status, economic resources, career objectives, personal values, and expectations of parenthood. Most of all, her reaction will depend on whether or not she wanted to be pregnant and how she feels about herself.

Negative feelings about a pregnancy, even when it is planned, are similar to the second thoughts we all have after taking a major step in our lives. Did I choose the right college? Is this really the person I wanted to marry? Why did I buy this car when that other one looks so good? Our initial uncertainties and hesitations do not necessarily predict how we will feel later on. The psychological impact of bringing a child into the world is immense and requires time for thought and acceptance.

At the same time, many women (especially those who have not yet had children) experience particularly vivid dreams about their pregnancy that are sometimes distressing to them. These dreams typically are full of anxiety: the baby has been born with a birth defect, for instance, or the baby was born but somehow was kidnapped from the nursery. Since dreaming seems to be a way in which the mind can deal with concerns that it doesn't want to think about consciously, such disturbing dreams are entirely normal (Todd and Tapley, 1988).

THE FATHER

While often neglected as a participant in the experience of pregnancy, men also have important feelings about this event. The man's initial reaction on learning of his partner's pregnancy may be elation, joy, surprise, uncertainty, or concern. Until he has time to adjust to the idea of pregnancy as a reality, he is likely to be somewhat ambivalent toward his partner. He may be anxious about her well-being and the developing baby's health until he can see his partner's bulging abdomen or feel the baby's movement (Grossman, Eichler, and Winickoff, 1980). His anxieties may also relate to the additional responsibilities (financial and emotional) that the pregnancy presents. Some men even have morning sickness along with their pregnant partners, perhaps a sign of their anxiety and wish to share in the pregnancy experience. In fact, one study recently found that 23 percent of a group of American expectant fathers had a condition called the **couvade syndrome,** in which husbands experience physical symptoms that are related to their wives' pregnancies and are not explained by other medical factors (Lipkin and Lamb, 1982).

Many men are uncertain about the effects of sex

couvade syndrome (koo vahd′) a condition in which a male experiences symptoms mimicking pregnancy and/or childbirth.

FOCUS IN BRIEF

Dealing with Morning Sickness

Many women can find relief from morning sickness by trying these tips:

- Eat five or six small meals throughout the day, rather than two or three large ones.
- Keep your protein consumption low and stress carbohydrates instead.
- Avoid fried foods and fatty dishes.
- Drink plenty of fluids to help neutralize stomach acids and to prevent dehydration from vomiting.
- Sucking on hard candy—lollipops, lemon drops, and so on—may help control feelings of nausea.
- Chewing on small pieces of ice or licking ice-pops (including the kind you can make yourself from natural fruit juices) is a good way to minimize problems for many women.
- Eat a snack at bedtime to help alleviate morning nausea the next day.

Source: Modified from Todd and Tapley, 1988, Table 7.1. Reprinted from THE COLUMBIA UNIVERSITY COLLEGE OF PHYSICIANS AND SURGEONS COMPLETE GUIDE TO PREGNANCY by permission of Crown Publishers, Inc.

during pregnancy (see p. 89) and believe that the woman must refrain from exercise or vigorous work so the baby will not be injured. Other men do not understand why a pregnant woman seems so sleepy and may become upset, especially if they imagine that this tiredness will progress relentlessly through the months ahead. Both partners are likely to react to pregnancy in a more relaxed fashion if they have already had a child and have some idea of what to expect.

In the early months of pregnancy, many couples draw closer together, both emotionally and physically. Pregnancy can be a very concrete manifestation of commitment and sharing, and a first pregnancy in particular provides good reason to plan and dream about the future.

Second Trimester

FETAL DEVELOPMENT

In the fourth month, the fetus develops lips, fingerprints, and hair on its head. Sucking motions begin, and the fetus swallows small amounts of amniotic fluid. The fetus moves and turns very actively within the amniotic sac (Figure 4–5). During the fifth month, the fetal heartbeat can be heard and the body becomes covered with tiny, downy hair. The fetus also responds to sound and spends part of its time being quite active and some being still. In the sixth month, the fetus opens its eyes and has long hair on its head. By the end of the second trimester, the fetus is 30 centimeters (12 inches) long and weighs 600 to 700 grams (1.3 to 1.5 pounds). If born at this time, the fetus has poor chances for survival.

FIGURE 4–5

A Sixteen-week Fetus

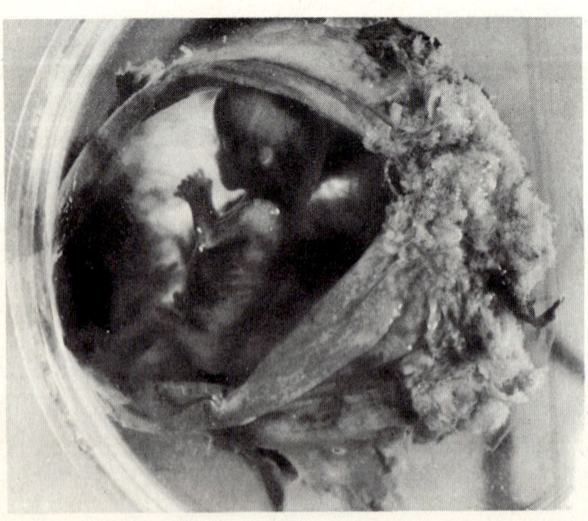

At this stage of development, although most major organs have formed, the fetus is unable to survive if born prematurely because its lungs are immature.

THE MOTHER

The second trimester is a time of many physical changes for the pregnant woman. Her waist begins to bulge, her abdomen protrudes, her bustline expands, and her regular clothes no longer fit very well. She may be troubled by these changes in her figure, or she may be happy with her body and anxious to let the whole world know that she is pregnant.

Late in the fourth month (between the sixteenth and eighteenth weeks), the woman can usually feel the fetus moving (**quickening**). This is often an exciting event and a moment of relief because the developing fetus "signals" that it is doing well. As the kicks and twists become more vigorous in the following weeks, the novelty and wonder may wear off and the sensations may become annoying. The mother may alternate between feeling love and tenderness and feeling resentment at being controlled by the fetus.

In the second trimester, the uterus grows considerably larger and pushes up inside the abdomen. This commonly leads to indigestion and constipation. The skin over the abdomen becomes stretched, and pink or reddish stretch marks may appear on its surface. The breasts increase prominently in size, the nipples become larger and more deeply pigmented, the areolae become broader, and **colostrum,** a thin yellowish fluid which is a precursor of milk, may drip out of the nipples. These changes are a result of the hormones produced by the placenta and prepare the breasts for later milk production.

Other physical changes may lead to minor problems. Varicose veins in the legs and hemorrhoids can start to form or be worsened because of the pressure of the growing uterus. Nose bleeds may occur because of a larger blood volume. Fluid retention can cause **edema,** swelling of the hands, wrists, ankles, or feet. On the other hand, the morning sickness of the first trimester usually disappears and the woman's appetite is apt to become hearty.

Psychologically, the second trimester is often a time of relative tranquility and confidence. Most women

Human Conception and Development

1 Photomicrograph showing a section of a human ovary with an egg (large pink circle) about to be released.

2 Scanning electron micrograph (SEM) of a human sperm.

3 SEM of many sperm attempting to penetrate an egg. Note the relative size of sperm and egg.

4 Close-up of sperm and egg. The sperm in the middle of the picture has penetrated the egg.

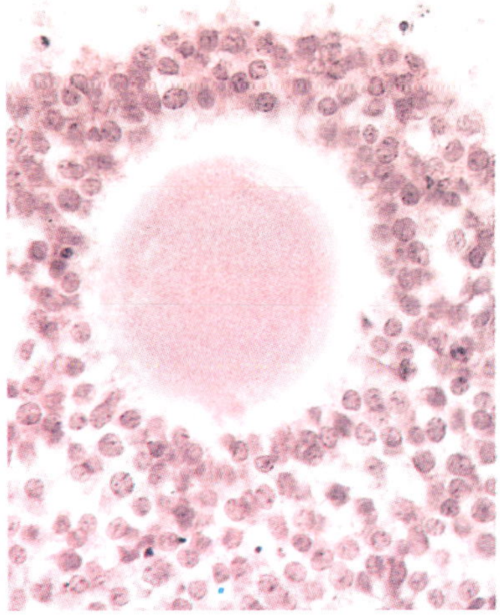

1

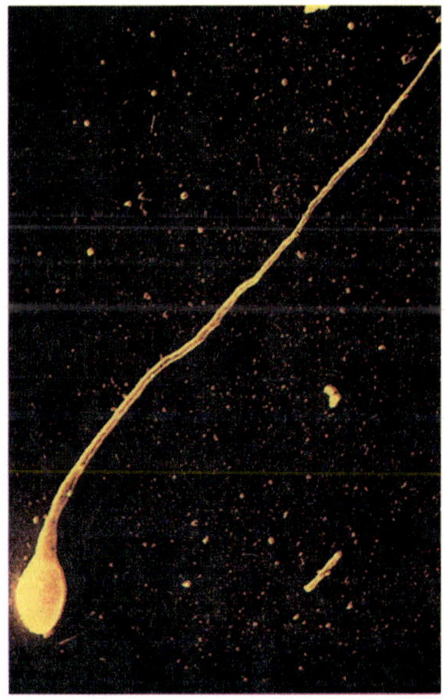

2

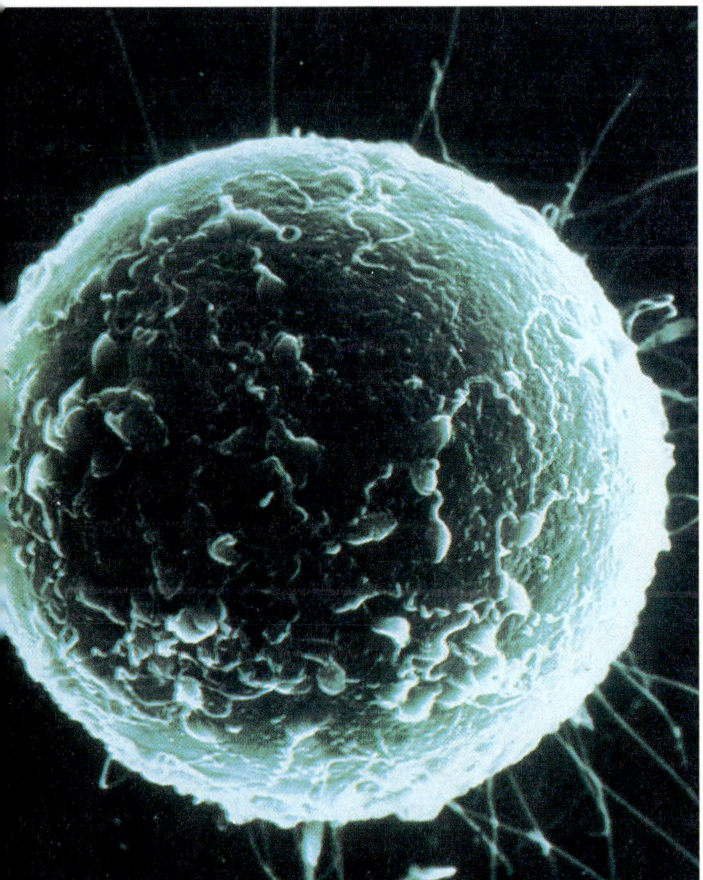

3

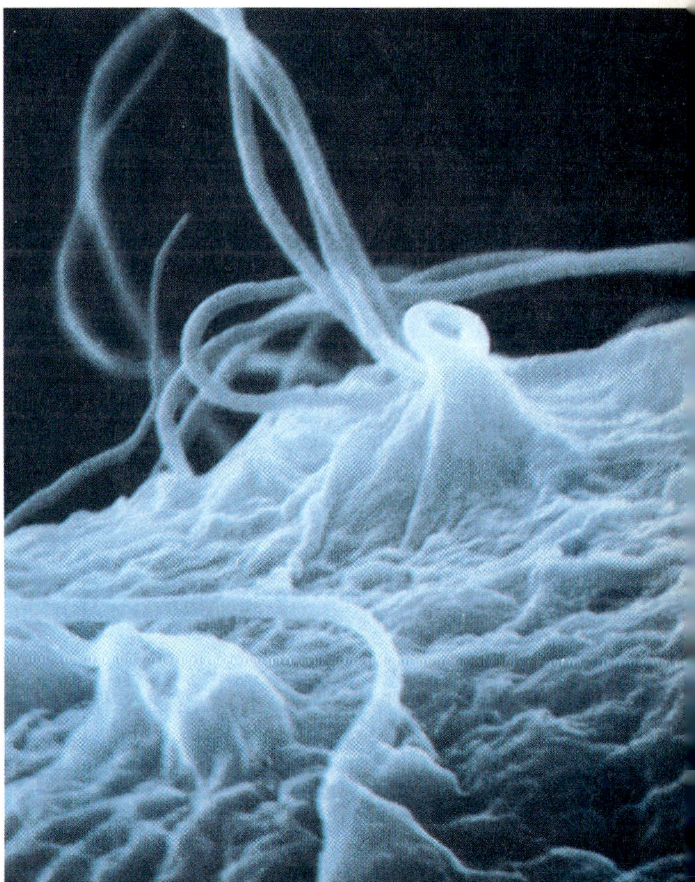

4

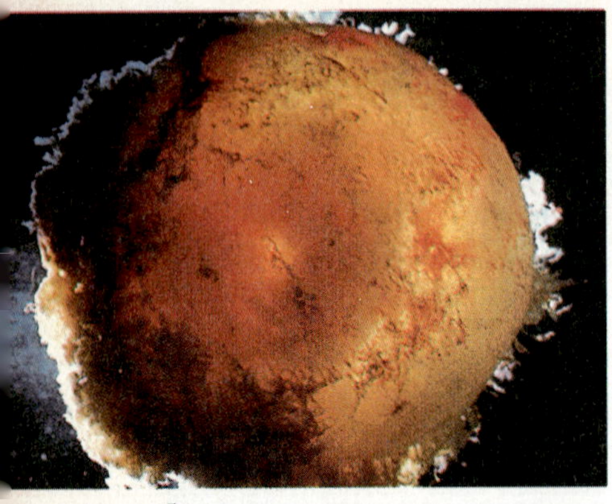

5

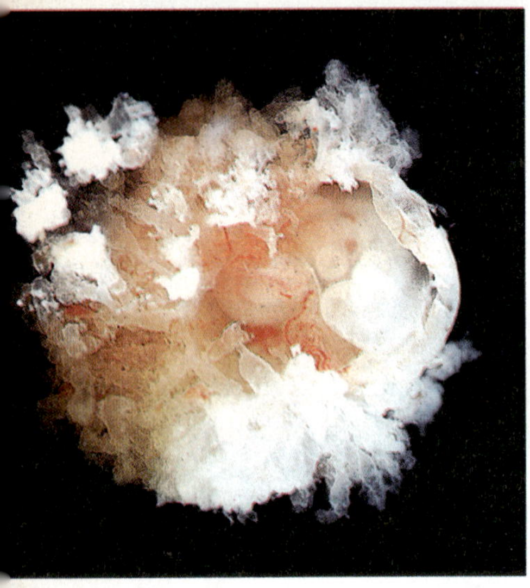

6

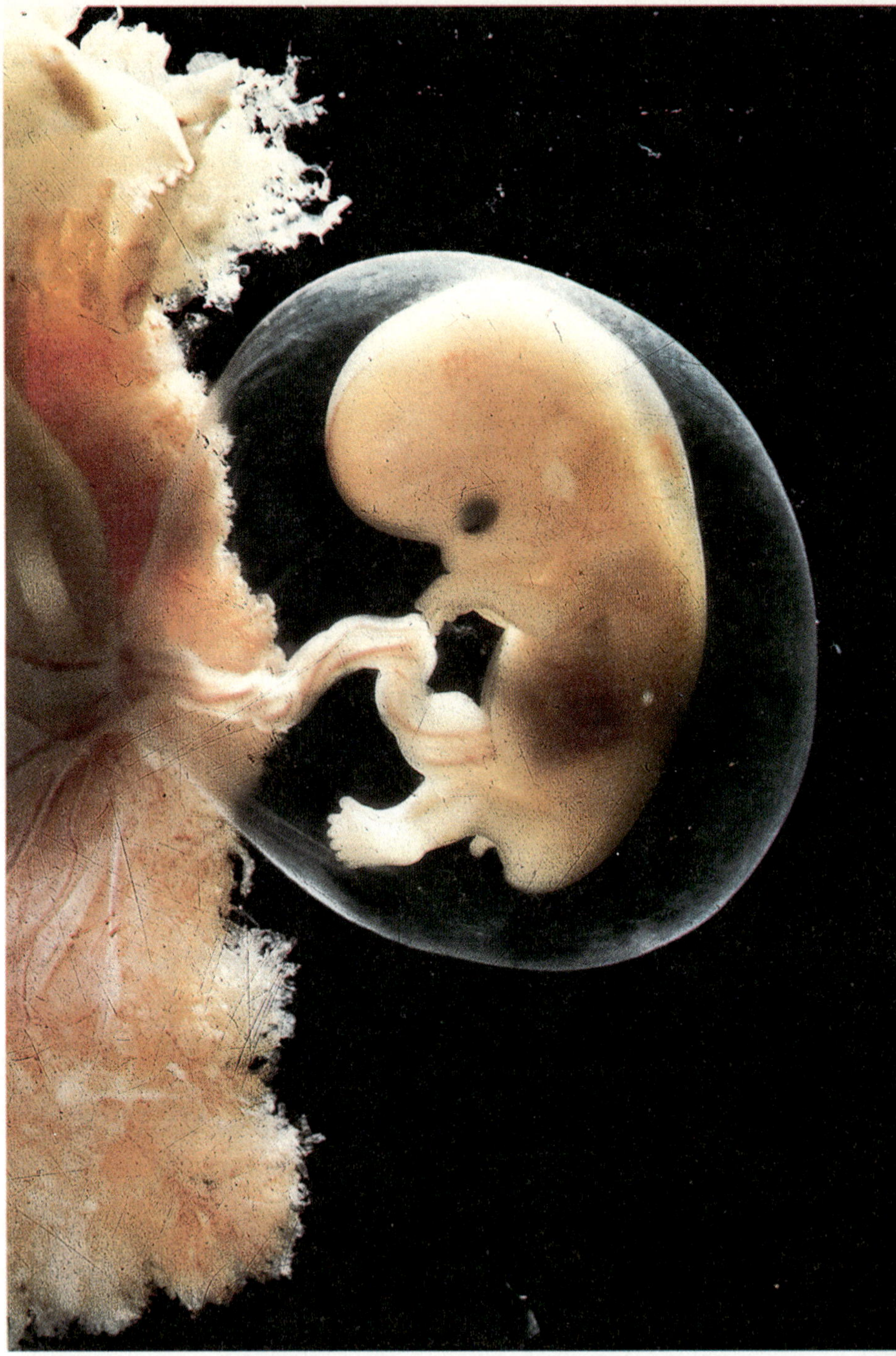

7

5 Fertilized human egg (embryo) at 4 weeks.

6 Human embryo at 4–5 weeks.

7 Human fetus at 9 weeks. The fetus (right) is connected to the placenta (left) by the umbilical cord. It is enveloped in the fetal membranes and suspended in the amniotic fluid.

8 Close-up of feet of human fetus at 8 weeks.

9 Human fetus (16 weeks) showing legs and feet.

10 Human fetus (20 weeks) showing close-up of feet.

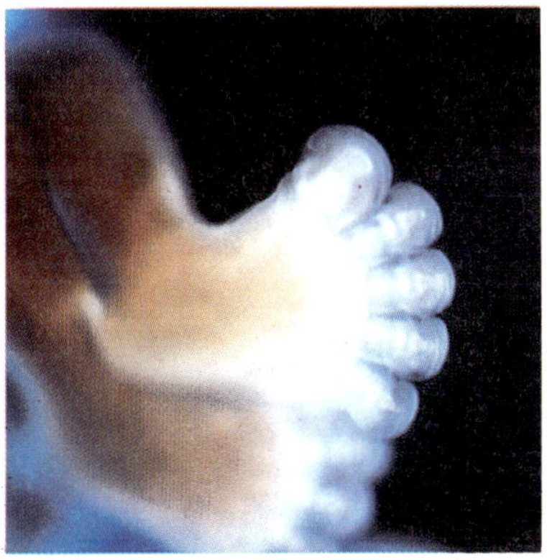

8

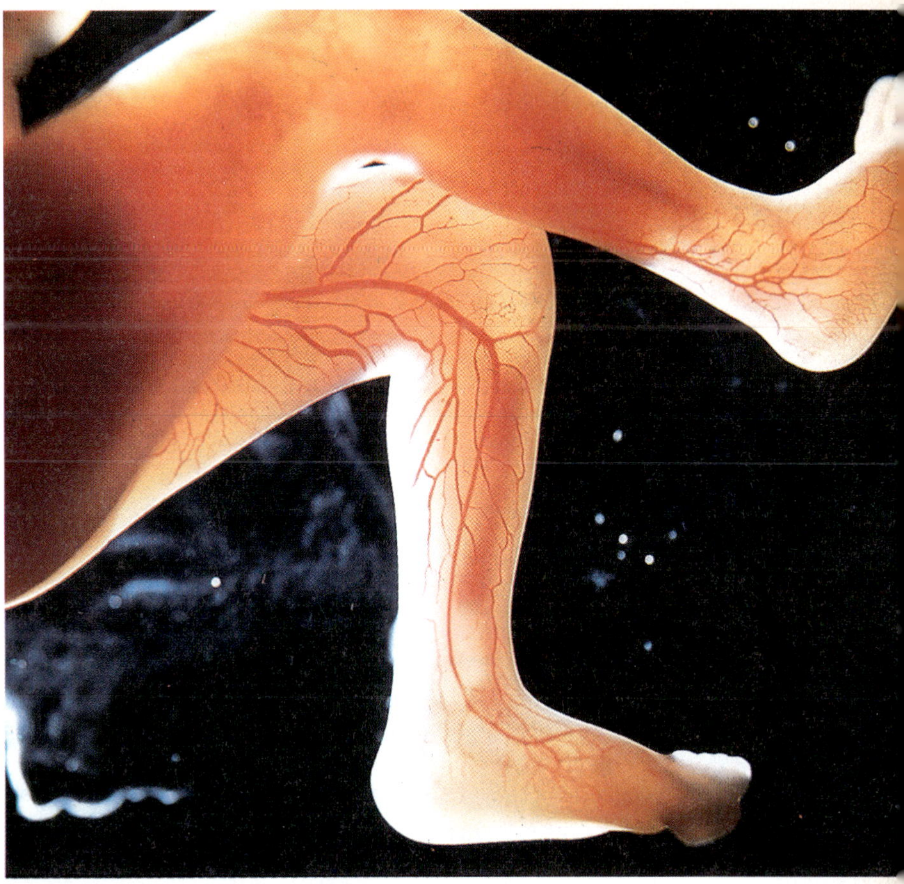

9

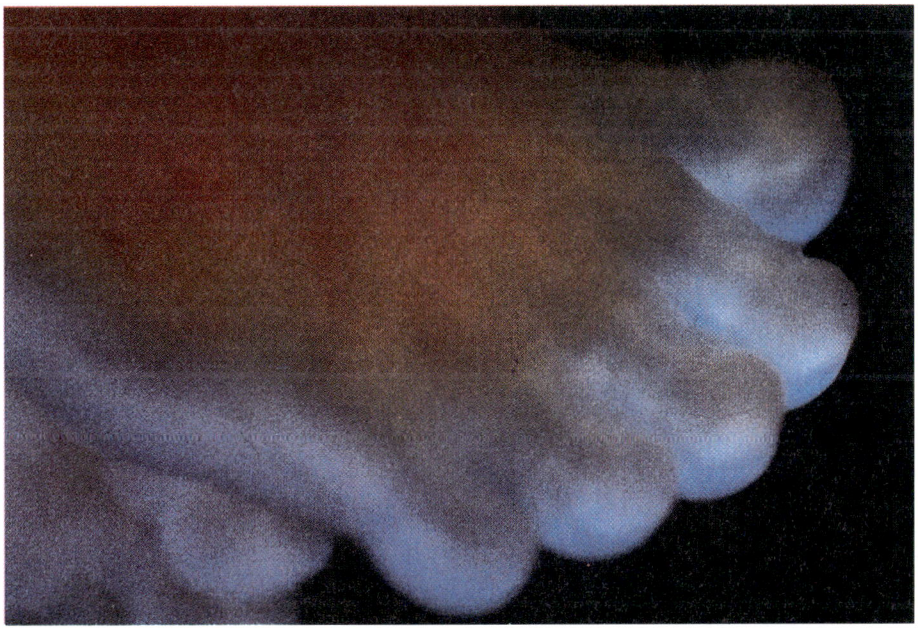

10

11 Fourteen-week human fetus in amniotic sac attached by umbilical cord to placenta.
12 Five-month-old female fetus.
13 Close-up of head of human fetus at five and a half months. Note the blood vessels in the scalp.

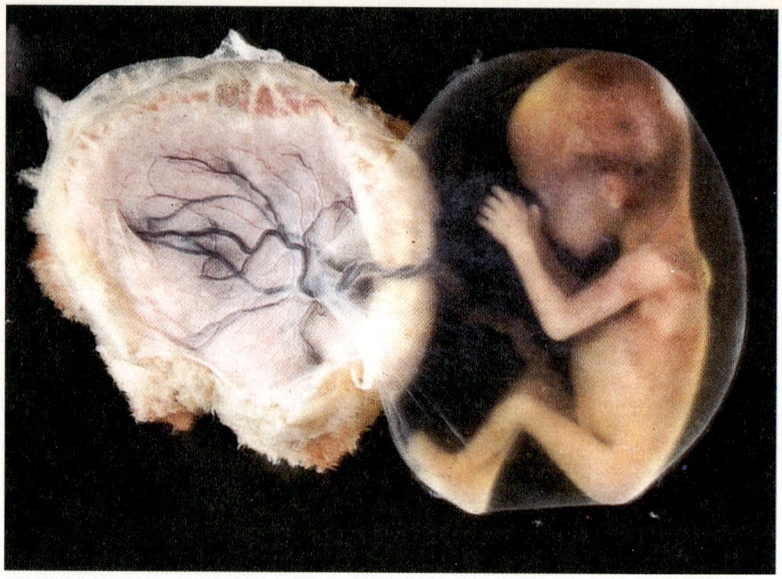

11

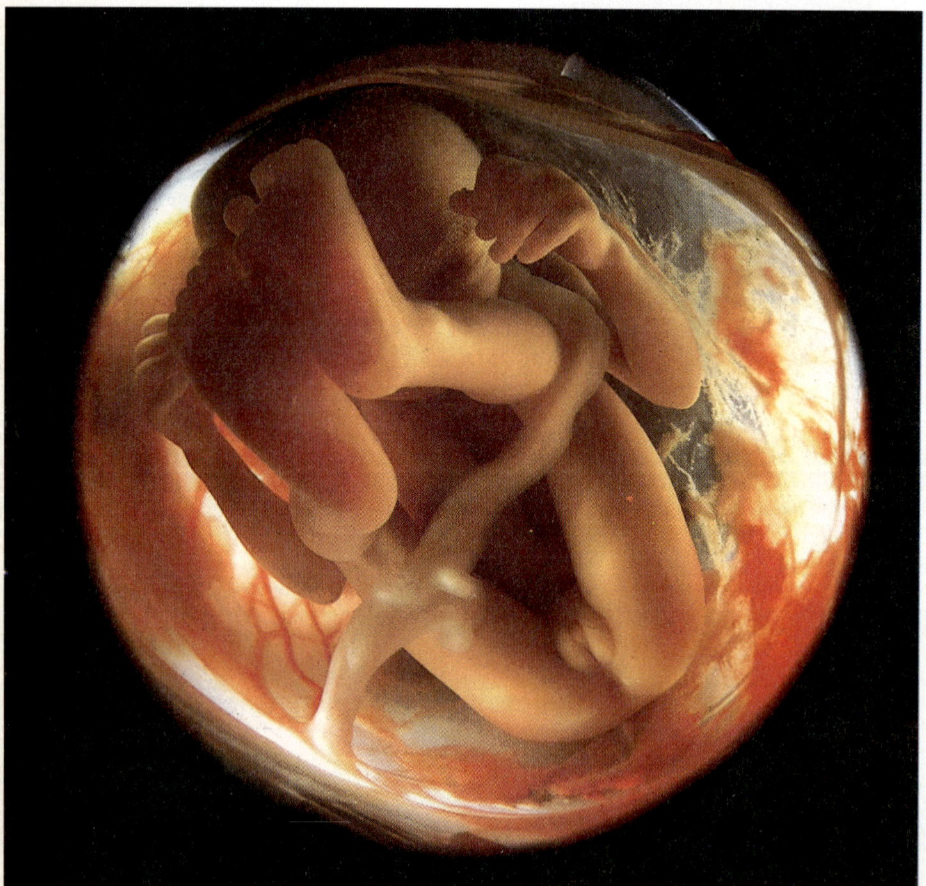

12

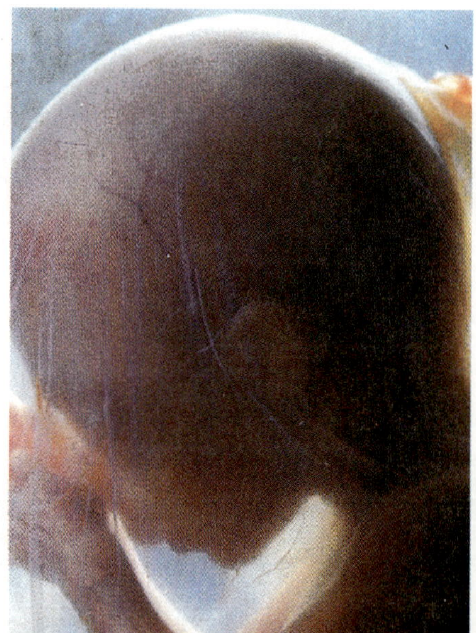

13

have adjusted to being pregnant and feel more energetic than they did in the first few months. Heightened sensuality at this time is often a pleasant bonus; it is not unusual for some women to first experience orgasm in the middle months of pregnancy (Masters and Johnson, 1966).

THE FATHER

With birth still far away, the father is likely to be drawn more closely into the experience of pregnancy in the second trimester. He is able to see obvious changes in his partner's body, but these changes occur gradually and give him time to adjust. Feeling the fetus kick or turn is likely to give him a greater sense of identification. His partner's renewed energy is also reassuring and gives the couple more time together—a pleasant interlude that will be gone all too soon when a newborn infant arrives. His earlier anxieties about the fragility of the developing fetus in the first trimester have been generally put to rest.

One of the more sensible developments of recent years has been a trend for fathers to become more involved in their partners' pregnancies in a variety of ways. For example, the father might attend prenatal checkups to get to know the nurse-midwife or physician before the actual delivery and to ask questions that might otherwise go unanswered. As a bonus, if ultrasound testing is done during such a checkup, the father gets to see an image of the developing fetus on the ultrasound monitor, which is often an exciting experience. Men can also be more active participants in the pregnancy if they read some of the books or articles their partner reads, so they can discuss them together, and if they prepare themselves by talking with other men about their experiences during childbirth.

In some instances, it may be possible for men to arrange for paternity leave so they can be at home with the mother and newborn baby once the big day comes. As a practical matter, if this seems like a desirable possibility, we suggest that the father-to-be begin inquiries about paternity leave at work during the second trimester, if he hasn't done so earlier. Even if your employer says that there is no official company policy on paternity leave, if you're persistent you may be able to make an arrangement that will work for you or you might actually get a new policy started—with you as the first beneficiary! If this attempt fails, you may be able to arrange for a paid vacation for a week or two after the baby's arrival, which can create a perfect opportunity for sharing in the baby's care from the earliest possible time.

EARLY PREGNANCY CLASSES

One of the newer developments to gain popularity in the last five years is the availability of early pregnancy classes that are typically held during the first three to six months of pregnancy. These classes are different from childbirth classes, which are usually offered later in pregnancy to help a couple prepare for labor and delivery. Early pregnancy classes focus, instead, on the couple's emotional adjustment to pregnancy, provide education about the physical changes affecting the mother, and help the couple prepare for the change from couple to family. Typically, these courses meet at a YMCA or community center and involve a group leader and four to eight pregnant couples meeting for three or four weekly sessions.

One of the main benefits of such a class is that the group setting helps couples talk about their feelings. Here is what one expectant father said about a course he attended:

> I wasn't too interested in going to this class at first, thinking it was just going to be a bunch of lectures. But it turned out, instead, to be more of a discussion group . . . and that gave me a chance to hear what a few other men who were in my same position were feeling. It was good to find out that many of the concerns I had were not that uncommon, and it was also useful to hear how other couples were dealing with these issues. The end result was that the classes brought me closer together with my wife. *(Authors' files)*

You can usually find out where and when early pregnancy classes are offered from a midwife, an obstetrician, a childbirth center, or your local hospital. If none exists in your community, you might consider recruiting a group leader to start one.

Third Trimester

FETAL DEVELOPMENT

During the seventh month, the brain and nervous system complete the major steps of their development,

quickening the time during pregnancy when a woman can first feel the fetus moving.

colostrum (kohl ah′ strum) a thin, watery fluid secreted by the breasts late in pregnancy as a precursor to breast milk.

edema (e dē′ muh) swelling due to fluid retention.

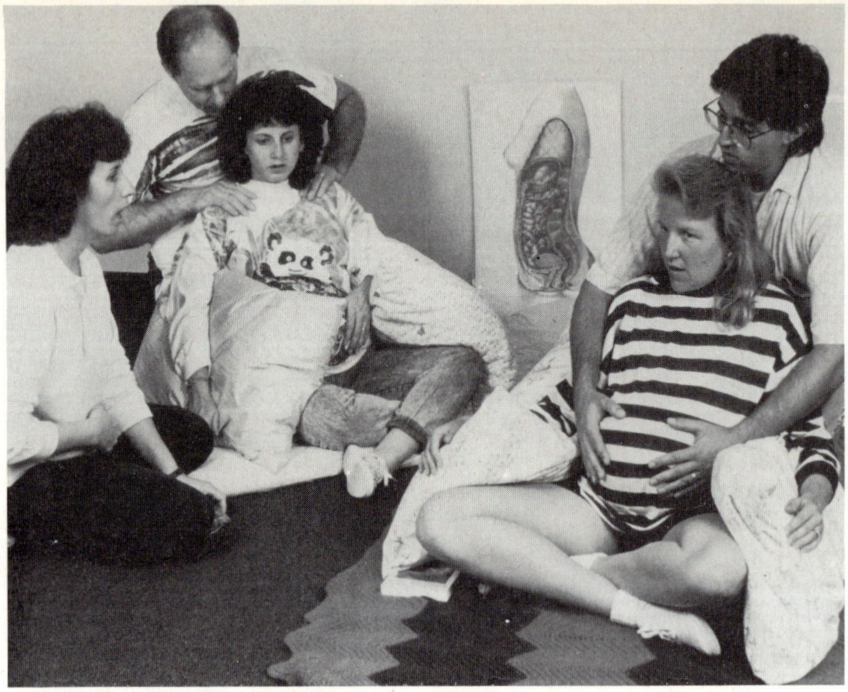

Both early pregnancy classes and later childbirth preparation classes, such as the Lamaze class shown here, help couples talk about their feelings and familiarize themselves with what's ahead.

fatty tissue grows under the skin, and the downlike hair on the fetus disappears in most places. A baby born prematurely at the beginning of the seventh month has a 20 percent chance of survival, but by the eighth month this increases to 85 percent (Pernoll and Benson, 1987). In the eighth month, the baby's skin has lost its wrinkled appearance and is pink in color. If it has not done so earlier, the baby is likely to assume a head-down position in the uterus. In the ninth month, the fetus usually is less active than it has been, partly because of its size and cramped quarters. Its eyes are blue, because other eye colors develop only after a period of exposure to light. The fetus has acquired antibodies from its mother that will help protect it against infection during early infancy. The average full-term baby is 50 centimeters (20 inches) long and weighs 3100 to 3400 grams (6.8 to 7.5 pounds).

THE MOTHER

The increasing size and firmness of the uterus are quite obvious. When the woman stands, it pushes forward, altering her center of gravity. To balance this, she may walk with her head and shoulders thrust backward and chest protruding, a position that can result in backache, a common occurrence in the last months of pregnancy. The enlarged uterus also puts pressure on the blood vessels in the lower part of the body, which may partly explain the common discomfort of leg cramps. Other problems caused by pressure changes include a frequent need to urinate because of pressure against the bladder and shortness of breath since the diaphragm is pushed upward against the lungs.

Many women have difficulty controlling their weight gain during pregnancy, especially during the third trimester. Physicians generally suggest that weight gain be limited to about 25 pounds because larger increases in weight increase the odds of medical problems. On the other hand, too little weight gained is potentially harmful to the fetus, since a gain of almost 20 pounds can be expected from normal physiological changes. This gain includes the weight of the baby (7½ pounds), placenta and membranes (1½ pounds), and amniotic fluid (2 pounds) as well as increases in the weight of the uterus (2½ pounds), blood (3½ pounds), and breasts (1 pound). Normal fluid retention is likely to account for another 2 or 3 pounds of weight gain.

In the last months of pregnancy, the uterus has more frequent **Braxton–Hicks contractions,** painless short episodes of muscle tightening that are not a sign of labor. In women who have not had a baby before, the head of the fetus lowers into the pelvis in the last few weeks of pregnancy. When the largest diameter of the head has settled firmly into position against the pelvic bones, it is engaged. **Engagement** (also called "dropping" or "lightening") usually occurs during labor in women who have had children.

The end of the last trimester is apt to be a time of physical discomfort and awkwardness. Each day may seem longer than the last. Sleeping is frequently interrupted by trying to find a comfortable position, by fetal movements, and by trips to the bathroom. Energy levels are low, irritability high. The first-time mother, especially, is likely to have anxieties about pain or problems with labor and delivery and may worry considerably about her baby not being normal. Her self-esteem may be on the wane as she seems, for now, to be at the mercy of the requirements of a body that does not seem really hers.

THE FATHER

The last trimester is not without its tribulations for the male. His partner's changing shape and physical discomforts may lead to a loss of his sexual desire for her, or his continued interest may not be matched by hers. Masters and Johnson (1966) found that for these reasons the last trimester is a time some men seek extramarital sex. Men may also feel aloof for other reasons. For example, the pregnant woman may become quite close to her own mother during pregnancy, with more discussions and time spent together as delivery nears. His partner's relation to her physician may also be a source of feeling "left out." Social events, recreation, and other details of everyday living are typically altered now, and the man may be understandably anxious for things to return to "normal."

At the same time, most men feel a strong sense of loyalty, closeness, and gratitude toward their very pregnant partner. They are usually glad not to be pregnant themselves, are concerned with making their partner comfortable, and, if a home delivery has not been chosen, are more than a little nervous about driving to the hospital once labor is under way. If this is their first child, and they have been asked to be present at the delivery, they may be somewhat queasy and unsure of "how they will do."

Prenatal Care and Planning

Most pregnancies progress smoothly for the mother and unborn child, but problems can also occur. **Prenatal** (prebirth) **care** not only increases the mother's chances of staying healthy but also protects the well-being of her developing fetus. Although most people think of prenatal care as something done by a doctor or nurse-midwife, it is a joint venture in which the mother and her physician or nurse collaborate. The mother's responsibilities are really more important than the health care provider's, since she lives with the pregnancy day in and day out. Prenatal care is mainly a means for preventing problems; secondarily, it is a way to detect complications as early as possible in order to minimize their impact.

NUTRITION

Good nutrition during pregnancy is an essential part of prenatal care. The mother requires more calories and extra nutrients such as vitamins and minerals to meet the needs of her body and her developing baby. Poor maternal nutrition can lead to slower fetal growth, premature delivery, and low-birth-weight babies. Prematurity and low birth weight both cause higher infant death rates, and malnourished babies with low birth weights may have brain damage and retardation.

Obviously, the woman's nutritional state before pregnancy is an important consideration. If previous dietary habits were poor, special steps must be taken to provide extra amounts of needed nutrients. Even when this is not a problem, pregnant women need about 300 extra calories and extra amounts of protein, calcium, iron, and vitamins A, B, C, and D compared to their ordinary daily intake. Protein (found in meat, fish, eggs, and dairy products) is important for the growth of the placenta, uterus, and the blood supply in the pregnant woman's body. Calcium (obtained mainly from dairy products and vegetables) is necessary for growth of the fetal skeleton and tooth buds; too little calcium can also cause muscle cramps for the mother. Iron (found in red meats, dried fruits, eggs, and enriched cereals) is needed for the manufacture of red blood cells to prevent maternal anemia; folic acid (found in leafy green vegetables) also helps pre-

Braxton–Hicks contractions painless short episodes of muscle tightening sometimes mistaken for the onset of labor.

engagement the settling of the fetal head into position against the pelvic bones for birth. It usually occurs during the last few weeks of pregnancy in women having their first child and during labor with subsequent pregnancies. Also called dropping or lightening.

prenatal care the combined efforts of doctor, nurse, and mother to see that the pregnant woman stays healthy and the unborn child has everything needed to grow and develop.

vent anemia. Necessary vitamins are usually provided by a balanced diet that includes milk, bread, fresh fruits, and vegetables.

DRUGS

Almost every drug used by a pregnant woman will cross the placenta and enter the circulation of the developing embryo or fetus. Because it is not always clear which drugs will have damaging effects, it is vital that drug use be restricted to situations of medical necessity, even for drugs that seem safe for the mother. Drugs that produce malformations in the embryo or fetus are called **teratogens.** The kind of effect a toxic drug produces depends partly on when it is used. Certain drugs act selectively on the formation of a particular organ in the embryo or fetus and do not cause damage after its formation is complete. For this reason, drug use in the first half of pregnancy is particularly likely to damage the fetus, since this is when organ formation occurs. The effects also depend on the duration and amount of drug use—taking a single pill is unlikely to be harmful, while repeated use may be a problem.

Medications

A wide variety of medicines can affect the fetus, including some that might surprise you. For instance, aspirin can cause fetal bleeding and, if used with large amounts of caffeine and phenacetin (in pills called APCs which are used to treat headache or pain), can lead to low birth weight, prolonged pregnancy, anemia, and lower infant survival rates after birth (Collins and Turner, 1975). Tranquilizers have also been reported to cause a variety of fetal malformations, including cleft palate (Valium) and heart defects (Librium and Equanil). Thalidomide, a tranquilizer widely used in Europe in the early 1960s (but no longer in use), resulted in severe malformations of the arms and legs of the fetus when taken during early pregnancy. Anticonvulsants, drugs used to control epilepsy, also can cause birth defects if they are used during pregnancy (see Chapter 10).

Hormones are also frequently teratogenic. Birth control pills used during pregnancy have been found to cause heart defects (Nora and Nora, 1973; Heinonen et al., 1977) and abnormalities of the limbs, spinal column, windpipe (trachea), and kidneys (Janerich, Piper, and Glebatis, 1974). Progesterone or testosterone can cause masculinizing changes in a female fetus and progestins or estrogens can cause improper formation of the penis in a male fetus. A form of estrogen called diethylstilbestrol (DES), which many mothers took to prevent miscarriage, may cause cancer of the vagina in girls whose mothers used this drug during pregnancy (see Chapter 10).

A drug used to treat severe acne, isoretinoin (trade name Accutane), is especially dangerous during pregnancy because it is likely to cause spontaneous abortions or major birth defects affecting the skull and face, the heart, the thymus, and the brain (Lammer et al., 1985). Medications that can damage the fetus are listed in Table 4–1.

Drug Abuse

Pregnant women who use drugs like cocaine, heroin, barbiturates, and amphetamines expose the fetus to a large number of problems. Low birth weight and prematurity are characteristic of such pregnancies. The fetus also may become addicted, in which case its first days as a newborn are likely to be a painful time of withdrawal symptoms. Convulsions and depressed breathing are commonly seen just after birth in infants born to addicted mothers. In addition, the mother's health may be compromised by poor nutrition, infections (particularly hepatitis B), and other medical difficulties caused by drug addiction or abuse. It is estimated that as many as 375,000 infants may be affected each year by maternal drug abuse during pregnancy (Silverman, 1989). In fact, one recent study found that 15 percent of pregnant women tested positive for substance abuse during pregnancy (Chasnoff, Landress, and Barrett, 1990). In many cases, the woman doesn't realize that her drug use poses a danger to her developing fetus.

Recent research shows that cocaine use in pregnancy, which had previously not been studied, has a number of major effects (Chasnoff et al., 1989; Zuckerman et al., 1989). Not only are the risks of miscarriage, premature birth, and stillbirth increased, maternal cocaine use impairs growth of the fetus. In addition to being small for their age, cocaine babies, as they are called in many hospitals, tend to have smaller heads than other babies; they also have a higher rate of malformations affecting their genitals or urinary tract (kidneys, ureters, bladder, and urethra). They are more prone to seizures than other babies and lag noticeably in development, showing increased jitteriness and irritability, abnormal sleep patterns, decreased interactive behavior, and poor organizational responses (Spear, Kirstein, and Frambes, 1989).

Researchers have not yet collected much data on the long-term effects of maternal drug use during pregnancy on children as they grow up, so little can be said on this matter. However, what is particularly distressing to some experts is that the overall effects of using combinations of drugs, which is common among drug abusers, may be even worse than the effects of using a single drug, which are bad enough to begin with.

Smoking

Dozens of studies show that cigarette smoking during pregnancy is associated with lower birth weights, shortened pregnancies, higher rates of spontaneous abortions, more frequent complications of pregnancy and labor, and higher rates of perinatal mortality (death of the fetus or newborn near the time of the birth) (see detailed reviews by Coleman, Piotrow, and Rinehart, 1979, and Rush and Callahan, 1989). In a more recent study, it was found that the link between maternal smoking during pregnancy and preterm delivery was especially strong, with a 60 percent increase in the risk of delivery before 33 weeks' gestation in women smoking at least a pack a day (Shiono, Klebanoff, and Rhoads, 1986).

A study involving 28,000 children found that children of mothers who smoke heavily during pregnancy have almost twice the risk of having hyperactive-impulsive behavior at age seven than children born to nonsmoking mothers; such children also have lower IQs, grade placement, and motor skills (Dunn et al., 1977).

The effects of marijuana smoking on fetal development are not clear. The active chemical ingredients of marijuana are known to cross the placental barrier (Harbison and Mantilla-Plata, 1972), and some animal studies have shown fetal damage and miscarriages with heavy marijuana use. However, these studies may not be applicable to humans. Because chronic, frequent marijuana smoking has been found to lower blood prolactin levels in women (Kolodny et al., 1980), it is possible that nursing might be affected by marijuana use. While data obtained on newborns during the first 30 days after birth have shown that prenatal marijuana exposure may "subtly depress the normal rate of development of the central nervous system," follow-up studies at one and two years of age did not demonstrate any negative effects (Fried, 1989).

FOCUS IN BRIEF

Warning Signs During Pregnancy

If pregnant women have any of the following problems, they should see a trained nurse-midwife or doctor immediately:

- Unusually heavy or smelly vaginal discharge.
- Very bad headaches, dizziness or blurred vision, persistent fatigue, or trouble breathing.
- Bleeding from the vagina.
- Swollen hands and face (especially in late second or third trimester).
- No signs of labor more than one day after membranes rupture.
- Seizures or blackouts.
- Marked decrease in urine output.
- Severe, unexplained pain in the shoulder.

Sources: Modified from *Population Reports*, Series L, Number 7, September 1988, and Todd and Tapley, 1988, Table 8.1. Reprinted from THE COLUMBIA UNIVERSITY COLLEGE OF PHYSICIANS AND SURGEONS COMPLETE GUIDE TO PREGNANCY by permission of Crown Publishers, Inc.

ALCOHOL

Heavy use of alcohol by a pregnant woman can cause considerable damage to the developing baby. The **fetal alcohol syndrome** includes growth deficiencies

teratogen (teh rat′ ō jin) a substance, such as a drug or chemical, that causes birth defects.

fetal alcohol syndrome the effects on the unborn child of heavy use of alcohol by the pregnant woman, including growth deficiencies, nervous system damage, and facial abnormalities.

TABLE 4–1

Medications that May Affect the Fetus If Taken During Pregnancy

Drug	Fetal Effect
Antibiotics (used to treat infections)	
Chloramphenicol	Vomiting, respiratory problems, circulatory collapse in newborns
Streptomycin	Deafness
Tetracycline	Stained teeth (common), cataracts (rare)
Anticancer drugs	
Aminopterin, Busulfan, Chlorambucil, Cyclophosphamide, Mercaptopurine, Methotrexate	Abortion, various malformations
Anticoagulant drugs (blood thinners)	
Dicumarol	Fetal bleeding or death
Warfarin	Facial deformities, mental retardation, fetal death or bleeding
Anticonvulsant drugs (used to treat epilepsy)	
Dilantin	Cleft palate, heart defects
Carbamazepine	Minor facial deformities, developmental delays
Paramethadione	Growth retardation
Trimethadione	Multiple defects
Phenobarbital	Bleeding
Hormones (various treatments)	
Birth control pills	Limb defects, genital malformations, possible heart or windpipe defects
Progestins	Masculinization for female fetus
Estrogens	Genital defects in male fetus
Diethylstilbestrol (DES)	Delayed effects: vaginal cancer in adolescent and young adult women; reproductive tract abnormalities in men
Testosterone	Masculinization of female fetus
Miscellaneous drugs	
Aspirin	Bleeding
Lithium	Heart defects
Tranquilizers (Librium, Valium, Equanil)	Various defects
Quinine	Deafness
Isoretinoin (Accutane)	Facial abnormalities, heart defects, nervous system abnormalities

Source: Data primarily from Wilson, 1977; Benson, 1978; Kalter and Warkany, 1983, and Jones et al., 1989.

before and after birth, damage to the brain and nervous system, and facial abnormalities, especially affecting the eyes (Ouellette et al., 1977; Clarren and Smith, 1978; Dorris, 1989). Mental retardation is sometimes found in the children of alcoholic mothers. There are also behavioral effects of the fetal alcohol syndrome, with irritability noted in infancy and hyperactivity in later childhood (Smith, 1979). Recent studies have shown that these major behavioral handicaps, including long-term deficits in academic achievement, last into adolescence and adulthood (Streissguth, Sampson, and Barr, 1989).

Moderate use of alcohol and "binge" drinking by pregnant women are viewed by some scientists as risky, although the evidence here is not complete. In 1984, in a study of almost 32,000 pregnancies, Mills and his co-workers (1984) found that having "at least one to two drinks a day was associated with a substantially increased risk of producing a growth-retarded infant" (p. 1875). It seems safest for pregnant women to abstain completely from alcohol. The less you drink during pregnancy, the better.

PHYSICAL ACTIVITY

Pregnancy should not be regarded as a time of incapacity and fragility. In healthy women, patterns of work and play do not usually need to change significantly during pregnancy. Many women continue working and engaging in some sports activities until the last month of pregnancy, when fatigue and discomfort may make such activity difficult. Common sense is the best guide to follow, since avoiding excessive fatigue is largely a matter of self-judgment. Activities that might be physically dangerous (skiing, diving, roller skating, mountain climbing, and so on) must be considered carefully by each woman in terms of her health and the length of her pregnancy. Proper amounts of sleep are also important but vary considerably from person to person. Women with health complications during pregnancy such as high blood pressure or vaginal bleeding will find that these conditions respond best to rest.

Sexual Activity During Pregnancy

Pregnancy has no uniform effect on sexual feelings or function. For some women, pregnancy is a time of heightened sexual awareness and sensual pleasure, while for others no changes are noticed or sexual feelings decline. Some couples find that late in pregnancy the awkwardness of a bulging belly and concern about the baby lead to voluntary abstention from sex. For others, adjustments in sexual positions or the use of noncoital sex play solves these problems fairly easily. It's important to remember that sex is not just intercourse: oral sex, sensual massage, and mutual masturbation are among the options for noncoital sex play that can be highly gratifying and can help keep a couple's sense of intimacy alive and well.

Masters and Johnson (1966) found marked variations in patterns of sexual behavior in the first trimester of pregnancy. Not surprisingly, women with morning sickness and high levels of fatigue reported losing interest in sex and a lower frequency of sexual activity, but other women experienced just the opposite effects. In the second trimester, however, 80 percent of the women noted heightened sexuality in terms of both desire and physical response. In the last trimester, there was a pronounced drop in the frequency of intercourse. The women thought this was because they were less physically attractive, but their husbands generally denied this explanation and instead voiced concern about injuring the fetus or their wife.

These findings have been verified in other studies that also showed an increased frequency of sexual activity in the second trimester (Falicov, 1973; Tolor and DiGrazia, 1976).

A few practical guidelines about sex during pregnancy are in order. Women with a history of previous miscarriages or whose pregnancy is in danger of miscarriage should abstain from any type of sexual activity that might result in their having orgasms, since contractions of the uterus during orgasm could be risky. If vaginal or uterine bleeding occurs during pregnancy, it is also wise to avoid all forms of sexual activity until receiving a medical okay. Air blown forcefully into the vagina during oral–genital contact can be dangerous for the pregnant woman, if it causes air embolism (air bubbles in the bloodstream). Cunnilingus *without* air blown into the vagina is not risky. If the membranes have ruptured, intercourse or cunnilingus should be prohibited because of the danger of fetal infection. Aside from these few cautionary notes, sex during pregnancy is quite safe for the fetus and the mother.

A few doctors have voiced concern about orgasms causing premature delivery. While it is possible that uterine contractions resulting from orgasm late in the third trimester may start labor in a small number of pregnant women (or that the prostaglandins contained in semen may trigger the same response), one report documents no statistical correlation between orgasm or intercourse and premature birth (Perkins, 1979). In fact, being orgasmic by intercourse or masturbation was associated with lower rates of prematurity.

BIRTH

Preparing for Childbirth

For the woman who has never had a baby, the process of childbirth may seem mysterious and frightening. Much of the mystery and fear can be relieved by attending childbirth classes held in hospitals or clinics and by obtaining accurate information from readings and discussions with her physician. Because friends and family are as likely to recite gruesome stories or incorrect "facts" as they are to be informative, what is heard from these sources must be taken with a large grain of salt. To get the most out of the experience, the pregnant woman and her husband or partner should attend childbirth classes together whenever possible.

Childbirth classes usually combine lectures and discussions with movies or slides showing a typical delivery. Participants are familiarized with medical terminology, labor room routines, and the operation of the hospital nursery. Most classes take a guided tour of the maternity ward and the nursery as well, so these rooms and their equipment will not seem unfamiliar to them during their labor, delivery, and hospital stay. In addition, most courses provide instruction in specific types of physical exercises designed to make labor and delivery easier.

If the decision has been made to have a home delivery, it is important to do some careful planning to assure that all necessary preparations have been made well in advance. Labor doesn't always begin exactly on schedule, and a baby's arrival can certainly come a week or two before the anticipated due date. While a few doctors are willing to participate in home deliveries, it is more typical to arrange for the services of a nurse-midwife or a lay midwife for the special event.

Lay midwives, known in some states as licensed midwives, come from varied backgrounds; some have graduate degrees, but others have little or no formal education. Nurse-midwives, in contrast, are all registered nurses with extensive health-care backgrounds. While nurse-midwives are legally permitted to perform deliveries throughout the country, lay midwives are legal in only 10 states, including Arizona, New Mexico, and Washington, and banned by law in 10 others, including California. In 21 states, there are no laws governing the practice, while in the remaining states lay midwifery is severely restricted but not banned entirely.

No matter who you choose to assist in an at-home birth, be sure to consult with them about what supplies should be on hand and about any special arrangements that might be required. For instance, many midwives suggest alerting a pediatrician to the impending birth so that he or she can visit the newborn infant shortly after its arrival.

Advocates of home birth feel that it provides a more natural, loving environment for the birth experience and allows women to exercise greater control over the process of having a baby. In addition, many couples believe that a home delivery allows for more personal sensitivity than a hospital birth (e.g., you don't have to deal with the bureaucracy) as well as a better system of social support from family and friends. But not all couples are willing to forego the extensive backup services that a hospital offers if something goes wrong, recognizing that in an emergency, precious time may be lost getting the mother and baby to a facility for necessary medical care.

Labor

Labor consists of rhythmic, regular contractions of the uterus that result in delivery of the child, the placenta, and membranes. Labor is usually preceded by several related events. As already mentioned, a few weeks before labor begins, women who are pregnant for the first time experience lightening. **Effacement,** or thinning of the cervix, and **dilatation,** opening of the mouth of the cervix, are also likely to begin about two weeks before the onset of labor. A very dependable sign of imminent labor is "show" (or "bloody show"), the discharge of a small amount of blood-tinged mucus.[2] Generally, labor begins a few hours or a few days after this occurs. About 10 percent of women experience a premature rupture of their membranes (the amniotic sac or "bag of waters") before labor starts. Warm fluid may trickle or gush from the vagina either running down their legs (if standing) or wetting the bed (if lying down). Labor typically begins within a day after this occurs. If it does not, it may be desirable to start labor artificially to protect the baby from infection since it is no longer isolated from the outside world.

HOW LABOR BEGINS

The exact biological forces that start labor are not clearly understood. For many years, it was thought that a rapid drop of progesterone at the end of pregnancy might stimulate the beginning of regular contractions of the uterus, but recent studies in humans do not support this explanation. **Oxytocin,** a hormone made in the pituitary gland, has been thought to play a role, but women whose pituitaries have been surgically removed are still capable of normal, spon-

[2] "Show" is not a reliable indication of labor if a pelvic exam was done in the preceding day or two, since this may have caused a slight amount of internal bleeding and disrupted the mucous plug guarding the cervix.

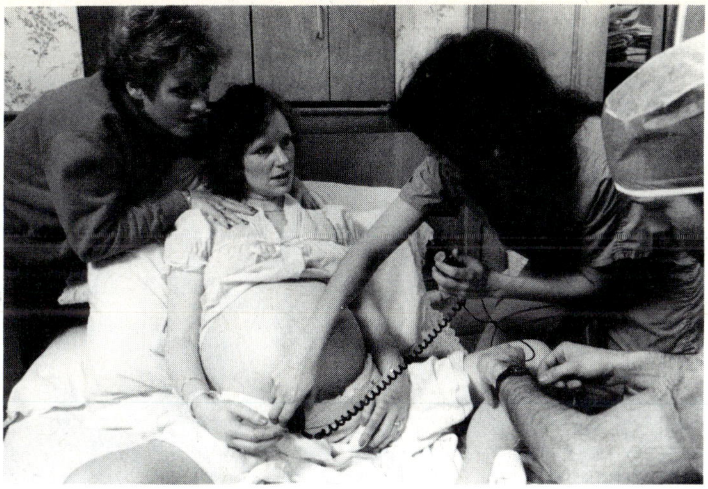

Monitoring the progress of labor and the heartbeat of the unborn child.

taneous labor. At present, evidence indicates that prostaglandins may be involved because (1) they can cause strong uterine contractions at any time during pregnancy, (2) the fetal membranes have high concentrations of the substances necessary for the manufacture of prostaglandins, and (3) drugs such as aspirin that inhibit prostaglandin formation can delay the onset of labor (Cunningham, MacDonald, and Gant, 1989).

THE STAGES OF LABOR

For descriptive convenience, labor is divided into three stages. The length and experience of these stages vary from woman to woman and for different pregnancies of the same woman.[3]

The **first stage of labor** begins when uterine contractions are strong enough, long enough, and frequent enough to begin effacement and dilatation of the cervix. In first pregnancies, complete effacement occurs before dilatation starts; in later pregnancies, the two occur simultaneously.

When the cervix is completely effaced, its thickness has decreased from about 2 centimeters (0.8 inch) to the thickness of a piece of paper. This process is measured in percentages. If the doctor tells a pregnant woman that she is 50 percent effaced, that means the thickness of the cervix is about 1 centimeter (0.4 inch).

When the opening of the cervix is 10 centimeters (4 inches), a width that must be reached for a baby to be born, dilatation is complete. Dilatation is caused by pressures from uterine contractions pushing the amniotic sac or the baby's head in wedgelike fashion into the cervix.

The first stage of labor is by far the longest: in first pregnancies, it averages 13 hours, and in later pregnancies, 8 hours. Early in first-stage labor, when dilatation is minimal, contractions are mild (lasting 20 to 40 seconds) and far apart, occurring at intervals of 10 to 20 minutes. The woman is usually comfortable and can be out of bed if she wishes. In fact, one recent study found that walking during early labor (instead of staying in bed) makes mothers more comfortable and less in need of pain relief. Walking also causes

[3] **False labor,** contractions that are simply an exaggeration of Braxton–Hicks contractions, may mimic the start of true labor. Although false labor can be convincing enough to result in a trip to the hospital, it can usually be differentiated from true labor. Its contractions tend to be irregular, the interval between them does not shorten, and the woman feels discomfort mainly in the lower abdomen and groin. True labor produces back and abdominal pain. Furthermore, false labor does not result in progressive effacement and dilatation.

labor the processes involved in giving birth, especially uterine contractions.

effacement (e fāce′ munt) the thinning or flattening of the cervix during labor.

dilatation (dil′ uh tā′ shun) opening of the mouth of the cervix in preparation for birth.

oxytocin (ahk′ sē to′ sin) a hormone made in the posterior pituitary thought to play a role in uterine contractions and lactation stimulation.

false labor irregular contractions that do not become regular. They are felt mainly in the lower abdomen and groin in contrast to true labor, which is felt in the back and abdomen.

first stage of labor the early portion of labor in which cervical effacement and dilatation occurs.

TABLE 4–2

Medications for Pain Reduction in Labor and Delivery

Analgesics	Effects on Mother	Effects on Fetus
Tranquilizers Valium, Vistaril, Sparine	Physical relaxation and reduced anxiety; takes the edge off pain but does not eliminate it entirely	Minimal
Barbiturates Nembutal, Seconal, Amytal	Drowsiness and reduced anxiety; may slow the progress of labor	Can depress nervous system and breathing
Narcotics Demerol, Dolophine, Nisentil	Reduce pain and elevate mood but may inhibit uterine contractions and cause nausea or vomiting	Can depress nervous system and breathing
Amnesics Scopolamine ("Twilight")	Does not reduce pain but causes the woman to forget her experience after it is over; may cause physical excitation and wildness	Minimal
Anesthetics	***Effects on Mother***	***Effects on Fetus***
Local		
Paracervical	Blocks pain in the uterus and cervix, but relatively short-lasting and ineffective late in labor; can lower mother's blood pressure	Causes a slowing of fetal heartbeat in about 20 percent of cases
Pudendal	Blocks pain from the perineum and vulva in about 50 percent of cases	Minimal
Regional		
Spinal, epidural, caudal	Blocks pain from the uterus, cervix, and perineum; highly effective but can cause serious drop in blood pressure or seizures	Generally does not affect fetus but requires forceps delivery more often than other methods
General		
Nitrous oxide (laughing gas), Halothane, Thiopental	Usually used only in the last few minutes of labor to eliminate pain completely but may cause vomiting or other complications and is a leading cause of maternal death	Can depress nervous system and breathing

stronger labor contractions, which may shorten the overall time until delivery.

In the first stage of labor, a woman may be discouraged by the length of time it takes to get even a little dilatation, but once she has gotten to 4 or 5 centimeters she has usually completed more than half of the time in this stage. At this more active part of the first stage, contractions are typically 30 to 60 seconds long and occur every 2 to 4 minutes.

The woman may obtain treatment to help deal with pain at this time, since medications given any earlier might slow the progress of labor. Various types of pain relief are available (see Table 4–2), and the woman should become familiar with them and discuss her options with her midwife or doctor well before labor starts. Although all medications have potential risks—including some negative effects on the baby—careful use under medical supervision can be important in allowing the mother to go through labor and delivery with less discomfort. This relief can have obvious psychological and physical benefits. Regrettably, some women feel guilty if they want pain relievers during childbirth. They may feel inadequate for needing such help, especially if a friend or relative had an easy delivery *without* drugs and is sure everyone else's experience should be the same. Others have been told that the medical "establishment" pushes medications primarily for its own convenience and income. While some doctors do this, most have the welfare and comfort of their patient and her baby uppermost in their minds.

The last part of the first stage of labor (8 to 10 centimeters dilatation) is usually the most uncomfortable. The woman's contractions last 45 to 60 seconds or longer, are only about 2 minutes apart, and are very strong. In first pregnancies, this part of labor usually lasts about 40 minutes and in later pregnancies it averages 20 minutes. Most often, the membranes rupture at this time. The first stage of labor ends when dilatation of the cervix is complete.

The **second stage of labor,** which goes from full dilatation to birth of the baby, is shorter (average length, 80 minutes in first pregnancies, 30 minutes in others) and is usually less stressful for the mother. She can now assist the baby's descent by pushing down with her contractions.

Once the baby's head is delivered, blood and mucus are wiped off and the nose and mouth are suctioned to aid breathing.[4] As soon as the rest of the baby is out (a process that is surprisingly quick in an uncomplicated birth), the newborn is held below the level of the mother's body and suctioning of the mouth and nose is repeated. The umbilical cord is clamped and cut about 3 centimeters (1¼ inches) from the baby's body (the stub dries up in a few days and falls off, leaving the navel behind as a souvenir). Although often shown in movies or television dramas, midwives or doctors rarely have to spank a baby to induce crying and breathing, since this usually happens spontaneously. As the baby takes his or her first breaths, the skin will become pink unless there is a medical problem.

The baby is shown to the mother and usually given to her to hold. To prevent eye infections after the passage through the vagina, the baby is almost always given eye drops (usually silver nitrate) or an antibiotic ointment. The baby is also given a vitamin K shot to prevent bleeding, since this vitamin cannot be manufactured in newborns immediately after birth. Finally, if the delivery has been conducted in a hospital or birthing center, the baby is given an identification bracelet, footprints are taken, and a medical exam is done to check for birth defects or other health problems.

The **third stage of labor** follows the baby's birth. At this point, the placenta separates from the wall of the uterus, and the placenta and membranes (the "afterbirth") are delivered. This usually requires only 10 to 12 minutes. If even small pieces of the placenta or membranes are retained in the uterus, bleeding problems may result.

Delivery

Over the years, many different schools of thought have emerged concerning the details and style of labor and delivery, and pregnant women and doctors are often bombarded with information "proving" that

[4] The baby's head is the first part to be delivered in about 95 percent of pregnancies. These are called **occiput, vertex,** or **cephalic presentations. Breech presentations** occur about 4 percent of the time; in this position, the buttocks or feet are delivered first. In the rarer cases, called **transverse positions,** the baby lies across the uterus and a shoulder or arm will present first. Breech or transverse presentations require either turning the baby or performing a cesarean section.

second stage of labor the portion of labor from full cervical dilatation to delivery of the baby.

occiput presentation the childbirth presentation in which the back part of the baby's head is the first part to pass through the birth canal.

vertex presentation (vur′ teks) the childbirth presentation in which the crown of the baby's head is first to be seen at the opening of the vagina.

cephalic presentation (se fal′ ik) the childbirth presentation in which the head is the first part of the baby's body to pass through the birth canal.

breech presentation the childbirth presentation in which the buttocks or feet are the first part of the baby to pass through the opening of the vagina.

transverse position the childbirth presentation in which the baby lies across the uterus and a shoulder or arm is first to be seen at the opening of the vagina. A cesarean section is often necessary if the baby cannot be turned.

third stage of labor the period immediately following delivery of the baby, concluding with separation and expulsion of the placenta.

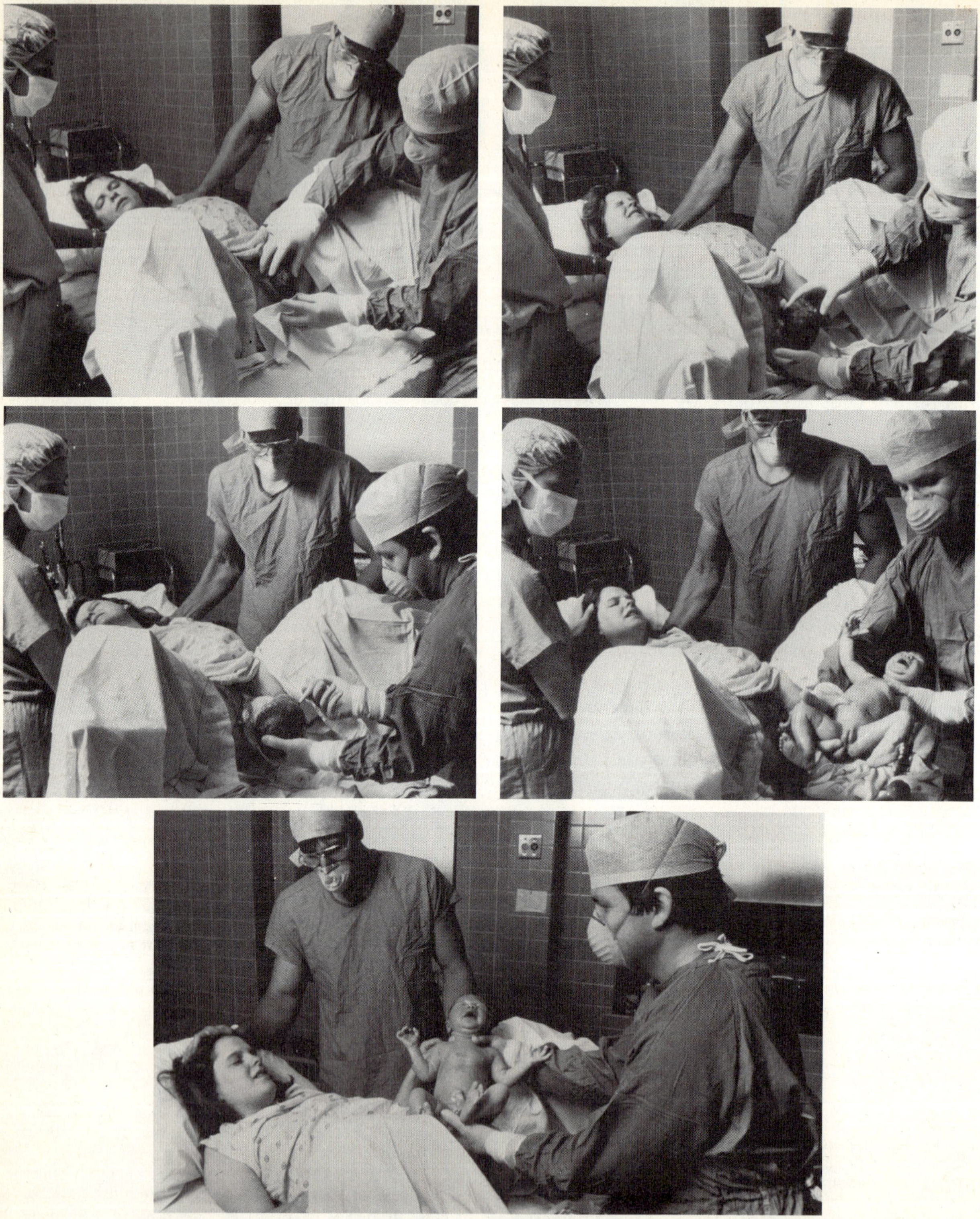

This sequence of photos of a hospital delivery shows the baby's head emerging, the doctor clearing mucus from the baby's mouth and nose, and the baby just delivered (and still connected to the mother by the umbilical cord). The bottom photo shows Mom taking her first good look at her baby, while a proud Dad looks on.

one way is undeniably the best. Usually, it is a matter of personal preference (or health considerations) between a woman and her midwife or doctor. Increasingly today, choices about the setting and style of delivery are made by the woman and her spouse or partner rather than leaving these up to the health care professional's choices alone. Here, we discuss some of the more popular methods of delivery.

HOSPITAL DELIVERY

A hospital delivery usually begins once the first stage of labor is under way. A nurse or doctor asks a series of questions to outline the history of the pregnancy and the sequence of events near the time of labor, and a vaginal examination is done to see how much dilatation and effacement have occurred. A blood sample and urine specimen are usually taken for a general health check, and a physical exam is performed to evaluate the mother's condition and that of the baby.

After this point, hospital procedures vary considerably. In many hospitals, sophisticated electronic equipment is used to check the progress of the baby **(fetal monitoring)** as well as the frequency, intensity, and duration of the mother's contractions. Watching the fetal heart rate is particularly important because a sustained change in rate may indicate fetal distress.

In some cases, a woman may be admitted to the hospital at, near, or past her due date to have labor started artificially. This procedure, called **induction** or **induced labor,** is usually done so that a well-rested woman can begin labor under planned conditions with her doctor present; this technique is also used in certain types of problem pregnancies where it can protect the health of the mother and child alike. Labor is usually induced by giving the mother oxytocin. Inducing labor is not without risk to the mother and fetus, but most physicians feel that the benefits outweigh the risks substantially. Some observers have claimed that the issue is really a matter of medical chauvinism, however, believing that induction is mainly done for the doctor's convenience (Hahn and Paige, 1980).

The woman's husband or partner is usually encouraged to be present during labor and delivery so that he can share the experience, give encouragement and support, and help make her comfortable. In the past, most hospitals did not permit other family members to be present. Fortunately, this situation is now changing rapidly, as many hospitals have altered their policy on this matter. Regardless of which members of the family are present, obstetrical nurses can provide close, continuing attention and information.

Doctors sometimes rupture the membranes to stimulate the progress of labor. An intravenous solution of sugar and water may be started to prevent dehydration and to allow for rapid administration of anesthesia or blood transfusions if something goes wrong. During the delivery, the baby's head may be assisted out of the vagina by the use of forceps if there is fetal distress, if the umbilical cord is wrapped tightly around the baby's neck, if the cord is being compressed so that the blood supply to the baby is cut off **(prolapsed cord),** or if anesthesia interferes with the mother's ability to push out her baby.

At the time of **crowning** (the first appearance of the baby's head at the opening of the vagina), many American physicians routinely perform an **episiotomy** to enlarge the opening for the baby's head. An episiotomy is an incision made through the skin and muscle of the perineum, the area between the vagina and the anus (see Figure 4–6). The episiotomy has several purposes: (1) it reduces the pressure against the baby's head, lessening the trauma of delivery; (2) it reduces the risk of tearing the perineum, which might cause more extensive tissue damage and might be ragged-edged and difficult to repair; and (3) it permits the use of forceps or vacuum devices if needed to assist in delivering the baby's head. Most women do not feel the incision being made because the perineum is numbed from the pressure of the baby's head.

Some people are opposed to routine episiotomies, noting that fewer than one-third of deliveries in Europe use this technique (Arms, 1975; Lake, 1976). Furthermore, they point out that the vaginal opening has the capacity to stretch widely without tearing in most circumstances and suggest that episiotomy should be done only in selected cases (Boston Women's Health Book Collective, 1984).

fetal monitor electronic equipment used during labor to check the progress of the baby, especially its heartbeat, and the duration, frequency, and intensity of uterine contractions.

induced labor labor started artificially, usually by infusing oxytocin into a vein.

prolapsed cord condition whereby the umbilical cord is compressed to the point where the blood supply to the baby is cut off.

crowning in childbirth, the appearance of the baby's head at the opening of the vagina.

episiotomy (e piz′ ē ot′ uh mē) during a vaginal delivery, the incision in the mother's perineum that gives the baby's head more room to emerge.

FIGURE 4–6

An Episiotomy Done During Labor

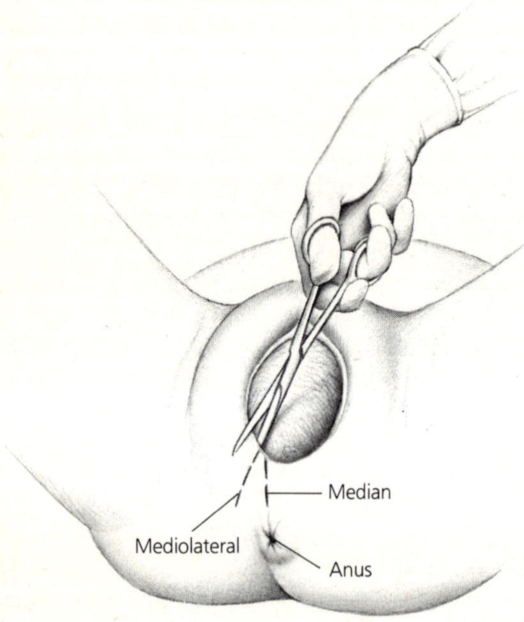

Although 80 percent of deliveries are straightforward and uncomplicated, there are specific advantages to hospital delivery. Sophisticated equipment is available for rapid diagnosis of problems affecting either mother or child, facilities for surgery are close at hand if emergency cesarean section is needed, blood is available for transfusion if maternal bleeding cannot be controlled, and the personnel and equipment of the nursery are specially geared to problems of the newborn infant. While some problems of labor and delivery are detectable in advance (e.g., breech presentation, transverse lie, maternal illness), others are not discovered until labor is far along.

NATURAL CHILDBIRTH

Natural childbirth refers to a method described by a British obstetrician, Grantly Dick-Read, in 1932 in a book titled *Childbirth Without Fear*. He objected to much of the medical intervention in delivery and believed that culturally imbued fear and tension were the principal causes of pain and difficulty in the childbirth experience. He felt that fear and anticipation of pain led to psychological and muscular tension, which opposed dilatation of the birth canal and became, in effect, a self-fulfilling prophecy.

To break the fear–tension–pain reaction, Dick-Read suggested eliminating fear through education and reducing tension by the use of relaxation techniques such as breathing and physical exercises. Prenatal classes were used to stress the positive side of childbirth and to teach exercises to increase elasticity in the pelvic muscles, flexibility in the joints of the pelvis and back, and improve circulation. Special breathing patterns to reduce pain and increase the effectiveness of contractions were taught.

Although some consider childbirth to be truly "natural" only if no painkilling medications are used at all, Dick-Read felt that painkillers were permissible but were to be avoided if possible.

LAMAZE

A similar approach to that of Dick-Read was advocated by Fernand Lamaze, a French obstetrician who traveled to Russia to study obstetrical practices. The Lamaze method, first publicized in this country in a book called *Thank You, Dr. Lamaze* (Karmel, 1959) and later described in *Painless Childbirth* (Lamaze, 1970), also depends on education and exercises to allow a woman to gain control over her labor.

The Lamaze method, taught in prenatal classes to both the wife and the husband (or to the woman and another friend acting as her "coach" if she is not married or her husband is not available), shows women how to relax all the muscles in their bodies and how to position themselves and breathe during different stages of labor. Other techniques are used to distract the woman from awareness of pain: these include **effleurage,** a light, circular stroking of the abdomen used when active labor begins, pressure on the front of the hip bones to reduce abdominal discomfort, and massage techniques to lessen backache. Both the coach and the mother are active participants in the labor, with a prearranged set of exercises to follow.

Neither natural childbirth nor childbirth by the Lamaze method is completely painless. Both approaches depend on personal awareness through education to reduce fear of the unknown and physical relaxation techniques that reduce tension and the anticipation of pain. In both methods, there is some distraction from the perception of pain, but pain is not eliminated.

CESAREAN SECTION

Cesarean section (C section) is an operation to remove the fetus through an incision in the walls of the abdomen and uterus. Cesareans are done when the woman cannot deliver vaginally without endangering her or the baby's life or health. Among conditions that usually require cesarean delivery are (1) a size difference between the baby's head and the mother's pelvis that makes it difficult or impossible for the baby to pass through the birth canal, (2) transverse position of the baby or another difficult presentation, (3) fetal distress from any cause (e.g., prolapsed cord), (4) premature separation of the placenta or abnormal positioning of the placenta so it blocks the opening to the cervix from within the uterus, and (5) long, difficult labor that is not progressing properly.

In the last decade, the cesarean birth rate in America has quadrupled, from 5.5 to almost 23 percent (Notzon, Placek, and Taffel, 1987; Myers and Gleicher, 1988). In fact, in many suburban hospitals, cesarean births now account for 30 to 35 percent of all deliveries and it has been predicted that, without a change in obstetrical trends, the national cesarean section rate could reach 40 percent by the end of this century (Placek, Taffel, and Liss, 1987).

This development has alarmed many medical experts and health-care consumer advocates, who contend that overuse of cesarean births reflects improper medical practice and that physicians who perform unnecessary cesareans are motivated by the higher fees they charge for this procedure as well as by the desire to avoid lawsuits (Danforth, 1985; Queenan, 1988; Gould et al., 1989; Goyert et al., 1989). After all, if obstetricians routinely perform cesareans in problem pregnancies, an attorney can legitimately ask why one wasn't done in a specific case. As an editorial in the *Journal of the American Medical Association* recently put it: "In our current litigious environment where patients expect a perfect obstetric outcome and physicians using available knowledge are eager to try new technologies to improve that outcome, is it surprising we have seen an escalation of cesarean delivery rates to a level that now appears unreasonable? (Jonas and Dooley, 1989, p. 1513)."

Rosen and Thomas (1989) point out that there are three assumptions that doctors and the public share that have also contributed to the torrent of cesarean births: cesareans are safe, they are required in a broad range of cases, and they produce healthier babies. The reality is quite different.

Although cesarean births have a low rate of complications, the maternal death rate (1 in 10,000) is double the rate for vaginal deliveries. In addition, a cesarean increases the risk of blood loss or infection during childbirth, and these complications may have long-term ramifications. Finally, there is no evidence that cesarean babies are healthier overall than those born by vaginal delivery (Gould et al., 1989; Rosen and Thomas, 1989): in fact, the opposite may be true (Battaglia, 1988).

In light of these facts, it is interesting to note that a 1980 task force sponsored by the National Institutes of Health recommended that many women who had cesarean deliveries can safely have subsequent normal vaginal deliveries, although in the past, 99 percent were automatically given cesareans for future childbirth (Kolata, 1980a). Confirming this, one study found that approximately two-thirds of women who had previously had a cesarean were able to have successful vaginal deliveries (Weitz, 1985). Furthermore, in a number of other countries, including Norway, Scotland, and Hungary, more than one-third of women who have had cesareans have vaginal births later on (Notzon, Placek, and Taffel, 1987).

The questions raised by the high rates of cesarean sections do not alter the need for this procedure as the proper treatment for certain obstetric problems, such as abnormal positioning of the placenta or fetal distress. But overuse of surgical delivery is part of the widespread American notion that doctors deliver babies, not that women give birth. In fact, one of the complaints that obstetricians have is that some women demand a cesarean—especially if they've had one before—which may reflect their feeling that a cesarean is an "easier" experience on the mother. As one 29-year-old woman explained it (Authors' files):

> I had heard a lot of stories from my friends about how painful vaginal delivery was, and to tell you the truth I'm not a person who's really good at dealing with pain. So I thought to myself, if you can have a C-section and be anesthetized so you don't feel anything at all, that's for me. So I just shopped around for a doctor who was willing to agree in advance to do it that way, and I was more than delighted with the result.

On the other hand, some couples who were not expecting a cesarean birth may feel cheated or disappointed by not going through labor and delivery as they had prepared for it, especially if they feel it is a

effleurage (ef' lu razh') the circular stroking movement used in massage of the abdomen during labor in the Lamaze method.

somewhat artificial, depersonalized kind of birth experience.

While it is possible to have a cesarean section while the woman is fully awake (using spinal anesthesia), if the operation is done on an emergency basis the woman is almost always put under general anesthesia. One final point about cesarean sections is a practical matter: there is usually a longer (and more expensive) hospital stay involved—four to five days, versus the two-day stay now common for uncomplicated childbirth.

HOME DELIVERY AND BIRTHING ROOMS

Not everyone views the hospital, with its authoritative atmosphere, complex rules, impersonality, and association with illness, as an ideal setting for childbirth. In some countries, such as France and Holland, some women go to special childbirth centers that are separate from hospitals (there are about 200 in the United States). The services of childbirth centers are usually covered by health insurance plans that include obstetrical benefits. In many societies, home delivery supervised by a midwife is common (Cavero, 1979). While two decades ago there were only 300 nurse-midwives in the United States, there are now more than 3000, with several hundred new nurse-midwives graduating annually from certified training programs. Although many work in hospitals, others are in private practice either in association with physicians or independently. Nurse-midwives generally emphasize prenatal counseling, family-centered childbirth, and a limited degree of intervention in the natural process of labor and delivery. Unlike most physicians, nurse-midwives typically stay with a woman throughout her labor and often encourage the woman to get up out of bed and move around through most of her labor. Today, a number of states (including New York, Pennsylvania, Alaska, Maryland, Mississippi, New Mexico, and Utah) have laws requiring that insurance companies provide coverage for the services of certified nurse-midwives who work under the guidance of physicians or hospitals, but in other states there is considerable resistance to the use of nurse-midwives, especially those who practice independently of hospitals. Only about 10 percent of certified nurse-midwives do home deliveries.

Having a baby at home offers a chance for a more relaxed experience in familiar surroundings, freedom from hospital routines, contact with the whole family (including children who can share in the process), and a less expensive medical bill. In addition, there is preliminary evidence that home delivery may be as safe as hospital delivery for uncomplicated pregnancies (Wertz and Wertz, 1977; Hahn and Paige, 1980).

Although many doctors are opposed to home births, some are willing to cooperate and a few are even enthusiastic about the practice. In any case, careful prenatal screening must be done to identify potential problem pregnancies or difficult deliveries, provisions must be made for appropriate supervision by an experienced midwife or doctor, and emergency ac-

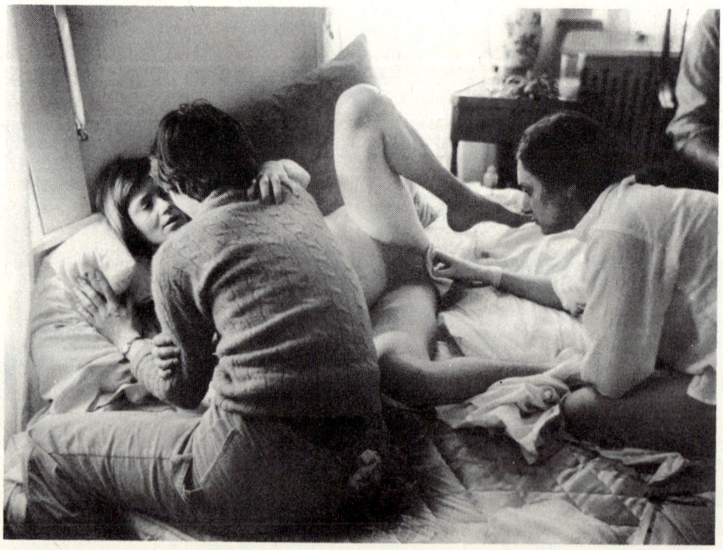

Birthing rooms have been added at many hospitals to provide a more homelike environment for labor and delivery while permitting the entire family to participate in the experience.

cess to a hospital must be available since prenatal screening is not infallible.

A relatively recent compromise designed to overcome the image of hospital austerity is the opening of birthing rooms at hundreds of hospitals across America. In these rooms, which are typically furnished in a comfortable, homelike fashion but are also equipped with oxygen and anesthesia, labor and delivery are possible in a more relaxed climate in which other family members, including children, can be part of the childbirth experience. In addition, the woman does not need to be moved from a labor room to a separate delivery room. If something goes wrong, however—for example, if a blood transfusion is needed—all necessary resources are at hand to take care of the emergency, thus circumventing what many see as the primary risk of home delivery. This is important because even among women who are prescreened to be at low risk for problems during childbirth, about one in five actually experience complications that require being transferred to the hospital (Petravage, 1983). Use of these birthing rooms usually costs about the same as a more traditional delivery in the hospital.

A recent survey of 11,814 deliveries at 84 freestanding childbirth centers involving women with a lower-than-average risk of a poor outcome of pregnancy found that one woman in six was transferred to a hospital but that overall birth centers offer a safe, acceptable alternative to hospital delivery (Rooks et al., 1989).

Psychological Aspects of Childbirth

Each woman brings her own personality style and ways of dealing with a new experience to the process of childbirth. Her initial anxieties may reflect concerns for her safety and the status of her baby, fear of the unknown, uncertainty about her capacity to love and care for a child, and a host of other questions (How will my husband react? What if the baby is not normal? Will I make a fool of myself?). The childbirth experience is also colored by the woman's relationship with her doctor, her feelings about the use of medications, the support she receives from her husband or partner, and the expectations she has of what it will be like. The relatively high rate of cesarean deliveries and other obstetrical complications means that childbirth is frequently not the experience it is expected to be (Grossman, Eichler, and Winickoff, 1980). No wonder it is difficult to talk about a "typical" experience.

In some cases, a woman may sacrifice personal choice about aspects of childbirth to medical routine or philosophical principles. For example, a woman may prefer to be given painkillers but may not allow herself to take them if friends or relatives discourage this practice. Certainly, competent obstetrical service must be available, but it should not preclude personal expression in having a baby. Childbirth is an intensely personal experience. The culmination of pregnancy in labor and delivery is ideally a time of intimacy, sharing, and fulfillment.

THE POSTPARTUM DAYS

The postpartum period, the time after the baby's birth, requires many adjustments for all concerned. Physical changes occur as the mother's body adjusts to no longer being pregnant. Both parents must also psychologically adjust to the new baby, parental roles and responsibilities, changes in family relationships, and looking ahead to the future. This is a complex time of ups and downs, new experiences, frustrations, and joys.

Physiologic and Anatomic Processes

After delivery, the uterus shrinks back to its normal size gradually, going from about 1000 grams (2.2 pounds) just after delivery to 50 to 70 grams (1.8 to 2.5 ounces) at the end of the sixth postpartum week. Once the placenta separates from the uterus, the levels of certain hormones in the mother's body (most notably, estrogen and progesterone) decline abruptly. It usually takes the woman several weeks to adjust to this rapid change, and some authorities believe that the emotional ups and downs of the early postpartum period are related to this phenomenon.

Immediately after childbirth, the cervix is collapsed and flabby but it quickly regains its tone, tightening so that by a week after delivery there is an opening of less than 1 centimeter (0.4 inch). During the first few postpartum weeks, as the lining of the uterus regrows, there is a discharge called lochia that changes in color from dark red to pinkish-brown to yellowish-white. The vagina, which was stretched considerably during birth, gradually gets smaller but usually does not return to the exact size it was before childbirth.

Psychological Reactions

The first day or two after childbirth is often a time of happiness and relief. The woman enjoys a feeling of accomplishment, family and friends congratulate her, and people around her attend to her needs without great demands on her time and energy. By the third or fourth day after delivery, many women experience a turn in their mood—feeling "down," being tearful, or having frightening thoughts or dreams—a phenomenon called "baby blues" or **postpartum depression.**

The irritability and vulnerability that also mark this emotional letdown probably stem from many sources: the hormonal changes previously mentioned, the effects of fatigue and physical stress, a sense of loneliness and separation, the strangeness of being in the hospital, and mixed feelings about the mother's role and viewing herself in a new light. In most cases, postpartum depression lasts for only a few days.

A recent study questions whether the unique mood changes that occur in both women and men during the postpartum period are actually depression at all (Quadagno et al., 1986). Husbands and wives in 21 couples completed daily questionnaires for 10-day periods during the third trimester, the postpartum period, and six months after birth. The moods that were experienced the most strongly during the postpartum period were not the ones usually associated with depression, such as feeling depressed, sad, discouraged, or pessimistic. Instead, the moods that were strongest during the postpartum days, for both men and women, were those related to anxiety and concern with coping ability (nervous, worried, helpless, anxious) and those associated with positive emotions (enthusiastic, happy). The authors of this study remarked, "Individuals may be nervous and worried about their ability to cope with the demands of a new infant, but yet, at the same time, they seem to feel very positively about the experience" (p. 1021).

Some women may feel guilty or troubled in the early postpartum period. Not all pregnancies result in normal children, and the mother of an infant with a birth defect or serious illness (as well as a woman whose child was stillborn) may try to "explain" what happened on the basis of something she did wrong. Women might also worry over their partner's welfare, over particular decisions such as nursing versus bottle-feeding, or over their ability to care for their child. For other women, there may be a personal sense of failure if, for example, they were unable to deliver vaginally and required a cesarean section. A woman who has previously decided to put her child up for adoption may have second thoughts at this time or may have a profound sense of loss even though she feels she's doing the right thing.

A new set of circumstances and a new set of adjustments occur immediately after leaving the hospital. The demands of the new infant (nighttime feedings, diaper changes, and so on) are thrown into the demands of everyday living. Older children and husband want attention, friends and family want to visit and talk, and the mother is apt to feel fragmented, confused, and exhausted. Some women receive considerable help during this time from their own mother, another relative, a friend, or someone they have hired. Husbands can help out, too, but do not always have the time, the interest, or the experience to be a major source of reliable assistance. The postpartum adjustment beyond the first week or two is primarily a reflection of the adjustment to parenting, a process that is now considered.

PARENTING

The first days after delivery can play a critical role in the development of an emotional link between parent and child, a process called **parent–child bonding.** Physical contact, cuddling, cooing, and eye contact in this period of the infant's life seem to have a major impact on the child's later behavior and psychological health (Trause, Kennel, and Klaus, 1977). One experiment showed that babies who received more early postnatal contact with their mothers were more attentive to them at four weeks of age (Klaus et al., 1972). Another study demonstrated that newborns were able to recognize differences in adult voices and to show a preference for their mother's voice within the first three days of life (DeCasper and Fifer, 1980).

Father–child bonding in the early postpartum period is also thought to be important. For one thing, fathers who have been present during birth and who have cuddled the newborn and spent some time talking or just making "goo-goo" noises to it do not seem to experience the sense of alienation that is often found among "waiting room fathers"; furthermore, research shows that the fathers who have bonded with the baby tend to spend more time with it later on (Todd and Tapley, 1988).

As already mentioned, arriving at home with a new baby is apt to be a trying time. Adjusting to the state of parenthood, with its restrictions on freedom, privacy, and self-indulgence, is not easy. No one can be the perfect parent—always patient, never angry, constantly available, forever exercising good judgment, and never making a mistake—but new parents often need a while to gain this perspective.

Nursing

Milk production (**lactation**) occurs two or three days after birth, replacing the colostrum previously secreted by the breasts. The breasts are prepared for lactation by large amounts of prolactin secreted by the pituitary during the second half of pregnancy. In response to the stimulus of suckling, which further increases prolactin secretion, the breasts become more distended until finally there is a milk flow reflex (ejection of milk from the breast), which is controlled by oxytocin. In the first day or two of nursing, the breasts may be uncomfortable because of congestion; the nipples may also be sore because the hungry baby's sucking grip is surprisingly powerful. This soreness can sometimes be limited if steps are taken to condition the nipples in the two months prior to childbirth.

Nursing has a number of advantages over bottle-feeding. Breast milk has natural ingredients that strengthen the baby's resistance to disease, is instantly available, does not require sterilization or heating as bottles do, and is self-replenishing. Nursing also provides a closeness that has psychological benefits for both child and mother. On the negative side, drugs and medications taken by the mother are usually secreted in her milk (Platzker, Lew, and Stewart, 1980), breast-feeding may be inconvenient if the mother works outside the home, and in some cases, if milk flow does not prove adequate to meet the baby's nutritional needs, the mother may experience a sense of failure.

Women often become sexually aroused during nursing; some women even have orgasms in this fashion. Erotic arousal in this context can create reactions ranging from pleasure to guilt or fear. Interestingly, Masters and Johnson (1966) found that women who breast-feed their babies have considerably higher sexual interest in the first three postpartum months than women who do not.

In the United States, there has been a definite trend toward breast-feeding in the past decade. Breast-feeding in hospitals after childbirth increased from 25 percent in 1971 to 58 percent in 1981, and the number of breast-fed five- and six-month-olds increased from 6 to 27 percent (Martinez and Dodd, 1982). While highly educated, relatively affluent mothers are most apt to nurse their babies, the greatest rate of increase in breast-feeding was found among less educated mothers.

Cultural factors also seem to affect breast-feeding, for reasons that are not entirely clear. According to data from the La Leche League, 62.2 percent of white mothers nursed their babies while in the hospital, compared to 50.6 percent of Hispanic mothers and 24.9 percent of black mothers (Leary, 1988a). In addition, black mothers tend to stop nursing sooner than whites do (Kurinij, Shiono, and Rhodes, 1988).

The individual woman's decision to nurse or to bottle-feed is influenced by many different factors. Jelliffe (1976) identified several social biases in this decision-making process: the Western world's tendency to overvalue manufactured products, overemphasis on the sexual rather than nurturing role of breasts, the changing role of women in terms of work outside the home, and pressures from the food industry via advertising. On the other hand, in recent years the arguments of breast-feeding advocates have often made women feel that bottle-feeding is a crime against nature and is a shirking of their duties as "good" mothers. Our suspicion is that if breast-feeding is undertaken out of a sense of obligation, the emotional benefits to mother and child probably diminish considerably. Bottle-feeding allows both parents to interact with the baby more freely and can certainly foster a close, loving relationship just as breast-feeding can.

Returning to Sexual Interaction

Most doctors advise women to abstain from coitus for a number of weeks after childbirth to allow healing of the episiotomy and restoration of the vagina and uterus. The exact timing of when sexual intercourse can be resumed is an individual matter, influenced by both medical factors (e.g., persistent bleeding, fatigue) and psychological considerations (e.g., post-

postpartum depression the letdown many women experience after giving birth. They are tearful and depressed and may have frightening dreams. Also called baby blues.

parent–child bonding the process of attachment and identification that usually occurs during early infancy.

lactation (lak tā′ shun) the production of milk by the breasts, usually beginning a few days after birth.

partum depression). By three to four weeks after delivery, most women find their sexual desire returning and can comfortably resume sexual activity. In circumstances where intercourse is still uncomfortable, alternative means of sexual expression can be used until full recovery takes place.

PROBLEM PREGNANCIES

Not all pregnancies go as planned or as described in textbooks. There are several common problems, which we discuss here.

Prematurity

A premature baby is one born any time before the thirty-sixth week of pregnancy. Babies born prematurely are more likely to have health difficulties than full-term babies; as a result, prematurity is a leading cause of newborn death. "Preemies" have a high rate of respiratory problems, seizures, and infections, which may lead to brain damage or other long-range handicaps. Premature births are associated with maternal illness, malfunction of the placenta, heavy smoking, and pregnancies in young teenagers, but in many cases no underlying cause can be found. Modern methods of caring for premature infants have significantly improved survival rates from just a few years ago (Working Group, 1990). Recently, a drug called ritodrine that inhibits labor by relaxing the muscles of the uterus has been found to be effective in stopping premature labor.

Toxemia

Toxemia of pregnancy is a disease marked by the sudden appearance of high blood pressure, severe edema, and protein in the urine after the twentieth week of pregnancy (**preeclampsia**), which in some cases progresses to convulsions and coma (**eclampsia**). Although 6 percent of pregnancies have this complication, its cause is not known. Toxemia is most frequent in first pregnancies, especially in the very young or in women over the age of 35. In later pregnancies, it may be associated with diabetes or vascular disease. Toxemia is most commonly found in women of low socioeconomic standing, and some evidence suggests that a tendency to this disorder is inherited. Untreated, toxemia can cause maternal or fetal death, but if properly treated it can usually be controlled.

Recent research on toxemia of pregnancy suggests that it may be prevented in many cases by the use of low doses of aspirin in the third trimester of pregnancy (Benigni et al., 1989; Schiff et al., 1989). Aspirin seems to work by suppressing the production of a prostaglandin-like substance from platelets (a type of blood cell) that causes spasms of the blood vessels and can lead to increases in blood pressure (Cunningham and Gant, 1989).

Birth Defects and Their Detection

Birth defects occur in approximately 3 percent of all live births and at a substantially higher rate in miscarried pregnancies. About 20 percent of birth defects are inherited, 3 to 5 percent reflect chromosome abnormalities, 2 to 3 percent are due to infections, and 5 percent are due to maternal drug use or exposure to environmental chemicals; but in the majority of cases no specific explanation can be discovered (Wilson, 1977).

Only two examples of birth defects will be mentioned here. **Down's syndrome** (also called trisomy 21 or mongolism) is a chromosome disorder that causes severe mental retardation and defects of the heart, kidneys, and intestines. Its incidence increases with advanced maternal age (see Table 4–3). Maternal infection with the virus that causes German measles (**rubella**) can also be dangerous to the developing baby. German measles causes serious defects in about half of exposed embryos during the first month of pregnancy, but this rate decreases to 25 percent in the second month and less than 15 percent in the third month. The fetal damage caused by rubella includes deafness, cataracts, heart defects, mental retardation, and retarded growth. Fortunately, as the number of cases of German measles in the United States has dropped dramatically—from 58,000 reported cases in 1969 to 225 reported cases in 1988—there has also been a major drop in cases of congenital rubella, with only 6 cases occurring in 1988 (*MMWR, 37*(54):Table 1, 1989).

Having a child with a birth defect can be frightening and disheartening. Our society emphasizes success and physical appearance, and the parents of a child with a defect may see their baby as a sign of a defect within themselves or as "punishment" for something they did wrong. Some parents react by rejection and denial, while others cope by bringing

TABLE 4–3

Risk of Chromosomal Abnormalities in Live Births, by Mother's Age

Maternal Age	Risk of Down's Syndrome	Risk of All Chromosome Abnormalities
20	1/1667	1/526
30	1/952	1/385
33	1/602	1/286
35	1/378	1/192
38	1/173	1/102
40	1/106	1/66
42	1/63	1/42
45	1/30	1/21

Source: American College of Obstetricians and Gynecologists, 1989.

extra love and care to their newborn and accepting the infant as a full-fledged family member. Some families find new strength and closeness after the birth of a child with a defect.

Fortunately, there are now several ways of detecting the presence of certain types of defects in the developing fetus. In the procedure called **amniocentesis** (Figure 4–7), a sample of amniotic fluid is obtained by inserting a needle into the uterus after first deadening the abdominal wall with a local anesthetic. Analysis of the fluid can identify a variety of genetic disorders (e.g., Down's syndrome and muscular dystrophy) as well as the sex of the fetus. If a serious abnormality is uncovered, the parents can consider terminating the pregnancy by abortion if this choice is consistent with their personal values. There is about a 1 percent risk that amniocentesis may result in loss of the fetus, but this risk must be balanced with the benefits of a highly reliable means of identifying serious genetic problems.

A newer technique, called **chorionic villi sampling (CVS)** is seen by some authorities as having even greater usefulness. This method, which involves insertion of a thin catheter through the vagina and cervix into the uterus (see Figure 4–8), takes a small sample of tissue from the chorionic villi—tiny threadlike protrusions on the chorion membrane that surrounds the fetus. But unlike amniocentesis, which cannot be done until the sixteenth week of pregnancy, CVS can be done at the eighth week—almost as soon as a woman knows she's pregnant. Furthermore, the results from CVS are available in two days, whereas it usually takes three to four weeks to get the results of an amniocentesis. Thus, if a birth defect is detected, a first-trimester abortion can be done, which is much safer than an abortion after 20 or more weeks of pregnancy. There is one drawback to CVS, however: there is a 3.8 percent rate of spontaneous abortion after it is done (Hogge, Schonberg, and Golbus, 1986). Since this rate is approximately the same as the spontaneous abortion rate found in women who do not undergo CVS (and have pregnancies of comparable lengths), it is not yet certain how many of

toxemia a complication of pregnancy marked by sudden increase in blood pressure, edema, and protein in the urine.

preeclampsia (prē′ e klamp′ sē uh) a condition occurring during the latter half of pregnancy characterized by high blood pressure, edema, and protein in the urine. May progress to **eclampsia.**

eclampsia (e klamp sē uh) a condition occurring during the latter half of pregnancy marked by high blood pressure, edema, protein in the urine, and convulsions, sometimes resulting in coma or death. Also known as **toxemia** of pregnancy.

Down's syndrome a chromosome disorder that causes mental retardation and defects of the heart, kidneys, and intestines. Also known as trisomy 21 or mongolism.

rubella (roo bel′ uh) German measles. If the virus crosses the placental barrier to the fetus, it can cause serious malformations including deafness, eye problems, and mental retardation.

amniocentesis (am′ nē ō sen tē′ sis) procedure used to obtain a sample of amniotic fluid from the uterus of a pregnant woman to be analyzed for a variety of genetic disorders and biochemical abnormalities in the fetus.

chorionic villi sampling (CVS) a method for diagnosing defects in the developing fetus; done by inserting a catheter through the vagina and cervix to take a small piece of tissue from the edge of the chorion, the membrane surrounding the fetus.

FIGURE 4–7

Amniocentesis

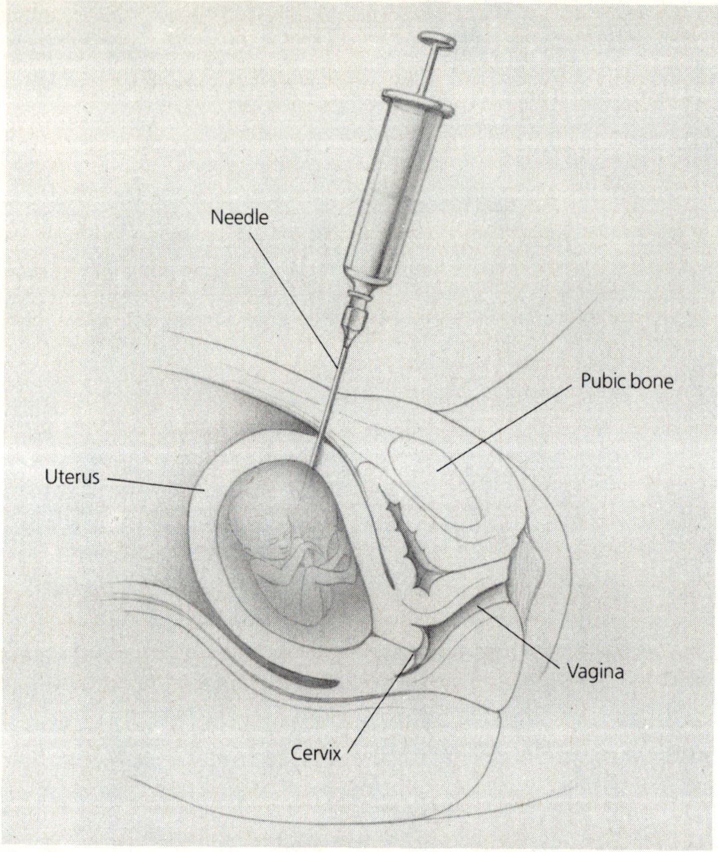

Amniocentesis involves removing a small amount of amniotic fluid from inside the pregnant uterus. The fluid is then analyzed in a laboratory to provide information about many types of birth defects or genetic conditions that may affect the fetus.

these pregnancies would have aborted even if the procedure had not been done. A more recent study of CVS done in more than 2200 women at seven different hospitals reported an excess rate of fetal loss of less than 1 percent compared to a group of women who underwent amniocentesis (Rhoads et al., 1989). Based on this difference, it appears that amniocentesis is slightly safer, but with the disadvantage of the delays involved, CVS will be the procedure of choice for many couples.

Another technique used to detect many birth defects (although it does not check for most genetic diseases that can be detected by amniocentesis or CVS) is the use of ultrasound examination. Ultrasonic waves are used to form a picture of the fetus. If a birth defect is detected it can sometimes be treated while the baby is still developing within the uterus, or this information may be used to plan for early delivery so the baby can receive corrective treatment (Hill, Breckle, and Gehrking, 1983). Ultrasound can also be used to evaluate the growth of the fetus, to determine if there is multiple pregnancy (twins, triplets, etc.), and to aid in the diagnosis of certain types of medical problems affecting the mother or baby.

FIGURE 4–8

Chorionic Villi Sampling

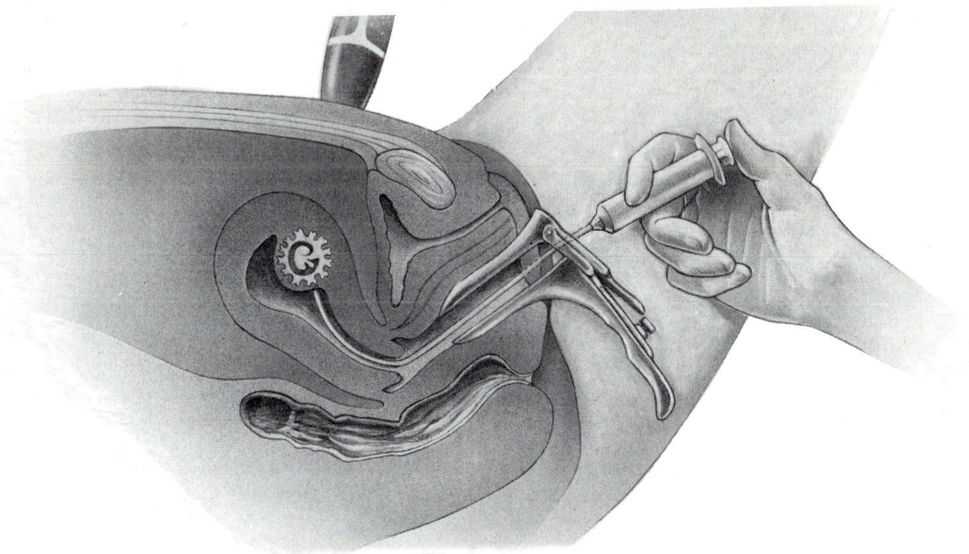

Although ultrasound studies are now done in more than half of all pregnancies (both for diagnostic purposes and to check the sex of the developing fetus), some have questioned the use of the procedure since there is no long-term data proving the safety of this technique.

Ectopic Pregnancy

Ectopic pregnancy (a pregnancy occurring outside the cavity of the uterus) occurs approximately once in every 100 pregnancies (Breen, 1970; Frankin and Zeiderman, 1973; Rubin, 1983). The number of ectopic pregnancies in the United States more than quadrupled from 1970 to 1986 (Figure 4–9), which probably reflects both improved diagnostic methods and an increased incidence of scarring of the Fallopian tubes as a result of pelvic inflammatory disease (see Chapter 7). The highest rates of ectopic pregnancy are in women 35 years of age or older and in women who are nonwhite (Centers for Disease Control, 1989a).

About 97 percent of ectopic pregnancies occur in the Fallopian tubes (tubal pregnancy); in the remainder of cases, the fertilized egg implants in the ovary, the abdomen, or the cervix. Ectopic pregnancies are usually caused by conditions that block or slow the passage of the fertilized egg into the uterus such as anatomical abnormalities, scar tissue resulting from surgery or infections, or tumors. The presence of an IUD (intrauterine device, a means of contraception) is also associated with an increased chance of ectopic pregnancy (Marchbanks et al., 1988).

Most ectopic pregnancies abort at a relatively early stage, but when growth of the embryo, placenta, and membranes occurs, there is a substantial risk of rupture and bleeding. Because it is difficult to diagnose this condition, ectopic pregnancy is the seventh leading cause of maternal death. The recurrence rate of an ectopic pregnancy in subsequent pregnancies is about 20 percent.

Until recently, ectopic pregnancies were treated by surgery requiring hospitalization (Ory, 1989). The surgery either involves making a small slit in the Fallopian tube to remove the ectopic pregnancy or excising the part of the tube containing the pregnancy. Now it has been found that some cases can be managed medically, on an outpatient basis, using injections of a drug called methotrexate (generally used to treat cancer) that causes the developing embryo to be resorbed before it gets large enough to rupture the Fallopian tube (Stovall, Ling, and Buster, 1989).

FIGURE 4–9

Ectopic Pregnancy Rates, by Year—United States, 1970–1987*

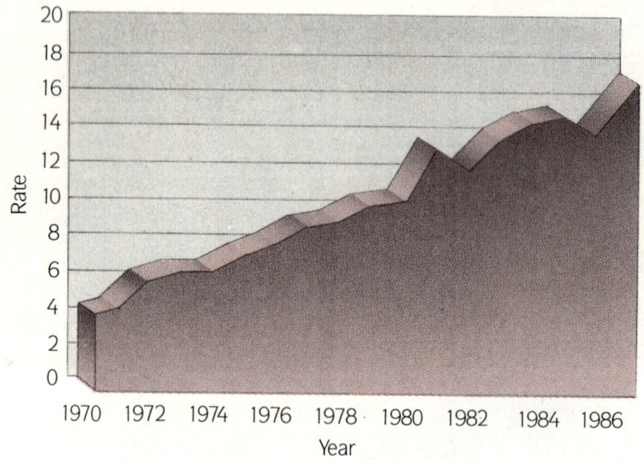

* *Per 1000 reported pregnancies.*
Source: Center for Disease Control, MMWR *39: 401, 1990.*

While this treatment approach is still in the experimental stages, it may prove useful since newer medical procedures, such as ultrasound, often lead to the earlier diagnosis of ectopic pregnancy than in the past.

Rh Incompatibility

Rh incompatibility refers to a condition in which antibodies (proteins that fight off foreign substances that invade the body) from the mother's bloodstream destroy red blood cells in the fetus, causing fetal anemia, mental retardation, or death. This problem occurs only when a mother whose blood does not have the Rh factor (Rh negative) has a fetus with the Rh factor (Rh positive), a combination that can occur only if the father is Rh positive. Even in this circumstance, the risk is usually not in the first pregnancy (since antibodies have not yet formed in the woman's circulation to the Rh factor) but applies to later pregnancies with an Rh positive fetus.

The development of Rh sensitivity can be prevented by the use of a medication called Rho-GAM, which neutralizes antibody formation. This must be given within 72 hours after delivery (or abortion) of an Rh positive fetus to an Rh negative mother. If sensitivity is already present, either from a blood transfusion or an earlier pregnancy, the fetus can be given a special blood transfusion while still inside the uterus.

INFERTILITY

People usually assume that reproduction happens almost automatically, but 10 to 15 percent of couples trying to have a baby do not succeed after a year or more without the use of contraception. This condition, known as **infertility,** has been greatly misunderstood. Often the source of considerable anguish and embarrassment, it rarely poses a direct threat to nonreproductive health or longevity.

Causes

Although the woman typically seeks medical help first, both partners in an infertile couple often have conditions that contribute to their inability to conceive. Thus, it is important that both the man and woman be seen by a physician, since proper treatment and an optimal chance for pregnancy depend on accurate testing. In about 85 percent of couples with infertility, a specific cause can be found.

FEMALE INFERTILITY

The two major causes of female infertility are failure to ovulate and blockage of the Fallopian tubes. Lack of ovulation (or infrequent ovulation) can be caused by ovarian disorders, hormone abnormalities, certain types of chronic illness, drug addiction or abuse, and poor nutrition. Rarely, ovulation is blocked by psychological stress.

Failure to ovulate may be detected by the use of **basal body temperature (BBT)** charts, hormone testing, or scraping the lining of the uterus to examine tissue under a microscope. The BBT chart is obtained by the woman's daily measurement of her temperature immediately after awakening and before getting out of bed. During the first portion of the menstrual cycle the BBT is low, but as progesterone production in the ovary increases just after ovulation, the temperature shifts upward and remains higher for 10 to 16 days (Figure 4–10). BBT increases just after ovulation; if no temperature shift is seen, it is an indication that ovulation did not occur.

Although keeping BBT charts was, until recently, the primary method used for predicting the timing or presence of ovulation, new do-it-yourself urine tests allow users to monitor levels of **luteinizing hormone (LH)** in their urine to identify the LH surge that precedes ovulation by 12 to 24 hours. Based on the same sort of monoclonal antibody technology used in some at-home pregnancy test kits, the LH tests are marked under trade names such as First Response, Ovutime, and OvuStick. While the tests must be done on four to six consecutive days for best accuracy and are expensive (usually costing $40 to $60 for a kit that permits testing for one month), they are much more precise than BBT patterns in identifying whether and when ovulation occurs (March, 1985).

Blocked Fallopian tubes may be caused by scarring after an infection in the pelvic tissues or abdomen. Blocked tubes can also result from **endometriosis,** a common disorder in which endometrial tissue (the tissue lining the uterine cavity) grows outside the uterus in other pelvic or abdominal organs, often leading to scar formation.

Endometriosis is usually diagnosed by inspecting the female reproductive organs through a procedure called **laparoscopy,** in which a thin, lighted telescope-like tube is inserted into the abdomen through a small incision next to the navel. If endometrial implants or cysts are found, a small piece of the abnormal tissue can be removed and thoroughly analyzed under a microscope.

The Fallopian tubes can be checked for obstruction by either **Rubin's test,** which involves inserting carbon dioxide into the uterus and seeing if this gas passes into the abdomen, or by x-rays of the uterus and tubes using a dye that outlines these structures. The x-ray method is preferred by most physicians because it is more accurate.

Other less frequent causes of female infertility include abnormal cervical mucus that impedes the passage of sperm, birth defects of the reproductive organs, tumors, infections (see Chapter 7), and allergy to sperm. In some cases, not having intercourse close to the time of ovulation may be a problem, and in other instances, the use of artificial lubricants like Vaseline or K-Y Jelly may be killing the sperm (but these preparations should not be considered as spermicides for birth control purposes).

MALE INFERTILITY

The primary cause of male infertility is a low sperm count. Less than 40 million sperm per cubic centimeter is below normal, but pregnancy is often possible with sperm counts of 20 million per cubic centimeter. With lower counts, the chances of impregnation are

Rh incompatibility condition in which antibodies from the mother's bloodstream destroy red blood cells in the fetus, causing anemia, mental retardation, or fetal death.

infertility the inability of a couple to achieve pregnancy, usually defined after a year or more of sexual intercourse without pregnancy.

basal body temperature (BBT) temperature taken immediately after awakening and used to predict ovulation.

luteinizing hormone (LH) (lū′ tē in īz′ ing) produced by the pituitary gland, LH triggers ovulation and stimulates the Ley dig cells to manufacture testosterone.

endometriosis the occurrence of endometrial tissue in locations other than the uterus; a frequent cause of female infertility.

laparoscopy an exploratory visualization of the pelvic and abdominal organs using a tube-like instrument.

Rubin's test a procedure to check for obstructed Fallopian tubes. Carbon dioxide is inserted into the uterus to see if it passes into the abdomen.

FIGURE 4–10

Basal Body Temperature (BBT) Patterns

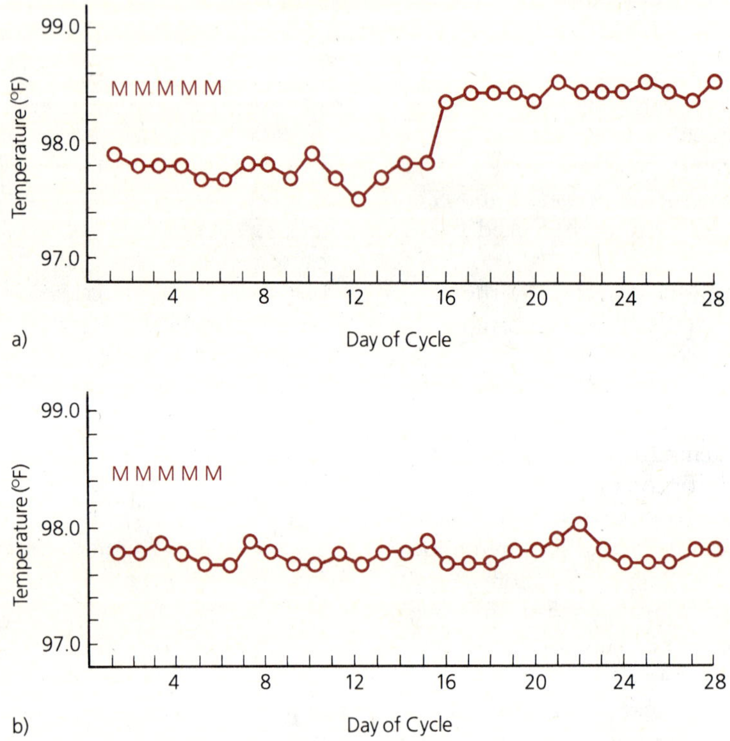

(a) The pronounced, sustained temperature rise beginning at day 16 indicates that ovulation occurred. (b) The absence of a sustained temperature rise suggests that ovulation did not occur in this cycle. (Days of menstrual flow are indicated by M.)

Source: From Robert C. Kolodny, William H. Masters, and Virginia E. Johnson, Textbook of Sexual Medicine, *© 1979 by Robert C. Kolodny, William H. Masters, and Virginia E. Johnson. Reprinted by permission of Little, Brown and Company.*

considerably reduced. Other factors that determine male fertility include the ability of sperm to swim, the number of abnormal sperm, and the volume of seminal fluid.

Low sperm counts can be caused by testicular injury, infection (especially mumps occurring after childhood, when it can spread to the testes), radiation, endocrine disorders, varicose veins in the scrotum, undescended testes, and birth defects. Drug use can also impair sperm production, with alcohol, cigarettes, narcotics, marijuana, and some prescription medications potential sources of such a problem (Kolodny, Masters, and Johnson, 1979). Some reports indicate that long-distance bicycle riding or tight-fitting underwear can lower sperm counts (Shane, Schiff, and Wilson, 1976). Since sperm production is sensitive to temperature, prolonged and frequent use of saunas, hot tubs, and steam baths may have a negative effect. A high frequency of ejaculation can also lower the sperm count (but not enough to be reliable as a contraceptive method!).

In the male, just as in the female, the reproductive tubing system may be blocked as a result of infection or birth defect. If the blockage is complete, no sperm will be in the ejaculate, even though sperm production in the testes is normal. Infertility can result if the male is unable to ejaculate, if he ejaculates outside the vagina, or if he is unable to have intercourse because of erectile difficulties. These conditions are discussed in Chapter 9.

Treatment

Women who do not ovulate can frequently be helped by treatment with clomiphene, a pill that induces ovulation by stimulating the pituitary to secrete LH and **follicle stimulating hormone (FSH).** About half of the women given this medication become pregnant. There is a modestly increased chance of having a multiple pregnancy (twins, triplets, etc.), which occurs about 8 percent of the time with clomiphene compared to 1.2 percent in routine pregnancies. Women who do not achieve a pregnancy with clomiphene may be treated with HMG (human menopausal gonadotropins), which is given in a series of injections. This medication acts directly on the ovaries, bypassing the pituitary gland, and induces ovulation in more than 90 percent of women with functioning ovaries. Pregnancy is achieved by 60 to 70 percent of women receiving this treatment, and 20 percent of these pregnancies are multiple (15 percent are twins, and 5 percent are triplets, quadruplets, quintuplets, or sextuplets). Neither clomiphene nor HMG causes a greater risk of abortion or birth defects than in naturally occurring pregnancies. These drugs, however, can overstimulate the ovaries, causing them to enlarge (sometimes to the size of grapefruit) and to leak fluid into the abdomen. This condition, which is more common with HMG than with clomiphene, usually requires hospitalization because there is a danger that the ovaries may rupture.

Blocked Fallopian tubes can sometimes be treated by microsurgery. Using a microscope for visual guidance, a surgeon removes the obstruction and then sews together the healthy portions of the tubes with tiny needles and suture material. Microsurgery is successful in only 30 to 50 percent of women with tubal problems at the present time (Jacobs et al., 1988). Women who have tubal damage beyond surgical repair or women without Fallopian tubes now have the possibility of being treated by *in vitro* fertilization, the dramatic "test-tube baby" procedure, which we discuss shortly.

When endometriosis is the cause of infertility, it is usually treated by surgery. One promising development is the use of laser technology, in which the surgeon focuses a laser beam to burn away endometrial implants or adhesions. Since the laser beam actually seals off small blood vessels in the surgical area as it burns away diseased tissue, there is very little blood loss with this procedure. Pregnancy rates after laser laparoscopy are in the 40 to 65 percent range (Berger, Goldstein, and Fuerst, 1989). Endometriosis can also be treated with drugs such as danazol.

The treatment of male infertility is considerably less developed. Surgical repair of varicose veins in the scrotum can improve the sperm count substantially, but most other conditions respond poorly to treatment. The use of testosterone to achieve a "rebound effect" after first suppressing sperm production is sometimes useful, but the results obtained from using clomiphene in men have been inconclusive. Proper medical management of infections, anatomical defects, or hormonal disorders is definitely helpful, but such cases are relatively few. In men with borderline sperm counts, daily ejaculation can actually lower fertility by reducing the number of sperm, and the chances for a pregnancy can be improved by decreasing the frequency of ejaculation to a minimum of 48 hours from one time to the next.

Two Canadian studies raise some important questions about the results currently attained in treating infertility. In the first, a two- to seven-year follow-up of 1145 infertile couples showed that the pregnancy rate in the treated couples (41 percent) was just slightly better than that in untreated couples (35 percent) (Collins et al., 1983). The second study showed that the cumulative pregnancy rate in untreated couples with unexplained infertility was 65 percent (Rousseau et al., 1983). Thus, since many cases of infertility achieve pregnancy spontaneously, it appears important for physicians to perform careful diagnostic testing to determine whether, and if, treatment is required. Likewise, couples contending with infertility should realize that pregnancy is quite possible in many cases even if medical treatment initially doesn't seem to be effective.

ARTIFICIAL INSEMINATION

Artificial insemination means placing semen in the vagina or uterus by a means other than sexual inter-

follicle stimulating hormone (FSH) a substance produced in the pituitary gland that prepares the ovary for ovulation and stimulates the production of sperm cells in the testes.

course. There are two basic types of artificial insemination: using semen from the husband (AIH) or using semen from a donor. For either method, the woman's fertility status must be relatively normal.

AIH can be tried if the husband's count is low but not zero. For practical reasons, successful AIH is infrequent if the count is less than 10 million per cubic centimeter or if the sperm motility is low. AIH is best done by inserting a fresh semen specimen in the vagina at the mouth of the cervix. Using frozen, thawed specimens reduces sperm motility, and combining several frozen specimens does not seem to improve the outcome. Injecting the semen into the uterus causes severe cramping and poses a risk of infection. AIH works by concentrating the husband's sperm at the mouth of the cervix; with coitus, only a small fraction of sperm get to this location.

Donor insemination is used when the husband's sperm count is zero or very low. A donor, selected on the basis of excellent health, good intelligence, and closeness of physical characteristics to the husband, provides a masturbated semen specimen (for which he is paid). The donor's identity is unknown to the couple. The legal status of donor insemination is uncertain in many states, although in California once the husband signs a consent form agreeing to use of a donor, he is the legal father of the baby. The pregnancy rate for donor insemination is about 60 percent using frozen semen obtained from a sperm bank.

The decision to undergo donor insemination must be made jointly by husband and wife; clearly this type of treatment is not psychologically right for everyone for whom it might be used. Some people equate this procedure with adultery, others have conflicts with their religious values, and some fear that the husband will reject or dislike the baby because it is not "his." Despite the latter concern, almost all couples who achieve a pregnancy using donor sperm find that the experience brings them very close together and that the husband's excitement at fatherhood is genuinely felt. In some locations, donor insemination is also being used by single women who want to become pregnant.

IVF: *In Vitro* FERTILIZATION

Late in the evening of July 25, 1978, a slightly premature 5 pound, 12 ounce baby girl was born by cesarean section to Lesley and John Brown of Oldham, England. They named their healthy, normal baby Louise, and since then her name and picture have made the pages of nearly every major newspaper in the Western world. The sperm and egg that united to conceive Louise met not in Lesley Brown's Fallopian tube, but in a test tube, *in vitro*, outside the mother's body. Louise Brown was the first baby ever born from *in vitro* fertilization techniques (see Figure 4–11).

The British doctors responsible for this remarkable achievement were Patrick Steptoe and Robert Edwards. Steptoe had been experimenting with ***in vitro* fertilization (IVF)** for more than a decade before meeting Lesley Brown, who was unable to conceive because of blocked Fallopian tubes. She had undergone surgery to unblock the tubes before coming to Steptoe. The surgery was not only unsuccessful, but when Steptoe did his exploration of her reproductive organs, he found the tubes so badly damaged ("mere remnants," he said) that they were removed.

Lesley was first given hormones to stimulate the maturation of eggs in her ovaries. Steptoe and Edwards then made a small incision near her navel and by using an instrument that magnifies and illuminates the tiny ovum, they withdrew a ripe egg and placed it in a laboratory dish. The dish contained a carefully mixed culture of nutrients designed to resemble the environment of the Fallopian tubes. As quickly as possible, John Brown's sperm (obtained through masturbation) were added to the culture, and the doctors waited for one of the sperm to impregnate the egg. Meanwhile, Lesley was given more hormones to ensure that her uterus would accept a fertilized egg. After the sperm and egg united in the laboratory dish and the pre-embryonic cells began to divide, the blastocyst (a hollow sphere of 60 separate cells) was inserted into Lesley's uterus. In about a week, the doctors knew the pre-embryo attached itself to a wall of the uterus and Lesley Brown was pregnant.

Steptoe and Edwards had made more than 30 attempts to implant eggs fertilized outside the mother before their success with the Browns. Two pregnancies had resulted, but both were spontaneously aborted—one because the membrane around the embryo ruptured and the other because of a genetic abnormality. This second case is a cause of concern by doctors working in this area. Who is responsible for a child born with genetic damage? Did the damage result from handling the pre-embryo outside the uterus, or would it have occurred even during normal fertilization? Is destroying a fertilized egg in a test tube abortion?

Since the initial breakthrough by Steptoe and Edwards, a large number of IVF clinics have opened

FIGURE 4–11

The Steps Involved in the In Vitro *Fertilization Process*

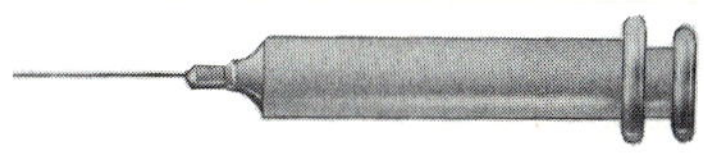

(a) Daily hormone injections stimulate egg production. About seven days later, a shot of the hormone HCG causes the release of eggs.

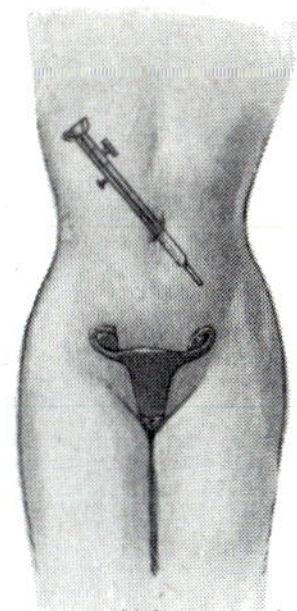

(b) A laparoscope is inserted at the navel to view the follicles, which hold the eggs. The eggs are retrieved using a hollow needle.

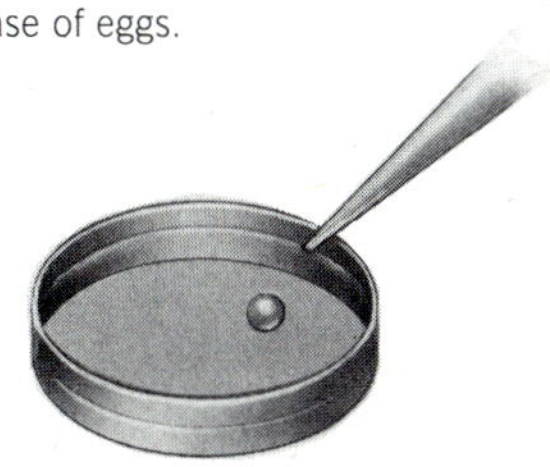

(c) Each egg is placed in a petri dish containing a culture medium that duplicates the chemical environment in the uterus. While incubation begins, sperm are collected.

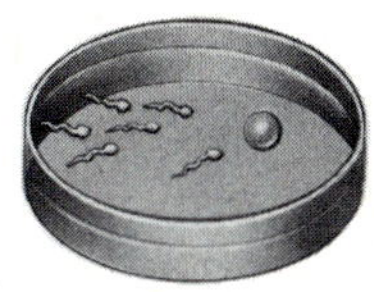

(d) Sperm are added 5 or 6 hours later. Only the most active sperm are used, reducing the number needed for fertilization.

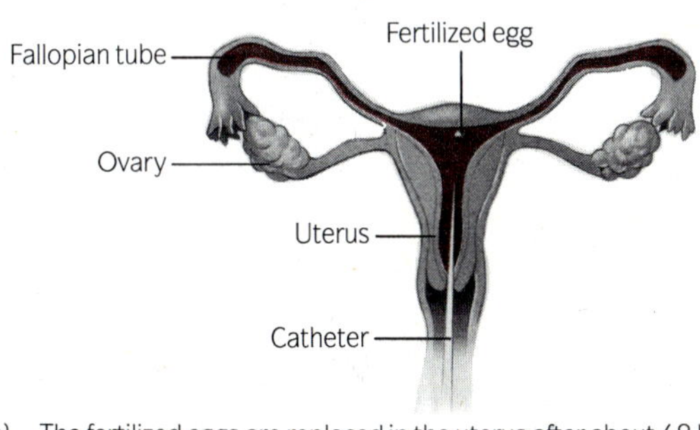

(e) The fertilized eggs are replaced in the uterus after about 48 hours of maturation. There implantation may take place.

around the world, including more than 200 clinics in the United States alone. More than 15,000 babies conceived *in vitro* had been born as of 1990, including 2627 live deliveries in 1988 in America (Medical Research International and Society for Assisted Reproductive Technology, 1990) and 3600 babies born in France in 1987 (*The New York Times*, April 11, 1989, p. C5). Aside from a higher rate of multiple pregnancies and a very high cesarean rate (50 to 60 percent

***in vitro* fertilization** a procedure involving removing eggs from a woman's body and fertilizing them with sperm in a laboratory. After successful fertilization, the embryo is surgically implanted in the woman's uterus.

in many clinics)—reflecting both older maternal ages and the "premium" nature of such pregnancies—the overall obstetrical experience with IVF is largely comparable to that expected in a similar group of women who had conceived by natural means (Andrews et al., 1986; Seibel, 1988). Particularly notable are several studies that show that there is no increased risk of birth defects or developmental difficulties for IVF children (Seibel, 1988; Morin et al., 1989).

The best candidates for IVF are women younger than 35 who have normal menstrual cycles and a husband with a normal sperm count (Berger, Goldstein, and Fuerst, 1989). (About 50 percent of IVF programs will treat women 40 or older, and most will also proceed if the sperm count is mildly to moderately reduced; if the sperm count is very low, or zero, then the couple can consider IVF using donor sperm.) IVF can overcome many of the causes of infertility, including blocked or absent Fallopian tubes, severe endometriosis, and immunologic infertility that in the past were almost insurmountable obstacles to pregnancy for hundreds of thousands of couples.

Like any complicated medical procedure, there are some drawbacks. For one thing, IVF is expensive, generally costing $4000 to $6000 for each attempt at pregnancy. This has led to charges of commercialism (especially directed at private, for-profit clinics) as well as some rancor toward health insurance companies that refuse to pay for such procedures. Another problem is that not all IVF clinics have comparable results: in fact, some have never had a successful pregnancy resulting in a live birth (Raymond, 1988). Since the IVF "industry" is essentially unregulated, even physicians involved in the field have been worried that there may be misleading claims and practices that may confuse, or even bilk, the public. This is especially troublesome since couples turning to IVF are often emotionally overwrought as a result of their lengthy efforts to have a child, so they are not apt to be as objective as consumers shopping for a new car. (A checklist of questions to ask to help you evaluate an IVF program can be found on page 113.) In addition, since live deliveries result from only about 12 percent of IVF stimulation cycles, it is clear that not every couple going through this physically and emotionally arduous procedure will wind up with a baby. [Some experts believe that ultimately only half the couples attempting IVF will be successful, with this success usually coming in the first four cycles in which IVF is attempted (Seibel, 1988; Seibel, Ranoux, and Kearnan, 1989).]

To put all this in perspective, it is helpful to remember that despite the expenses and problems involved, IVF is in many ways a miracle come true. As one happy father said:

> We had basically given up on ever getting pregnant after more than ten years of treatment. When an IVF program opened up at the university nearby, we decided to give it one more shot. Now we have two-year-old twins who are a testimonial to the skill of the team at the clinic. What better reward could persistence ever have? *(Authors' files)*

OTHER ASSISTED REPRODUCTIVE TECHNIQUES

A number of related procedures have been developed as outgrowths of IVF. These are briefly summarized here.

1. **GIFT (Gamete Intrafallopian Transfer)** involves the direct placement of a mixture of sperm and eggs into the Fallopian tube. Fertilization takes place naturally, in the Fallopian tube, rather than in the laboratory, as it does with IVF. A woman must have at least one normal Fallopian tube to be a candidate for GIFT, but this procedure generally has somewhat higher success rates than IVF: an overall 21 percent live delivery rate was reported for 135 clinics in the United States in 1988, with some centers having rates of 30 percent or more (Medical Research International and Society for Assisted Reproductive Technology, 1990). GIFT is particularly useful in dealing with endometriosis, unexplained infertility, and cervical factor infertility (where the chemical environment of the cervix seems to kill sperm). It ensures that the ovum and a large number of motile sperm reach the physiologic fertilization site—the Fallopian tube. [GIFT can be combined with donor insemination if the male has a poor sperm count; this method has a high rate of success (Cefalu et al., 1988).]
2. **ZIFT (Zygote Intrafallopian Transfer)** combines IVF with GIFT. The wife's eggs are fertilized by her husband's sperm *in vitro*. The zygote (the fertilized egg) is then transferred to the Fallopian tube within 24 hours. The advantage to this procedure is that the medical team can be certain that fertilization has occurred. If fertilization doesn't take place, then the couple can decide if they want to try donor insemination.
3. **Egg donors** are used in some programs for women who are unable to ovulate or who don't have ovaries. Egg donation—although only re-

QUESTIONS TO ASK ABOUT AN IVF/GIFT PROGRAM

With any medical treatment, patients should ask questions to determine how appropriate the treatment is for them, how qualified and experienced the personnel are in providing the treatment, what to expect in terms of costs and time, and perhaps most important, how successful the treatment may be. When it comes to highly technical procedures such as those involved in IVF or GIFT, the importance of these queries cannot be stressed enough when it comes to gathering the information needed to make an informed decision.

The following list provides 11 key questions to ask when evaluating an IVF/GIFT program. As a practical matter, if you don't get straight answers to these questions, or if the doctor or program director you're discussing them with seems annoyed at your inquisitiveness, it is usually wisest to find a different program.

1. When was your program started?
2. When did the program perform its first IVF (or GIFT) procedure?
3. How many babies have been born as a result of this program's IVF (or GIFT) procedures? How many babies have been born in the last two years in this program from IVF or GIFT?
4. What is your clinical pregnancy rate per IVF (or GIFT) procedure? What is your clinical pregnancy rate for couples our age with our particular type of problem?
5. Do you freeze eggs or embryos as part of your program? If so, what is done with them after we've had a baby?
6. Do you offer an egg donation program? If so, do we provide the donor or do you?
7. Does your program report its results to the IVF Registry?
8. Are any of your doctors board certified in Reproductive Endocrinology?
9. How much does the entire procedure cost per cycle, including the cost of drugs?
10. Do we need to pay in advance? (If so, how much?)
11. Do you have an age limit for patients?

---

cently undertaken—is somewhat like sperm donation. The donor in some programs is completely anonymous but matched for physical characteristics with the recipient (Kennard et al., 1989). In other programs, only donors selected by the woman wishing to conceive are used (Sauer et al., 1989). Most commonly, a sister or close relative is the egg donor, but personal friends and sometimes people paid for the egg donation serve as donors. Egg donation may be particularly useful for women who want to avoid passing on a genetic disorder in the wife's family, like hemophilia, to their children. Once the eggs are obtained from the donor, fertilization with the husband's sperm is usually done in the laboratory; the fertilized egg can then be placed by ZIFT into the Fallopian tubes or handled as a straightforward IVF procedure. (The recipient must be prepared by hormonal stimulation so her uterus is ready to accept a pregnancy.) Just as

gamete intrafallopian transfer (GIFT) the direct placement of a mixture of sperm and eggs into the Fallopian tube as a treatment for infertility.

zygote intrafallopian transfer (ZIFT) a technique of assisted reproductive technology in which the woman's eggs are fertilized *in vitro*, after which the zygote is placed in the Fallopian tube.

egg donors women who volunteer to provide their eggs for the purposes of treating anovulatory infertility or avoiding the transmittal of a genetic disorder in another woman.

with sperm donation, ethical and religious concerns about egg donation abound, as might be expected with a relatively new technology of this sort. Results obtained with egg donation are about the same as with assisted reproductive techniques using the wife's own eggs.

4. **Embryo transplant** is a more controversial method that uses the husband's sperm to artificially inseminate a woman who is not his wife. Five days later the embryo is flushed out of the donor's uterus, where it is in the earliest stages of implantation, and transplanted into the wife's uterus. If it implants successfully, a normal pregnancy typically ensues. (A key element to this procedure is synchronizing the recipient's menstrual cycle with the donor's by hormone injections so that the recipient's endometrium is properly "primed" to accept the transferred embryo and to allow it to implant.) Potential problems with this method include the need to be certain of the donor's health and guaranteeing that she abstain completely from using drugs or alcohol during the cycle in which she conceives. There may also be legal difficulties in some states, so couples should check with an attorney before undertaking this approach to having a baby.
5. **Embryo freezing** is another very recent development; the first human birth from a frozen embryo (actually, a frozen pre-embryo) was in 1985 (Fugger, 1989). One of the major reasons for freezing pre-embryos is to reduce the risk of multiple pregnancy when the woman has "superovulated"—produced a large number of eggs—in response to the hormonal stimulation given in an egg retrieval cycle as part of IVF. In addition, freezing the extra pre-embryos cuts down the costs of future treatment cycles, since it isn't necessary to retrieve more eggs. Prior to 1989, approximately 2000 patients had a total of more than 7000 eggs and pre-implantation embryos frozen at 25 clinics across the country, and 48 live births have already occurred after thawing (Fugger, 1989). However, thawing doesn't always work; there are still some concerns that freezing and thawing might damage the fertilized egg, with unknown consequences; and ethical and legal questions abound. For instance, who "owns" the pre-embryo if a couple divorces or if the couple dies? Who determines when, or if, to destroy the frozen pre-embryo?

SURROGATE MOTHERHOOD

Some couples composed of an infertile wife and a fertile husband have hired a woman to act as a "surrogate mother." Such a stand-in is artificially inseminated using the husband's sperm and carries the pregnancy to term, at that point giving the baby for adoption to the couple who had hired her. In at least one case, a surrogate mother was implanted with an ovum from an infertile woman that was fertilized *in vitro* by sperm from the infertile woman's husband (Utian et al., 1985). The infertile woman had previously undergone surgical removal of her uterus and Fallopian tubes and so was unable to carry her own pregnancy, but she still had functioning ovaries, which allowed one of her own eggs to be used for transfer to the surrogate mother after IVF

It is currently estimated that hundreds of surrogate mothers have contracted with couples to bear a child for them for pay (ranging from $2000 to $20,000), with legal fees in the neighborhood of $5000.

In January 1983, the public's attention was drawn to this previously little-known practice by headlines announcing "Surrogate Infant Left Unclaimed." As the complicated story unraveled, what became clear was that the 26-year-old surrogate mother, Judy Stiver of Michigan, had given birth to a deformed and probably mentally retarded baby, only to have 46-year-old Alexander Malahoff of New York, who had contracted for the child, reject the child on the grounds that he was not the father. Although medical tests eventually supported Mr. Malahoff, the entire episode was an unsavory one in many respects, including a tasteless, prearranged television confrontation between the Stivers and Malahoff in which accusations seemed more important than the welfare of the child. Although the Stivers eventually agreed to keep the baby, who may need to be institutionalized, this case raises a number of difficult issues about the ethical implications of our new reproductive technologies.

What would have happened if Malahoff, or some future Malahoff, had proved to be the infant's father? Could he, as one journalist suggested, try to send the child back and demand a refund?

> Technological parenthood may have the trappings of a business, but it is not a business; it is the answer to someone's most personal prayers. So it should be seen and handled. If the answer to a particular prayer happens to emerge deformed, it is no less the prayer's answer; and, as so many parents of such "damaged goods" have discovered, they sometimes give more contentment to a family than whole and healthy children and thus provide answers to different prayers entirely. *(Rosenblatt, 1983, p. 90)*

This viewpoint seems laudable, but in the real world people don't always behave in kindhearted ways. What will become of deformed children born not only to surrogate mothers but to unmarried women using the services of a sperm bank? If a baby conceived by *in vitro* methods turns out to be defective, will lawsuits follow and financial repercussions ensue? Or are we on the verge of an era of government regulation of reproductive decisions along the lines envisioned by George Orwell in *1984* or Aldous Huxley in *Brave New World?*

Another twist in the surrogate mother story occurred in 1986, when Mary Beth Whitehead of Brick Township, New Jersey—who had contracted to bear a child for William and Elizabeth Stern, using Mr. Stern's sperm for artificial insemination—decided after the birth of a baby girl that she didn't want to give her up to the Sterns. Mrs. Whitehead and her husband fled to Florida with the baby, but in a much-publicized trial in 1987, a New Jersey court awarded custody to the Sterns and upheld the legality of the contract Mrs. Whitehead and the Sterns signed. Both the trial and the judge's decision provoked a great deal of controversy, with many observers feeling it was improper to enforce a contract that required Mrs. Whitehead to give up her baby.

Although as of mid-1990 no states have passed legislation barring the practice of surrogate motherhood, a number of states are considering such bills. But there is also a growing acceptance of the practice among the public, physicians, and attorneys. A representative of the American Bar Foundation noted:

> The movement has to be seen in the perspective of the strong autonomy our society puts on the child-bearing decision. Legislation banning surrogate motherhood would be held unconstitutional, infringing on a couple's procreative autonomy under the right of privacy. So, we have to think about a public policy to make the experience a better one for everyone involved. We can't take an ostrich-like approach to this anymore. *(Lawson, 1986, p. C18)*

On the other hand, a report from an expert panel on ethics and reproduction from the American Fertility Society raised a number of questions about the ethical propriety of permitting surrogate motherhood.

Adoption and Infertility

Adopting a child is another way of becoming a parent, although this option is far less available today than it was 20 years ago because of legalized abortion. Adoption is the only route to having a child if both partners are infertile. It is a common misconception that many women of infertile couples conceive shortly after adopting a child—presumably because the couples' pressure to reproduce is lessened (Lamb and Leurgans, 1979). While the conception certainly attracts attention, such couples were obviously not infertile.

The Impact of Infertility

Infertility is rarely an expected problem. Not being able to have a child when you want to can be frustrating, confusing, and depressing. Pressures may be felt from peers and family, spouses may blame each other for the failure to conceive, and sex may become work rather than fun as a couple "tries harder" to achieve a pregnancy. Many women feel empty and unfulfilled as they deal with a situation of infertility, and men often experience anxiety or depression because they incorrectly equate virility with the ability to father a child. Many men are so unwilling to deal with the issue of possible infertility (or afraid of what might be discovered) that they refuse to participate in medical testing. It is no wonder that marital tensions often flare up in this situation.

Being treated for infertility is frequently a source of sexual problems, since there are time pressures ("the doctor says to have intercourse Monday, Wednesday, and Friday this week"), restrictions ("not tonight, dear, I have to have my sperm count checked tomorrow"), and pressures to perform ("I'm ovulating today and we *have* to have intercourse. *Why* can't you get an erection?"). When sex becomes highly focused on the goal of reproduction, couples often dispense with aspects of sexual play that they previously enjoyed in an effort to "get down to business," thereby creating a hurried, unimaginative, and often emotionally detached experience. Under these circumstances, it is not surprising that sexual pleasure and responsivity both diminish.

SUMMARY

1. Conception occurs when sperm and egg meet in the Fallopian tube. This leads to a single fertilized cell called the zygote, which has 46 chro-

embryo transplant a method of treating female infertility that involves artificially inseminating a donor female, then removing the pre-implantation pre-embryo and transplanting it to the infertile woman's uterus.

embryo freezing a technique of freezing pre-embryo (usually zygotes or blastocysts) for use in subsequent menstrual cycles so as to reduce the risk of multiple gestations and reduce the cost of treating infertility.

mosomes, including two sex chromosomes (XY = male, XX = female). The zygote divides into a blastocyst that implants in the uterus.

2. The development of the embryo or fetus depends on the placenta, which transmits nourishment and filters wastes between the mother's body and her unborn child's. The embryo is protected by two membranes (the amnion and chorion) and the amniotic fluid. In the first trimester, all major organs develop in the fetus; in the second and third trimesters, these organs mature and the fetus undergoes considerable growth.
3. Early pregnancy is usually marked by missing a period, nausea, breast tenderness, and fatigue. Pregnancy tests, which are 95 to 98 percent accurate, depend on detecting human chorionic gonadotropin (HCG) in urine. The emotional reactions to pregnancy vary considerably from person to person, and even when a pregnancy is wanted it may be a source of uncertainty or worry.
4. The second trimester is a time of prominent physical changes for the pregnant woman: the uterus enlarges, making the abdomen bulge, and quickening occurs. It is usually a time of emotional tranquility and heightened sexual interest.
5. Physical discomfort becomes prominent in the third trimester, as the abdomen is occupied by a growing "resident" who kicks and turns a lot. Backache, leg cramps, shortness of breath, and frequent urination are common.
6. Proper prenatal care is important to the health of mother and fetus alike. This includes regular medical check-ups, proper nutrition, avoidance of unnecessary drugs, and prompt treatment of pregnancy complications such as toxemia. Attendance at childbirth classes and appropriate reading can help familiarize the parents-to-be with what lies ahead.
7. Sexual activity during pregnancy usually is possible without difficulty or risk. Although controversial, one study shows that sexual activity may reduce the frequency of premature labor.
8. Labor is divided into three stages. In the first (and longest) stage, the cervix effaces and dilates as a result of regular contractions of the uterus. In the second stage, the baby passes through the birth canal, and in the third stage, the placenta and membranes are delivered.
9. Different styles of childbirth are possible, including hospital or home delivery, induction of labor versus spontaneous labor, and use of natural childbirth or Lamaze techniques. None of these methods can guarantee a "painless" childbirth. In certain situations, cesarean section may be required to protect the child's or the mother's health.
10. The postpartum period, marked by an abrupt drop in hormone levels, is a time of adjustment. Postpartum depression is common but usually transient; adjusting to parenthood takes a while longer. Early parent–child bonding is thought to be of special significance to the child.
11. Lactation occurs because of hormone actions on the breasts. Breast-feeding provides an opportunity for a satisfying psychological experience as well as health benefits to the newborn child, but bottle-feeding has advantages of convenience and flexibility.
12. Problem pregnancies—prematurity, toxemia, birth defects, improper implantation, and Rh incompatibility—were outlined briefly.
13. Approximately one out of seven couples is affected by infertility, with the majority of cases due to failure to ovulate and blocked Fallopian tubes in women and low sperm count in men. While treatment with drugs can often induce ovulation, treating the other two problems is less successful at present. Artificial insemination using a donor's semen may be done if the husband's sperm count is poor; *in vitro* fertilization techniques (including egg donation and the use of frozen embryos) are now being used increasingly to treat women with infertility due to blocked Fallopian tubes; and hiring a surrogate mother is also sometimes done.

Thought Questions

1. Should a woman be prosecuted for child abuse if she uses an illegal substance during pregnancy? What if she drinks alcohol? Smokes cigarettes?
2. Is it correct to refer to an embryo as an "unborn baby"? "Unborn child"? "Unborn teenager"? "Unborn senior citizen"? Where do you draw the line, and why?
3. How would our society change if parents could reliably choose the sex of their children? Would most people do this? Ultrasound can tell the parents what the sex of the fetus is. Do most parents want to know? Would you?
4. How does having a first baby typically affect a couple in terms of their romantic relationship and their sex lives? Do their roles tend to change from "lovers" to "parents"? What can be done about this? Should anything be done about this?

5. What is the source of the commonly experienced let-down feeling following childbirth—the so-called postpartum blues? Do you think it is primarily physiological in nature or more a result of the increased workload that a baby represents? How can family and friends best help new parents?
6. Since amniocentesis and chorionic villi sampling are expensive procedures that are not totally without risk, should they be available for women who would be unwilling to have an abortion? Why would a woman have amniocentesis or CVS for the purpose of discovering if her fetus has a genetic defect, if she believes abortion is morally wrong?

Suggested Readings

Ashford, Janet. *The Whole Birth Catalog: A Sourcebook for Choices in Childbirth*. Trumansburg, NY: The Crossing Press, 1983. A most impressive collection of material about the various options for different styles of childbirth available today. Lots of diagrams, lists of suggested readings, and practical pointers throughout.

Berger, G. S.; Goldstein, M.; and Fuerst, M. *The Couple's Guide to Fertility: How New Medical Advances Can Help You Have a Baby*. New York: Doubleday, 1989. This is an outstanding resource book for any couple contending with infertility, explaining with great clarity the technical side of the latest medical advances and also offering many practical pointers regarding consumer awareness, legal issues, and costs. As a bonus, it has an extensive directory of leading fertility specialists and clinics.

Brown, Judith. *Nutrition for Your Pregnancy*. Minneapolis: University of Minnesota Press, 1983. A well-done, practical guide to nutrition during pregnancy and in the first three months of postpartum months. Answers almost every imaginable question in a readable but authoritative style.

Chesler, P. *Sacred Bond: The Legacy of Baby M*. New York: Times Books, 1988. A carefully thought through analysis of the Baby M surrogate mother case along with reflections on the social, legal, and ethical ramifications of surrogate parenthood and related issues.

Cunningham, F. G.; MacDonald, P. C.; and Gant, N. F. *Williams Obstetrics*, 18th edition. East Norwalk, CT: Appleton and Lange, 1989. This is the definitive medical textbook on obstetrics. We wouldn't call this easy bedtime reading, but it has all the facts as well as many detailed drawings that are useful. (Please note: Because this text has lots of information about problem pregnancies, it is not for worry-prone readers!)

Gilman, Lois. *The Adoption Resource Book*. New York: Harper & Row, 1987. A thorough overview of the process and options in adoption, including ample attention to the emotional aspects of raising adopted children. Includes useful discussion of international adoptions.

Grad, Rae; Bash, Deborah; Guyer, Ruth; Acevedo, Zoila; Trause, Mary Anne; and Reukauf, Diane. *The Father Book—Pregnancy and Beyond*. Washington, DC: Acropolis Books, 1981. A fine forum for answering questions and clearing up uncertainties for the expectant father.

Messenger, Maire. *The Breastfeeding Book*. New York: Van Nostrand Reinhold, 1982. The best book we've ever seen on this topic.

5

Birth Control and Abortion

- Without the use of birth control, 80 to 90 percent of fertile couples will conceive within one year of sexual activity (Ross, 1989).
- Although birth control pills are used by many young women in America, their use drops dramatically among women in their 30s and, often unnecessarily, is virtually nil among those over 35 (Potts, 1988; Kaeser, 1989).
- Although the popularity of condoms has increased considerably in the last decade—in part because they offer some protection against sexually transmitted diseases such as AIDS—many otherwise well-educated people are unaware of key facts about how to use them properly (Richwald et al., 1988; Pugh, 1989; Voeller, 1989).
- New national estimates of contraceptive failure rates indicate that spermicides alone are far less reliable than many other birth control methods (Jones and Forrest, 1989).
- Women who profess no religion have a higher abortion rate than do women with some religious affiliation; among the latter, Catholics are about as likely to have an abortion as are all women nationally, while Protestants and Jews are less likely to do so (Henshaw and Silverman, 1988).

TABLE 5–1

Current Contraceptive Method for Sexually Active U.S. Women Aged 18 to 44, 1987[a]

Method	*Percentage*
Sterilization, female	22
Sterilization, male	16
Pill	32
Condom	16
IUD	3
Diaphragm	4
Foam	1
Cream/jelly	0.5
Suppository	1
Sponge	3
Rhythm	5
Withdrawal	5
Douche	1
No contraception	7

[a] Does not include women who are pregnant or trying to become pregnant, women who have had hysterectomies, or women who are infertile.

Source: Modified from Forrest and Fordyce, 1988, Table 5.

Methods for preventing unwanted or unintended pregnancy either are not used, are misused, or are used sporadically by many people. Those who rely on "faith" and "hope" as their primary contraceptives are playing a risky form of reproductive roulette, as many discover to their surprise. Others depend on unreliable contraceptive techniques like douching, using Saran wrap, or using tampons. Contrary to common misbelief, female orgasm is not a requirement for conception, and making love while standing up or crossing your fingers doesn't prevent sperm from reaching the egg.

Not too long ago, contraceptive products could not be displayed or sold in certain states, abortions were illegal, and birth control methods were not very reliable. (The landmark case of *Griswold* v. *Connecticut* that established the legality of selling contraceptive products occurred in 1965.) Although times have changed remarkably, people are now faced with a vast number of birth control products or methods, each with its own advantages and disadvantages (Table 5–1). In trying to make a personal choice, people may have a number of questions: Why use contraception? How does each method work? How well does it work? What are the medical risks? How might each method affect my sexuality? What possibilities do I have if I'm already pregnant? In the following pages, we examine the currently available methods of birth control in an effort to answer some of these questions.

WHY USE CONTRACEPTION?

An individual's or couple's decisions about birth control depend on many factors including age, future plans, marital or relationship status (including trust and cooperation), finances, religious beliefs, sexual attitudes, health, and prior experiences. *Not* using birth control if you are sexually active is a specific kind of personal decision, just as choosing to use birth control, whatever the reason, is a personal decision.

The main reason for using birth control is to prevent an unwanted pregnancy. Not only is an unwanted pregnancy likely to cause emotional turmoil and health risks, it also may present financial burdens. Often, unwanted pregnancies occur in young teenagers or women over 35, times when health risks during pregnancy are highest. The social and economic costs may also be high at these same ages.

Of the 1.2 million teenagers who become pregnant in the United States each year, more than 400,000 obtain abortions (Henshaw and O'Reilly, 1983). Many others drop out of school and enter into hasty marriages where the odds of divorce are high, the chances of getting a good job are low, and ending up on welfare is common (Furstenberg, 1976; Fielding, 1978). Others try to raise a child alone or with assistance of relatives, but this plan often proves more difficult than it might seem. An unplanned pregnancy at any age may also disrupt career plans, and economic costs are created by terminating the pregnancy or raising the child. There is also an emotional cost to an unwanted pregnancy. Feelings of foolishness, guilt, anger, or helplessness may strain or break a relationship ("It was *all your fault!*") or may create later sexual problems.

Of course, there are other reasons for using contraception, including the wish to space pregnancies, limit family size, avoid potential genetic disorders or birth defects, protect the mother's health, and allow women more control over planning their lives. Contraception also permits people to enjoy a sexual relationship without making commitments to marriage or parenthood. Limiting reproduction also has major social and philosophical consequences in a world of limited natural resources where overpopulation exerts political and psychological effects and environmental issues are of prominent concern.

Finally, there is a compelling health reason today for many people to consider using certain forms of contraception—condoms and spermicides—for a purpose that has nothing at all to do with birth control. The reason is that these contraceptive products offer some protection against the risk of many sexually transmitted diseases, including protection against infection with HIV, the AIDS virus.

EVALUATING CONTRACEPTIVE EFFECTIVENESS AND SAFETY

The decision to use contraception and the choice of one method over another depend primarily on two practical matters: how well it works (its effectiveness) and its health risks (its safety).[1] Evaluating these two issues is complicated. *No one contraceptive is always best or safest.*

When evaluating effectiveness and safety, remember that information from various sources may be biased. The popular media, for instance, are eager to report the latest "news" about the real or suspected hazards of a contraceptive method. Yet the story is usually condensed to a few paragraphs in the newspaper or is crammed into less than 60 seconds of TV or radio broadcast time. Scientific accuracy or caution is often lost in a process of oversimplification, misinterpretation, and unwarranted conclusions. In addition, much of the research on the effectiveness and safety of birth control methods is funded by the drug companies that manufacture them. These companies have an obvious interest in presenting their merchandise in a way that will boost sales. Finally, all scientific studies are not equivalent in their applicability to *you*. In general, studies about people close to your age, cultural background, and socioeconomic status are more meaningful than studies about other groups. For example, if you are a 22-year-old single American woman, you cannot put much faith in the findings of a study about 35-year-old married women in China.

Understanding some other aspects of evaluating effectiveness can also be helpful. First, it is important to distinguish between two factors: theoretical versus actual effectiveness. The **theoretical effectiveness** of a particular method is how it *should* work if used correctly and consistently, without human error or negligence. The **actual effectiveness** is what occurs in real life, when inconsistent use or improper technique ("user failure") combines with failures of the method alone ("method failure"). For example, if a couple runs out of condoms on a week-long camping trip yet continues to have intercourse, the woman's subsequent pregnancy is not counted as a method failure. But if she conceives even though she has used a contraceptive foam exactly according to instructions each time she had intercourse, her pregnancy qualifies as a method failure.

Second, for most types of contraception, the longer a person uses a particular method, the more effective it becomes. That is, with practice and experience, the actual failure rate decreases and becomes closer to the theoretical failure rate. (Actual effectiveness rates for the first year of use of the most common methods of birth control are shown in Table 5–2.)

Third, effectiveness rates for almost every nonsurgical contraceptive method vary depending on whether a couple uses the method to *prevent* pregnancy or to

[1] The choice of method may also depend, in individual cases, on factors such as cost, availability without a prescription, aesthetic preferences, and sometimes even the ease of concealment.

TABLE 5–2

Actual Contraceptive Failure Rates During First Year of Use[a]

Pill	5.6%	Rhythm	19.1%
Condom	15.7%	Spermicides	30.0%
Diaphragm	18.3%	IUD	6.0%

[a] These figures are standardized by age, race, and marital status and are corrected to allow for underreporting of abortion.

Source: Modified from Jones and Forrest, 1989, Table 5.

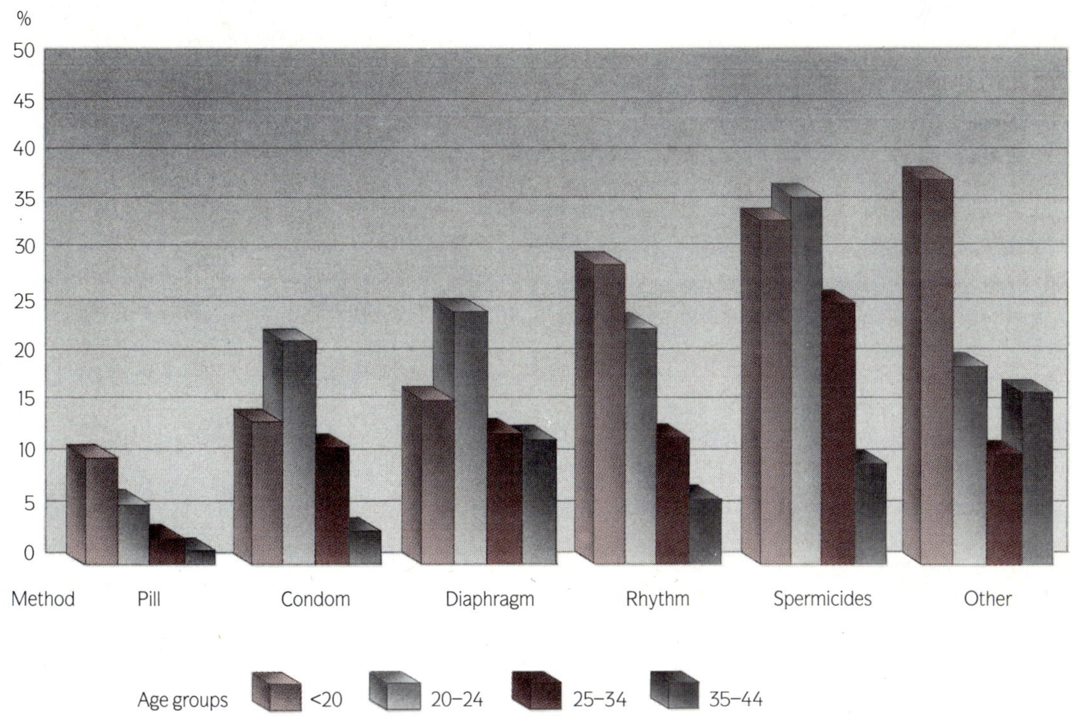

Percentage of women experiencing contraceptive failure during the first 12 months of use, by age and method, standardized by race and marital status.

delay (space) pregnancy. Failure rates are generally 50 to 100 percent higher for delay compared to prevention, since there seems to be less consistency in method use (Ryder, 1973).

There are other difficulties in assessing the safety of contraceptive methods. First, there are often wide differences in the frequency of side effects reported by different investigators. Their results reflect differences in research design, choice of control groups, different characteristics in the populations studied (such as age, health, socioeconomic status), and the methods investigators use to identify a problem (self-administered questionnaire, personal interview, laboratory testing). Second, there are some relative aspects to the safety question. How important is avoiding pregnancy? Are the side effects of a contraceptive method more or less serious than the risks of pregnancy and childbirth? How do the risks of a contraceptive

theoretical effectiveness the ideal effectiveness of a contraceptive method when used correctly and consistently.

actual effectiveness the observed effectiveness of a contraceptive method in real life, including user failures and method failures.

method compare with other health risks (such as the risk of getting cancer or having high blood pressure) or with risks of everyday life? These questions are addressed in more detail as we review the safety and side effects of each method of contraception.

METHODS OF CONTRACEPTION

Birth Control Pills (Oral Contraceptives)

The introduction of birth control pills in 1960 revolutionized contraceptive practices around the world. Millions of women turned enthusiastically to this convenient and effective method of preventing pregnancy, but within a decade reports of serious side effects of the pill began to appear and the popularity of this method declined substantially. Now, after more than 30 years of observation, what are the facts about the pill?

There are two types of oral contraceptives currently in use: a **combination pill,** which contains a synthetic estrogen and a progesterone-like synthetic substance called progestogen, and a **minipill** with progestogen only in low dosage. This discussion focuses on combination pills (unless otherwise specified) because they are the most commonly used.

The most popular pill used today, accounting for 85 percent of the oral contraceptives used in America and Europe, is the low-dose combination pill. This has one-fourth or less the estrogen and about one-tenth the progestogen that earlier birth control pills contained. The lower hormone concentrations cause fewer annoying side effects; in addition, it is believed that they are less likely to cause serious complications than earlier, higher-dose forms of the pill (Wharton and Blackburn, 1988; Mishell, 1989).

Among the numerous types of low-dose combination pills on the market are some that have a constant dose of hormones in each pill and some that are *multiphasic*, meaning that the amount of hormones in each pill varies at different times in the monthly cycle. In biphasic pills, for example, the amount of progestogen increases around midcycle; in triphasic pills, the amount of hormones is changed three times. Women using the multiphasic pills should note that taking their pills in an incorrect sequence may lessen contraceptive effectiveness considerably.

FIGURE 5–1

Serum Gonadotrophin Levels During the Menstrual Cycle

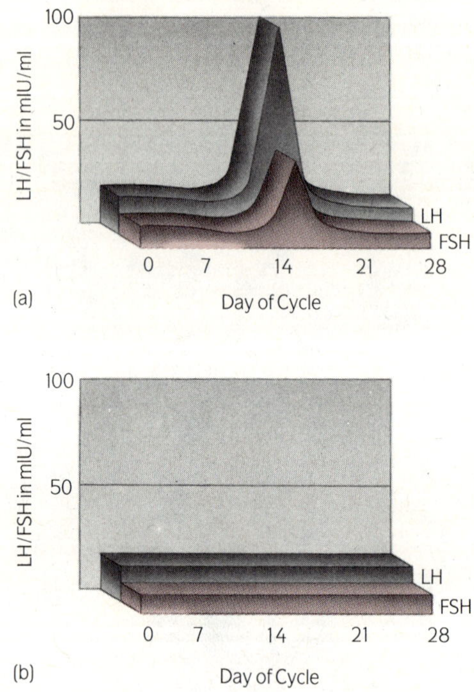

(a) Women not using oral contraceptives. (b) Women using combination oral contraceptives.

HOW BIRTH CONTROL PILLS WORK

Birth control pills prevent pregnancy primarily by blocking the normal cycle output of **follicle stimulating hormone (FSH)** and **luteinizing hormone (LH)** by the pituitary, thus preventing ovulation (Figure 5–1). In addition, the progestogen makes implantation difficult by inhibiting the development of the lining of the uterus and also thickens the cervical mucus, decreasing the possibility that sperm can get through.

USE AND EFFECTIVENESS

Birth control pills are taken one per day for 21 days beginning on the fifth day of the menstrual cycle (i.e., 4 days after a period begins). Some brands of birth control pills are packaged with seven inactive pills (usually of another color) that the woman takes on a daily basis to complete the cycle, whereas with other brands the woman must remember to resume her pills one week later. Multiphasic pills come in several different colors within each monthly packet, with each color corresponding to a different dose of hormones.

If a pill is missed, two pills should be taken the next day. If two pills in a row are missed, the woman should take two pills as soon as she realizes it and take two pills again the next day; after that, she should continue to take one pill each day. Since it is likely that birth control pills will not work properly in such a cycle, an *alternative* form of contraception must be used to prevent pregnancy. If a woman misses more than two pills in a row, or misses pills three or more times during one cycle, she should stop taking pills entirely and use another method of contraception for the rest of the cycle. She can begin a new cycle of oral contraceptives at the start of her next period. If her period is late, she should continue using her other contraceptive method and get a pregnancy test before resuming birth control pills.

Birth control pills are the most effective nonsurgical method of contraception. Among women who use the pill consistently, only one pregnancy will occur among 200 women during a year. Among all women using the pill—including those who sometimes forget to use it—three to six pregnancies will occur in 100 women annually.

The minipill, which is taken every day, even during menstruation, is less effective than the combination pill. If used perfectly, one or two pregnancies will occur in 100 women during a year. In actual conditions—including the occasional forgotten pill—five to ten pregnancies occur in 100 women using the minipill for a year.

SIDE EFFECTS AND SAFETY

Birth control pills have now been used by more than 180 million women around the world and have probably been studied more intensively than any other medication in history. Despite scare stories that appear regularly in the press, the evidence shows that the pill has more health benefits than risks for many users. For example, there is no reliable evidence that birth control pills cause cancer (Drill, 1975; Lipsett, 1977; Rinehart and Piotrow, 1979; Kols et al., 1982), and they actually protect against cancer of the ovaries (Newhouse et al., 1977; Centers for Disease Control, 1983) and of the uterine lining (Weiss and Sayvetz, 1980; Kaufman et al., 1980; Centers for Disease Control, 1983a).[2] Furthermore, women who use birth control pills are only one-fourth as likely to develop benign (noncancerous) breast tumors as nonusers, one-fourteenth as likely to develop ovarian cysts, one-half as likely to develop rheumatoid arthritis, and two-thirds as likely to develop iron deficiency anemia (Ory, Rosenfeld, and Landman, 1980).

Other beneficial effects of the pill have also been

FOCUS IN BRIEF

Health Benefits of the Pill

- Reduced risk of ovarian cancer.
- Reduced risk of endometrial cancer.
- Reduced risk of benign breast tumors.
- Reduced risk of ovarian cysts.
- Reduced risk of pelvic inflammatory disease.
- Reduced risk of iron deficiency anemia.
- Reduced risk of rheumatoid arthritis.
- Reduced risk of ectopic pregnancy.
- Increased bone density in the spine.
- Often relieves premenstrual symptoms.

[2] Two points should be made: (1) An earlier type of birth control pill, the sequential pill, was banned because it *was* found to cause cancer of the uterus. (2) As it may take decades for certain types of cancer to develop, it cannot be concluded that the combination pill *does not* cause cancer. However, more than 2000 cases of endometrial cancer are prevented each year by use of the pill (Centers for Disease Control, 1983a).

combination pill a birth control pill containing both estrogen and progesterone.

minipill a contraceptive pill containing only progesterone in low dosage.

follicle stimulating hormone (FSH) a substance produced in the pituitary gland that prepares the ovary for ovulation and stimulates the production of sperm cells in the testes.

luteinizing hormone (LH) (lū′ tē in īz′ ing) produced by the pituitary gland, LH triggers ovulation and stimulates the Leydig cells to manufacture testosterone.

noted. Many women find that the pill reduces the amount of menstrual flow and produces more regular cycles with less menstrual cramping (Mishell, 1989). Acne can be improved by the pill (although sometimes it is worsened), premenstrual tension can be reduced, and pelvic inflammatory disease—a serious cause of infertility—is only half as common in pill users as in nonusers (Wharton and Blackburn, 1988). In addition, the pill seems to cause an increased bone density in the lumbar spine, which may help to prevent the thinning out of bone called osteoporosis that occurs in many women after the menopause (Mishell, 1989).

The most common bothersome side effects of the pill mimic those encountered in pregnancy: nausea, constipation, breast tenderness, minor elevations in blood pressure, edema (swelling), and skin rashes (including brown spots on the face called **chloasma**). Other relatively minor side effects include weight gain or loss, an increased amount of vaginal secretions, and an increased susceptibility to vaginal infections.

Less common but more troublesome problems caused by the pill include high blood pressure, diabetes, migraine headaches, and, rarely, jaundice or liver tumors (Mishell, 1989). In addition, if taken during pregnancy, the pill may cause birth defects (Nora and Nora, 1978; Kasan and Andrews, 1980).

The most serious risks to women using birth control pills are disorders of the circulatory system. Three different types of circulatory problems are involved. The most common is the formation of a blood clot in a vein (usually in the legs), which typically results in only minor discomfort caused by inflammation and swelling. Infrequently, a piece of the clot may break off and circulate to the lungs or the brain, where it can cause serious damage or death. These problems, called thromboembolic diseases, were two to four times more common among pill users than other women in the 1960s and 1970s (occurring in about 1 out of 1000 pill users in a year) but are thought to occur less often today with the considerably lower dose of estrogen contained in the pills currently being used (Wharton and Blackburn, 1988). The same observation (lower estrogen dose = lower rates of complication) applies to the other two forms of circulatory disorders linked to use of the pill, heart attacks and stroke. Earlier studies found that oral contraceptives increased the risk of heart attacks in women who smoked and/or women over age 35 (Mann and Inman, 1975; Jick et al., 1978; Rosenberg et al., 1980). A heightened risk of stroke (bleeding into the brain, or blockage of blood flow in the brain) was also found in early studies of pill users.

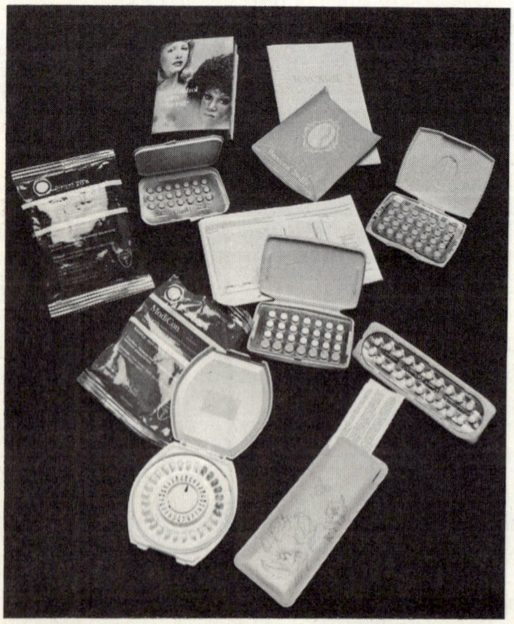

Birth control pills come in different brands and packages, each accompanied by a package insert describing their use and potential side effects.

Based on data from these early studies, the pill was not usually prescribed for women over age 35. More recent research indicates that use of low-dose combination pills by healthy, nonsmoking women up to age 45 does not cause any increased risk of serious cardiovascular disease (Mann et al., 1987; Mishell, 1989; Upton, 1990).

For several decades, there has been a persistent concern that the pill may cause an increased rate of breast cancer in users, with just enough conflicting research reported from time to time to keep the matter unresolved (Vessey, 1987; Johnson, 1989). Most studies have not identified any link between birth control pills and breast cancer. For example, one recent investigation found no evidence that use of oral contraceptives, even over many years, increased the risk of subsequent breast cancer in women with a family history of the disease (Murray et al., 1989.) Likewise, a ten-year study of a total of 118,273 female nurses concluded, "overall past use of oral contraceptives is not associated with a substantial increase in the risk of breast cancer" (Romieu et al., 1989). Other studies have been inconsistent, however (Kay and Hannaford, 1988; Miller et al., 1989).

An FDA panel convened in 1989 to examine all the available evidence concluded that there was no need

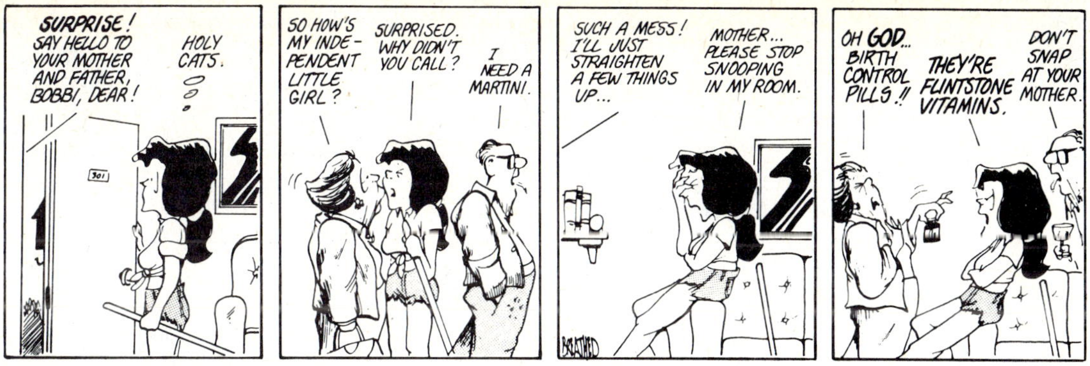
SURPRISE! SAY HELLO TO YOUR MOTHER AND FATHER, BOBBI, DEAR!
HOLY CATS.
SO HOW'S MY INDE-PENDENT LITTLE GIRL?
SURPRISED. WHY DIDN'T YOU CALL?
I NEED A MARTINI.
SUCH A MESS! I'LL JUST STRAIGHTEN A FEW THINGS UP...
MOTHER... PLEASE STOP SNOOPING IN MY ROOM.
OH GOD... BIRTH CONTROL PILLS.!!
THEY'RE FLINTSTONE VITAMINS.
DON'T SNAP AT YOUR MOTHER.

Bloom County by Berke Breathed. © 1987 Washington Post Writers Group. Reprinted by permission.

for recommending changes in the use of birth control pills or in their warning labels (*The New York Times*, January 6, 1989, pp. A1 and A13). The panel noted that the small number of studies suggesting a heightened risk of breast cancer in women who have used the pill are inconsistent with each other and plagued with methodological problems. [These problems have been thoroughly reviewed elsewhere (Wharton and Blackburn, 1988; Johnson, 1989), so we do not go into further detail here.] Nevertheless, because the risk of breast cancer occurring long after use of the pill (20 years or more) has not yet been conclusively examined, the final word on a possible relationship between the pill and breast cancer cannot be given at this time. As a practical precautionary matter, we suggest that people whose mothers or sisters have had breast cancer should probably avoid use of the pill until more conclusive studies have been completed.

A few final words about the safety of oral contraceptives are in order. Safety is a relative matter, not just a statistical equation. For example, a woman who has frequent intercourse receives more contraceptive protection from the pill than one who does not. While other contraceptive methods may seem "safer," she may choose to risk certain health problems to be more certain of not becoming pregnant. Another example applies to women in developing countries, where maternal death rates during pregnancy and childbirth are much higher than in countries with advanced medical care systems. In this situation, oral contraceptives are far safer than no birth control, even with their attendant side effects. The safety of birth control pills should also be looked at in comparison with risks of everyday living such as auto accidents or sports injuries. In this case the figures may seem somewhat different: only one pill-related death occurred in 46,000 women under 35 who were nonsmokers in 200,000 *woman-years* (one woman-year is equivalent to a woman using a particular contraceptive method for 12 calendar months) of use of the pill (Royal College, 1977). By contrast, nine deaths from auto accidents would be expected in a group of this size over this period of time. Confirming this view, the largest prospective American study of pill users found that, overall, the risks of oral contraceptive use appear to be minimal (Ramcharan, 1981). Today, with the widespread use of low-dose forms of the pill, it is likely that oral contraceptives are safer than they have ever been by a considerable margin (Wharton and Blackburn, 1988; Mishell, 1989). However, women who rely on the pill for birth control should recognize that it provides no protection against HIV, the virus that causes AIDS.

SEXUAL EFFECTS OF BIRTH CONTROL PILLS

Evaluating the effects of birth control pills on sexuality is tricky. Older research generally noted that long-term use of the pill had negative sexual effects (Masters and Johnson, 1970; Herzberg et al., 1971), but later studies do not support this view (Bragonier, 1976; Gambrell et al., 1976). There is no research available as yet on the sexual effects of today's low-estrogen pills.

There are many individual reasons that the pill helps or hinders a woman's sexual feelings and function. Some reasons are biological: a woman who develops a vaginal infection may have sexual problems as a result, or a woman who has less premenstrual and menstrual cramping may feel better physically and

chloasma (klō as′ muh) brown pigmented spots, usually on the face, caused either by birth control pills or hormones produced naturally during pregnancy.

thus may be more sexually receptive and responsive. Some reasons are psychological. If a woman expects to have sexual side effects from the pill, her prophecy becomes self-fulfilling. Some women may feel guilty about using the pill because of religious beliefs or conflicts between wanting children and using contraception. Alternatively, the psychological security of using a highly effective method of contraception reduces the fear of pregnancy and may therefore improve sexual interest and enjoyment (after all, it is harder to enjoy something when you are afraid). One woman told us, "After switching to the pill, I found that sex became more fun. I had my first orgasm during intercourse less than two months later" (Authors' files). Since the pill also requires no interruptions at the time of sexual activity, it permits a degree of spontaneity and intimacy that other methods may not.

Most women using oral contraceptives today do not report significant changes in sexual interest, behavior, or enjoyment. Approximately 10 percent experience improved sexuality, which is about the same as the percent who note decreased sexual interest or responsiveness.

IUDs

The **IUD,** or **intrauterine device,** is a small plastic object that is inserted into the uterus through the vagina and cervix and then is continuously kept in place. As of early 1990, there were only two models of IUDs available in the United States: a progesterone-releasing device (called Progestasert) and a copper-containing device (called the Copper T380A). These are shown in Figure 5–2.

In the mid-1980s, major IUD manufacturers withdrew from the U.S. market because of a substantial number of lawsuits over infections in the upper part of the female genital tract—especially infection of the Fallopian tubes, known as salpingitis or pelvic inflammatory disease (PID)—which is particularly serious because it can cause permanent sterility, increases the chances of having an ectopic pregnancy, and can cause abscesses around the ovaries that may require surgery to be corrected (Mishell, 1985). The older IUD devices have now been replaced by substantially safer versions, but their popularity in the United States is considerably lower than it was a decade ago.

While IUDs became popular in this country only in the last 25 years, they are a modern application of an ancient concept. For centuries, Arab and Turkish camel drivers put a large pebble into the camel's uterus for contraceptive purposes, since a pregnant camel on a long desert trek would not be very helpful. The first IUD designed for humans, a ring made of silkworm gut, did not gain much attention when introduced in 1909. In the late 1920s a ring of gut and silver wire was developed by Grafenberg, a German physician, and enjoyed some popularity. Early models of the IUD, however, were condemned because of the risk of pelvic infection and fell into disrepute.

By 1978 about 6 percent of married women of reproductive age in America used the IUD, while about 20 percent did in Scandinavia and approximately half of all women using contraceptives adopted it in China (Piotrow, Rinehart, and Schmidt, 1979). On a worldwide basis, approximately 60 million women use the IUD.

HOW IUDs WORK

The exact way the IUD works is not known. In the past, it was thought that the major effect was by interfering with the implantation of the fertilized egg in the lining of the uterus by a local inflammatory reaction. Now it appears that IUDs also act to block sperm from fertilizing the egg (Alvarez et al., 1988; Treiman and Liskin, 1988; Mishell, 1990). This spermicidal action is thought to be a result of white blood cells engulfing or damaging sperm before they reach the egg as well as because of chemical reactions caused by enzymes in the Fallopian tubes. IUDs containing progesterone also alter the development of the lining of the uterus so that implantation is unlikely.

USE AND EFFECTIVENESS

The IUD must be inserted into the uterus (Figure 5–2) by a trained health care professional after determining that the woman is not pregnant and does not have chlamydia, gonorrhea, or other pelvic infections. Inserting an IUD can cause abortion in a pregnant woman and can push bacteria from an infection into the uterus or Fallopian tubes. Insertion is usually done during a menstrual period, since it is a fairly reliable sign that the woman is not pregnant, but it can be done at other times.

Inserting an IUD usually causes only brief discomfort, but some women prefer to be given a short-acting painkiller. Taking two or three aspirin tablets about an hour before insertion provides some pain relief and may theoretically decrease cramping because it blocks release of prostaglandins. The woman must

FIGURE 5–2

The IUD

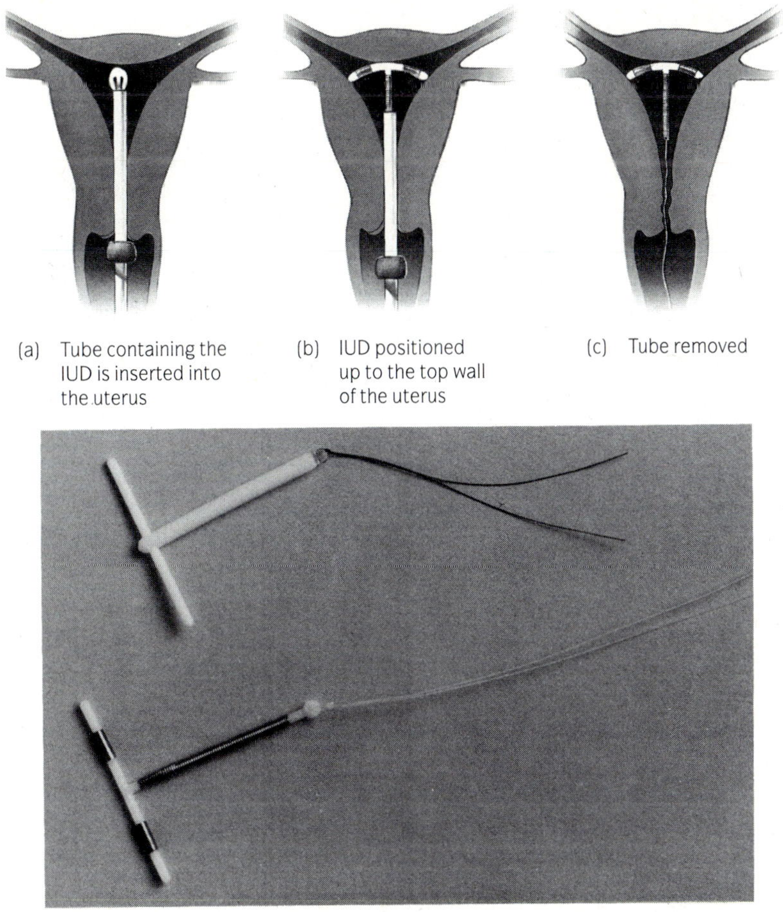

Insertion of an IUD (a–c) and photographs of the Progestasert and Paraguard IUDs currently in use in the United States.

be shown how to check the plastic thread that comes through the mouth of the cervix to be sure the IUD is in place. If this thread cannot be located, or if it seems longer than it was before, the woman must return for a check-up, because contractions of the uterus can push the IUD downward, causing it to be partly or completely expelled from the uterus. Expulsion rates for the copper- or progesterone-containing IUDs are about 7 per 100 women during a year, with most of the expulsions occurring in the first three months after insertion (Treiman and Liskin, 1988; Cole, 1989). Expulsion rates are higher in younger women and in women who have never had children.

Even though they may be expelled, IUDs are highly effective. A number of studies show fewer than 1 pregnancy occurring in 100 women using the Copper T380A for one year, while the Progestasert IUD has a pregnancy rate of about 3 per 100 women in one year (Cole, 1989). (Adjusting the effectiveness data for abortions resulted in an actual failure rate of 6 percent in the first year of use, as shown in Table 5–2). The Progestasert device must be replaced after one year of use because its progesterone supply is depleted by that time; the Copper T380A is currently approved for four years of continuous use.

intrauterine device (IUD) (in truh ū′ ter in) a small object, either plastic or metal, placed inside the uterus for birth control.

FIGURE 5–3

The Diaphragm

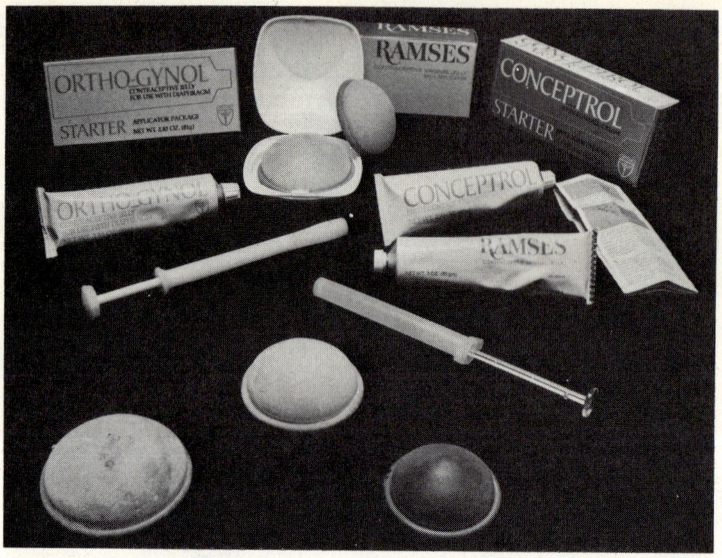

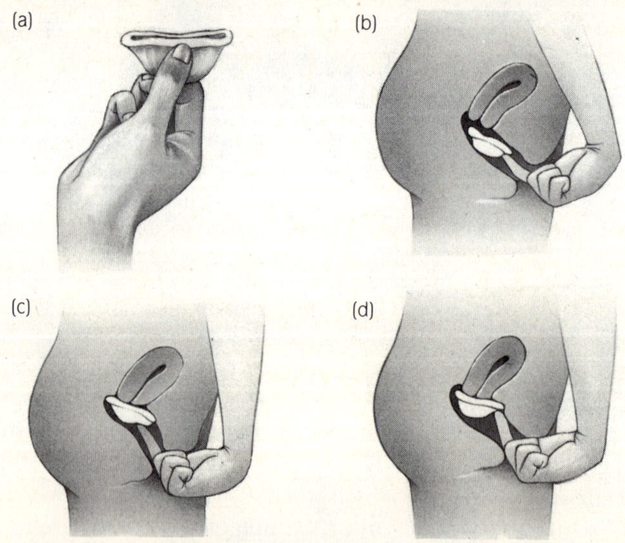

Proper use of a diaphragm: (a) After inserting spermicidal jelly or cream, the rim of the diaphragm is pinched between the fingers and thumb. (b) The folded diaphragm is gently inserted into the vagina and pushed downward and backward as far as it will go. (c) To check for proper positioning, feel the cervix to be certain it is completely covered by the soft rubber dome of the diaphragm. (d) A finger is hooked under the forward rim to remove the diaphragm.

SIDE EFFECTS AND SAFETY

Perforation of the uterus (puncturing the wall of the uterus) is the most serious risk of using an IUD. If it occurs, it is almost always at the time of insertion. This problem, which occurs in about 1 in 1000 insertions, can cause sudden pain and bleeding or, more rarely, may be without immediate symptoms. Perforation usually requires surgery to prevent damage to the intestines, since the IUD usually perforates through the uterus into the abdomen. Inserting an IUD while a woman is breast-feeding causes a tenfold increase in the risk of perforation of the uterus (Merz, 1983), so it seems advisable to choose a different method of birth control during this time.

The most common side effects of the IUD are increased bleeding from the uterus and cramping pain. Menstrual periods are typically heavier and longer (except in women using IUDs with progesterone, which decreases menstrual flow), and there is more likely to be spotting between periods. This increased blood loss can cause anemia. Cramps and bleeding can be serious enough to have the IUD removed (about 10 percent of women find this necessary) but usually lessen after the first three months.

IUD users have about a four times higher risk of pelvic infection than other women. This risk is present not only at the time of insertion but also with continued use of the device. Bacteria, viruses, or fungus infections may enter the uterus by "climbing" the tail of the IUD, and there is a chance that such an infection will spread to the Fallopian tubes and ovaries, which can cause permanent scarring and infertility (Vessey et al., 1981; Beerthuizen et al., 1982). However, it should be noted that for women in monogamous sexual relationships, IUDs pose little risk of infection except in the first few months after they are inserted (Lee, Rubin, and Borucki, 1988).

If a pregnancy occurs in a woman with an IUD, there is about a 5 percent chance that the pregnancy will be ectopic (misplaced) (Cole, 1989). This is because IUDs protect better against intrauterine pregnancies than against ectopic ones. Since pregnancies are infrequent in IUD users, the rate of ectopic pregnancy is relatively low: less than 1.5 ectopic pregnancies per 1000 woman-years of use (Treiman and Liskin, 1988), about one-tenth the rate of ectopic pregnancies overall.

If a uterine pregnancy occurs in an IUD user, approximately half will abort spontaneously (usually in the second trimester) unless the IUD is removed. There is no evidence, however, that IUDs cause birth defects.

The IUD is well suited to women who want a highly effective contraceptive method that requires no active participation on their part and is easily and promptly reversible. It may be particularly appropriate for women who cannot use birth control pills for medical reasons and for the mentally retarded who may not be able to remember to take a pill or use a mechanical method of birth control. IUDs should not be used by women who are pregnant or who have active pelvic infection, bleeding disorders, anatomical abnormalities of the uterus or cervix, or abnormal pelvic bleeding. Women who have had an ectopic pregnancy, severe menstrual disorders, or any disease that suppresses normal immunity to infection should not use IUDs. Likewise, women who have multiple sexual partners or who have had repeated genital infections should not use IUDs.

SEXUAL EFFECTS OF IUDs

Like birth control pills, the IUD is effective in preventing pregnancy and does not interfere with sexual spontaneity or mood. Yet the IUD can cause pain during intercourse. The woman may experience pain if the IUD is not in the right position or if there is a pelvic infection or inflammation; the man may have pain at the tip of the penis or along the shaft because of irritation from the tail of the IUD in the vagina. Both abdominal cramping and persistent bleeding can lessen a woman's interest in sexual activity, but these side effects occur in only about 10 percent of users. Infrequently, women who use IUDs find that orgasm may cause intense, unpleasant cramping because of uterine contractions around the IUD.

Anyone using an IUD should also realize that it provides no protection against infection with HIV, the virus that causes AIDS.

Diaphragms

The **diaphragm** is a round, shallow dome of thin rubber stretched over a flexible ring (Figure 5–3). After a spermicidal (sperm-killing) jelly or cream is applied inside the dome and around the inner part of

diaphragm (dī′ uh fram) a dome-shaped rubber contraceptive device that is positioned inside the vagina so that it blocks the cervix; it must be used with a spermicide to be effective.

the rim, the diaphragm must be inserted inside the vagina and positioned so that it completely covers the cervix. Before the introduction of birth control pills, the diaphragm was the most widely used method of contraception, and it is still popular today.

HOW DIAPHRAGMS WORK

The diaphragm is a mechanical barrier that blocks the mouth of the cervix so that sperm cannot enter. Because this blocking effect is not very reliable by itself, the use of a spermicide is required to kill sperm that manage to swim inside the rim of the diaphragm.

USE AND EFFECTIVENESS

Diaphragms come in different sizes and must be properly fitted by a trained health care professional to match the anatomy of the user. The size and position of the cervix and the size and shape of the vagina must be taken into account to achieve a proper fit; the actual fitting is done using a set of graduated flexible rings to select the right size. After the fitting, the woman is shown how to insert the diaphragm either manually or with a plastic inserter (see Figure 5–3). Some clinicians recommend that a woman be refitted if she gains or loses ten pounds. However, one study found that more women whose weight was stable needed refitting (Fiscella, 1982), so the matter is not a clear one. We recommend that women be refitted for a diaphragm after a pregnancy or annually. If there is a weight change of 15 pounds or more, it also may be advisable to be refitted.

The diaphragm can be inserted up to two hours before intercourse and should remain in place at least six hours afterward. If it is worn for more than two hours before intercourse, the effectiveness of the spermicide may drop. For this reason, a second, full application of spermicidal jelly, cream, or foam should be placed in the vagina before intercourse in these circumstances. If the diaphragm is removed less than six hours after intercourse, it is possible that live sperm in the vagina may reach the cervix and swim up into the uterus.

The effectiveness of this method is not as high as that of birth control pills or IUDs, with failure rates in most reports ranging from 6 to 20 pregnancies in 100 women using the device during a year (Sherris, Moore, and Fox, 1984). During the first year of use, the actual failure rate for diaphragm use is 18.3 percent (see Table 5–2) (Jones and Forrest, 1989).

Since the effectiveness of this method depends on the regularity of its use, the woman's motivation and memory are important factors. A woman who leaves her diaphragm at home and finds herself unexpectedly in a sexual situation might have a "user" failure rather than a "method" failure. In one study with a highly motivated, experienced population of users, the failure rate was only 1.9 per 100 woman-years (Vessey, Lawless, and Yeates, 1982). Another problem that influences effectiveness is that the diaphragm may slip out of position during sexual play because of improper insertion, a poor fit, or expansion of the inside of the vagina and movement of the uterus during excitation. Johnson and Masters (1962) found that even a well-fitted and properly inserted diaphragm can become dislodged during intercourse when the woman is on top of the man or if the penis is removed and reinserted into the vagina during plateau levels of arousal. Even a tiny hole in the dome of the diaphragm will permit sperm to enter, so it is important to inspect it carefully and to avoid use of Vaseline or similar products on it, since this can cause deterioration of the latex. Despite these problems, there are some advantages, too. The diaphragm seems to offer protection against cervical cancer (Wright et al., 1978) and against some sexually transmitted diseases (Sherris, Moore, and Fox, 1984). Another benefit of the diaphragm is that it offers considerable protection against damage to the Fallopian tubes from infection (Cramer et al., 1987). Furthermore, if consistently used in combination with a condom, the rate of effectiveness is comparable to that of birth control pills.

SIDE EFFECTS AND SAFETY

The only potential side effects of diaphragm use are (1) possible allergic reactions to the rubber in the diaphragm or to the spermicide itself and (2) the chance of introducing infection into the vagina if the diaphragm is not clean. Both problems are infrequent. In addition, it is not advisable to wear a diaphragm for more than 12 hours at a time because this seems to cause an overgrowth of bacteria in the vagina and cervix that is linked to the toxic shock syndrome (see Chapter 10). The diaphragm has no effects on hormones or physical processes of the body and poses no danger to later fertility.

Women who have pelvic disorders affecting the vagina or cervix or who do not like to touch their genitals should not use the diaphragm.

SEXUAL EFFECTS

The primary sexual difficulty with use of the diaphragm is inconvenience. For example, either partner may experience loss of sexual arousal while the woman takes time to insert and check the diaphragm if she did not insert it before sex play began. Some couples solve this problem by making the insertion of the diaphragm a part of their sexual play preliminary to intercourse. Either partner may find the diaphragm or the process of its insertion messy and unaesthetic. (Some users are annoyed by the "gloppiness" after removal of the diaphragm, when the spermicidal jelly may drip out of the vagina for several hours.) In addition, a diaphragm that is too large may cause pain during intercourse and some men complain that intercourse feels "different" with the diaphragm in place. For people who don't like to have intercourse during menstrual periods, the diaphragm can be used to provide a "reverse barrier" that contains flow during sexual activity.

The Cervical Cap

A device related to the diaphragm is the **cervical cap,** which fits snugly over the cervix and stays in place by suction (see Figure 5–4). After enjoying considerable popularity for the past three decades in Europe, the device was finally approved for use by the U.S. Food and Drug Administration in 1988 (*The New York Times,* May 24, 1988, pp. A1 and C8).

There are several types of cervical cap, although only one—the Prentif cavity-rim cap—has been approved by the FDA so far. This thimble-shaped version is made of soft, pliable latex and is a bit less than half the size of a diaphragm. Other types are made of a harder plastic material.

HOW THE CERVICAL CAP WORKS

Like the diaphragm, the cervical cap is a mechanical barrier that blocks the mouth of the cervix so that sperm cannot enter. In fact, this blocking action is more efficient than that of the diaphragm because the cervical cap fits on the cervix more tightly than the diaphragm.

USE AND EFFECTIVENESS

The Prentif cap is made in four different sizes and must be fitted properly in order to be effective. It is somewhat more difficult for the user to learn how to insert the cap correctly than it is to learn how to use a diaphragm (Mishell, 1989). At the present time, the FDA has approved the cap for only 48 hours of continuous wear, although data suggest it can safely be worn for longer periods of time (Klitsch, 1988).

The FDA recommends that a spermicide should always be placed inside the cap before use, but this is apt to only be an effective "back-up" for the first six hours of use; after that, the sperm-killing action of spermicides decreases considerably. In fact, members of the National Women's Health Network, which led the drive to obtain approval for the device, believe that spermicide is unnecessary for the cap's effectiveness (Klitsch, 1988).

The effectiveness of the cervical cap seems to be generally comparable to the diaphragm. In several different studies, pregnancy rates ranged from 8 to 20 per 100 woman-years (Boehm, 1983; Cagen, 1986; Powell et al., 1986). In the largest U.S. study of the cap, involving around 1500 women who were randomly assigned to either the cap or a diaphragm, one-year pregnancy rates were roughly the same for both devices—17.4 per 100 women using the cervical cap, compared to 16.7 per 100 diaphragm users (Bernstein et al., 1986).

SIDE EFFECTS AND SAFETY

There is only one major questionmark about potential adverse effects of the cervical cap. The cap has been linked to abnormal Pap smears in a small number of users. In one study, for instance, 4 percent of women who used the cervical cap for three months developed changes in their Pap smears, an incidence about twice as high as in diaphragm users (*The New York Times,* May 24, 1988, pp. A1 and C8). It is unclear if these cervical abnormalities are minor microscopic changes resulting from inflammation or if they may be precancerous.

There is also a small risk that if the cap is worn too long it may cause an overgrowth of bacteria linked to toxic shock syndrome (see Chapter 10). As with the diaphragm, very infrequently women may have an allergic reaction to the latex in the cap.

One of the principal safety advantages of the cap is that it does not influence a woman's hormone production or cause any changes in the functioning of a woman's body.

cervical cap (ser' vi kul kap) a small plastic or rubber contraceptive device worn on the cervix to provide a barrier to sperm.

FIGURE 5–4

Cervical Caps

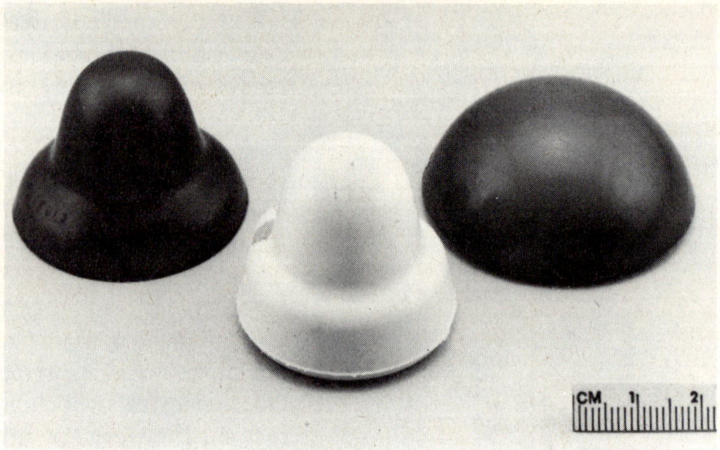

Three different types of cervical caps currently used for contraception.

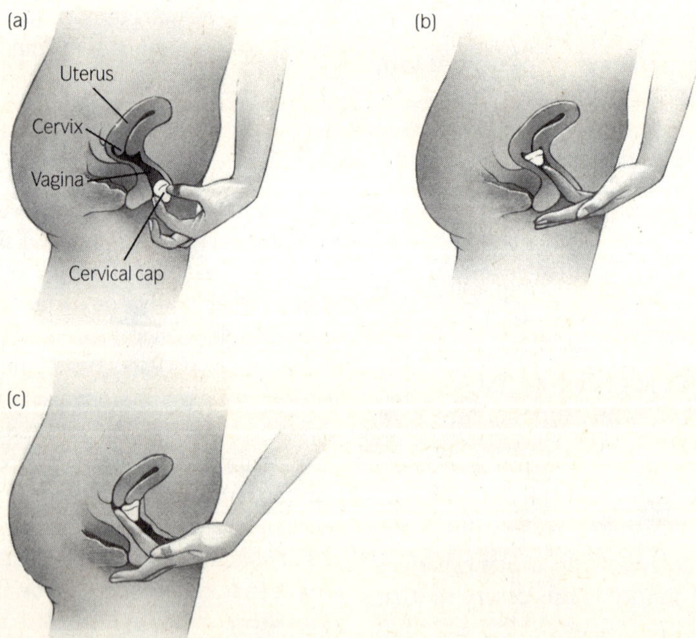

Women who have abnormal Pap smears or anatomical abnormalities of the cervix should not use the cervical cap.

SEXUAL EFFECTS

Most women who have switched to the cervical cap after experience with a diaphragm say that it is advantageous in two ways: it permits more sexual spontaneity and it is considerably less messy (Klitsch, 1988). In a small number of cases, the cap has been reported to cause discomfort to the male during intercourse, but in our experience, this problem is quite infrequent. On the other hand, about one out of five women complains of vaginal odors caused by the cervical cap (probably the result of a backup of cervical secretions), which can be embarrassing. One other drawback is that the cap can be dislodged from the cervix, especially during deep penile thrusting. In one large study, this occurred at least once in 40 percent of women using the cap (Bernstein et al., 1986).

Condoms

The condom (also called a rubber, safe, or prophylactic) is a thin sheath of latex rubber or tissue from a lamb's intestine that fits snugly over the penis. Currently, it is the only effective nonsurgical birth control method for males, and it does not require a prescription. Condoms can be purchased in drug stores, by mail order, at family planning clinics, and, in some locations, from coin-operated vending machines in men's rooms of bars and gas stations. In addition, many colleges now provide condom dispensers in dormitories and student health centers.

Condoms are usually rolled up into plastic or foil packets (Figure 5–5) and come in different styles. Some are lubricated, some come in a variety of colors, and some have tiny ribs or bumps on their surface that supposedly provide more stimulation to the female as intravaginal thrusting occurs. One of the more recent innovations in condom design is the introduction of a condom coated with a spermicide combined with a lubricant. Condoms are designed with either a round end or a reservoir end, a small receptacle to catch the semen.

Although condoms were somewhat ignored in the 1960s and 1970s because they were viewed as cumbersome and old-fashioned, there has been a marked increase in their popularity in the past few years for several different reasons. First, the condom's effectiveness as a barrier to the spread of the AIDS virus (as well as to the spread of other bacteria and viruses that cause sexually transmitted diseases) has brought it into the spotlight. This focus on the condom's usefulness as a preventive health measure (as well as a birth control device) has been the main reason for a resurgence of its use. Second, in addition to the positive publicity about condoms contained in the U.S. Surgeon General's Report on AIDS (Surgeon General, 1986) and similar sets of recommendations by other governmental and scientific groups, condom manufacturers have increased their advertising of this product, generating additional consumer awareness and interest. One interesting by-product of these changes is that several brands of condoms are now being marketed primarily to women, and condom sales to women surged by an estimated 300 percent between 1980 and 1989 (in one ad for Lifestyles condoms, a young woman proclaims, "I'll do a lot for love, but I'm not ready to die for it"). Finally, increasing attention to the role and responsibilities of teenage males in the high rates of unintended pregnancy in America has led to a greater emphasis on recommending condom use as a relatively inexpensive, accessible, nonprescription form of birth control that is safe and effective if properly used.

USE AND EFFECTIVENESS

The condom, which works by preventing sperm from entering the vagina, must be unrolled onto the erect penis shortly before intercourse. If it is put on too early, it may tear if rubbed against the sheets (or dirt, sand, or car seat) or it may be accidently punctured by a fingernail. If put on shortly before ejaculation, some drops of preejaculatory fluid containing live sperm might have already entered the vagina. If a round-end condom is used, a little extra space should be left at the tip to catch the ejaculate. After ejaculation, the condom should be held at the base of the penis so it does not slip or spill while being withdrawn. If leakage occurs for any reason, it is wise to put a spermicidal foam or cream in the vagina immediately. A condom should not be tested before use by inflating, stretching, or being filled with water. It is impossible to detect microscopic holes that would be large enough to allow sperm to pass through, and you *may* inadvertently damage the condom while you are trying to check it.

An important aspect of condom use that has received relatively little attention is that latex condoms deteriorate rapidly and are liable to break if they are in contact with oil-based lubricants such as Vaseline, baby oil, vegetable oil, many hand creams, or some of the exotic massage oils sold in sex shops. In one recent experiment, it was found that exposure of the condom to such products for just ten minutes at body temperature causes a significant weakening in the strength of the condom—a weakening that is pronounced enough to be "likely to cause the product [the condom] to fail during use" (Pugh, 1989). Voeller (1989) reported that a large fraction of college-educated men who reported having condoms break on more than 10 percent of the occasions they used them mistakenly believed that these types of sexual lubricants were water-based because they washed off easily with water. (True water-based lubricants include K-Y Lubricating Jelly, Today Personal Lubricant, and Corn Huskers Lotion.)

FIGURE 5–5

The Condom

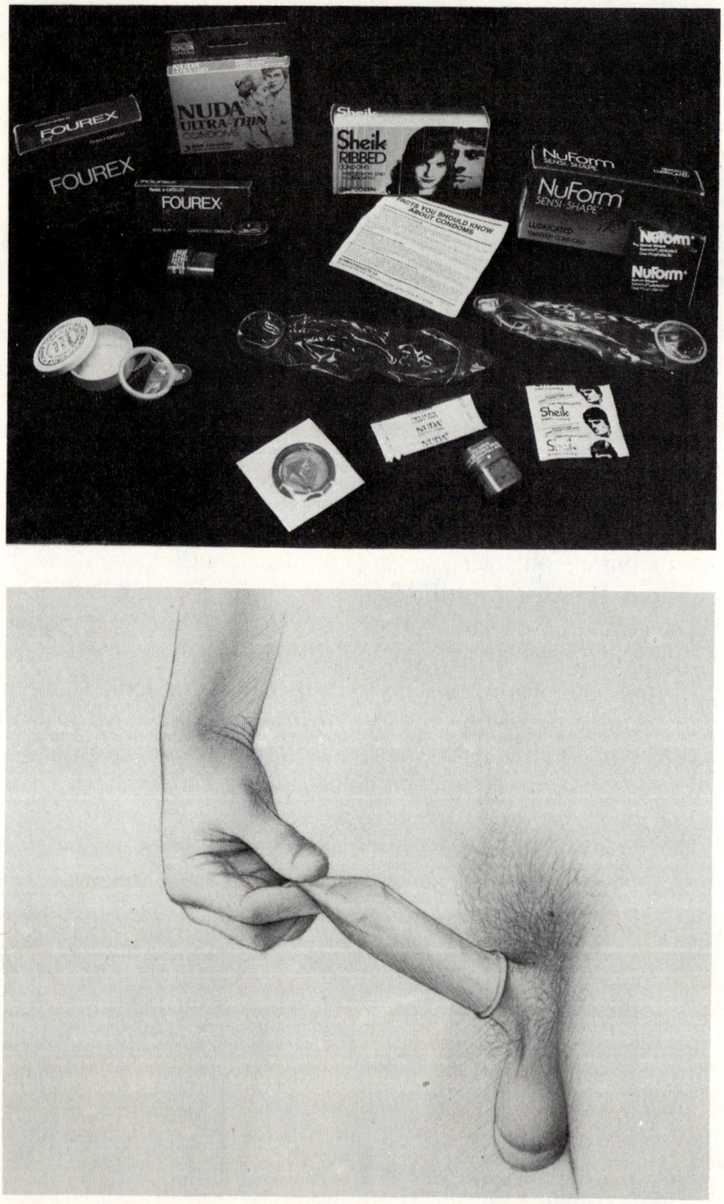

The photo shows an assortment of condoms and their packages. The drawing shows the proper method of pinching the tip of the condom without a reservoir end to leave some room for the semen.

In theory, the condom is a very reliable method of birth control—when used properly and consistently. Fewer than 5 pregnancies should occur in 100 couples using condoms for a year. Furthermore, if condoms are consistently used in combination with a vaginal spermicide, the theoretical effectiveness is even better, becoming almost as good as the pill. In actual practice, however, couples using the condom as their only

GUIDELINES FOR USE OF CONDOMS

1. Latex condoms should be used rather than natural membrane condoms because they offer greater protection against HIV and other viral STDs.
2. Condoms should be stored in a cool, dry place out of direct sunlight.
3. Condoms in damaged packages or those that show obvious signs of age (e.g., those that are brittle, sticky, or discolored) should not be used, since they may be defective.
4. Condoms should be handled with care to prevent punctures or rips.
5. Condoms should be put on before any genital contact to prevent exposure to fluids that may contain infectious agents.
6. Only water-based lubricants should be used. Petroleum or oil-based lubricants such as Vaseline, cooking oils, shortening, and most lotions should not be used because they weaken the latex and may cause breakage.
7. Use of condoms containing spermicides may provide some additional protection against STDs. However, vaginal use of spermicides along with condoms is likely to provide even better protection.
8. If a condom breaks, it should be replaced immediately. If ejaculation occurs after condom breakage, the immediate use of spermicide may be of some utility.
9. After ejaculation, care should be taken so that the condom does not slip off the penis before withdrawal; the base of the condom should be held throughout withdrawal. The penis should be withdrawn while still erect.
10. Condoms should never be reused.

Source: Centers for Disease Control, MMWR *38:S-8, Table 2, 1989.*

method of contraception often have unwanted pregnancies: overall failure rates of 10 to 20 per 100 couple-years are commonly reported. The main problem is not defective condoms (they must meet rigorous testing standards of the Food and Drug Administration[3]) or improper use, but *inconsistent* use. Many people using this method sometimes "take chances" instead of using condoms during every act of intercourse.

One other aspect of condom use that is increasingly important today is that latex condoms provide considerable protection against many sexually transmitted diseases. Condoms made of natural membranes sometimes have pores large enough to allow viruses such as hepatitis B or HIV (the AIDS virus) to pass through (Minuk, Bohme, and Bower, 1986; Goldsmith, 1987).

A recent experiment confirmed that latex condoms effectively block the transmission of HIV (Rietmeijer et al., 1988). In this study, 30 condoms (20 of them coated with the spermicide nonoxynol-9) were

[3] In 1987, the FDA reported that one out of five sample lots of latex condoms failed the stringent standards that they employ in testing: in other words, they leaked (*American Medical News,* September 4, 1987, p. 37). While the failure rate was highest in brands of imported condoms, roughly one out of 10 domestically manufactured condom batches were defective. (The March 1989 issue of *Consumer Reports* contains a ratings guide to latex condoms that includes data on their failure rates.)

mounted on hollow dildos and were then put into cylinder-shaped containers with a liquid culture medium. After a solution containing HIV was put inside each condom tip through a small hole in the end of the dildo, the dildo was pumped up and down in the container and then the condom was deliberately ripped. Before the condoms were ruptured, none of the 30 allowed HIV to pass into the surrounding culture medium. After the condoms were ripped, 7 of the 10 without spermicide allowed HIV to leak out, but no leakage of HIV was detected in the 20 condoms treated with nonoxynol-9.

SIDE EFFECTS AND SAFETY

Very infrequently, the material the condom is made from can cause burning or irritation to the genitals. Otherwise, condoms have no health risks at all.

SEXUAL EFFECTS

There are several sexual disadvantages to using condoms. Putting the condom on may interrupt sexual spontaneity, although some couples make this a shared moment of sexual play. Many men complain of lessened sensations in the penis while wearing a condom (one student told his class, "It's like playing the piano wearing mittens"), and some men have difficulty maintaining an erection while trying to put on the device. The condom is a poor contraceptive choice for a man having problems with erection, since it calls attention to the degree of erection and may seriously increase "performance anxiety" (see Chapter 9). Also, unless the penis is removed from the vagina soon after ejaculation, loss of erection makes spillage of semen more likely. This can certainly interfere with the intimacy and mood of the moment.

There are also some sexual advantages to the condom. The female may be pleased because her partner is not leaving the responsibility for birth control to her. Lubricated condoms can make intercourse more comfortable if vaginal lubrication is a problem. There is little or no postcoital drippiness for the woman whose partner uses condoms. And use of a condom may help many men who have difficulty controlling the rapidity of ejaculation.

One of the most notable sexual benefits of condom use is that it can help give a person a sense of security about protection from sexually transmitted diseases such as genital herpes or HIV infection in a new sexual relationship. For this reason, many women who use other methods of birth control such as the pill or an IUD insist that their partners use condoms for greater personal safety.

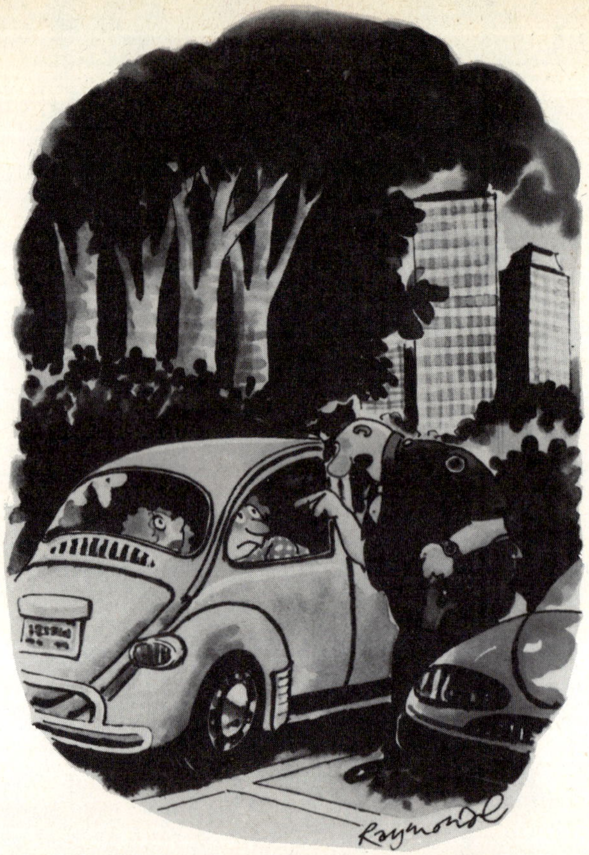

"Hear me, and hear me good, kid. Unroll the condom all the way to the base of the erect penis, taking care to expel the air from the reservoir at the tip by squeezing between the forefinger and thumb . . ."

Spermicides

Spermicides, or vaginal chemical contraceptives, come in many varieties, including foams, jellies, creams, and tablets or suppositories. They do not require a prescription and are available at drug stores and family planning clinics. Spermicides should not be confused with feminine hygiene products, often displayed beside them, which have no spermicidal effectiveness.

HOW SPERMICIDES WORK

Spermicides work in two ways: their active chemical ingredient kills sperm, while the material containing this ingredient provides a mechanical barrier that blocks the entrance to the cervix.

FIGURE 5–6

Vaginal Spermicides

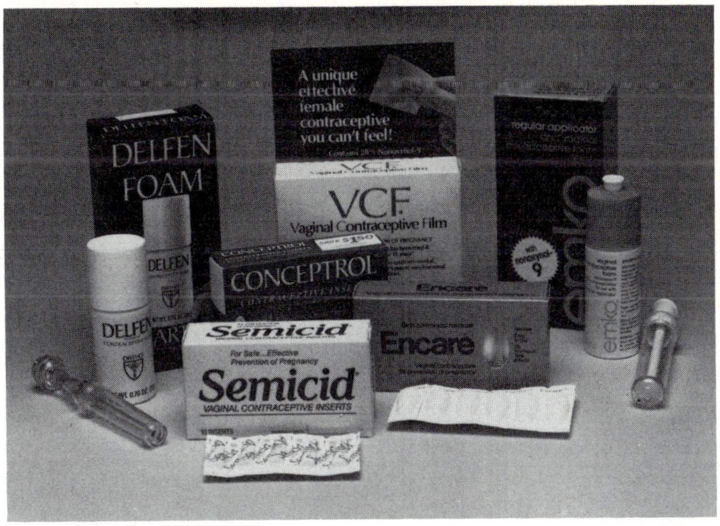

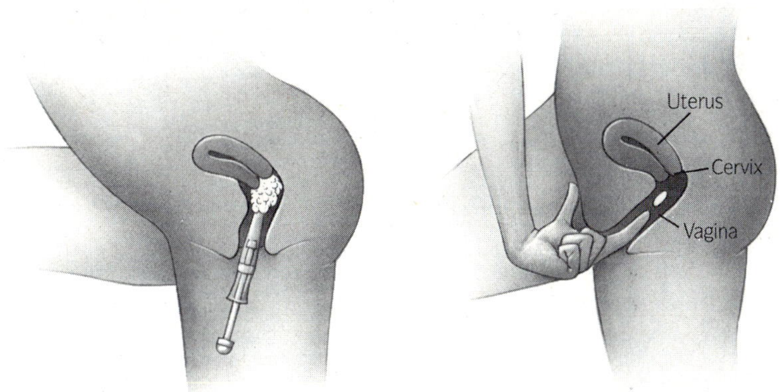

(a) Correct foam placement

(b) Correct suppository placement

Use of vaginal spermicides: (a) When contraceptive foam is inserted with a plastic applicator, it must be placed well within the vagina so it completely covers the cervical mouth. (b) Spermicidal suppositories must be removed from their wrapper and inserted high in the vagina; the manufacturer's instructions on the timing of intercourse must be followed carefully since these products may require up to ten minutes to dissolve.

USE AND EFFECTIVENESS

Because of the individual differences in the many products on the market, the manufacturer's instructions regarding use and effectiveness must be consulted. This information is given in the package insert that comes with each product. *These products are not identical in how they are used or in their reliability in preventing pregnancy.* In general, foams and suppositories are much more effective than creams or jellies, which should be used only with another method of birth control such as a diaphragm or condom. All spermicides require proper placement in the vagina, as shown in Figure 5–6. If used properly and regularly, some spermicidal products can be very effective. In several studies, less than five pregnancies occurred for every 100 couples using these methods for one year (see Coleman and Piotrow, 1979). Failure rates tend to be about three to six times higher than this in actual practice as a result of inconsistent use of the method and improper following of the manufacturer's instructions. Failures occur when a couple inserts the spermicide in the vagina incorrectly, has intercourse a second time without using more of the product, or overlooks the time limits of product effectiveness. In addition, failures can occur if the spermicide has become outdated; for this reason, users should check the expiration date stamped on the spermicide package prior to use.

SIDE EFFECTS AND SAFETY

Burning or irritation of the vagina or penis occurs in about 1 in 20 people using spermicides, but this problem can often be alleviated by changing to a different product. There are no other adverse side effects, which is one of the major advantages spermicides offer.

Despite earlier concerns, spermicides do not cause birth defects (Shapiro et al., 1982; Bracken, 1985; Watkins, 1986; Louik et al., 1987). However, it appears that women who use spermicides after becoming pregnant are more likely than other women to have miscarriages (Scholl et al., 1983).

On the positive side, there is mounting evidence that spermicides provide some protection against sexually transmitted diseases such as gonorrhea and also protect against pelvic inflammatory disease (Jick et al., 1982; Cates, Weisner, and Curran, 1982; Sherris, Moore, and Fox, 1984). Another positive is that spermicides reduce a woman's risk of developing certain types of vaginal infections (bacterial vaginosis and trichomoniasis, conditions discussed in Chapter 7) (Feldblum, Bernardik, and Rosenberg, 1988). Perhaps most important of all is early laboratory evidence that spermicides containing nonoxynol-9 offer some protection against infection with HIV, the AIDS virus (Hicks et al., 1985).

SEXUAL EFFECTS

The use of spermicides may require interrupting the spontaneous flow of sexual activity, but insertion can be made a part of sexual play. With spermicidal suppositories, unlike aerosol foams, 10 to 15 minutes must elapse before vaginal distribution of the product has occurred (depending on the brand) and intercourse is "safe"—so these should not be used if you are in a hurry! Vaginal chemical contraceptives may discourage cunnilingus (oral stimulation of the vulva and vagina) because most products do not have a very pleasant taste. Finally, some people find that these products are messy and provide too much vaginal lubrication (one woman described the sensation as "sloshy").

The Contraceptive Sponge

The newest type of birth control device to become widely available (approved by the Food and Drug Administration in April 1983) is a soft, disposable contraceptive sponge that is inserted into the vagina. Now sold exclusively under the Today brand name, the 2-inch-by-1-inch round product is made of polyurethane permeated with the commonly used spermicide nonoxynol-9 (see Figure 5–7). The contraceptive sponge is sold over the counter in drugstores and doesn't require a prescription or need to be fitted by a physician. Its early reception by consumers was enthusiastic.

HOW THE SPONGE WORKS

There are three different ways in which the sponge functions. First and most important, it carries the spermicidal effect of nonoxynol-9 (which is the active chemical ingredient in many contraceptive creams, foams, and gels). Second, the sponge also functions as a mechanical barrier, partially preventing sperm from entering the mouth of the cervix. Finally, the sponge is also thought to trap and absorb sperm, although the importance of this action is uncertain.

USE AND EFFECTIVENESS

The contraceptive sponge is inserted into the vagina before intercourse. The sponge is first dampened with about two tablespoons of water and then squeezed gently until foam appears (this activates the spermicide in the sponge). Many users report that it is considerably easier to insert than a diaphragm or a cervical cap and, since it can be inserted up to 18 hours before intercourse, it is convenient as well. (Insertion can be done either manually or with an applicator.) As another major advantage, the sponge retains its contraceptive effectiveness for 24 hours without any need for the reapplication of spermicide, so it provides contraceptive protection regardless of how many times the user has intercourse. The sponge is removed by pulling on a small ribbon attached to one of its sides. It should be kept in place for at least six hours

FIGURE 5–7

The Contraceptive Sponge

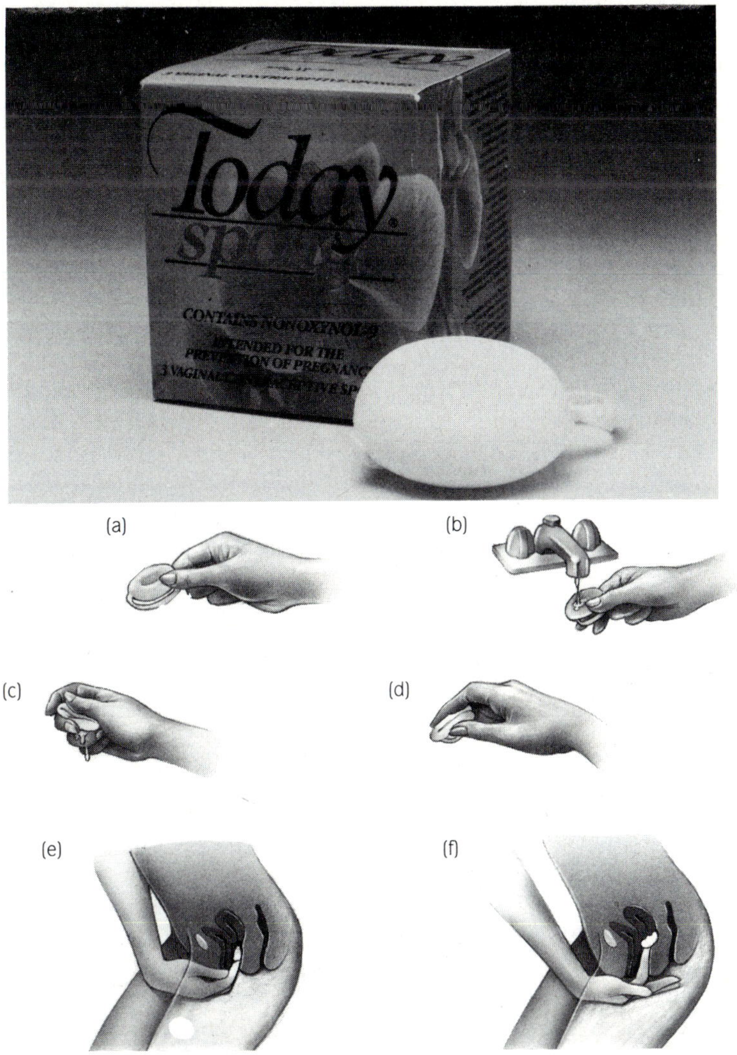

Proper insertion of the sponge: (a) Remove the sponge from the inner pack and hold with dimple side up. The loop should dangle under the sponge. (b) The sponge will feel slightly moist. Wet it further with a small amount of clean water (about two tablespoons). (c) Squeeze the sponge gently to remove excess water. It should feel moist and soapy, but not dripping wet. (d) Fold the sides of the sponge upward with a finger along each side to support it. The sponge should look long and narrow. Be sure the string loop dangles underneath the sponge from one end of the fold to the other. (e) From a standing position, squat down slightly and spread your legs apart. Use your free hand to spread apart the lips of the vagina. You may also stand with one foot on a stool or chair, sit cross-legged, or lie down. The semisquatting position seems to work best for most women. Slide the sponge into the opening of the vagina as far as your fingers will go. Let the sponge slide through your fingers, deeper into the vagina. (f) Now use one or two fingers to push the sponge gently up into your vagina as far as it will go. Be careful not to push a fingernail through the sponge. Check the position of the sponge by sliding your finger around the edge of the sponge to make sure your cervix is not exposed. You should be able to feel the string loop.

after intercourse, with a maximum time of insertion of 30 hours.

One of the major disadvantages of the sponge is a relatively high actual failure rate of 17 per 100 woman-years during its first year of use, compared with a rate of 13 for the diaphragm (Grimes, 1986). However, the actual failure rate in the second year of use was found to be much lower—5 per 100 woman-years (North and Vorhauer, 1985). As with the diaphragm or spermicides, many of the failures are due to improper use—such as removing the sponge too soon after intercourse (i.e., less than six hours after intercourse)—and the user's motivation also seems to play a role. The effectiveness rate can be materially improved by combining use of the sponge with use of a condom.

Women who have used the sponge report a number of distinct advantages over use of the diaphragm. In addition to mentioning how easy it is to insert (which is nearly a universal reaction), many women are pleased to have an inexpensive, disposable contraceptive method that is unobtrusive, tasteless, and odorless and lasts for 24 hours. In addition, the sponge reportedly isn't as messy or drippy as some spermicidal products.

SIDE EFFECTS AND SAFETY

The commonest side effect of the sponge is mild irritation of the vagina or penis, which occurs in about 3 to 5 percent of users. Although the sponge hasn't been in widespread use for a long enough time to assess its safety fully, the only serious health risk to come to attention at the time of this writing is the rare occurrence of toxic shock syndrome (TSS) in a few women who used the sponge. A recent study found that, while there have been a small number of confirmed cases of toxic shock syndrome associated with the use of the contraceptive sponge, the overall risk is exceptionally low (Faich et al., 1986). According to this study, there had been 13 confirmed cases of TSS related to sponge use as of November 1, 1984, which was estimated to be equivalent to 1 case of TSS in 4 million nonmenstrual days of use. The risk of dying of nonmenstrual TSS for a contraceptive sponge user is "in the range of 0.1 to 0.6 per 100,000 woman-years," which is far below the risk of dying from all birth- and contraception-related causes (Reingold, 1986). Thus, while there is a clear-cut association between the sponge and TSS, it is not a large relative risk.

One recently discovered benefit of the sponge is that it protects women against becoming infected with chlamydia and gonorrhea, which are the two most common sexually transmitted pathogens (Rosenberg et al., 1987). However. the sponge offers little protection against infection with HIV.

SEXUAL EFFECTS

Because the sponge can be inserted either hours before sexual activity or at the last moment before intercourse, convenience makes it especially advantageous from a sexual viewpoint. In addition, men and women who have tried the sponge almost invariably say they don't feel it during intercourse, and many couples also report that it doesn't interfere with cunnilingus. But the sponge's most noticeable sexual benefit may be that once it is inserted, it provides protection for multiple acts of intercourse. As one woman told us, "That means we can make love at night and then again in the morning without my having to get up and get ready all over again."

Rhythm

Rhythm methods of contraception depend on periodic abstinence from intercourse during times of the menstrual cycle when fertility is most likely. These methods are the only methods of birth control approved by the Roman Catholic church, which considers them "natural" rather than "artificial."

CALENDAR METHOD

The **calendar method** involves identifying "safe days" in the menstrual cycle (days where intercourse will not lead to pregnancy) based on the lengths of previous cycles. The underlying assumption is that ovulation will occur approximately 14 days before the start of the next menstrual period. Careful hormone studies of the menstrual cycle, however, indicate that this assumption is not always correct (Kolodny and Bauman, 1979).

To calculate the "unsafe" (fertile) period, a record must be kept of the length of each menstrual cycle for a minimum of six months. The first day of the unsafe period is determined by subtracting 18 from the length of the shortest cycle, and the last day of the unsafe period is found by subtracting 11 from the number of days in the longest cycle. For example, if a woman's shortest cycle is 26 days and her longest is

32 days during her "record-keeping" time, she must abstain from intercourse beginning on cycle day 8 (26 − 18 = 8) and continue abstention until day 21 (32 − 11 = 21). Thus, the unsafe days would be days 8 to 21, inclusive, a time of 14 days when intercourse would not be permitted.

THE TEMPERATURE METHOD

The **temperature method** involves daily recording of the basal body temperature (BBT) to pinpoint the time of ovulation. Intercourse is not allowed from the day menstrual flow stops until two to four days after the temperature rises. (If no temperature rise is detected in a full menstrual cycle, which sometimes happens, users of this method must observe total abstinence from sexual intercourse.)

THE OVULATION METHOD

The **ovulation method,** also known as the Billings method or as "natural family planning," depends on changes in cervical mucus to indicate the probable days of fertility during the menstrual cycle. The start of the fertile time is signaled by the appearance of a mucus discharge within the vagina which is whitish or cloudy and of tacky consistency. A day or two before ovulation, greater amounts of mucus are produced in a clear and runnier form with a stretchy consistency very similar to egg white. Intercourse is thought to be "safe" four days after the clear mucus begins, when the mucus has returned to a cloudy color.

EFFECTIVENESS OF THE RHYTHM METHODS

The overall effectiveness of the rhythm methods leaves a great deal to be desired. The calendar method is unquestionably the least reliable among this group (failure rates are approximately 15 to 45 per 100 woman-years; Ross and Piotrow, 1974), and unless the woman's cycle is very regular, long periods of abstinence from intercourse will be required. Temperature methods are inaccurate because they are difficult to interpret (Lenton, Weston, and Cooke, 1977; Bauman, 1981), and in about 20 percent of ovulatory cycles, the BBT chart does not indicate ovulation (Moghissi, 1976; Bauman, 1981). The World Health Organization (1978) found that the ovulation method was "relatively ineffective for preventing pregnancy" based on carefully designed studies done in five different countries, with an overall failure rate of 19.4 per 100 woman-years. This is probably because many women have difficulty noting the cyclic changes in their cervical mucus, and women who have a vaginal infection (which may itself create a discharge) usually cannot use this method. In another study of 725 women, an overall failure rate of 22.3 per 100 woman-years was noted (World Health Organization, 1981).

To keep these data in perspective, it should be noted that the standardized actual failure rate of women using the rhythm method (19.1 per 100 woman years) is almost identical to the failure rate for the diaphragm and is considerably better than the failure rate for spermicides (see Table 5–2). However, a recent report points out that couples who do not use the rhythm method properly—taking risks on occasion—actually have an 86 percent chance of pregnancy (Trussell and Grummer-Strawn, 1990).

The availability of a number of home-use ovulation detection kits, based on identifying the preovulatory LH surge in urine, may eventually be shown to increase the effectiveness of periodic abstinence as a method of birth control, but research documenting this type of use has not yet been conducted (Corsan, Ghazi, and Kemman, 1990).

SEXUAL EFFECTS OF THE RHYTHM METHODS

Most couples using the rhythm methods do not experience major sexual difficulties. However, some couples may develop sexual problems because the need for abstinence creates unusual pressures to have intercourse on "safe" days regardless of whether they feel like it or not. Fear of pregnancy may also lead to sexual difficulties.

calendar method a technique of determining the days in the menstrual cycle when the risk of pregnancy is low; a form of the rhythm method.

temperature method a technique of determining the part of the menstrual cycle when pregnancy is likely to occur so that intercourse can be avoided then. Involves daily recording of basal body temperature to pinpoint ovulation. Intercourse is not allowed from the day menstrual flow stops until two to four days after a temperature rise. Failure rate is high.

ovulation method a method that depends on changes in the cervical mucus thought to indicate the time of ovulation. The mucus changes from cloudy, white, and tacky to clear and stretchy at the time of ovulation. Intercourse is thought to be safe four days after the ovulatory mucus begins and when the mucus has returned to a cloudy, tacky consistency. Failure rate is high.

FIGURE 5–8

Two Types of Tubal Ligation

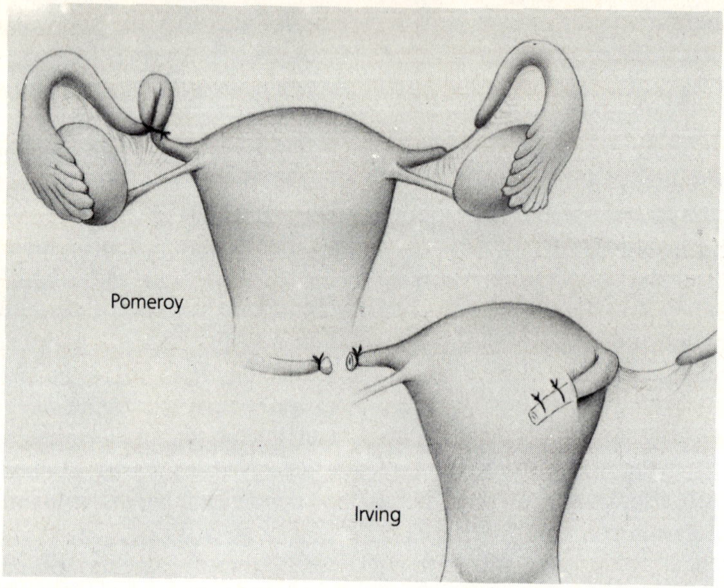

Sterilization

The highest degree of contraceptive protection currently available short of absolute abstinence is found in the use of **sterilization,** surgical procedures to prevent pregnancy. The popularity of these operations for both men and women has increased considerably in America in the last 20 years. One estimate indicates that among all married American couples, about one-quarter will use sterilization within two years after the birth of their last wanted child; by ten years after their last child, more than half will undergo sterilization (Westoff and McCarthy, 1979).

Sterilization procedures are appealing because they are safe, effective, and permanent. Their permanence can be a drawback, however, if there is a change in feelings or circumstances (e.g., death of a child or spouse, divorce) that leads a person to want more children. Although there is some possibility of reversing the sterilization, these procedures are far from guaranteed. Anyone thinking about sterilization as a method of birth control should assume that it will not be reversible. One way of retaining the option to reproduce after male sterilization is to use a sperm bank to store several samples of frozen semen produced before sterilization. If reproduction becomes desirable at a later time, the semen samples are thawed and used in artificial insemination.

FEMALE STERILIZATION

More than 100 different types of operations can be used to achieve female sterilization. Almost all block the Fallopian tubes to prevent the union of sperm and egg. **Tubal ligation** (tying the tubes) is rarely done by itself today, since it is not as effective as other methods that also cut, clip, or otherwise block the tubes (Figure 5–8). Many of these operations are still called "tubal ligation" even though more is done.

Tubal ligation is frequently achieved by using a laparoscope, a tubelike instrument with lights and a viewer that is inserted through the abdominal wall. The tubes are cut and cauterized (burned) through this instrument. If laparoscopy can be done through the navel, no scar is visible; as only a 1-inch incision is required for this operation, it is often called "Band-Aid sterilization." A similar instrument can be inserted through the back end of the vagina or through the vagina and uterus to perform a tubal ligation.

Laparotomy, an operation involving a 4 or 5-inch incision through the abdomen, can also be used to perform a tubal ligation. It is rarely used for sterilization unless there is another reason for abdominal surgery, a technical difficulty, or a danger to the woman because of a medical problem. Female sterilization also results from **hysterectomy** (removal of the uterus) or **ovariectomy** (removal of the ovaries), but these operations are generally done for other reasons with sterility occurring as a by-product.

Female sterilization by most techniques offers almost foolproof protection against pregnancy. In rare instances, the cut ends of the tubes may rejoin, leading to a pregnancy, but the most common cause for "method failure" is when the woman is already pregnant (but no one knows it) when the operation is performed (Wortman and Piotrow, 1973). Side effects are infrequent (less than 5 percent) and are usually limited to the first few days after surgery, when infection or bleeding may be a problem.

Most women have no sexual difficulties after sterilization, which affects neither their hormones (since their ovaries are intact) nor their sexual anatomy. A few women may run into problems. If a woman undergoes sterilization involuntarily (e.g., if it was a decision she was pushed into by her husband or by health or economic circumstances), she may develop a reduced interest in sex for psychological reasons. Some women find that after sterilization they no longer feel the same way about sex (or have lowered sexual responsiveness) because they feel "incomplete" or "less than a woman." This reaction is particularly possible in a woman whose religious background considers sex unnatural or sinful if it is separated from its reproductive potential. On the other hand, some women show increased sexual interest after sterilization due to no longer fearing pregnancy.

MALE STERILIZATION

Vasectomy is a simple surgical procedure that consists of cutting and tying each **vas deferens** (the tube that carries sperm) (see Figure 5–9). The operation is usually done using local anesthesia in a doctor's office or clinic and requires only about 15 or 20 minutes. The man can then go home, although it is usually advisable to avoid strenuous physical activity for a day or two afterward. Occasionally, a man will experience pain in the scrotal area for a week or ten days after a seemingly uncomplicated vasectomy.

Vasectomy does not stop sperm production; it blocks the passage of sperm from the testes to the upper part of the vas deferens. Sperm then accumulate in the **epididymis** (a mass of tubes at the back of each testis), where they are engulfed and destroyed by cells called phagocytes. Some sperm appear to leak out into the scrotum, where they disintegrate. Because some sperm are already above the point where the vasectomy was done, it usually takes six to eight weeks (about a dozen ejaculations) after this operation before the ejaculate is sterile (contains no sperm). For this reason, the man and his sex partner should use another method of birth control until at least two consecutive semen exams show that no sperm are present. [Very rarely, vasectomies fail even after one semen exam has been negative (Alderman, 1988).]

Vasectomy does not affect hormone production and does not interfere in any physiological way with erection or ejaculation. The amount of the ejaculate is almost unchanged, since secretions from the testis and epididymis account for less than 5 percent of the volume of seminal fluid.

In the 1970s, there was some concern that vasectomy might lead to later health problems, especially in light of research in monkeys that showed that vasectomy produces hardening of the arteries years after the operation (Clarkson and Alexander, 1980). But several more recent large-scale studies provide convincing evidence that vasectomy does not lead to any long-term health problems in humans. Massey and his colleagues (1984) studied more than 10,000 vasectomized men and a matched nonvasectomized control group. They found that vasectomized men had fewer cancers, fewer cancer deaths, lower rates of heart disease, and fewer deaths from heart attacks or strokes than the men in the control group who had not had

sterilization surgical procedure performed on men (vasectomy) or women (tubal ligation; hysterectomy) to prevent union of sperm and egg.

tubal ligation (tū′ bull lī gā′ shun) literally, tying the tubes—cutting, cauterizing, and blocking the Fallopian tubes to prevent conception.

laparotomy (lap uh rot′ uh mē) any operation involving an incision through the abdominal wall. Now used for sterilization only if other surgery is required in the abdomen.

hysterectomy (his′ tur ek′ tuh mē) partial or total removal of the uterus.

ovariectomy (o vuh′ re ek′ tuh mé) surgical removal of the ovaries.

vasectomy (vas ek′ tuh mē) surgical procedure for sterilization of the male consisting of cutting and tying each vas deferens. The operation does not stop sperm production but blocks its passage from the testes.

vas deferens (vas def′ ur enz) one of two long, tubelike structures that convey spermatozoa from the testes.

epididymis (ep′ i did′ i mis) the tightly coiled tubing network folded against the back surface of each testis in which sperm cells spend several weeks maturing.

FIGURE 5–9

Vasectomy

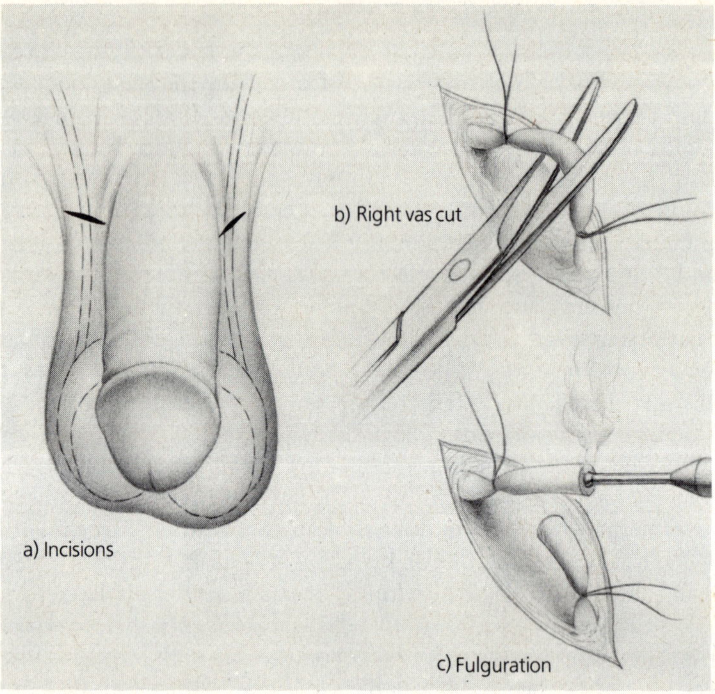

A vasectomy must completely prevent sperm from traveling out of the scrotum higher into the male reproductive system. Drawing (a) shows the site of the small incision in the scrotum used to perform a vasectomy; (b) shows the vas being cut with surgical scissors; and (c) shows the cut end of the vas being burned with a controlled electric current so that scar tissue forms to block the passage of sperm.

vasectomies. Perrin and co-workers (1984), in a study with an average follow-up interval of 15 years, also found no indication that vasectomy predisposes to arteriosclerosis or heart disease.

Vasectomy is the simplest and safest form of surgical contraception: the failure rate is a very low 0.15 percent. Failures occur because of unprotected intercourse before all sperm have disappeared from the ejaculate, mistakes in performing the operation, or, very rarely, because the cut ends of the vas have grown back together. The rate of medical complications such as bleeding or infection is less than 5 percent, although minor swelling, pain, and temporary skin discoloration due to bruising occur in about half of men after this procedure. Postoperative ice packs and a well-fitted athletic supporter can reduce discomfort.

Less than 1 man in 20 reports decreased sexual pleasure after a vasectomy, while close to half claim increased pleasure and about a quarter report an increased frequency of intercourse (Wortman, 1975). In fact, many couples find that sex is more spontaneous and fun after a vasectomy since they don't need to worry about becoming pregnant. Men with a history of sexual problems are not always good candidates for vasectomy, since they may be more prone to developing psychological impotence or other difficulties after surgery. For some couples, there may be a drop in marital harmony after a vasectomy because the man expects gratitude from his wife in return for having the surgery (Rodgers and Ziegler, 1973) or because the wife resents not being able to have more children. A man who has been well adjusted to a vasectomy may become impotent (usually temporarily) if he divorces and then remarries, particularly if he and his new wife would like to have children. More typical, however, is this comment from a 30-year-old man six months after his vasectomy: "It was simple and quick and did the trick. Now sex is *really* making love, without worrying about 'accidents'" (Authors' files).

Other Methods of Contraception

Withdrawal (coitus interruptus) is the removal of the penis from the vagina before ejaculation occurs. This is a difficult form of birth control in which even perfect timing (which is not always possible) does not give perfect results. If ejaculation occurs before the penis is withdrawn completely, or if drops of semen spurt into the opening of the vagina, pregnancy can occur. Because live sperm can also be in the preejaculatory fluid long before ejaculation (or even if the male doesn't ejaculate), this method of contraception is chancy at best, with a failure rate of 20 to 25 percent. This method can also be a frustrating form of birth control for both parties, who may find that it seriously interrupts the spontaneity of sexual interaction. However, it is clearly better than not using any contraceptive when nothing else is available.

Douching, using a liquid to flush the vagina, is a poor method of contraception, since sperm can quickly penetrate the cervical mucus, where they are unaffected by douching. The failure rate is more than 40 percent.

Breast-feeding inhibits ovulation in some women (possibly via the effect of high prolactin levels on the ovaries), but this method of birth control is very unreliable. Women who do not want to become pregnant soon after childbirth should begin using a more effective means of contraception right away. Some studies of nursing mothers not using any other method of birth control indicate pregnancy rates of over 50 percent (Buchanan, 1975).

Abstinence from intercourse is, needless to say, a highly effective way to prevent pregnancy if practiced consistently. Some couples voluntarily limit their sex lives to noncoital acts, but this does not seem to be a very popular choice for most heterosexual couples.

POSTCONCEPTION METHODS OF BIRTH CONTROL

The "Morning After" Pill

Various types of estrogen used in high doses shortly after conception can prevent implantation and provide a form of after-the-fact birth control. This approach can be useful in special situations (such as rape or leakage of a condom) but is not suitable for routine contraceptive use. Most commonly, diethylstilbestrol (DES) is given to the woman for five days, beginning as soon after unprotected intercourse as possible but, at the outside, within 72 hours. The effectiveness of using this timetable is extremely high: the pregnancy rate is less than 1 percent (Rinehart, 1976). Another form of the "morning after" pill uses only two doses of ethinyl estradiol (a type of estrogen) and a progestogen taken 12 hours apart. In a study involving nearly 900 women who received this treatment within 72 hours of unprotected intercourse, there was a 2 percent failure rate (Percival-Smith and Abercrombie, 1987).

The primary side effects are nausea (sometimes accompanied by vomiting), breast tenderness, and alterations in the menstrual cycle. Used on a short-term basis, as just outlined, DES or other forms of estrogen are unlikely to have any lasting effect on the woman or on a fetus if a pregnancy occurs. Although DES used during later stages of pregnancy (as it used to be, to prevent miscarriage), has been linked to abnormalities in the reproductive systems of children of mothers receiving this drug (see Chapter 10), there is no indication that this effect applies to its use in preventing pregnancy. Nevertheless, the risks of "morning after" pills are not entirely known at present, and it should not be assumed that they are completely safe.

Menstrual Extraction

This technique has been pioneered by the women's self-help movement. Just when a period is expected, a thin, flexible plastic tube is inserted through the cervix into the uterus, and suction (using either a syringe or a pump) is applied to draw out the endometrial lining. If the woman is pregnant, the tiny embryo is easily withdrawn. There may be mild cramping, but no anesthetic is usually used. Menstrual extraction should not be performed more than eight weeks after a missed period because complete evacuation of the embryo and its support system (the placenta) is more difficult after this point.

Although further research is required, there do not

withdrawal (coitus interruptus) the removal of the penis from the vagina before ejaculation occurs. When used as a birth control method, failure rate is high.

douching (dŭsh′ ing) using a liquid to flush the vagina.

abstinence the act of voluntarily not engaging in some act, such as sexual intercourse. A highly effective method of birth control if practiced consistently.

seem to be any major side effects when done under proper conditions by a health care professional. In some instances, however, when menstrual extraction has been done as a self-help procedure by women without proper health care training, there have been complications such as uterine perforation, infection, or incompletely extracted uterine contents, requiring subsequent surgery (Perrone, 1990).

Abortion

Abortion is the termination of pregnancy before the embryo or fetus is able to survive outside the uterus (Tietze, 1977). Abortion can be either **spontaneous,** that is, when a medical problem ends a pregnancy, or **induced,** when the contents of the pregnant uterus are removed intentionally. On a worldwide basis, it has been estimated that 30 to 40 million induced abortions are performed legally each year, with a similar number of illegal abortions (Baulieu, 1989).

Today, the abortion issue is argued heatedly by various groups. The "right-to-life" movement opposes abortion on the grounds of protecting the rights of the unborn, while "pro-choice" advocates want women to have freedom of choice in controlling their own bodies and futures. Public opinion on these issues is divided. The complex aspects of rights and responsibilities as they affect individuals and society are not simple or easily summarized; they are not discussed here because of space limitations.

WHO HAS ABORTIONS: POPULATION PATTERNS

In 1985, there were approximately 1.3 million legal abortions performed in the United States (*MMWR* 38:SS-2, 1989). This corresponded to a national abortion rate of 24 abortions done per 1000 females aged 15 to 44. The national abortion ratio, which is stated in terms of the number of abortions per 1000 live births, was 354 in 1985.

A study conducted by the Alan Guttmacher Institute in 1987 showed that teenagers had 26 percent of all legal abortions (Henshaw and Silverman, 1988). Women 20 to 24 years old accounted for one-third of all abortions, while women aged 30 or over had 19 percent of the abortions that were performed that year (see Figure 5–10).

FIGURE 5–10

Selected Characteristics of Women Who Have Abortions

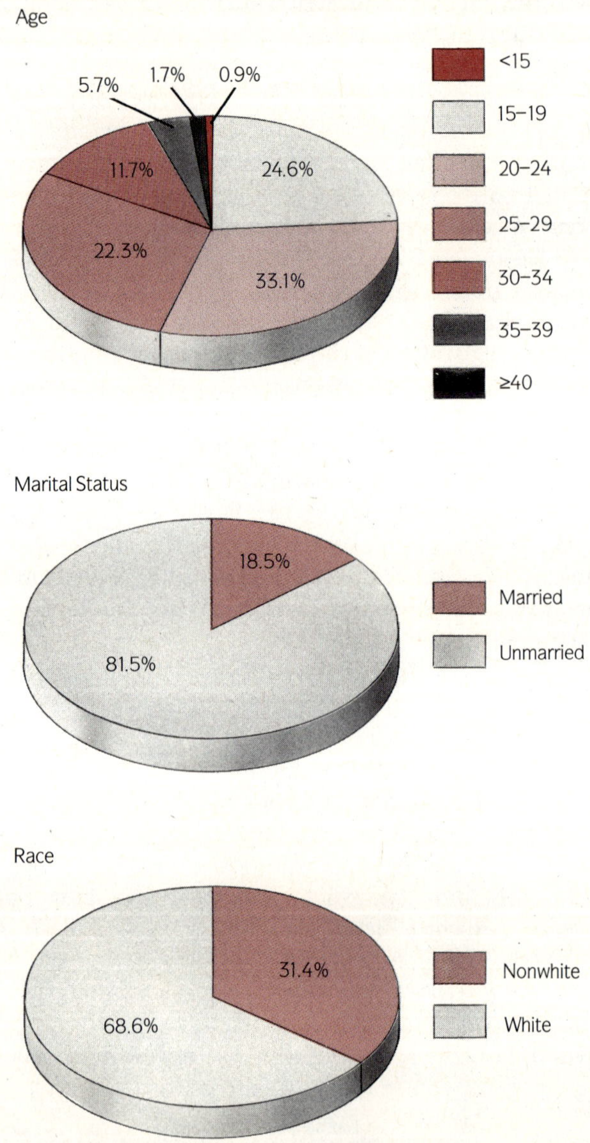

Source: Adapted from Henshaw and Silverman, 1988, Table 1.

Only 18.5 percent of women who had abortions were married. Close to two-thirds had never been married, while the balance were either separated (6.4 percent), divorced (11.2 percent), or widowed (0.6 percent). Not surprisingly, a disproportionately high percentage of women who obtained abortions had family incomes of under $11,000 a year, while abortions were far less common among women whose family income was $25,000 or more.

Both U.S. government figures and the Alan Guttmacher Institute study show that approximately two-thirds of the women who obtain legal abortions are white (*MMWR* 38:SS-2, 1989; Henshaw and Silverman, 1988). However, it is noteworthy that the abortion ratio is much higher among minority women than for white women: 472 versus 277 abortions per 1000 live births in 1985 (*MMWR* 38:SS-2, 1989).

Looking at the religion of women who had legal abortions in 1987 revealed that 42 percent were Protestant, 32 percent were Catholic, 1 percent were Jewish, 3 percent were adherents of other religions, and 22 percent indicated that they had no religious affiliation (Henshaw and Silverman, 1988). This is of some interest since it shows that many Catholic women are willing to disregard the Church's teachings that prohibit abortion.

Another notable point made by the Alan Guttmacher Institute survey was that half of all females who had abortions in 1987 said that they were practicing contraception during the month in which they conceived. This is in sharp contrast to the idea that most women who have abortions are either uninformed about contraception or unwilling to make an effort to practice birth control, as the following comment makes clear:

> *A 23-year-old female graduate student:* When I was a college junior I was involved in a live-in relationship with a guy I cared a lot about. We had a great sex life, but we were careful about it, with me using a diaphragm and him using a condom. You can imagine our shock—and dismay—when I turned out to be pregnant. We had never "forgotten" to use birth control; in fact, we were using two separate kinds of birth control. Still, when I told my best friend about it, she insisted that there must have been one time we slipped up and forgot. "Maybe," she said, "you were both drunk and you don't remember it." I really resented that attitude and realized how easy it is to make assumptions about people's behavior that just may not be true. (Authors' files).

As Table 5–3 shows, the majority of women who had an abortion in 1985 had never had a live birth. Likewise, most had never previously had an induced abortion. Less than one in 20 women who have abortions have had three or more abortions in the past. This strongly suggests that very few women rely on abortion as a means of birth control, although some who are opposed to legalized abortion claim that this is a common practice.

ABORTION METHODS

The abortion method chosen depends mainly on the length of the pregnancy. During the first trimester, the most common method is called **vacuum aspiration** or suction. After the mouth of the cervix is widened (dilated), a small plastic tube is inserted into the uterus. The tube is connected to an electric pump that

FOCUS IN BRIEF

What Happens to Unintended Pregnancies?

When an unintended pregnancy occurs, there are three possible outcomes: birth, abortion, or miscarriage. The following data show the percentage of unintended pregnancies that fall into each of these three categories for American women in different age groups.

Age	*Birth*	*Abortion*	*Miscarriage*
15–19	41.7%	45.4%	12.9%
20–24	44.8%	42.0%	13.2%
25–29	43.5%	43.5%	13.0%
30–34	45.0%	41.8%	13.2%
35–39	38.0%	49.5%	12.5%
40–44	17.3%	72.0%	10.7%

It is interesting to note that the percentage of women choosing abortion is remarkably similar over the 20-year span from age 15 to 34.

Source: Jacqueline Darroch Forrest and Sushella Singh, "Public Sector Savings Resulting from Expenditures for Contraceptive Services." FAMILY PLANNING PERSPECTIVES, volume 22, number 1, January/February 1990) p. 9.

abortion termination of a pregnancy before the fetus can survive outside the uterus. **Spontaneous** abortions occur naturally due to medical problems; **induced** abortions are done intentionally.

vacuum aspiration the method usually chosen for abortion during the first trimester. The cervix is dilated and the contents of the uterus are removed through a plastic tube connected to a pump.

TABLE 5–3

Percentage Distribution of Reported Legal Abortions in the United States, by Number of Previous Live Births and by Number of Previous Induced Abortions, 1985

Previous Live Births						
0	*1*	*2*	*3*	*≥4*	*Unknown*	*Total*
55.1%	21.4%	14.4%	5.1%	2.5%	1.5%	100%

Previous Induced Abortions					
0	*1*	*2*	*≥3*	*Unknown*	*Total*
56.8%	25.0%	9.6%	4.7%	3.8%	100%

Source: Modified from data in *Morbidity and Mortality Weekly Report* 38:SS-2, Tables 15 and 16, September 1989.

removes the fetal tissue, placenta, and membranes from the uterus by suction (Figure 5–11). The procedure usually requires only 10 to 15 minutes.

During the fourth and fifth months of pregnancy, the safest method for abortion is **dilatation and evacuation (D&E),** a method that is similar to vacuum aspiration. After the mouth of the cervix is widened, vacuum suction is applied to partly remove the contents of the uterus. However, because at this later stage of pregnancy not all the tissue can be removed by suction alone, a forcep is used to remove additional material until the uterus is completely empty. In addition, a metal instrument called a curette may be used to gently scrape the walls of the uterus to ensure that all remnants of extra tissue have been removed.

Second-trimester abortions are also sometimes done by using chemicals to stimulate contractions of the uterus, causing expulsion of the fetus and membranes. **Prostaglandin-induced abortions** are done by injecting prostaglandins into the amniotic sac, dripping them slowly into a vein, or placing them in the vagina. In **saline-induced abortions,** 7 ounces of a saline (salt) solution are injected into the amniotic fluid. Both methods require hours before completion, have the disadvantages of physical and emotional discomfort during contractions of the uterus, and require vaginal delivery of the dead fetus.

Less commonly, surgical procedures are used for abortion. **Dilation and curettage (D&C)** involves dilating the cervix and then gently scraping the lining of the uterus with a metal instrument (the curette) to extract the fetal tissue, placenta, and membranes. A D&C can be done until about 15 weeks after the last menstrual period and, unlike previously mentioned methods, requires the use of general anesthesia. A **hysterotomy** is an operation like a cesarean section that can be used throughout the second trimester. It also requires general anesthesia and is rarely used.

Although some people believe that eating certain foods, vigorous exercise, or other do-it-yourself techniques will lead to abortion, this is not true. Attempts at inducing abortion by inserting objects such as a wire coathanger or knitting needle into the uterus are *extremely dangerous* and can lead to fatal infections or bleeding.

SAFETY

Modern abortion techniques are less risky to the mother than a full-term pregnancy: less than 4 deaths occur per 100,000 induced abortions compared to approximately 14 deaths per 100,000 live births (Grimes and Cates, 1980; Koonin et al., 1988). In fact, among healthy women (those with no serious preexisting medical problems) the risk of dying from a legal abortion in the United States is less than 1 per 100,000 procedures (LeBolt, Grimes, and Cates, 1982). Abortions done during the first trimester are simplest and safest; after this, complications such as bleeding, infection, and perforation of the uterus are more common. There is no solid evidence that having a properly done abortion causes later infertility. Several reports indicate that having two or more induced abortions leads to a higher rate of miscarriages in subsequent pregnancies (Harlap et al., 1979; Levin et al., 1980; Madore et al., 1981) and may increase the rate of prematurity and low-birth-weight infants (World Health Organization, 1978).

FIGURE 5–11

Vacuum Aspiration Abortion

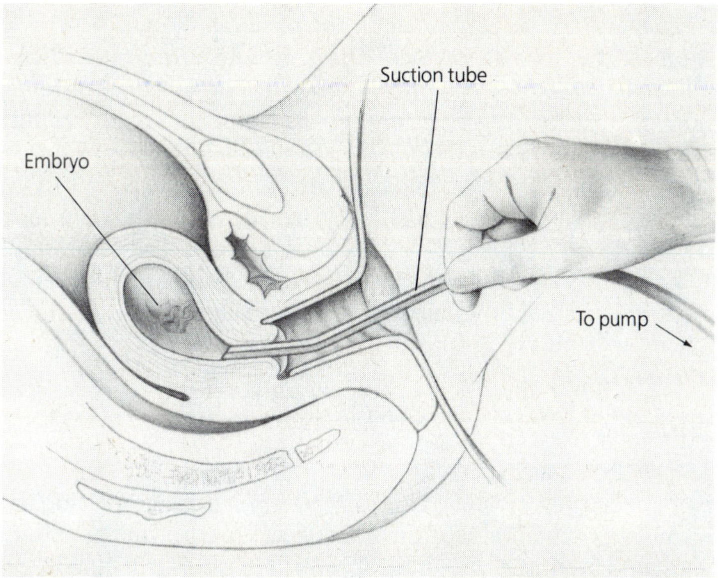

Vacuum aspiration for abortion involves suctioning the embryo and membranes within the uterus.

PSYCHOLOGICAL ASPECTS OF ABORTION

The emotional benefits of abortion outweigh the psychological risks for most women (Osofsky et al., 1971; Niswander, Singer, and Singer, 1972; Nadelson, 1978). Except for case studies, which usually involve problem abortions, none of the scores of studies of women following abortion reveals a high degree of psychiatric distress (Holden, 1989). In fact, serious psychological problems after abortions are far less common than postpartum depression.

Not surprisingly, many women report considerable relief after an abortion (H. P. David, 1978). As one woman explained, "When I found out I was pregnant, I felt like there was a dark cloud over my future. Once I had my abortion, I could feel the sunlight again" (Authors' files). Nevertheless, short-lived feelings of guilt, sadness, and loss are common in women who have had abortions. Pre- and post-abortion counseling are usually effective in helping women deal with these reactions.

The right-to-life camp was dealt a serious and unexpected setback when U.S. Surgeon General C. Everett Koop (who personally opposed abortion) issued a letter to President Reagan on the health effects of abortion that failed to identify serious psychological aftereffects. Koop wrote that "at this time, the available scientific evidence . . . simply cannot support either the preconceived beliefs of those pro-life or pro-choice" (Koop, 1989). Koop's basic position was that because of methodological flaws, such as the absence of control groups, very low follow-up rates, and non-representative samples, good scientific evidence is not available on the psychological or physical effects of abortion. However, it later became known that

dilatation and evacuation (D&E) a method for abortion involving widening the mouth of the cervix, followed by removing the products of conception by a combination of suction and scraping.

prostaglandin-induced abortion evacuation of the contents of the pregnant uterus produced by infusion of prostaglandins.

saline-induced abortion evacuation of the contents of the pregnant uterus produced by infusion of a salt solution into the amniotic fluid.

dilatation and curettage (D&C) (kyur e tazh′) process involving dilating the cervix and then gently scraping the lining of the uterus with a metal instrument. Sometimes used as a form of abortion.

hysterotomy (his tur ot′ uh mē) incision of the uterus. Infrequently used for abortion during the second trimester.

Koop's actual report had been more favorable in its conclusions about the relative safety of abortions but had been censored by higher government figures (*The New York Times*, 1989; *Science*, 1989). For this reason, the American Psychological Association organized a blue ribbon panel to review studies on the psychological responses of U.S. women after legal abortions. This group concluded "the weight of the evidence from scientific studies indicates that legal abortion of an unwanted pregnancy in the first trimester does not pose a psychological hazard for most women" and that "severe negative reactions after abortion are rare" (Adler et al., 1990).

One relatively neglected aspect of the abortion experience is the *male's* reaction. An interesting survey of the impact of abortion on men shows that many men try to approach the abortion decision in an abstract, intellectual way but later find themselves having to deal with feelings of hurt, guilt, or anger (Shostak, McLouth, and Seng, 1984). Few abortion centers offer counseling services for men, perhaps reflecting the view of one abortion counselor who told us: "The imperial male attitude is just too hard to deal with in many cases. It's the woman who's pregnant, and it's her feelings I worry about. Let the men go find a psychiatrist on their own if they need to." While not all abortion counselors share this view, many say that men don't seem interested in their services.

THE PSYCHOLOGY OF CONTRACEPTIVE USE

Why do some people who do not want a pregnancy avoid the use of contraception or misuse the form of birth control they have selected? One common reason is inadequate knowledge. Illustrating this point, Zelnik and Kantner (1979) found that about half of sexually active teenage women aged 15 to 19 thought they could not become pregnant (see Table 5–4). Similarly, a survey of urban mothers showed that only one-third knew when during the menstrual cycle a woman is most likely to become pregnant, and for mothers under age 21, only 10 percent were correct in their knowledge (Presser, 1977).

Inadequate knowledge does not explain why many people who understand the techniques and risks of conception still do not use birth control or use it haphazardly. This phenomenon raises a fundamental question about personal motivation and contraceptive practice. Clearly, some people avidly want to avoid pregnancy, while others only want to delay the timing of a pregnancy or do not mind if they happen to conceive (in this discussion, we do not deal with couples wanting a pregnancy, since contraceptive use does not really apply). In general, the more motivated a person is to avoid pregnancy, the more likely he or she will choose and consistently use a highly effective birth control method. But this motivation may also be affected by other factors, such as forgetfulness, denial ("it can't happen to me"), dissatisfaction with a particular method, wanting to please a partner, or concern about medical risks. This comment from a 23-year-old woman illustrates a commonly encountered situation:

> I'd been using the pill for about two years, but I read about its risks so I decided to switch. I got pregnant the third time I used a diaphragm. I'm back on the pill now, older but wiser. *(Authors' files)*

Not using contraception is sometimes a sign of personal embarrassment about sexuality in general or about a particular method. One 24-year-old woman told us that she had tried to insert a diaphragm for a half hour and finally just gave up because she felt foolish about it. Other people worry that someone may discover their contraceptive devices, giving away that they are, or plan to be, sexually active. While this concern obviously affects teenagers who may be afraid of a parent finding out that they use contraception, it may also apply to a woman whose date accidentally discovers a container of foam in her purse. She may have no intention of having intercourse or *any* sexual activity with him, but the "discovery" may be taken to mean that she is willing or even expecting to.

For other people, it is okay to have sex in the heat of passion, but *planning* for it makes it immoral, mechanical, or unromantic (these people are often called parents). Many people also use contraceptives on a fairly regular basis with only occasional lapses into sexual brinksmanship. In these instances they decide to indulge their soaring sexual feelings (and not call Time Out) or to forgo contraception to "have more fun" or "make it more natural." For example, couples using rhythm methods may find sex more enticing on the days when abstinence is expected.

In some cases hostility, power struggles, or differences in the reproductive goals of two sexual partners may lead to disuse or misuse of contraception. The man who insists on using withdrawal may make sex unpleasant and even threatening to his partner. The

TABLE 5–4

Percentage Distribution of Women Aged 15–19 in 1976 Who Had Premarital Intercourse More than Once Without Contraception

Intention and Reason for Last Nonuse	*Total*	*White*	*Black*
All nonusers	(*N* = 590)	(*N* = 339)	(*N* = 251)
Pregnant	15.0	15.0	15.2
Trying to become pregnant	5.2	4.1	9.2
Not pregnant or trying	79.8	80.9	75.6
Total	100.0	100.0	100.0
Not pregnant or trying	(*N* = 452)	(*N* = 261)	(*N* = 191)
Thought they could become pregnant	49.0	46.7	58.4
Did not expect to have intercourse	20.3	19.3	24.3
Wanted to use something but could not under the circumstances	7.2	7.7	5.2
Partner objected	1.9	1.4	4.2
Believed it was wrong or dangerous to use contraception	4.9	4.4	6.9
Did not know about contraception or where to get it	3.1	3.2	2.7
Sex was not much fun with contraception or contraception was too difficult to use	3.8	2.6	8.5
Other	7.8	8.1	6.6
Thought they could not become pregnant	51.0	53.2	41.6
Had intercourse at time of month when could not become pregnant	22.6	24.3	15.7
Too young to become pregnant	5.3	5.3	5.2
Had intercourse too infrequently to become pregnant	4.1	3.4	6.7
Other	19.0	20.2	14.0
Total	100.0	100.0	100.0

Source: Zelnik and Kantner, 1979, p. 292. Reprinted with permission from *Family Planning Perspectives*, Volume 11, Number 5, 1979.

woman can attempt to manipulate her partner by limiting her sexual availability ("My IUD is cramping" or "I have an infection") or by seeking a pregnancy to entrap her partner in marriage or to prevent separations or divorce (Sandberg, 1976). Who assumes responsibility for contraception may be a heated issue, particularly if the woman has done so for a long while and then wishes to turn this job over to her partner.

One last aspect of the psychology of contraceptive use will be mentioned. When sexual problems exist in a relationship, couples frequently become sloppy in their attention to birth control or stop using contraception altogether. Sometimes they believe their sexual difficulty results from or is worsened by their contraceptive method. In other cases, they think that when sex is a problem, conception is unlikely (of course, they *may* be mildly shocked to discover how wrong they are). In yet other instances, discontinuing the use of birth control may be used as a psychological ploy to symbolize that "sex really is not so important" or, conversely, to attempt to make sexual contact more intimate and exciting.

FUTURE TRENDS IN CONTRACEPTION

There is general agreement that currently available contraceptive methods are less than perfect from the viewpoints of safety, reversibility, effectiveness, and ease of use. To improve the range of choices, considerable research is under way.

New Directions in Male Contraception

Not surprisingly, the most intense interest focuses on the possibility of developing a male birth control pill. In theory, this could be accomplished by using drugs to (1) block sperm production in the testes, (2) interfere with sperm maturation in the epididymis, (3) impair sperm transport at any point along their journey from testis to epididymis to vas deferens to urethra, or (4) reduce sperm motility or ability to undergo capacitation. Various drugs have already been found to accomplish each task, but so far they have either proved to have incomplete effects or to have unacceptable side effects. For example, combinations of estrogen and progestogen (as used in the "female" pill) are effective in blocking sperm production but cause a profound drop in sexual interest in most males and frequently lead to impotence. Pills combining testosterone and a progestogen are currently under investigation, since they do not seem to cause the circulatory side effects estrogen does and do not usually interfere with sexual function. However, these pills are not highly effective in inhibiting sperm production for long periods of time (Segal, 1979).

A report from China indicates that an extract from cottonseed oil called gossypol suppresses sperm production (National Coordinating Group for Male Contraceptives, 1978). Gossypol acts on sperm metabolism, either immobilizing sperm cells or killing them (Tong, Zhou, and Zhou, 1982). While the incidence of short-term side effects with gossypol seems to be acceptable, with only about 10 percent of men developing minor problems such as dizziness, fatigue, dry mouth, and digestive tract difficulties and only 5 percent reporting decreased libido or potency problems, it is not clear if gossypol's effects on sperm production are completely reversible (Liskin, Pile, and Quillin, 1983). Furthermore, one report found that 10 to 20 percent of the men taking gossypol remained irreversibly infertile even after they had stopped use of the drug (Ziporyn, 1984). This condition would severely restrict the appeal of such a birth control measure.

A more promising development has been the creation of a synthetic form of inhibin, a protein substance made in the testes that provides feedback to the hypothalamus and pituitary gland controlling the production of FSH (Sairam et al., 1984). Since it is thought that inhibin suppresses sperm production without affecting sexual function, clinical trials with this substance may provide the ultimate breakthrough in the search for an effective, reversible male contraceptive.

The search for additional methods of male contraception also includes several other possibilities:

1. Developing a vaccine or drug to block production of FSH in the pituitary, since this hormone controls sperm production but has no known effects on sexual function.
2. Developing a vaccine to impair the enzymes released by the acrosome (chemical reservoir) of the sperm, since these enzymes are required for the sperm to penetrate the egg.
3. Using ultrasound to produce temporary sterility by blocking sperm production.

New Directions in Female Contraception

Improvements in methods of female fertility control are being studied currently by many groups of scientists. One of the most promising approaches is the attempt to develop an antipregnancy vaccine that is activated only in the event of conception and that works in a reliable and unobtrusive fashion. Vaccines directed against HCG, a hormone secreted by the placenta (and the hormone detected by pregnancy tests), are among those being tested; they seem to prevent pregnancy without interfering with ovarian or menstrual cycles.

An attempt is also under way to identify a compound that could block progesterone production by the corpus luteum (the part of the ovarian follicle that produces hormones in early pregnancy). This compound would prevent implantation and induce menstruation whether or not pregnancy occurs. Closely related to this concept is a new drug discovered in Europe that both blocks and terminates pregnancies. Known currently as RU 486, this drug is a progesterone antagonist: that is, it blocks the effects of progesterone, the hormone that is needed to prepare the lining of the uterus for implantation of a fertilized egg and that also maintains pregnancy. In one study, it was found that RU 486 led to abortion in 85 percent of pregnant women who took this medication with ten days of a missed period (Couzinet et al., 1986). Now, after being used on thousands of women, the utility of RU 486 has been widely confirmed, with complete success in more than 95 percent of seven-week pregnancies (Baulieu, 1989a; Cherfas, 1989). Furthermore, given in combination with a prostaglandin-like medication called sulprastone, it seems to be even more effective. This means that if a woman wants to avoid pregnancy after unprotected intercourse or if she has already missed a period and thinks she may be pregnant, she can take a pill that would either block pregnancy from occurring or end the pregnancy in its earliest stages without requiring a surgical abortion. While government approval of RU 486 is undoubtedly some time away in the United States, it became available in France and China in 1988 (*The New York Times*, September 24, 1988, pp. 1 and 8).

The inventor of RU 486, Dr. Etienne-Emile Baulieu, now spends much of his time engaged in a political campaign to increase the acceptance of this controversial drug. Although it currently is often called the "abortion pill," Baulieu objects to the connotation of this label, saying that the word abortion is automatically negative: "I resent when people present the very early interruption of pregnancy as killing a baby, morally or physically," Baulieu observes (Greenhouse, 1989). Instead, he suggests calling it a "contragestive"—a phrase he has coined to denote blocking gestation.

Although there are no indications of when, or whether, RU 486 will become available in the United States, it is important to realize that the drug has potential for many uses other than for abortion. In addition to potential medical uses such as in treating breast cancer and certain brain tumors, the drug has a strong potential as a contraceptive in the conventional sense. Taken during the first part of the menstrual cycle (the follicular phase), RU 486's anti-progesterone action may be effective in blocking ovulation, which might eventually prove to be its most important use (Cherfas and Palca, 1989).

Research is also being conducted to develop a pill, liquid, or vaginal tampon that could be self-administered at the expected time of menstruation to induce menstrual flow and evacuate the contents of the uterus. Various synthetic analogues of prostaglandins that cause uterine contractions are being investigated for this purpose, but while they appear to be at least 90 percent effective, they are typically accompanied by an unacceptably high rate of negative side effects. Another idea is to block signals from the hypothalamus to the pituitary gland that trigger LH release. An important step in the initiation of ovulation would thereby be disrupted. Theoretically, blocking tubal transport of the fertilized egg could also reduce the chances of implantation, but this possibility has not been thoroughly studied.

Attention has also been focused on improving hormonal methods of female birth control. These include developing pills without estrogen (to avoid unwanted side effects) and using long-acting forms of contraceptive hormones. These hormones are either injected or placed in small implants under the skin or in plastic vaginal rings that slowly release hormones. In fact, it is currently possible for a woman wishing long-term contraceptive protection to carry a five-year supply of hormonal birth control with her all the time in an implant placed under the skin in the upper arm. This implant, called the NORPLANT system, actually consists of six small silastic capsules packed with the hormone levonorgestrel—the same progestogen used in many minipills—which are thought to provide about the same degree of contraceptive effectiveness as the pill. The contraceptive, which is slowly released from the capsules, doesn't always block ovulation but instead prevents pregnancy in two ways: by thickening the cervical mucus (making it difficult for sperm to swim up the Fallopian tubes) and by blocking implantation. The major drawback at this time is that many users experience abnormal menstrual bleeding (but this problem generally decreases after about one year of use).

A synthetic form of progesterone called medroxyprogesterone acetate (MPA) is currently used as a long-acting contraceptive in other countries. (In the United States, its trade name is Depo-Provera.) It is given by injection once every three months (so the woman does not need to remember to use it) and is about as effective as combination birth control pills. Its drawbacks include possible infertility after long-term use, reported toxicity in animal studies, and the finding that MPA may cause cancer of the uterus (Maine, 1978; *Family Planning Perspectives,* 1979). However, two other studies found no evidence to support a definite link between MPA and any form of cancer in humans (Liang et al., 1983; Rosenfield et al., 1983).

Various techniques for developing a nonsurgical method of female sterilization are also being explored.

WHY THE UNITED STATES LAGS IN CONTRACEPTIVE DEVELOPMENT

Since the pill and IUD came on the market, no fundamentally new form of birth control has been introduced in the United States. In fact, research related to new contraceptive methods has slowed. The following factors help explain why this is so:

- All but one major U.S. pharmaceutical company have fled the field of contraceptive research because of lawsuits (some of which have wound up with multimillion dollar verdicts) and a difficult regulatory climate that makes contraceptive testing very time-consuming and expensive.
- Foundation support for contraceptive research, which has traditionally been a major source of funding in this area, has declined noticeably in the past decade, and federal support has languished, barely keeping pace with inflation.
- Economic factors are stacked against private industry playing a more major role, since the market for a successful contraceptive vaccine or a "once-a-month" pill is not large enough to make it a big moneymaker.
- Drug companies are also hesitant about entering the contraceptive market because of the political and economic clout of the anti-abortion movement, including the threat of consumer boycotts.

What can be done to change things? In addition to the obvious solution—more federal and foundation grants for innovative contraceptive research—a joint committee of the National Research Council and the Institute of Medicine has proposed two vital steps (Mastroianni, Donaldson, and Kane, 1990):

1. The FDA should streamline its procedures for evaluating new contraceptive products and "should be prepared to approve a contraceptive drug or device even if that drug or device presents a risk, *if* it can be shown that the new contraceptive also offers a safety advantage for an identifiable group of users."
2. A new federal product liability law should be implemented that would give contraceptive manufacturers protection against large liability claims if they met all the FDA requirements in developing and testing a new drug or device and if they provide proper warnings for consumers.

A similar law has already been passed to protect manufacturers of vaccines given to children to prevent diseases like measles and mumps. But because contraception is a political "hot potato," it is not very likely that such a measure will be put in place in the foreseeable future.

A special summary of the committee's overall report concluded by saying: "Unless immediate steps are taken to change public policy, the choice of contraceptives in the United States in the next century will not differ appreciably from what it is today" (Mastroianni, Donaldson, and Kane, 1990, p. 484). That is a sad state of affairs for a country that boasts the world's most sophisticated medical and scientific technology.

Sources: Committee on Contraceptive Development, 1990; Mastroianni, Donaldson, and Kane, 1990.

TABLE 5–5

Summary of Contraceptive Methods

Method	Effectiveness Rating	Ideal Failure Rate	Actual Failure Rate	Advantages	Disadvantages
Birth control pills (combination)	Excellent	1%	3–6%	Highly reliable; coitus independent; has some health benefits	Side effects; daily use; continual cost
IUD	Excellent	1–3	5–6	No memory or motivation required for use; very reliable	Cramping, bleeding, expulsion; risk of PID
Condom and diaphragm	Excellent	1	3–5	Highly reliable with no major health risks	See separate discussions of condom and diaphragm below
Condom and foam	Excellent	1	3–5	Highly reliable with no major health risks	See separate discussions of condom and foam below
Diaphragm and cream or jelly	Good–very good	3	15–20	No major health risks; inexpensive	Aesthetic objections
Condom	Very good	3	15	Protects against STDs; simple to use; male responsibility; no health risks; no prescription required	Unaesthetic to some; requires interruption of sexual activity
Sponge	Good–very good	3	15	24-hour protection; simple to use; no taste or odor; inexpensive; effective with several acts of intercourse	Aesthetic objections
Cervical cap	Good	3	10–20	Can wear for weeks at a time; coitus independent; no major health risks	May be difficult to insert; may irritate cervix
Spermicides	Poor to fair	3	20–30	No major health risks; no prescription required	Unaesthetic to some; must be properly inserted
Rhythm	Poor to fair	13	20–40	No cost; acceptable to Catholic church	Requires high motivation and periods of abstinence; unreliable
Withdrawal	Fair	9	20–25	No cost or health risks	Reduces sexual pleasure; unreliable
Douching	Poor	?	40+	Inexpensive	Extremely unreliable
Breast-feeding	Poor	15	50+	No cost; acceptable to Catholic church	Extremely unreliable
Vasectomy	Excellent	0.15	0.25	Permanent and highly reliable	Expensive; relatively irreversible; possible complications
Tubal ligation	Excellent	0.40	0.40	Permanent and highly reliable	Expensive; relatively irreversible; possible complications

Source: Based on data from Hatcher et al., 1982, Jones and Forrest, 1989, and *Population Reports* research reviews (see Suggested Readings).

These methods, which are irreversible, involve plugging up the place at which the Fallopian tubes open into the uterus. Material that causes thick scar tissue to form at the tubal openings is inserted through the vagina and cervix with a special instrument that doesn't require making an incision or using anesthesia. Studies of the effectiveness of this approach have been under way for the last decade but are inconclusive to date.

SUMMARY

Table 5–5 summarizes the various contraceptive methods that we have discussed in this chapter.

Thought Questions

1. Describe your idea of an ideal contraceptive method. What are the most essential criteria? What are additional desirable features? Do any methods exist which approximate this ideal?
2. Do most men behave as if they have as great a responsibility as women do regarding the consistent and careful use of birth control techniques? Do they in fact have an equal responsibility? Why is there essentially only one reliable method for reversible male contraception (i.e., the condom)?
3. The IUD is a convenient and effective method of birth control that is safe for most women. However, fear of litigation has been acknowledged as causing companies to be unwilling to market them. Is this fair to American women? What could be done about this problem? Or should market forces control the availability of contraceptive devices like they control other commodities in our society?
4. Do most men and women respond negatively to using condoms during sex? Do you have any advice as to how condoms can be made more attractive to those who say they would rather not use them?
5. In your experience (among your friends and acquaintances), to what extent is abortion used as a method of birth control? That is, how widespread is the practice of not using contraception because "You can always get an abortion"?
6. Do you believe that RU 486—the so-called abortion pill—should be legalized in the United States (as it already has been in some other parts of the world)? Why or why not?

Suggested Readings

Committee on Contraceptive Development. *Developing New Contraceptives: Obstacles and Opportunities*. Washington, DC: National Academy Press, 1990. An important look at the political and policy issues involved in contraceptive research and development in the United States.

Djerassi, C. *The Politics of Contraception*. New York: W. W. Norton & Co., 1979. One of the inventors of the pill provides an authoritative look at the ethical, social, and political sides of birth control.

Dornblaser, C., and Landy, U. *The Abortion Guide: A Handbook for Women and Men*. New York: Berkley, 1982. A readable, comprehensive guide to all aspects of abortion, including its aftereffects.

Henshaw, S. K., and Van Vort, J. *Abortion Services in the United States*. New York: Alan Guttmacher Institute, 1988. The most complete national, state, and local information on abortion practices in the United States available anywhere. Loaded with statistical tables, as well as discussions of survey methodologies.

Population Reports. Published by the Population Information Program, Johns Hopkins University, Hampton House, 624 North Broadway, Baltimore, Maryland 21205. A series of in-depth review articles on all aspects of contraceptive technology and policy, with major subjects updated annually.

Shapiro, Howard I. *The New Birth-Control Book: A Complete Guide for Women and Men*. Englewood Cliffs, NJ: Prentice-Hall, 1988. One of the most thorough and understandable guides to current contraception methods available for consumers.

Interested persons may also find useful literature at any Planned Parenthood office.

6

Developmental Sexuality: A Biological View

Sexual development is a complex process that starts at conception and continues throughout the life cycle. Before birth, in the **prenatal period,** sexual development is controlled mainly by biological forces. But from the moment the doctor says, "It's a girl" or "It's a boy," the rest of our sexual development is profoundly influenced by psychosocial factors interacting with our biological heritage.

In this chapter, we consider developmental sexuality from a biological viewpoint. Some behavioral observations are discussed when they help to clarify biological principles, but the influences of learning on our sexual development are not considered here to any significant degree.

TABLE 6–1

Homologous Sex Organs

Male	Female
Testes	Ovaries
Penile glans	Clitoral glans
Penile shaft	Clitoral shaft
Foreskin	Clitoral hood
Scrotum	Labia majora
Underside of penile shaft	Labia minora
Cowper's glands	Bartholin's glands

Note: Homologous structures are those that develop from the same embryonic tissue.

PRENATAL DEVELOPMENT

At the moment of conception, the combination of genetic material from each parent starts a process called **sexual differentiation** that leads to the specific physical differences between females and males. The process of prenatal sexual differentiation is largely controlled by genetic and hormonal mechanisms. We examine these mechanisms and the events they control in two ways. First we examine normal development patterns of prenatal sexual differentiation, and then we consider several examples of altered or abnormal development that can occur.

Normal Prenatal Differentiation

At fertilization, when the male sperm and female egg unite to form a zygote, the initial programming for sexual differentiation is set in place. Remember that the sperm carries an X or Y sex chromosome while the egg always has an X chromosome. When the 23 chromosomes of the sperm combine with the 23 chromosomes of the egg, the zygote has a total of 46 chromosomes. Under ordinary circumstances, a 46,XX chromosome pattern is the genetic code for a female and a 46,XY pattern programs for a male.

Regardless of the genetic coding, during the first weeks of development male and female embryos are anatomically identical. Two primitive gonads form during the fifth and sixth weeks of pregnancy, first as ridges of tissue and then as more distinct structures. At this point, the gonads are bipotential, meaning that depending on events to come, they can differentiate into either testes or ovaries (Table 6–1). There are also two paired primitive duct systems that form in both male and female embryos during this time, the **Müllerian ducts** and the **Wolffian ducts** (Figure 6–1).

For the testes to develop, there must be one further step in genetic control. The H-Y antigen, a chemical substance of uncertain identity (controlled by the Y chromosome), starts the transformation of the primitive gonads into testes. If this testis determining factor is not present, the primitive gonads will always develop into ovaries.

From this point on, sexual differentiation occurs at three different levels—the internal sex structures, the external genitals, and the brain—and is largely controlled by hormones. Even if the sex chromosome pattern is 46,XY, without enough testosterone produced at the right time anatomic development will be female rather than male (Jost, 1953; Jost, 1972; Money and Ehrhardt, 1972; Wilson, George, and Griffin, 1981).

prenatal period the time from conception to birth.

sexual differentiation the process that begins at the moment of conception to create a normal male or female.

Müllerian duct (mew ler' ē un) one of two pairs of embryonic genital ducts. In females, this duct system develops into the Fallopian tubes, uterus, and inner part of the vagina. In males, a substance secreted by the embryonic testes causes the Müllerian duct system to shrink and practically disappear.

Wolffian duct (wool' fē un) one of two primitive duct systems in the embryo. Develops in the male to form the epididymis, vas deferens, seminal vesicles, and prostate; it shrinks in the female to nonfunctioning remnants.

FIGURE 6–1

The Stages of Internal Fetal Sex Differentiation

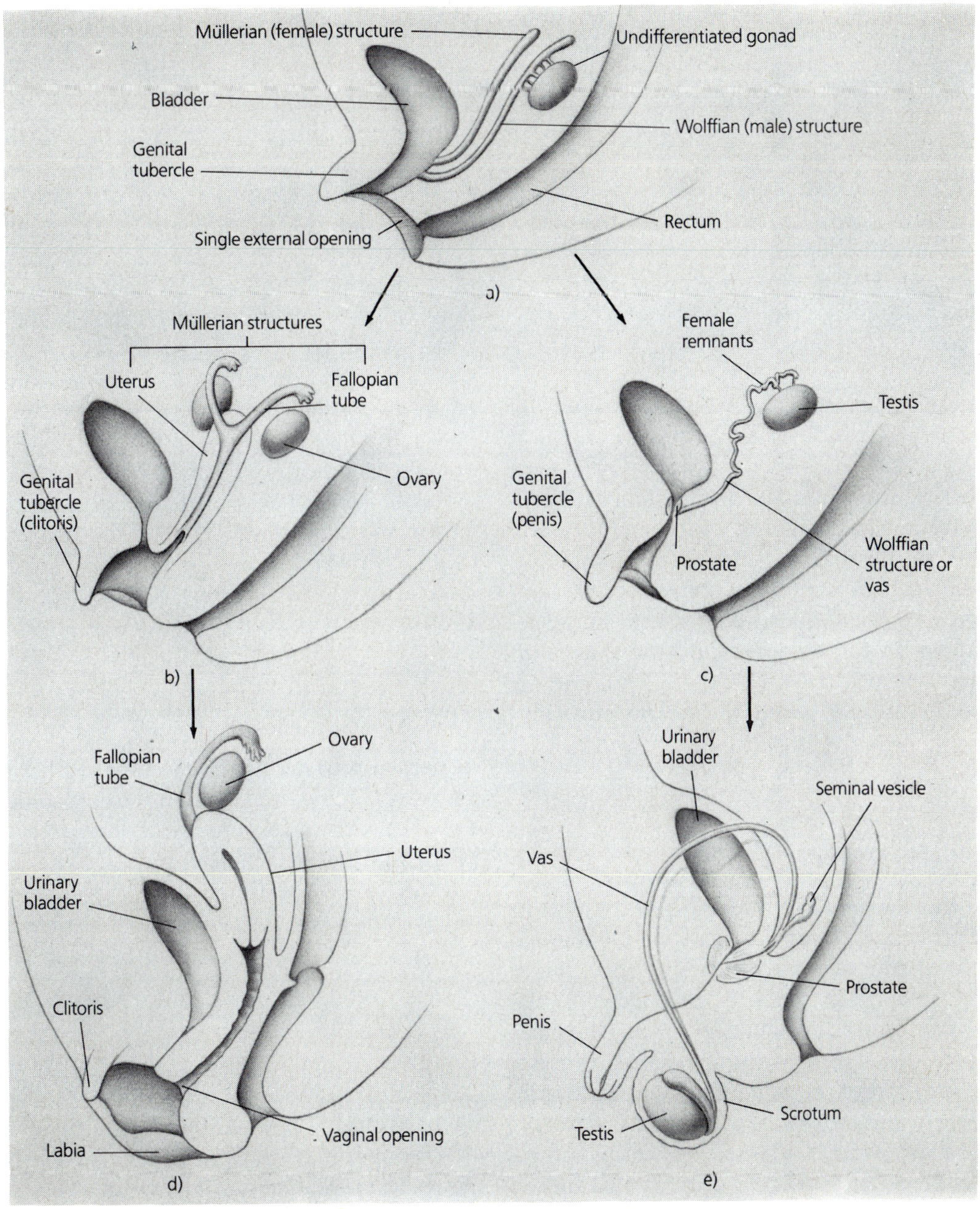

(a) The undifferentiated stage at approximately 6 to 7 weeks of development. (b) The pattern of female internal differentiation at approximately 14 weeks. (c) Male differentiation at approximately 14 weeks. (d) Female differentiation at approximately 40 weeks. (e) Male differentiation at approximately 40 weeks.

INTERNAL SEX STRUCTURES

If the embryo is a male, the newly formed testes begin secreting two different products by the eighth week after conception. A chemical called Müllerian duct inhibiting substance causes the Müllerian ducts to shrink and practically disappear instead of forming female internal sex organs. At the same time, testosterone is also produced, stimulating the development of the Wolffian ducts into epididymis, vas deferens, seminal vesicles, and ejaculatory ducts (Figure 6–1). In addition, testosterone is converted in some tissue to another form, called **dihydrotestosterone,** which stimulates development of the penis, scrotum, and prostate gland (Imperato-McGinley and Peterson, 1976). Testosterone and dihydrotestosterone are both **androgens,** hormones that cause masculinization.

In contrast, female sexual differentiation does not depend on hormones. Ovaries generally develop at about the twelfth week after conception, but even if they do not, the Müllerian duct system will proceed to develop into the uterus, Fallopian tubes, and inner third of the vagina (Money and Ehrhardt, 1972). Without high amounts of testosterone to stimulate its growth, the Wolffian duct system in the female shrinks into tiny remnants. By the fourteenth week of development, there is a clear difference in the internal sex structure of a male and female fetus (Figure 6–1b, c).

EXTERNAL GENITALS

In the seventh week of development, the external genitals look the same in both sexes. If there is little androgen present, as we expect in a female embryo, a clitoris, vulva, and vagina will form in six to eight weeks (Figure 6–2). In the male, androgen stimulation causes the folds that would develop into the inner vaginal lips in the female to grow together, forming the cylindrical shaft of the penis. The genital tubercle, which develops into the clitoris in the female, becomes the glans of the penis in the male. The labioscrotal swellings differentiate into the outer vaginal lips in the female and the scrotum in the male.

Both ovaries and testes first develop inside the abdomen during fetal life. Later, the ovaries move into the pelvis and the testes migrate down into the scrotum.

BRAIN DIFFERENTIATION

Intriguingly, hormones in the blood of the fetus also affect the development of the brain and pituitary gland. The best-documented structural differences between male and female brains are in the number and location of certain types of nerve cell connections (synapses) in the **hypothalamus** (Goldman, 1978; Carter and Greenough, 1979). As in other aspects of prenatal sex differentiation, with androgen stimulation the brain develops in a male pattern; without it, the brain develops in a female direction (Plapinger and McEwen, 1978; McEwen, 1981; MacLusky and Naftolin, 1981). This prenatal hormone programming determines the pattern of function of the hypothalamus and pituitary gland during and after puberty. As a result, girls have cyclic sex hormone production and menstrual cycles, while boys have a relatively constant level of sex hormone production. Female fertility is also cyclic whereas male fertility is not. Prenatal hormone effects on the brain may also influence later behavior patterns, including sexual behavior and aggressiveness, but the exact nature of these effects remains uncertain (Reinisch, 1974; Hutchison, 1978; Rubin, Reinisch, and Haskett, 1981).

Abnormal Prenatal Differentiation

Abnormal prenatal sexual development has three major causes: sex chromosome disorders, other genetic conditions, and exposure of the fetus to drugs given to the mother. A complete catalogue of such abnormalities would require an entire book, so we briefly discuss only a few conditions that illustrate important principles of sexual development. Table 6–2 is a summary.

SEX CHROMOSOME DISORDERS

We have already pointed out that normally there are 46 chromosomes, including two sex chromosomes (XX or XY). Sometimes, however, a person may be born with extra sex chromosomes or one sex chromosome may be missing. These conditions have variable effects on a person's physical appearance, health; and behavior. Two of the most common sex chromosome abnormalities are described below.

FIGURE 6–2

The Stages of External Fetal Sex Differentiation

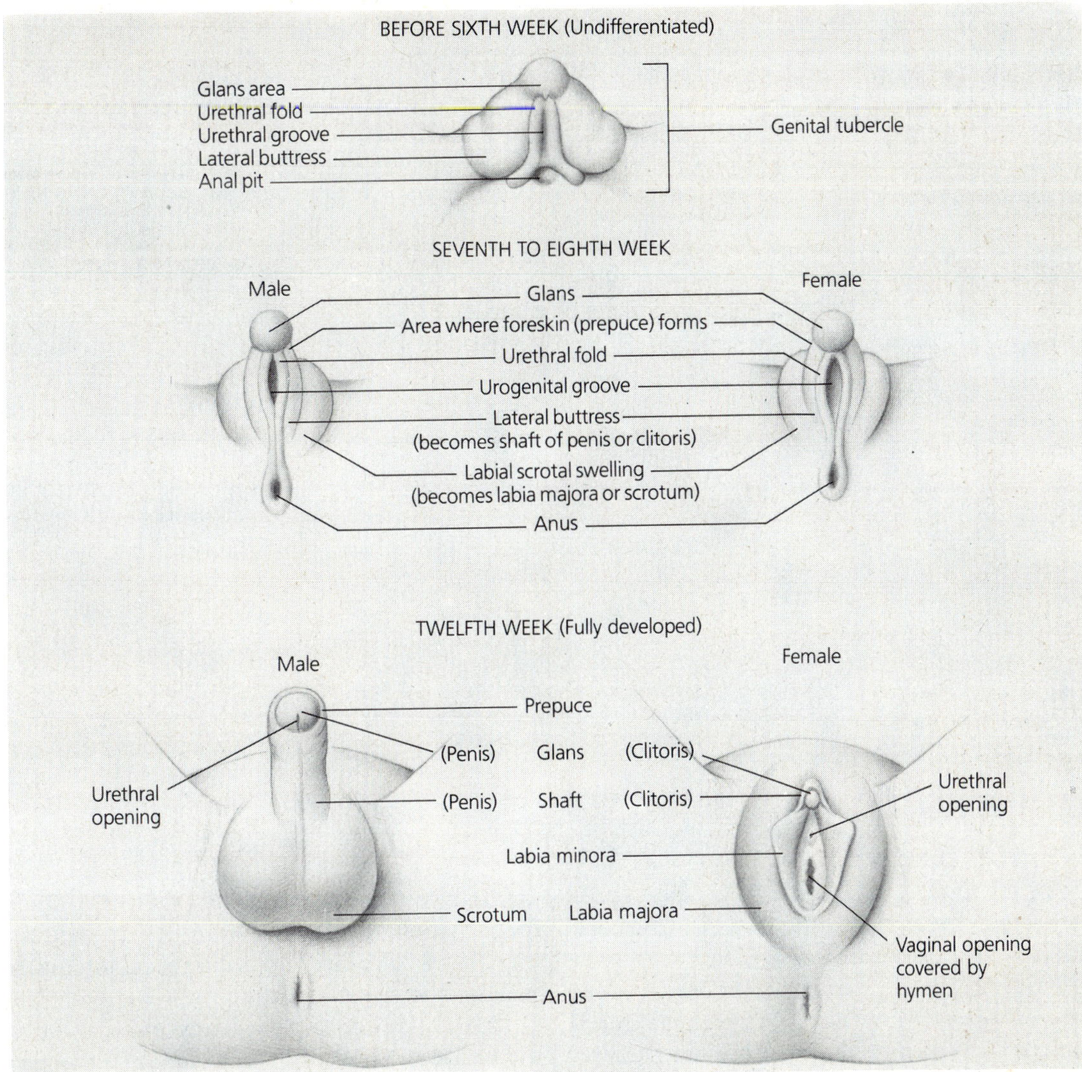

Klinefelter's syndrome occurs when a genetic male has an extra X chromosome (a 47,XXY pattern). This condition occurs about once in every 500 live male births but is usually not detected until adulthood. As a result of the extra X chromosome, the microscopic

dihydrotestosterone (dī hī′ drō tes tos′ ter ōn) a hormone similar to testosterone that stimulates development of the penis, scrotum, and prostate gland in the embryo.

androgens (an′ dro jinz) hormones such as testosterone that develop and maintain secondary sex characteristics in males and, if in large quantities, promote masculinization in females.

hypothalamus (hī′ pō thal′ uh mus) the portion of the brain that has primary control over most endocrine pathways. It reacts to the level of hormones in the blood supply which regulate many sexual responses and direct their production.

Klinefelter's syndrome a sex chromosome abnormality marked by an extra X chromosome in a genetic male, giving a 47, XXY pattern. Most of these men tend to be tall with poor muscular development and small testes. Sexual desire is often low and impotence common.

TABLE 6–2

Summary of Abnormalities of Prenatal Sex Differentiation

	Chromosome Pattern	Gonads	Genitals	Internal Sex Structures	Fertility	Comments
Klinefelter's syndrome	47,XXY	Testes	Male	Normal male	Sterile	Low testosterone (80%) impotence is common
Turner's syndrome	45,X	Streak ovaries	Female	Uterus and Fallopian tubes	Sterile	No spontaneous menstruation or breast development due to estrogen deficiency
True hermaphroditism	46,XY or 46,XX	Testes and ovaries	Variable	Variable male and female combinations	Usually sterile	Exceedingly rare
Pseudohermaphroditism;						
Female adrenogenital syndrome	46,XX	Ovaries	Ambiguous male	Normal female	Fertile	Requires medical management and surgical revision of genitals; tomboy pattern in childhood; increased rate of lesbian fantasy
Testicular feminization syndrome	46,XY	Cryptorchid testes	Female (short vagina)	No uterus or tubes; no prostate	Sterile	Spontaneous breast development at puberty but no menstruation; female psychosexual orientation
Dominican Republic syndrome	46,XY	Cryptorchid testes	Ambiguous female	Vas deferens, epididymis, and seminal vesicles, but no prostate	Fertile but unable to inseminate	At puberty, voice deepens, muscles develop in male pattern, penis grows, testes descend and enlarge, male gender identity is assumed.

structure of the testes is abnormal and no sperm production occurs, leading to infertility. Testosterone production is also usually reduced. These men tend to be tall and may have poor muscular development and enlarged breasts. Low sexual desire and impotence are common in this condition but are likely to improve if the man is given regular injections of testosterone (Kolodny, Masters, and Johnson, 1979). Of particular interest is the observation that men with Klinefelter's syndrome tend to be passive and have relatively low ambition or drive, which may be related to their testosterone deficiency.

Turner's syndrome is an example of a missing sex chromosome: the pattern is 45,X. Because one X chromosome is missing, the ovaries of a woman with Turner's syndrome never develop properly. The external genitals, however, are normal. The usual features of Turner's syndrome, which occurs in about one in 2500 live female births, include shortness, absence of menstruation, infertility, and a variety of abnormalities that may involve facial appearance and internal organs such as the heart and kidneys. Girls with Turner's syndrome who do not have any physical limitations usually develop normally as children. Yet when other girls begin to menstruate, develop breasts, and have an "adolescent growth spurt," these girls do not because of their nonfunctioning ovaries. Although menstruation and breast development can be induced by hormone treatment, the problems of height and infertility cannot be solved by any currently known approach.

GENETIC CONDITIONS

A true **hermaphrodite** is a person born with both testicular and ovarian tissue. In some cases, there is one ovary and one testis; in others, the gonads are mixtures of ovarian and testicular tissue. In this rare condition, a uterus is almost always present. There is either a Fallopian tube on one side of the body and a vas deferens and/or epididymis on the other, or male and female duct systems are on both sides. The **pseudohermaphrodite** is born with gonads that match their sex chromosomes but a genital appearance that resembles the opposite sex. A female pseudohermaphrodite has ovaries, a uterus, Fallopian tubes, and a 46,XX chromosome pattern but masculinized genitals. The appearance of the genitals can range from mild enlargement of the clitoris to the formation of a penislike phallus, and the labia may be fused together, looking like a scrotum. Sometimes the genitals seem so obviously male that the gender of the newborn child is misidentified by the physician.

The most common cause of female pseudohermaphroditism is the **adrenogenital syndrome (AGS),** an inherited disorder in which excessive amounts of androgens are produced during fetal development. Although babies with this condition may look like boys, their internal sex structures are completely female, with normal fertility potential. When proper medical treatment is begun in early childhood, the abnormal androgen output of the adrenals can be brought under control, and plastic surgery can correct the appearance of the genitals.

There is some evidence that girls with AGS treated at an early age show a high rate of tomboyishness, a preference for having boys instead of girls as playmates, and little interest in doll play, grooming, attractiveness, caring for infants, or rehearsing adult roles of mother or wife (Money and Ehrhardt, 1972). (Of course, many girls *without* AGS would also rather climb trees or play ball than play house or mother.) Girls with AGS, however, are not at all ambivalent about their female gender identity. In adolescence, their dating behavior is often delayed and they commonly have difficulty in forming close erotic relationships (Money and Schwartz, 1977). In addition, there are reports that bisexual and lesbian fantasy or experience is relatively common in this syndrome (Ehrhardt, Evers, and Money, 1968; Money and Schwartz, 1977). However, it is not clear whether these findings are solely the result of prenatal androgen effects on the brain.

Male pseudohermaphrodites have testes and a 46,XY chromosome pattern but female genitals. The most common form of this disorder is the **testicular feminization syndrome,** an inherited condition in which testosterone and other androgens have no effect on body tissues. Thus, even though normal levels of testosterone are produced, differentiation proceeds as if no androgen were present at all: a clitoris, labia, and vagina develop. Yet since the fetal testes also

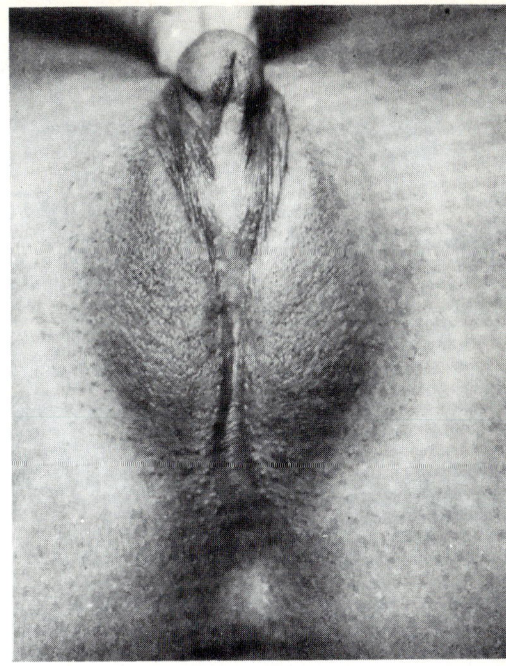

Untreated female with adrenogenital syndrome. This severe case has resulted in the fusion of the labia and marked enlargement of the clitoris.

Turner's syndrome a sex chromosome abnormality caused by a missing chromosome. The individual has a 45, X chromosome pattern and may appear fairly normal until puberty, when nonfunctioning gonads prevent development of the secondary sex characteristics and the adolescent growth spurt. May also be accompanied by webbing of the neck, heart defects, and other abnormalities.

hermaphrodite (hur maf′ rō dīt) a person with both testicular and ovarian tissue.

pseudohermaphrodite (sue′ dō hur maf′ rō dīt) an individual born with gonads matching the sex chromosomes but a genital appearance that resembles the opposite sex.

adrenogenital syndrome (AGS) (a drē′ nō jen′ i tul) an inherited disorder involving an enzyme block in the adrenal glands. Females born with this condition frequently have masculinized genitals because of excess androgen exposure prenatally. In males, genital appearance is usually unaffected.

testicular feminization syndrome an inherited condition in which tissues are insensitive to the effects of testosterone. The individual is born with a 46, XY chromosome pattern (male) but with female genitals.

RESEARCH SPOTLIGHT

The Nature–Nurture Argument

Scientists have argued for years about the relative importance of nature (biological forces) versus nurture (learning and the environment) in controlling human development. The complexity of this issue can be highlighted by reviewing two fascinating situations.

The first is one of the most famous cases in the annals of modern sexology, which was reported by John Money (Money and Ehrhardt, 1972; Money, 1975). When identical twin brothers underwent circumcision at 7 months of age, an operating error led to the loss of the penis of one twin. After considerable anguish and consultation with various medical experts, the parents were finally referred to Johns Hopkins University, and a joint decision was made that the twin missing a penis would be raised as a girl. At 17 months, the child's name, clothing, and hairstyle were changed, and 4 months later the first of a series of surgical procedures designed to reconstruct the genitals as female was started. Family members were provided with the best available advice about ways of coping with this gender reassignment.

The parents took great care to treat their twins as son and daughter even while knowing that both were biologically male. As a result, the daughter quickly began to prefer dresses to slacks and showed other "typical" signs of femininity, such as a desire for neatness. When the twins were 4½, the mother remarked: "One thing that really amazes me is that she is so feminine. . . . She just loves to have her hair set; she could sit under the drier all day long to have her hair set" (Money, 1975). The twins were encouraged to develop play patterns and interests in toys along traditional lines—dolls for the girl, cars and tools for the boy. The mother also reported that her son and daughter imitated their parents' behavior differentially, the son following his father's example and the daughter imitating what the mother did. According to Money, these two children achieved normal (and different) gender identities and roles although they both had identical chromosomal, anatomic, and hormonal sex during prenatal development and for the first 7 months of life.

The case subsequently took a new twist, however, and the "girl" twin's adjustment to a female gender identity may not be as straightforward as Money previously suggested. According to interviews with the girl's psychiatrist conducted by the British Broadcasting System, she is having many problems as a teenager and is so unfeminine in appearance and behavior that classmates taunt her by calling her "cave-woman" (Diamond, 1982). While a final picture of her psychosexual development has not been reported as yet—and while her problems as a teenager may have reflected a need to adjust her estrogen dose properly—it is now difficult to use this case to support the position that gender development depends primarily on learning.

---

produce Müllerian duct inhibiting substance (which is not impaired in this syndrome), the Müllerian ducts shrink and no uterus or Fallopian tubes develop. Because the inner third of the vagina normally is formed from the Müllerian system, the vagina in this syndrome is short and ends in a blind pouch.

A newborn baby with testicular feminization looks like a normal baby girl unless the testes have de-

Another research study claims to support just the opposite conclusion. In 1974, 38 male pseudohermaphrodites were discovered in four rural villages of the Dominican Republic. Although these subjects have normal sex chromosomes, an inherited enzyme defect causes improper formation of the external genitals, even though prenatal testosterone production is normal. The testes and internal sex organs are completely male. But at birth, the affected babies have an incompletely formed scrotum that looks like labia, a very small penis that looks like a clitoris, and a partially formed vagina. As a result, many of them are raised as female. Then, during puberty, normal male testosterone production starts, and definite masculine changes occur. The voice deepens, male-pattern muscles develop, the "clitoris" grows into a penis, and the testes descend into the scrotum. Normal erections occur and intercourse is possible.

Of the 18 genetically male children with this condition who were raised as girls, 17 changed to a male gender identity and 16 of 18 shifted to a male gender role during or after puberty (Imperato-McGinley et al., 1979). The authors of this report believe that these findings show that when sex of rearing is contrary to the biological sex, the biological sex will prevail if normal hormone production occurs during puberty.

So far it all sounds very neat and convincing. Biology is "obviously" more important than learning, since these "girls" seem to easily discard the gender roles they learned in the first 10 or 12 years of life in order to become boys. A closer look at some of the reasons that may be behind this switch may give us a different message, however.

First, girls in these rural areas have to stay at home after age 7 and do chores, while boys have "freedom to romp and play." After age 11 or 12, the boys can go to bars or cock fights, which girls are not permitted to do. Adult women are also supposed to stay home and be faithful, while men can seek entertainment and enjoy the services of prostitutes. Given these social restrictions, why wouldn't a young teenager with a choice choose to be the free and fun-seeking male? In addition, people usually define who or what they are by the reality of their physical appearance. Seeing a penis grow and a scrotum form and *knowing* that other such cases have occurred in the same village, the child would probably choose to live as a male. If he were to continue to live in a female role, he probably would not attract any male sex partners. Thus, this study does not "prove" anything about nature versus nurture, except that our sexual development is probably determined by an interaction of the two.

---

scended into the labia or can be felt in the groin. These children are raised as girls and their development proceeds in a normal feminine pattern. This condition is usually not diagnosed until age 16 or later, when the lack of menstrual periods is investigated medically. Interestingly, at puberty female breast development occurs because some testosterone is broken down into estrogen (as it is in all males). Although there is a male chromosome pattern, normal testes, and no ovaries or uterus, these girls are quite feminine in appearance and behavior (Money and Ehrhardt, 1972). Their sexual behavior is also that of a normal female, although fertility is not possible.

In cases of complete testicular feminization, the child must be raised as a girl even if the diagnosis is made at birth. Neither surgery nor hormone treatment can create a functioning penis or alter the female appearance of the body. This syndrome is contrasted with another type of male pseudohermaphroditism in the Research Spotlight, "The Nature–Nurture Argument" (pp. 164–165). The comparison raises some intriguing questions about prenatal hormone effects.

PRENATAL DRUG EXPOSURE

Hormones given to a pregnant woman for medical reasons cross the placenta and enter the circulation of the developing fetus. Depending on when in the pregnancy the drug is taken and how much is taken, such hormones may affect sexual anatomy. As examples, androgens can enlarge the clitoris, creating a condition very similar to AGS, and synthetic female hormones can cause malformation of the penis (Aarskog, 1979). Research interest at present, however, centers on the behavior of children exposed to synthetic hormones during their prenatal development.

One report found that teenage boys born to diabetic mothers who had received estrogen and progesterone during pregnancy were rated as lower in general masculine behavior, assertiveness, and athletic ability than other boys of the same age (Yalom, Green, and Fisk, 1973). In another study, adolescent males 16 to 19 years old who had been exposed prenatally to high levels of progesterone were found to have less physical activity and participation in heterosexual activity than control group subjects (Zussman, Zussman, and Dalton, 1975, 1977). Another study investigating adolescents who received lower hormone doses did not find such effects (Meyer-Bahlburg, 1978). And in girls exposed prenatally to estrogens or progesterone, there seems to be a mild "enhancing effect" on femininity (Ehrhardt, Grisanti, and Meyer-Bahlburg, 1977).

Although these studies are far from conclusive, they suggest that in certain cases prenatal hormone exposure may influence later patterns of behavior. The relative importance of such prenatal influences is still a matter of controversy (Ehrhardt and Meyer-Bahlburg, 1981; Rubin, Reinisch, and Haskett, 1981).

INFANCY AND CHILDHOOD

From birth on, learning is ordinarily more important than biology in shaping sexuality. However, it is impossible to completely separate learning and biology. For instance, a baby "learns" about the physical sensations of various body parts, but this type of learning is impossible without biological responses. For any learning to occur, events and their meanings must register in the brain, where they are probably coded and stored in chemical form (Money, 1980; Parsons, 1980). Individuals grow and change throughout their lives in a fashion determined by an interaction between biology and experience.

There is a surprisingly full range of physical sexual responsiveness in the first year of life. Kinsey and his colleagues reported orgasm during masturbation in nine baby boys under a year old, describing the physiological changes as "development of rhythmic body movements with distinct penis throbs and thrusts, an obvious change in sensory capacities, a final tension of muscles . . . a sudden release with convulsions, including rhythmic contractions—followed by the disappearance of symptoms" (Kinsey, Pomeroy, and Martin, 1948, p. 177). Orgasm has also been noted in girls during infancy and childhood (Kinsey et al., 1953; Bakwin, 1974). Although boys do not ejaculate prior to puberty, it appears that all other mechanisms of sexual response are present from infancy on.

There are only minor hormone differences between young girls and boys. In childhood, the gonads are relatively nonfunctional, and the major source of testosterone and estrogen is the adrenal glands. Because the adrenals are the same in both boys and girls, sex hormone production is the same too. The pituitary gland is, sexually speaking, not yet active because it receives no major signals from the hypothalamus.

In approximately 3 percent of newborn males (and 30 percent of premature male babies), the testes have not descended into the scrotum and are said to be **cryptorchid** (hidden). In most cases, descent occurs automatically within the first few months of life. If this does not happen, medical treatment with hormones or corrective surgery is advisable, since prolonged positioning of one or both testes in the abdomen can damage their sperm-producing capacity and creates an increased risk of cancer (Lattimer et al., 1974).

PUBERTY

Puberty is a period of change from biological immaturity to maturity. In this transition, dramatic physical changes occur such as the adolescent "growth spurt," the development of secondary sex characteristics, the onset of menstruation (**menarche**), and the ability of the male to ejaculate. In addition, this is a time when fertility for both sexes is achieved and important psychological changes occur.

Some people think that puberty happens overnight—as a student put it, "One morning, you wake up with pimples"—but actually, the maturing process lasts anywhere from one and one-half to six years (Grumbach, 1980). The blueprint for the physical changes that occur during puberty was actually established before birth, when the hypothalamus and pituitary gland were programmed by hormones for a later "awakening."

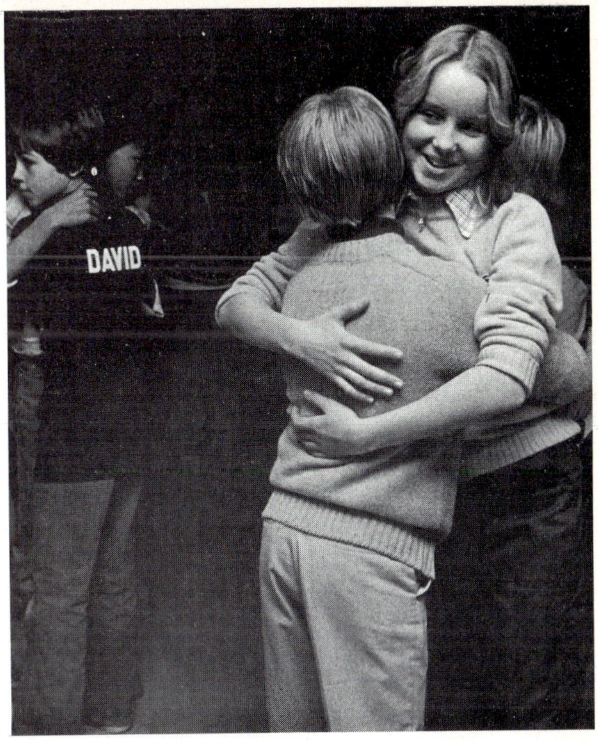

Around age 12, girls are often taller than boys because they have an earlier adolescent growth spurt.

Physical Growth and Development

CHANGES IN BODY SIZE

Everyone probably remembers a teenage friend who went away over a summer and came back much taller. This was not a result of sunshine, exercise, or clean living—it was simply the **adolescent growth spurt**. The explanation of this explosive growth rate is simple: it occurs because rising sex hormone levels in puberty temporarily cause bone growth.

The adolescent growth spurt typically occurs two years earlier in girls than in boys (on average, age 12 versus 14) (Marshall, 1977). As a result, girls are usually taller than boys of the same age from about age 11 to 14. (Remember those seventh grade dances where girls seemed to tower over their partners, especially if they wore heels?) The self-consciousness this may cause fortunately lessens by mid-adolescence as males "catch up" and usually go on to become somewhat taller than females.

The adolescent growth spurt does not always start at the same time in all parts of the body. For example, growth of the foot typically begins about four months before growth in the lower leg, so an adolescent's feet may seem disproportionately large (Marshall, 1975). Not realizing that more harmonious relative proportions will be restored, some teenagers are upset at this pattern.

There is no correlation between an "early" growth spurt and final adult height (which is partly controlled by genetics). This finding should comfort a young teenager who is the class "shrimp"; by age 16 or 17 the "shrimp" may be as tall as or taller than his or her classmates.

SEXUAL MATURATION IN GIRLS

The first physical sign of puberty in girls is usually the beginning of breast development, which occurs as early as age 8 or as late as age 13. In the earliest stage of breast growth, there is only a small mound of tissue (the "breast bud"), but gradually the nipple and areola enlarge and the contour of the breast becomes more prominent (see Figure 6–3). Some girls have fully mature breasts before their twelfth birthdays, but

cryptorchid (krip tor′ kid) undescended testes.

menarche (me nar′ kē) the onset of menstruation.

adolescent growth spurt a period of fast bone growth usually occurring in the early or middle teens caused by the rising sex hormone levels of puberty.

FIGURE 6–3

Stages of Female Breast Development During Puberty

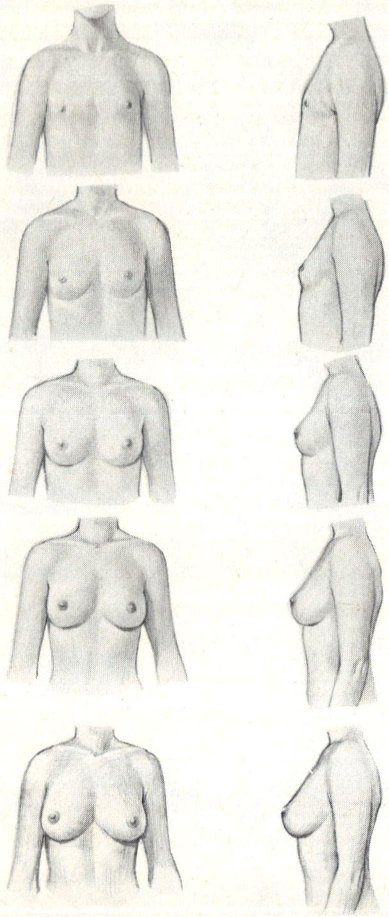

others do not reach this stage until age 19 or even later. Breast growth is controlled by estrogen levels and heredity.

The appearance of pubic hair (first lightly pigmented and sparse, gradually becoming darker, coarser, curlier, and more abundant) usually starts shortly after breast growth begins. By this time, the vagina has already begun to lengthen and the uterus is slowly enlarging. Menarche usually occurs as breast growth nears completion and almost invariably comes after the peak growth spurt (Marshall and Tanner, 1969).

In the United States, the average age at menarche is 12.8 years for whites and 12.5 for blacks (U.S. Department of Health, Education, and Welfare, 1973). It is interesting to note that a century ago, menstruation first occurred at an average of 16 or older; since then, the age at menarche has been consistently decreasing decade by decade (Zacharias and Wurtman, 1969) (Figure 6–4). Socioeconomic factors, climate, heredity, family size, and nutrition all influence the age of menarche. Most recently, this decrease has leveled off, perhaps reflecting more uniform nutritional conditions.

An interesting idea has been proposed by a research team studying the onset of menstruation. They believe that menarche occurs only when a minimum percentage of body fat is present (Frisch and McArthur, 1974). In support of this theory, female long-distance runners and ballet dancers have been noted to have delayed menarche or to actually stop having periods when they are in rigorous training (Frisch, Wyshak, and Vincent, 1980).

The age of menarche varies widely from one girl to another, occurring as early as age 8 and as late as 16 or later. In the first year after menarche, menstrual cycles are frequently irregular and ovulation usually does not occur. It is possible, however, to begin ovulating with the very first menstrual cycle, and young adolescents who engage in intercourse need contraception.

One other aspect of female puberty not mentioned often is that vaginal secretions are likely to increase because of the changing hormone status. Some vaginal lubrication occurs because of sexual excitation whether this results from daydreams, reading, or sexual activity. But vaginal lubrication can also appear spontaneously, without a direct connection to sexual thoughts or acts. The sensations of vaginal wetness may be curious, pleasing, shameful, or alarming to the young teenager.

SEXUAL MATURATION IN BOYS

The physical signs of puberty in boys are also controlled by hormone changes, but puberty usually starts one to two years later than in girls. The earliest change during puberty is growth of the testes, resulting from LH stimulation and subsequent testosterone production. The increasing levels of testosterone also stimulate growth of the penis and the accessory male sex organs (prostate, seminal vesicles, and epididymis). Ejaculation is not possible before puberty because the prostate and seminal vesicles do not begin to function until they receive appropriate hormone signals.

FIGURE 6–4

Declining Age of Menarche in Various Countries

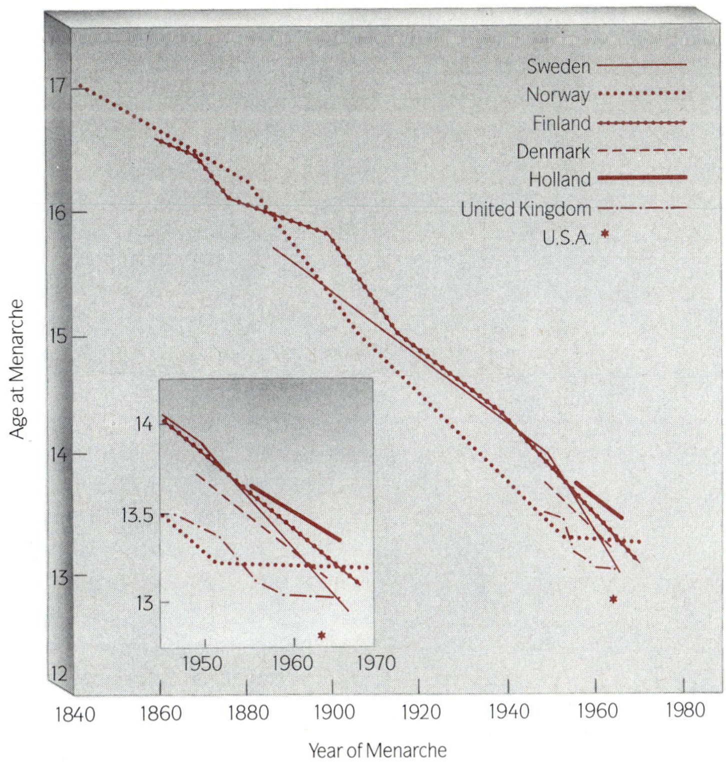

Source: From J. M. Tanner, in Endocrine and Genetic Diseases of Childhood and Adolescence *(L. I. Gardner, Ed.) W. B. Saunders, 1975, pp. 14–64.*

Boys begin to undergo genital development at an average age of 11.6 years, and the genitals reach adult size and shape at an average age of 14.9 (Marshall and Tanner, 1970) (Figure 6–5). In some boys, genital development occurs rapidly (in about a year), while in others it may take up to five and one-half years (Tanner, 1974). Sperm production (which begins in childhood) becomes fully established during puberty so fertility is present.

There is no exact counterpart in male puberty to menarche, but wet dreams seem to have a parallel degree of psychological importance. Kinsey, Pomeroy, and Martin (1948) reported that one-quarter of 14-year-olds and nearly two-thirds of 17-year-olds had this experience, yet many pubertal boys are not told about the possibility of nocturnal emissions and are surprised, puzzled, or frightened upon discovery of the event. The ejaculatory experience itself or the resulting sensation of wetness or stickiness may awaken the boy having a nocturnal emission, and—just as uninformed girls may view their initial menstrual flow as a sign of illness—he may become anxious about disease or injury. Whether informed or not about this experience, the pubertal boy may attempt to "hide the evidence" of a stained sheet or pajamas to avoid embarrassment or questioning by his parents.

Growth of pubic hair begins around the time of genital development and is usually followed a year or two later by the appearance of facial and axillary hair. Facial hair growth is an important event because the earlier changes of male puberty are usually less visible than breast development in the female and beard

FIGURE 6–5

Stages of Male Genital Development During Puberty

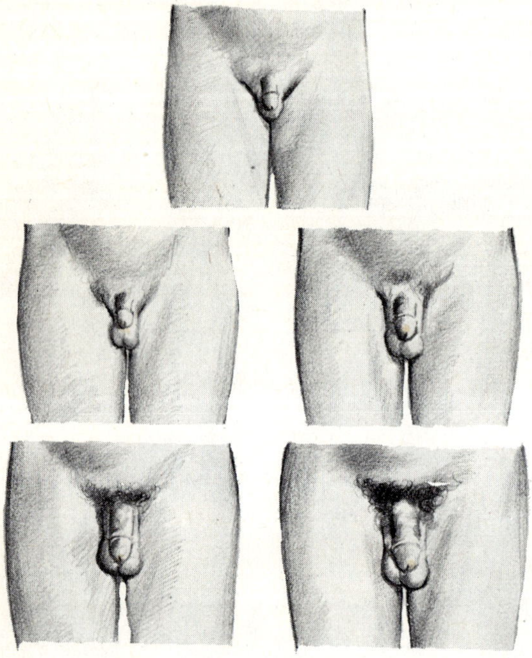

growth is a visible sign of "becoming a man." Facial hair growth begins at the corners of the upper lip with a fine, fuzzy appearance and then spreads to form a mustache with coarser texture. Hair next appears on the upper cheeks and just below the lower lip and last of all on the chin. Body hair also appears during puberty, and chest hair continues to grow for a decade or more after this time.[1]

Deepening of the voice is another change of puberty and is caused by testosterone stimulation of the voice box, or **larynx.** As the larynx grows, the boy's voice may go through an awkward period of breaks and squawks, which may be a source of embarrassment. Like age at menarche, the average age of this voice change in boys has decreased, from 18 years in 1749 to about 13.5 years today (Grumbach, 1980). Transient breast enlargement or gynecomastia is commonly seen in male puberty but typically disappears a year or two after it starts.

Hormone differences between adolescent boys and girls also cause differences in body shapes. For instance, the average 17- or 18-year-old boy has a leaner body and more muscle mass than his female counterpart. This is because estrogens cause accumulation of fat under the skin, while testosterone stimulates muscle growth. The structure of pelvic bones is also different in males and females, with the wider female pelvis creating a properly sized birth canal.

Pubertal Hormones and Sexuality

During puberty, rising hormone levels contribute to an activation of sexual sensations and erotic thoughts and dreams for boys and girls. John Money has described the role of hormones as follows: "The correct conception of hormonal puberty is that it puts gas in the metaphorical tank and upgrades the model of the vehicle, but it does not build the engine nor program the itinerary of the journey" (Money, 1980, pp. 36–37).

The relationship between pubertal hormones and sexual behavior is shown in the finding that boys who undergo "late" puberty (around age 15 or 16) generally have less and later teenage sexual activity—including masturbation and intercourse—than boys who have "early" puberty (around age 12 or 13). Kinsey and his colleagues pointed out this pattern (Kinsey, Pomeroy, and Martin, 1948), and we have some preliminary data showing it is probably true. If testosterone levels of the pubertal boy increase the frequency or intensity of erections, for example, he may possibly have a heightened awareness of sexual sensations. Increased testosterone in the blood may also influence the brain itself to activate sexual feelings or thoughts or to lower the threshold for external triggers that activate such feelings or thoughts. Boys with higher testosterone levels, then, are more likely to be more physically developed and sexually active. Shorter, less muscular, later-maturing boys may experience a social handicap. While having sexual feelings, they may feel less confident about their abilities and therefore "lag" in sexual behavior.

In parallel fashion, girls who undergo "late" puberty seem to have a lower rate of early adolescent

[1] The degree of facial and body hairiness in both sexes is controlled by genetic factors in addition to hormones. As a result, some people are hairier than others. This is often a source of embarrassment to women who compare themselves to the apparently "hairless" women in *Playboy* or *Vogue* or to men who are exposed to macho figures of heavily mustached men with an abundant crop of chest hair in various advertisements.

sexual activity than girls who complete puberty at age 12 or 13. Although a lower frequency or later age of participation in sexual activity might be explained by purely psychological or social factors (e.g., less physically developed girls may be more shy or self-conscious about sex with a partner), it appears that masturbation is less frequent and occurs later in late-maturing compared to early-maturing adolescent girls. A large cross-cultural study found similar evidence. According to Udry and Cliquet (1982), data from five different countries show that girls who are younger at menarche tend to have intercourse and to give birth at earlier ages than girls with later menarche.

In contrast to the findings linking sexual activity to "early" puberty, when pubertal changes occur before age 9—a condition called **precocious puberty**—there is usually no accompanying change in sexual behavior (Kolodny, Masters, and Johnson, 1979). This is probably because the hormonal stimulation alone is not enough to initiate new behavior patterns without a state of psychosexual readiness that the younger child simply hasn't attained.

THE MENOPAUSE

With aging, all women reach an end to their fertility. First, there is a gradual decline in female reproductive capacity from age 30 on, reflecting both a drop in fertility and a higher rate of miscarriages (Schneider, 1978; Schwartz, 1982). In addition, abnormalities of the menstrual cycle become more frequent over 35 as the aging ovaries respond less efficiently to luteinizing hormone (LH) and follicle stimulating hormone (FSH) from the pituitary gland. After age 40, the frequency of ovulation generally begins to decrease, and around age 48 to 52, menstrual flow stops entirely in a process called **menopause.**[2] However, since deciding when the menopause has occurred can be done only retrospectively—by convention, after one year without further menstrual flow—women who are sexually active at this stage of their lives should continue to practice birth control until it is certain they cannot become pregnant.

The timing of the menopause and the symptoms that accompany it vary greatly from one woman to another. Although the ovaries stop producing all but a minute amount of estrogen, and ovarian progesterone production ceases entirely, small amounts of these hormones are still present because of continued activity of the adrenal glands. LH and FSH levels typically become elevated after menopause.

Symptoms

Although about 80 percent of women experience symptoms due to their changing hormone levels, only a minority of menopausal women seek treatment for symptom relief (Weideger, 1977; Perlmutter, 1978). This is probably because the majority of symptoms are of a relatively minor nature and tend to disappear with time.

The most common symptom in the menopause is the **hot flash,** which affects 75 to 80 percent of menopausal women (Bates, 1981; Erlik et al., 1981). Typically, the hot flash appears suddenly as a feeling of warmth over the upper part of the body (very much like a generalized blushing) and is accompanied by reddening, sweating, and, occasionally, dizziness. In some women, hot flashes are infrequent (once a week or less) but others have them every few hours. Hot flashes may last just a few seconds and be quite mild, or they may last for 15 minutes or more in the most severe cases (experienced by less than 10 percent of

[2] The term **menopause** correctly refers only to a woman's last natural menstrual period. Many people incorrectly use the word menopause to refer to a time more correctly called the **climacteric** or the **perimenopausal years,** that is, the several years immediately before and after the menopause.

larynx the voice box.

precocious puberty (pree koh' shus pew' burr tee) physical changes of puberty occurring before age 9 in girls or age 10 in boys.

menopause (men' ō paws) the period during which menstruation gradually stops, usually occurring in the late forties. Sometimes called female climacteric.

climacteric (klī mak' tur ik) syndrome experienced by about 5 percent of men over 60, marked by weakness, fatigue, poor appetite, decreased sexual drive, reduction or loss of potency, irritability, and impaired ability to concentrate. Also see *menopause*, which is sometimes called the female climacteric.

perimenopausal years (perry men oh paws' uhl) the years immediately before and after menopause.

hot flash sudden sensations of warmth, blushing, and sweating, sometimes with dizziness, that occur commonly in menopausal women.

women). One particularly disturbing feature of the hot flash is that it occurs more often during sleep than in the daytime, in which case it is liable to awaken the woman abruptly and contribute to insomnia.

Current evidence suggests that hot flashes are due to a malfunction of temperature control mechanisms in the hypothalamus (Casper, Yen, and Wilkes, 1979; Bates, 1981; Erlik et al., 1981). Although estrogen deficiency seems to be a necessary condition for hot flashes to occur, and estrogen therapy effectively combats this symptom, hot flashes generally disappear spontaneously within a few years after the menopause even without treatment. In approximately 20 percent of affected women hot flashes persist for at least five years beyond the onset (Perlmutter, 1978). Since this symptom is sometimes severe enough to interfere with everyday functioning and there is no test that can predict when hot flashes will disappear spontaneously, deciding whether to obtain treatment or not is very much a subjective decision for the woman.

Other changes also reflect prolonged estrogen deficiency (Soules and Bremner, 1982; Speroff, Glass, and Kase, 1983). Lowered levels of circulating estrogen predispose women to shrinking and thinning of the vagina, a loss of tissue elasticity, and lessened vaginal lubrication during sexual arousal, all of which may sometimes lead to painful intercourse. Other physical changes that may occur in the postmenopausal years include thinning of the breasts and the vulva and loss of mineral content in bones, resulting in a more brittle structure (a condition that is called **osteoporosis**).

Treatment

Although there has been considerable controversy in the last decade about the risks and benefits of estrogen replacement therapy (ERT) in the menopause and postmenopausal years, strong scientific evidence shows that the symptoms we have discussed can be significantly alleviated by its use (Soules and Bremner, 1982; Council on Scientific Affairs, 1983; Barrett-Connor, 1989). In fact, ERT plays a preventive role in slowing the occurrence of osteoporosis rather than just alleviating symptoms once they occur. Because there is also evidence that ERT increases the risk of cancer of the uterus (Greenblatt and Stoddard, 1978; Antunes et al., 1979) and an unsubstantiated but realistic concern that it may increase the risk of breast cancer (Gambrell, 1982; Bergkvist et al., 1989), caution is certainly in order. The consensus of medical opinion seems to favor ERT for several different reasons:

1. Adding a progestin to the latter part of the estrogen cycle materially reduces the increased risk of cancer of the uterus that arises from estrogen use (Gambrell et al., 1979; Council on Scientific Affairs, 1983).
2. Osteoporosis has now been recognized as a disorder of great seriousness, since it often leads to hip fractures in elderly women, and in 20 to 30 percent of cases these women die due to the fracture or its complications (Speroff, Glass, and Kase, 1983).

   Fortunately, ERT in postmenopausal women has now been shown quite conclusively to provide significant protection against bone loss and fractures associated with osteoporosis (Ettinger et al., 1985; Riis, Thomsen, and Christiansen, 1987). In fact, the Food and Drug Administration approved the use of ERT for this purpose in 1986. Now ERT is available in several different versions: either in standard pill form, in the form of a cream, or by a new method that involves using a patch that sticks to the skin, like a Band-Aid, slowly releasing estrogen over time in a manner that more closely mimics the way estrogen is released naturally by the ovaries (Padwick et al., 1985).
3. ERT provides protection against certain forms of heart disease (Colditz et al., 1987; Sullivan et al., 1988).

Most authorities caution that ERT should not be used indiscriminately and that it should be employed in the smallest effective dose for the shortest period of time compatible with the therapeutic need. However, Horsman and his co-workers (1983) found that the dose of estrogen needed to produce the greatest protective effect on bone (preventing osteoporosis) is greater than the dose needed to control other menopausal symptoms. On the other hand, estrogen is not the entire answer to the osteoporosis problem, since exercise and calcium intake are also related to preventing this disorder (Raisz, 1988).

Psychological Aspects

In the past, just about every problem that could befall a woman was inaccurately attributed to the menopause. In eighteenth- and nineteenth-century Europe, for instance, physicians thought women decayed at menopause (Stearns, 1975), and "nervous irritability" was diagnosed in nine out of ten menopausal women

TABLE 6–3

Incidence of Increased Sexual Interest and Capacity for Orgasm During Preceding Five-Year Period, by Age

Age (years)	Increase in Sexual Interest		Increase in Capacity for Orgasm	
	%	N	%	N
38	16	93	21	91
46	12	225	18	215
50	4	204	13	188
54	2	62	6	52

Source: Modified from Hallstrom, 1979, Table 2, p. 167.

(Ballinger, 1981). Mistakenly blaming emotional instability, depression, and other psychological problems on the hormonal changes of the menopausal years has not just been a practice of ancient history; it is a relatively common error in modern times that continues even today.

Ballinger (1981) finds no evidence for an increased rate of depression or major psychiatric disorders in the years following the menopause and points out that "emotional symptoms at this time of life, as at any other time, are influenced by a multitude of environmental and personality factors." Others contend that menopausal discomfort has been greatly exaggerated, that the menopause may actually be an adaptive, positive event, and that "the mythology surrounding the menopause is based less on the reality of the female experience than on the sexist interpretations of the female experience" by male physicians (Alington-MacKinnon and Troll, 1981). Bart and Grossman (1978) also point out that much of the research on the menopause is methodologically flawed, particularly the portion related to psychological aspects of the menopausal years. They suggest that a woman's response to the menopause is in large part a function of her "premenopausal personality and life patterns" and note that menopausal depression (when it occurs) is far more a result of lack of meaningful roles for women and poor self esteem at this stage in their lives than a reflection of hormonal changes.

While there is some disagreement about the impact of the menopause on female sexuality, several studies suggest there is characteristically a decline in sexual interest and possibly a loss of female orgasmic responsivity in the immediate postmenopausal years (Pfeiffer, Verwoerdt, and Davis, 1972; Zussman et al., 1981; Dennerstein and Burrows, 1982). Hallstrom (1979) studied 800 women in Sweden and found considerable evidence to support this premise; for example, the prevalence of weak or absent sexual interest increased progressively from age 38 to 54, and a declining capacity for orgasm was reported for these same ages. However, Hallstrom also found that some postmenopausal women showed increased sexual interest and capacity for orgasm (see Table 6–3). On the other hand, several reports (Masters and Johnson, 1966, 1970; Kaplan, 1974; Starr and Weiner, 1981) have noted that sexual interest may increase in the postmenopausal years. The discrepancy in these findings may be the result of inadequate research design that does not take into account factors such as the health status of study subjects and their spouses or sexual partners.

LATE ADULTHOOD

In America, sex is generally regarded as something for the young, healthy, and attractive. Thinking of an elderly couple engaging in sexual relations usually provokes discomfort in young adults. The idea of sexual partners in a nursing home seems shocking and immoral to most people. Despite these cultural myths, the psychological need for intimacy, excitement, and pleasure does not disappear in old age, and there is nothing in the biology of aging that automatically shuts down sexual function.

osteoporosis (ah stee oh pohr oh′ sis) a condition in which the bones become thin and brittle due to mineral loss; a common occurrence in postmenopausal women.

Biological Considerations

FEMALE AGING

Aging alone does not diminish female sexual interest or the potential of the woman to be sexually responsive if her general health is good. Specific physiological changes do occur, however, in the sexual response cycle of postmenopausal women. These changes do not appear abruptly or in exactly the same fashion in each woman (Masters and Johnson, 1966).

Typically, there is little or no increase in breast size accompanying sexual arousal, although breast sensitivity to stimulation continues. The sex flush occurs less often and less extensively than at younger ages, but this change has absolutely no effect on sexual feelings or functioning. Less muscle tension develops during sexual arousal, particularly in the plateau phase, which is not surprising since this corresponds to the usual decrease in muscle size and strength that occurs with aging. This reduced muscular tension may account (at least in part) for the reduced intensity of orgasm that is sometimes experienced by women in late adulthood.

While clitoral response is not affected by aging, vaginal function changes in two different ways. First, reduced elasticity in the walls of the vagina leads to less expansion during sexual arousal. Second, vaginal lubrication generally begins more slowly than at younger ages, and vaginal dryness may create some problems as the quantities of lubrication are somewhat reduced. This condition can be overcome if it causes discomfort either by estrogen replacement therapy or by the use of an artificial lubricant such as K-Y Jelly.

The decrease in vaginal lubrication in postmenopausal women is the direct result of diminished vaginal blood flow that, in turn, is caused by low estrogen (Semmens and Wagner, 1982). Leiblum and co-workers (1983) found that sexually active postmenopausal women had less shrinkage of the vagina and higher levels of androgens and pituitary gonadotropins (LH and FSH) than sexually inactive women. This suggests that regular sexual activity may provide at least some protection against the physiologic changes of aging in relation to female sexual anatomy.

MALE AGING

The normal pattern of reproductive aging in men is quite different from that in women because there is no definite end to male fertility. Although sperm production slows down after age 40, it continues into the eighties and nineties. Similarly, while testosterone production declines gradually from age 55 or 60 on, there is usually no major drop in sex hormone levels in men as there is in women.

About 5 percent of men over 60 experience a condition called the male *climacteric*, which resembles the female menopause in some ways. (Using the term "male menopause" to describe the male climacteric is incorrect since men do not have menstrual periods.) This condition is marked by some or all of the following features: weakness, tiredness, poor appetite, decreased sexual desire, reduction or loss of potency, irritability, and impaired ability to concentrate (Greenblatt et al., 1979; Kolodny, Masters, and Johnson, 1979). These changes occur because of low tes-

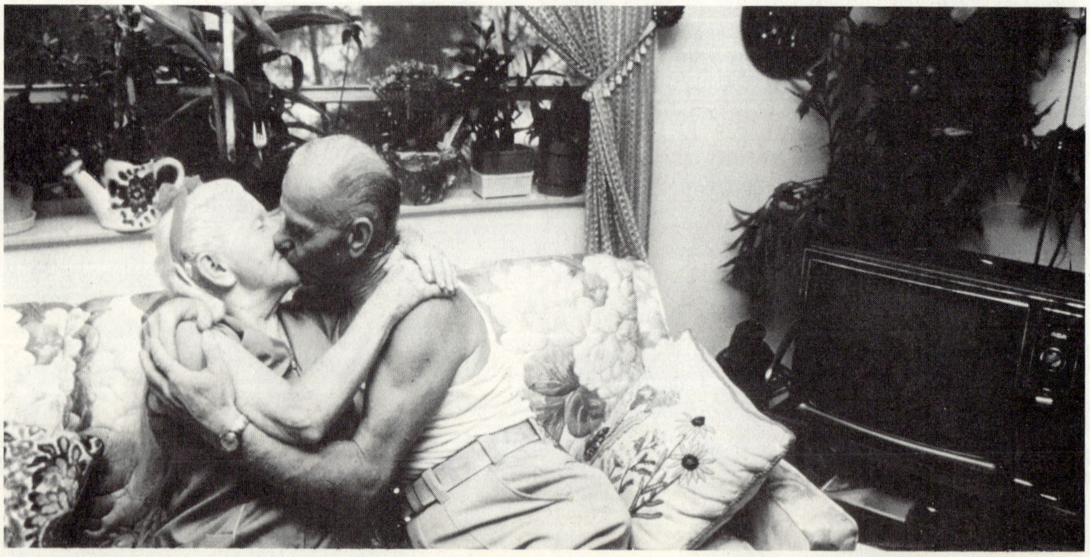

tosterone production, and they can be reversed or improved by testosterone injections. It should be stressed that *most* men do not have a recognizable climacteric as they age.

The physiology of male sexual response is affected by aging in a number of ways. The following changes have been noted in men over 55:

1. It usually takes a longer time and more direct stimulation for the penis to become erect.
2. Erections tend to be less firm, on average, than at earlier ages.
3. The testes elevate only partway up to the perineum and do so more slowly than in younger men.
4. The amount of semen is reduced, and the intensity of ejaculation is lessened.
5. There is usually less physical need to ejaculate.
6. The refractory period—the time interval after ejaculation when the male is unable to ejaculate again—becomes longer (Masters and Johnson, 1966).

In addition, the sex flush usually does not occur in aging men, and muscle tension during sexual arousal is reduced, as in women, since muscle mass and strength generally decrease with aging.

Although the changes in male sexual physiology do not usually occur abruptly or represent an impairment of function, men who are uninformed about these patterns may be frightened into thinking something is wrong with them. In other instances, a man's partner may be the one to become alarmed. For example, while many men find that they enjoy sex in their later years without ejaculating at every opportunity, partners who don't realize this may think it reflects poorly on their attractiveness or skill as lovers.

Some men have completely unrealistic expectations about what their sex lives *should* be as they age. While they wouldn't expect to run a mile as fast at age 65 as they did at age 25 (or to recuperate from their exertion as quickly), they expect to get rock-hard erections instantly in all sexual situations and are worried when they can't make love twice in one evening. The aging male, by misinterpreting these changes, is particularly vulnerable to performance anxiety.

Psychosocial Considerations

In part, our cultural negativism about sex and romance in the geriatric years is a reflection of an attitude called **ageism,** a prejudice against people because they are old, that is similar to the more familiar prejudices of racism and sexism in our society. As Butler and Lewis (1976, p. 4) point out: "The ageist sees older people in stereotypes: rigid, boring, talkative, senile, old-fashioned in morality and lacking in skills, useless and with little redeeming social value." These same authors observe that ageism in relation to sexuality is the ultimate form of desexualization: "if you are getting old, you're finished" (p. 5).

Ageism is not restricted to heterosexuals, either, as this quote from *Gay and Gray: The Older Homosexual Male* (Berger, 1982) shows:

> Many older gay men believe that younger gays react negatively to them. Most older gays feel that young people sometimes take advantage of them, do not welcome their company in bars, clubs, and bathhouses, do not care to associate or form friendships with them, and think they are dull company. *(p. 191)*

It is interesting to note that in one study, college students estimated that married couples in their sixties had intercourse less than once a month and expected that married couples in their seventies had intercourse even less often (Zeiss, 1982). As we will see, these are underestimates of actual behavior, showing that young adults are susceptible to ageism in their thinking—at least when it comes to sex.

Kinsey and his colleagues (1948, 1953) were the first to examine systematically the effect of aging on sexual behavior. Although their studies indicated that sex continued well into late adulthood, they also described a general decline in the frequency of sexual activity for both men and women across the adult age range. A number of other studies confirmed these overall trends (Newman and Nichols, 1960; Pfeiffer and Davis, 1972; Martin, 1977), with most reports suggesting that the decrease in sexual activity is partly due to diminished health and partly a reflection of cultural attitudes and expectations.

More recently, a longitudinal study done at Duke University found that patterns of sexual activity actually remained relatively stable over middle and late adulthood, with only a modest decline appearing in most individuals (George and Weiler, 1981). For example, men who were 66 to 71 years old at the start of this study had no overall decline in sexual activity scores over the next six years, and a majority of men and women in the 56 to 65 age bracket at the beginning of the study had stable rates of sexual activity during this same time period. However, in those over

ageism an attitude of prejudice against the elderly.

TABLE 6–4

Sex Problems[a] in the Old Old

Men (N = 43)	%	Women (N = 20)	%
Fear of poor performance	37	Orgasms too infrequent	30
Inability to maintain erection	33	Partner's erection problems	30
Inability to reach orgasm	28	Lack of vaginal lubrication	30
Inability to achieve erection	28	Worry about nonsexual problems	25
Not enough opportunities for sexual encounters	23	Not enough opportunities for sexual encounters	25
Partner's vaginal pain or lack of lubrication	23	Low sex drive	25

[a] Problems of men and women aged 80 or older who were in good health and who had a regular sex partner or partners.

Source: Bretschneider and McCoy, 1988, Table V.

age 65, 18 percent of the men and 33 percent of the women completely stopped sexual activity with their partners over a six-year period.[3]

Data regarding sexual interest and behavior in a previously neglected subgroup of the aged, the "old old," were recently collected by Bretschneider and McCoy (1988), who studied a sample of 202 healthy men and women between the ages of 80 and 102 (see Table 6–4). Sixty-two percent of the men and 30 percent of the women indicated that they were still having sexual intercourse, but for both sexes the most common form of sexual activity was touching and caressing without intercourse. Notably, the past importance and frequency of sexual activity earlier in life correlated significantly with the frequency and enjoyment of sexual intercourse and touching and caressing without intercourse in "old old" age.

Various studies of sexual behavior in late adulthood indicate that the male's declining interest seems to be the major limiting factor to continued sexual activity (Kinsey et al., 1953; Pfeiffer and Davis, 1972; Martin, 1977; George and Weiler, 1981). This declining interest, however, may say more about cultural expectations that become self-fulfilling prophecies than about anything else. While the pattern of sexual activity among aged people varies considerably, coital frequency in early marriage and overall quality of sexual activity in early adulthood correlate significantly with the frequency of sexual activity in late adulthood (Masters and Johnson, 1966).

On the other hand, a recent report noted that 35 percent of a sample of men over 60 had difficulty getting or maintaining erections, with more than half of the married men over 70 affected by this problem (Diokno, Brown, and Herzog, 1990). Many of these cases were linked to medical difficulties. The same conclusion has been reached in several other recent studies (Kaiser et al., 1988; Mulligan and Katz, 1988; Mulligan et al., 1988), suggesting that the real problem is not just declining sexual interest, but declining health. Both hormonal and vascular factors appear to be frequently involved (Kaiser et al., 1988; Diokno, Brown, and Herzog, 1990). One plausible explanation is that the health problems cause erectile difficulties and that male sexual interest wanes only after the erectile problems have been firmly established.

It is interesting to note that most researchers who claim to be studying sexual activity rates in the elderly have actually restricted themselves to studying coital behavior, as though other forms of sexual activity "don't count." As Table 6–5 shows, many adults over 60 continue to masturbate (Catania and White, 1982; Bretschneider and McCoy, 1988), although these are almost entirely individuals who masturbated when they were younger. Not surprisingly, elderly people without sexual partners tend to masturbate more frequently (Catania and White, 1982). In couples over 60, other forms of sexual stimulation continue to be utilized (e.g., oral sex and manual stimulation); they

[3] The George and Weiler (1981) study was particularly well designed in ways that represent an important advance over prior studies of geriatric sexuality. In addition to being longitudinal rather than cross-sectional (so that each person's behavior could be tracked over time), they also included only married subjects, since marital status is a determinant of sexual opportunity and sexual behavior in old age.

not only provide some variety but also can be a source of pleasure and closeness even if the male is unable to obtain or maintain erections (Starr and Weiner, 1981; Turner and Adams, 1988). Here is what one 78-year-old man told us:

> In my mid-sixties, I had a real problem getting it up. Sexual intercourse became impossible and I got very upset over it at first. But my wife just found other ways to excite me, and after a while—when I relaxed more, I guess—my problem disappeared. Now, even though she doesn't always want to have intercourse when I do, we still use our mouths and tongues on each other, and we plan to keep doing it, too. *(Authors' files)*

In late adulthood, the longer life span of women combined with their tendency to marry men who are their age or slightly older frequently creates a situation of widowhood. At the same time that fewer men of the same age are available as new sexual partners, younger men tend to focus their attentions on women under 40. Thus, sexual opportunities and social contacts with men are often extremely limited for these mature women who might otherwise be enthusiastic sexual partners.

In the past decade, a new trend has emerged in which not all women 60 or older who find themselves widowed or divorced are passively accepting their fate. Some women in this situation are using their ingenuity to find new partners, as shown by the following ad from the personal classified section of a well-known magazine.

> Tall, handsome intelligent man sixty to sixty-five, wanted for attractive, lively sixty-two-year-old widow with fantastic figure and modern values. If you're interested in romance more than golf, send a photo and your phone.

Although a 65-year-old widow (or widower) may have an interest in sexual activity, social pressures may prevent sexual opportunities or belittle their meaning via snide jokes (e.g., only "dirty old men" are interested in sex, and "dirty old women" should "act their age"). As prolonged abstention from sexual activity in old age leads to shrinking of the sexual organs (just as a healthy arm loses strength and coordination if put in a sling for four months), the older adult is truly faced with a sexual dilemma—"use it or lose it."

An often-neglected aspect of aging in our society is that many elderly persons are relegated to nursing homes or other long-term care facilities for health reasons, to "protect" themselves, or for the convenience of their children. Although research on sexual behavior in this population is understandably sparse, a number of authorities have spoken out in favor of making provisions in such facilities (such as making private rooms available) for those who desire sexual interaction (Kassel, 1976; McKinley and Drew, 1977; D. B. Miller, 1978; Wasow and Loeb, 1979). While most nursing home administrators seem opposed to this notion, and some facilities actually insist on seg-

FOCUS IN BRIEF

Marital Status of Population 65 and Over by Sex, 1987

	Males		Females	
Marital Status	*65–74*	*75+*	*65–74*	*75+*
Total[a]	7608	3970	9624	6773
Never married	4.7%	4.3%	4.8%	6.4%
Married, spouse present	79.7%	65.9%	51.0%	22.4%
Married, spouse absent	0.7%	1.9%	0.8%	0.9%
Widowed	9.0%	23.6%	36.7%	67.0%
Separated	1.1%	1.0%	1.2%	0.6%
Divorced	4.8%	3.3%	5.5%	2.7%

[a] Number expressed in thousands.

Source: U.S. Bureau of the Census, 1989.

TABLE 6–5

Current Incidence of Masturbation in Older Adults

Age	*Male*	*N*	*Female*	*N*
60–69	52.6%	152	47.1%	281
70–79	29.5%	95	49.1%	161
80–91	45.8%	24	34.5%	29

Source: Copyright © 1981 by Bernard D. Starr, Ph.D. and Marcella Bakur Weiner, Ed.D. from the book THE STARR-WEINER REPORT ON SEX AND SEXUALITY IN THE MATURE YEARS. Originally published by Stein & Day, Inc., reprinted with permission of Scarborough House/Publishers.

regating men and women even if they're married, both ethical considerations for protecting the rights of the elderly and more practical considerations having to do with maintaining self-esteem and personal well-being lead us to advocate change in this area. However, it should be noted that permitting sexual expression in the institutionalized elderly is not the entire solution to their plight. Additional steps must be taken to overcome loneliness and boredom in the nursing home environment so that these facilities are not unintentional prisons for our older adults.

In the United States, where there is little preparation or education for aging, it is not surprising that many people are uninformed about the physiological changes in their sexual function in their sixties and seventies. They may mistakenly view these normal "slowing down" processes as evidence that loss of function is imminent. Brief preventive counseling during middle age might result in significant change in this area, but changed attitudes toward sex and aging seem even more necessary. What people must recognize is that given good health and the availability of an interested and interesting partner, there is no reason that sexual enjoyment should have to come to an end in late adulthood. Perhaps the ultimate test of whether we have lived through a sexual revolution will be if attitudes toward sexuality in old age are transformed.

SUMMARY

1. Sexual development begins before birth and continues throughout the life cycle. Sex chromosomes (XY = male, XX = female) provide the initial programming for sex differentiation.
2. Growth of the testes begins at about the sixth week after conception. The testes then produce testosterone (stimulating growth of the Wolffian ducts) and Müllerian duct inhibiting substance, which causes the structures that would develop into a female reproductive system to shrink. *For male sexual differentiation to occur, both the testis determining factor and testosterone must be present in adequate amounts at the right time of development.*
3. Female sexual differentiation does not require hormone stimulation. The ovaries develop at the twelfth week of pregnancy, and the Müllerian duct system gives rise to the uterus, Fallopian tubes, and inner third of the vagina.
4. Prenatal sex differentiation in both sexes involves the genitals, the internal reproductive structures, and the brain itself.
5. Disorders of prenatal sex development include sex chromosome problems (47,XXY = Klinefelter's syndrome; 45,X = Turner's syndrome), conditions of male or female pseudohermaphroditism (such as adrenogenital syndrome and the syndrome of testicular feminization), and problems caused by hormones given to a pregnant woman.
6. In infancy and childhood, the sexual reflexes for males and females are all present except for the ability of the male to ejaculate. Sex hormone levels are low.
7. With puberty, as sex hormone levels are activated, there is a growth spurt, maturation of the gonads and genitals, and development of secondary sex characteristics. Girls begin menstruation and have breast and pubic hair growth; boys become able to ejaculate and have voice deepening, growth of facial and body hair, and development of muscle mass. There is great variability to the timing and duration of puberty.
8. The menopause, which typically occurs around age 48 to 52, is the cessation of menstrual periods. Dramatic decreases in estrogen production in the ovaries in the perimenopausal years can cause a variety of symptoms, including hot flashes, shrinking and thinning of the vagina, decreased vaginal lubrication during sexual arousal, and osteoporosis. These symptoms can generally be prevented or alleviated by estrogen replacement therapy combined with cyclic use of progestin (to minimize the risk of cancer of the uterus).
9. Although many psychological problems have been attributed to the menopause, current research finds no evidence of an increased rate of emotional problems in the postmenopausal years.
10. About 5 percent of men over 60 have a male climacteric, marked by symptoms such as decreased sexual desire, weakness, tiredness, and poor appetite. This condition is the result of a testosterone deficiency that can be corrected by testosterone injections.
11. In late adulthood, there are a number of biological changes in the sexual response cycle, such as decreased vaginal lubrication in women and slower erectile response in men. In both sexes, muscle tension is reduced. However, these changes do not generally prevent sexual functioning.

12. Sexuality in late adulthood is profoundly influenced by ageism and other cultural stereotypes that deny the normality of sexual feelings and capabilities at this stage of the life cycle. While health problems and lack of a partner may complicate sexual functioning, there is no inherent reason most elderly persons must stop enjoying sex.

Thought Questions

1. The parents of the identical twin boys decided on the best advice available to reassign the damaged twin to be a girl. They decided it would be better to raise the child as a girl who would need surgeries, hormones, and be unable to have children, rather than as a boy without a penis. Setting aside the outcome in this particular case, do you agree with the values expressed by this decision? Why or why not? What problems would the child and the parents have had if the twin without a penis had been raised as a boy?
2. The trend in our society has been to reduce the stigma associated with birth defects and to accept with sympathy rather than horror that some babies are born with defects that may or may not be correctable. However, if the defects involve the sex organs, people seem still to regard such errors as embarrassing and shameful. Do you agree that this is true, and, if so, can you explain why?
3. Children who are born with the "Dominican Republic syndrome" are reported to change their gender identity from female to male when the penis grows at puberty. Why might this be so, when, in general, other pseudohermaphrodites are reported to maintain the gender identity of their sex of rearing, regardless of bodily changes at puberty?
4. Suppose you found that your apparently normal friend or lover was an XY individual with testicular feminization syndrome: would this change your feelings toward this woman?
5. How do girls typically feel about having their first menstrual period? How do boys typically feel about the first few times they have a "wet dream"? How should parents respond to evidence of these events?
6. What are the implications of the fact that the fetal sex hormones produce brain differentiation? How might it signify that males and females have anatomically different brains?
7. Most readers of this text would probably deplore prejudice on the basis of race or sex. However, prejudice against the elderly is also very common and probably more socially acceptable in our culture. Why is prejudice against the elderly a *particularly* foolish form of prejudice? Do younger people really mean it when they say things such as "I hope I die before I get old"?

Suggested Readings

Golub, Sharon, ed. *Menarche: The Transition from Girl to Woman*. Lexington, MA: Lexington Books (D. C. Heath), 1983. The first book-length treatment of this important developmental event is an excellent, multidimensional collection of essays.

Katchadourian, H. *The Biology of Adolescence*. San Francisco: W. H. Freeman, 1977. A fine review of all biological aspects of puberty. Numerous charts, tables, and diagrams aid the reader in using this book.

Money, J., and Ehrhardt, A. E. *Man & Woman, Boy & Girl*. Baltimore: Johns Hopkins University Press, 1972. A comprehensive, readable account of the principles of sex differentiation amply illustrated and filled with intriguing case reports.

Starr, Bernard D., and Weiner, Marcella B. *The Starr–Weiner Report on Sex and Sexuality in the Mature Years*. New York: Stein and Day, 1981. Results of a survey of 800 people over age 60, presented clearly and nontechnically.

7

Sexually Transmitted Diseases and Sexual Infections

Infections that are spread by sexual contact are referred to as **sexually transmitted diseases,** or **STDs**. STDs include infections that were formerly known as venereal diseases (VD)—those almost always transmitted by sexual contact—as well as various other infections that are sometimes transmitted by nonsexual routes. In addition to describing a broader category of infections, the term STD has not yet acquired the stigmatizing sound that the label VD carries. The following sections will describe the symptoms, diagnosis, and suggested treatment of sexually transmitted diseases, as well as similar information about several other types of sexual infections. Because of the complex influence the human immunodeficiency virus (HIV, the virus that causes AIDS) has had on sexuality and society in recent years, HIV infection and AIDS are discussed separately in the following chapter even though they too are STDs.

GONORRHEA

Gonorrhea is the oldest and one of the most common forms of STD. In the Old Testament, Moses spoke about its infectivity (Leviticus 15); it was also mentioned in the ancient writings of Plato, Aristotle, and Hippocrates. Its modern name was coined by Galen, a Greek physician in the second century A.D. In 1879 Albert Neisser discovered the bacterium that causes it, which was named after him (*Neisseria gonorrheae*).

Although the discovery of penicillin as an effective treatment for this disease slowed its spread in the 1940s and 1950s, the incidence of gonorrhea had grown to epidemic proportions by 1980. However, there has been a relatively slow but steady decline in cases since that time (see Figure 7–1), with the one million cases of reported gonorrhea of 1980 having dropped to approximately 750,000 cases reported in 1989 (Handsfield, 1984; Centers for Disease Control, 1989). A significant portion of this drop has been due to declines in the occurrence of gonorrhea in homosexual and bisexual men, presumably as a result of safer sex practices linked to concerns about AIDS (Judson, 1983; Holmes et al., 1989). Most authorities agree that fewer than half of all cases of gonorrhea are actually reported, so there are probably some two million cases annually in the United States (Handsfield, 1984).

Gonorrhea is transmitted by any form of sexual contact, ranging from sexual intercourse to fellatio, anal intercourse, and, infrequently, cunnilingus or even kissing (Barlow, 1979; Robertson, McMillan, and Young, 1980). A woman who has intercourse once with an infected man has a 50 percent chance of getting gonorrhea (Platt, Rice, and McCormack, 1983), while a man who has intercourse once with an infected woman has a lower risk, probably around 20 to 25 percent, of becoming infected (Handsfield, 1984). The old excuse "I caught it from a toilet seat," which was previously laughed at by scientists, has now been shown to be at least theoretically possible since the infective bacteria can survive for up to two hours on a toilet seat or on wet toilet paper (Gilbaugh and Fuchs, 1979). However, it is unlikely that this form of transmission is more than a rare occurrence.

Symptoms

Most men with gonorrhea develop a yellowish discharge from the tip of the penis and painful, frequent urination as the first indications of gonorrhea. These symptoms usually appear within two to ten days after infection but may sometimes start as much as a month later (Schofield, 1979). The symptoms are produced by infection in the urethra which leads to inflammation (urethritis). The puslike discharge (which often stains the underwear) is part of the body's reaction to this infection. In about 10 percent of cases in men, there may be no symptoms from the infection, which means that the man can spread gonorrhea without realizing it.

Men with symptoms from gonorrhea usually seek treatment promptly and are cured. For men who do not receive treatment, the infection may move up the urethra to the prostate, seminal vesicles, and epididymis and can cause severe pain and fever. If untreated, gonorrhea can lead to sterility (Holmes et al., 1989), but this is a relatively infrequent complication in men.

Since less than half of the women with gonorrhea have any visible symptoms, they are likely to have their infection for a longer time before treatment is begun. This delay exposes women to a greater risk of complications. In addition, symptomless women may unknowingly spread their infections to their sexual partners. Many women do not find out they are in-

sexually transmitted disease (STD) infection spread mainly by sexual contact.

FIGURE 7–1

Gonorrhea—By Sex, United States, 1960–1989

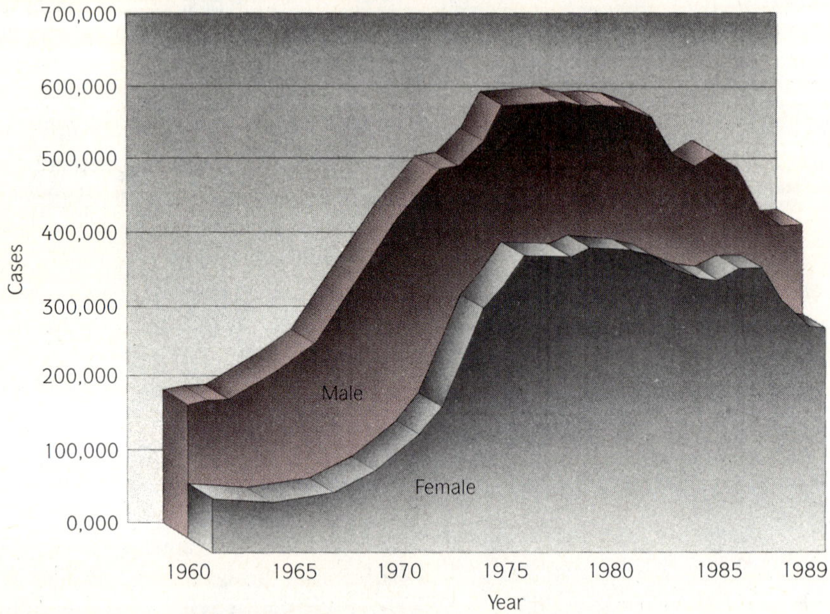

Source: CDC, *MMWR* 38 (54): 1989 (published Oct. 5, 1990).

fected until their partner's penile discharge or burning appears.

Even when symptoms occur in women, they may be very mild and tend to go unnoticed or are misdiagnosed. The symptoms include increased vaginal discharge, irritation of the external genitals, pain or burning with urination, and abnormal menstrual bleeding. In women, infection is most commonly found in the cervix (90 percent of cases) but can also be present in the urethra (70 percent), the rectum (30 to 40 percent), the throat (10 percent), or any combination of these sites.

Women who are untreated may develop serious complications. Gonorrhea commonly spreads from the cervix to the uterus, Fallopian tubes, and ovaries, causing pelvic inflammatory disease (PID). PID, although not always caused by gonorrhea, is the most common cause of female infertility because it can produce scarring that blocks the Fallopian tubes. The early symptoms of PID are lower abdominal pain, fever, nausea or vomiting, and pain during intercourse.

In both sexes, gonorrhea can spread through the bloodstream to other organs, causing infection and inflammation of the joints (gonococcal arthritis), the heart (gonococcal endocarditis), or the covering of the brain (gonococcal meningitis). Fortunately, these complications are rare and treatable. Eye infections with gonorrhea occur (rarely) in adults, where they are caused by touching the eye with a contaminated hand. Newborn children may develop eye infections during birth if their mother's cervix is infected. Because this can produce blindness, infection-preventing drops, usually silver nitrate, are routinely put in every newborn baby's eyes.

Diagnosis and Treatment

Gonorrhea in men is diagnosed by examining the urethral discharge under a microscope after staining it with a specially colored dye. As this method is only about 90 percent accurate, it may also be necessary to try to grow the infecting bacteria in a laboratory by a culture test that takes several days. Men who have had homosexual contacts should have cultures of the throat and rectum as well as the urethra.

In women, culture tests are the only reliable means of establishing the diagnosis. Swabs should *always* be taken from the mouth of the cervix *and* the rectum, even if the woman has never had anal intercourse, because a vaginal discharge may drip onto the anus and cause infection there. If the woman has experience with fellatio, a throat swab should also be taken. There is no blood test that can identify gonorrhea reliably at the present time.

The most effective treatment for gonorrhea used to be an injection of penicillin G given along with a pill called probenecid that blocked excretion of the penicillin in the urine, keeping a high concentration in the body. Unfortunately, some strains of gonorrhea that are resistant to penicillin evolved and have now become so common that they account for over 4 percent of gonorrhea cases in the United States (Handsfield et al., 1989). As a result, the U.S. Public Health Service and the CDC now recommend that nonpregnant adults with gonorrhea be treated with a combination of an injection of an antibiotic called ceftriaxone *plus* the use of doxycycline pills (Centers for Disease Control, 1989). This regimen also has the advantage of simultaneously treating the chlamydial infections that often coexist with gonorrhea (see p. 188).

It is also recommended that ALL people with gonorrhea should have a blood test for syphilis and should be offered confidential testing and counseling for HIV infection. In addition, anyone exposed sexually to gonorrhea within the previous 30 days should be examined, cultured, and treated as above on the presumption that they are infected (Centers for Disease Control, 1989).

In *any* case of gonorrhea, it is important to abstain from sexual activity with a partner until you have been rechecked after treatment to be certain you are cured. *It is also extremely important to notify anyone with whom you had sexual contact, including the person you know or suspect gave you the infection, to insist that he or she see a doctor for proper diagnosis and treatment.*

SYPHILIS

Syphilis first came to public attention at the end of the fifteenth century, when it swept across Europe, decimating armies and towns as it traveled. The source of this widespread outbreak is unclear. Some authorities believe that a particularly infectious type of syphilis was imported from America by Columbus and his crew (*The New York Times,* October 10, 1989, p. C13), while others believe that it was already present in Europe (Catterall, 1974). The spiral-shaped microorganism that causes syphilis, *Treponema pallidum,* was identified in 1905.

Syphilis is far less common than gonorrhea today. Unfortunately, the sudden upsurge in the use of crack cocaine (a smokeable form of cocaine that is intensely addictive) has been tied to a tremendous increase in rates of heterosexually transmitted syphilis in the United States in the past few years because many women trade sex with numerous partners for drugs (Goldsmith, 1988; Centers for Disease Control, 1989). In 1989, the overall number of reported syphilis cases exceeded 40,000, a level not seen for more than 40 years (see Figure 7–2). Most experts believe that this represents less than half of the actual cases that occur each year.

Syphilis is usually transmitted by sexual contacts, but it can also be acquired from a blood transfusion or can be transmitted from a pregnant mother to the fetus. In New York City alone, cases of transmission from a pregnant woman to her baby grew by over 500 percent between 1986 and 1988; nationwide, a corresponding increase is occurring as we enter the early 1990s (Centers for Disease Control, 1989).

Symptoms

The earliest sign of syphilis in its *primary stage* is a sore called a **chancre** (pronounced "shanker"). The chancre generally appears two to four weeks after infection. The most common locations for the chancre, which is painless in 75 percent of cases, are the genitals and anus, but chancres can also develop on the lips, in the mouth, on a finger, on a breast, or on any part of the body where the infecting organism entered the skin. The chancre typically begins as a dull-red spot which develops into a pimple. The pimple ulcerates, forming a round or oval sore usually surrounded by a red rim. The chancre usually heals within four to six weeks, leading to the erroneous belief that the "problem" went away.

chancre (shan′ ker) a painless sore that appears in the primary stage of syphilis.

FIGURE 7–2

Syphilis (primary and secondary)— By Sex, United States, 1956–1989

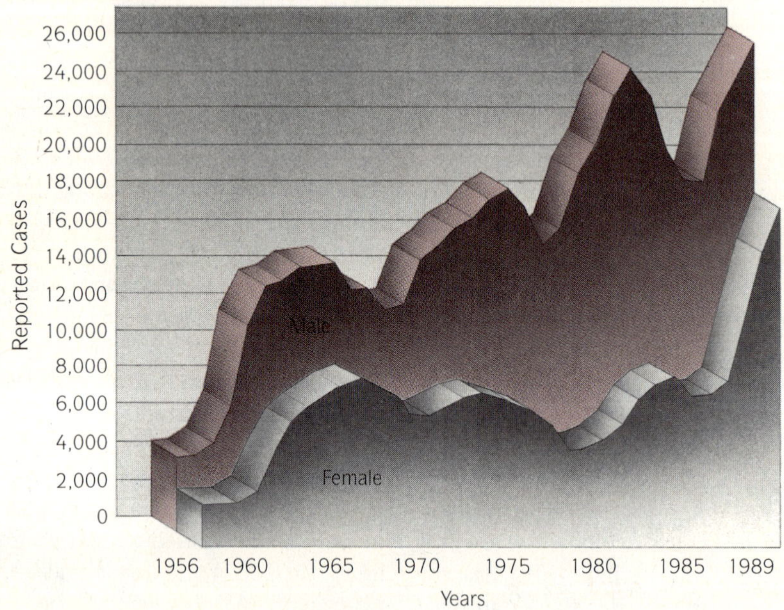

Source: CDC, *MMWR* 38 (54); 1989 (published Oct. 5, 1990).

Secondary syphilis begins anywhere from one week to six months after the chancre heals if effective treatment was not received. The symptoms include a pale red or pinkish rash (often found on the palms and soles), fever, sore throat, headaches, joint pains, poor appetite, weight loss, and hair loss. Moist sores called *condyloma lata* may appear around the genitals or anus and are highly infectious. Because of the diversity of symptoms, syphilis is sometimes called "the great imitator." The symptoms of the secondary stage of syphilis usually last three to six months but can come and go periodically. After all symptoms disappear, the disease passes into a *latent stage*. During this stage, the disease is no longer contagious, but the infecting microorganisms burrow their way into various tissues, such as the brain, spinal cord, blood vessels, and bones. Fifty to 70 percent of people with untreated syphilis stay in this stage for the rest of their lives, but the remainder pass on to the *tertiary stage,* or late syphilis. Late syphilis involves serious heart problems, eye problems, and brain or spinal cord damage. These complications can cause paralysis, insanity, blindness, and death.

Syphilis can be acquired by an unborn baby from its mother if the infecting microorganisms are in her bloodstream, since they cross the placenta. The resulting infection, called **congenital syphilis,** produces bone and teeth deformities, anemia, kidney problems, and other abnormalities. Congenital syphilis can be prevented if a pregnant woman with syphilis is treated adequately before the sixteenth week of pregnancy (Holmes, 1980).

Diagnosis and Treatment

Syphilis is usually diagnosed by a blood test. Several different tests are available, including some that are most suitable for screening and others that are more time-consuming and expensive but also more accurate. Although none of these tests is completely foolproof in detecting the primary stage of syphilis, secondary syphilis can be diagnosed with 100 percent accuracy. Diagnosis also depends on a carefully performed physical examination looking for signs of primary or secondary syphilis. Chancres of the cervix or vagina may be detected only by a pelvic examination, since they are usually painless. An examination under a special microscope of the fluid taken from a chancre will usually show the characteristic spiral-shaped organisms.

Syphilis can easily be treated with one injection of penicillin in its primary or secondary stages. Latent, tertiary, or congenital syphilis requires larger doses over a period of time, but the treatment is usually successful in these cases too. Patients who are allergic to penicillin can be given tetracycline or erythromycin.

Persons sexually exposed to someone with proven early syphilis should promptly be evaluated. The CDC recommends that if exposure occurred within the previous 90 days, the person should be treated with penicillin even if blood tests are negative, since the person could be infected but not yet have developed a positive blood test (Centers for Disease Control, 1989).

CHLAMYDIAL INFECTIONS

Infections caused by the bacteria *Chlamydia trachomatis* have been surprisingly overlooked until recently although they are now known to be the most common bacterial STD in the United States, with an estimated 3 to 4 million cases annually (Sanders et al., 1986). Furthermore, because it has been difficult to grow *C. trachomatis* in the laboratory, the disease often went undetected as a cause of nonspecific medical symptoms. In addition, because chlamydial infections are not reportable diseases nationally, physicians may have been lulled into thinking that they are less important or less transmissible STDs than others. Unfortunately, however, the health problems caused by chlamydial infections are serious, so being properly informed about this group of STDs is important. In fact, the U.S. Centers for Disease Control estimates that the direct and indirect cost of complications from chlamydial infections in women and newborns is one billion dollars annually (*American Medical News,* February 24, 1989, p. 34).

The number of new cases of chlamydial infections has been growing rapidly over the last decade and has now reached an alarming incidence. Data from several different surveys show the extent of this problem. Among several thousand sexually active women attending family planning clinics, 9 percent were found to have chlamydial infections (Schacter, Stone, and Moncada, 1983; Handsfield et al., 1986). This figure is similar to the prevalence rate of 10 percent found in men in military settings. Some college health services are reporting rates of chlamydial infection as high as 17 percent in undergraduate women (Goldsmith, 1986). At STD clinics, an average of 20 to 40 percent of all people tested are found to have chlamydial infections (Thompson and Washington, 1983; Stamm et al., 1984; Jones et al., 1986). The prevalence of chlamydial infections in adolescents is especially noteworthy: 15 percent of teenage girls and 8 percent of teenage boys are infected with this STD (Shafer et al., 1989).

Many diseases and medical complications are caused by *C. trachomatis*. In men, about half of all cases of nongonococcal urethritis (infection of the urethra not due to gonorrhea) is caused by this organism (Stamm, 1988). This condition alone—chlamydial urethritis—has an incidence about 2.5 times that of urethritis caused by gonorrhea (Centers for Disease Control, 1985). In addition, *Chlamydia trachomatis* causes about half of the 500,000 annual cases of acute epididymitis (infection of the epididymis) in the United States. Both of these conditions are more common in younger males: chlamydial urethritis is most prevalent in males aged 15 to 24, while chlamydial epididymitis is predominantly found in males under 35 years of age. Chlamydial urethritis is only one-third as common in homosexual males as in heterosexuals, but 6 to 8 percent of homosexual males have evidence of chlamydial infections of the rectum (Centers for Disease Control, 1985). Based on current knowledge, there do not seem to be major long-term consequences to males from chlamydial infections, even if they recur or are chronic (Holmes et al., 1989). However, relatively little research has been done on this topic, so it should not be presumed that it is safe for men to ignore such an infection. Furthermore, men who are not properly treated will almost inevitably transmit their infections to their sex partners, which can have dire consequences for females.

congenital syphilis syphilis contracted by the fetus from an infected mother, causing various abnormalities in the unborn child.

In females, *C. trachomatis* causes a number of different problems at various levels of the reproductive tract. The female version of chlamydial urethritis is a condition called the urethral syndrome. In addition, chlamydia causes cervicitis (infection of the cervix) and accounts for an estimated 250,000 to 500,000 cases of PID (pelvic inflammatory disease) annually. If you recall that many cases of PID eventually progress to the point where they cause scarring of the Fallopian tubes, you will see why this complication is a major cause of female infertility as well as a major factor in some ectopic pregnancies (Centers for Disease Control, 1985; Sanders et al., 1986; Holmes et al., 1989). In many cases chlamydial infection also involves the endometrium (inner lining) of the uterus. In one study, it was found that 41 percent of women infected with *C. trachomatis* had chlamydial endometritis (Jones et al., 1986).

Another major problem in females is that maternal chlamydial infections during pregnancy are commonly passed to the newborn during childbirth, presumably from the infant coming in contact with infected secretions in the birth canal. Up to 50 percent of infants born to infected mothers develop conjunctivitis (a type of eye infection), and 3 to 18 percent develop chlamydial pneumonia (a lung infection) before they are four months old (Centers for Disease Control, 1985; Schacter et al., 1986). While chlamydial pneumonia is not usually serious, chlamydial conjunctivitis can sometimes cause chronic eye disease (Holmes et al., 1989). (This is not the same type of eye infection as trachoma, another form of chlamydial disease and a major cause of blindness in developing countries. Trachoma is spread primarily by flies, not by sexual transmission.)

A number of studies also link chlamydial infections with various complications of pregnancy, such as premature rupture of the fetal membranes, premature delivery, and postpartum endometritis (Holmes et al., 1989; Handsfield et al., 1986). However, the data are not conclusive.

Chlamydial infection can also be a cause of pharyngitis (sore throat), although the strain that causes this problem is a different one, just recently recognized, called *Chlamydia pneumoniae* (Komaroff et al., 1989).

A different strain of *C. trachomatis* also causes an STD called lymphogranuloma venereum (LGV), which is rare in North America and Europe but common in South America, Africa, and Asia. LGV is about four times as common in males as in females. Like syphilis, this disease has three stages. The primary lesion is a small, hardly noticeable ulcer or pimple on the genitals that appears after an incubation period of 3 to 12 days and then heals rapidly. While this lesion is usually painless, if it occurs in the urethra it may cause pain or burning.

The secondary stage of LGV, which occurs several months after the primary lesion, is marked by painful swelling of lymph nodes in the groin (usually on one side of the body), with accompanying fever, chills, and generalized aching. While almost all males with LGV have such a reaction in the secondary stage, only 20 to 30 percent of females do. Another one-third of women have lower abdominal and back pain. In addition, both men and women may experience symptoms of rectal infection that include a mucuslike discharge, rectal bleeding, and abscess formation. While the great majority of people recover from LGV after the secondary stage, even if untreated, late complications of this STD are serious. They include genital elephantiasis (large swellings of the genitals) and severe scarring of the rectum, sometimes leading to partial bowel obstruction.

Transmission

Chlamydial infections (except for trachoma) are most commonly sexually transmitted. As a STD, chlamydial infections follow a pattern that is quite similar to that of gonorrhea, although with a lower degree of transmissibility. In one study, male sexual partners of women who had either gonorrhea or chlamydial cervicitis were found to have chlamydial infections less often than gonorrhea: 28 percent versus 81 percent (Lycke et al., 1980). In the same study, male partners of women who had dual infections of gonorrhea and chlamydia also got chlamydial infections much less often than they got gonorrhea (28 percent versus 77 percent).

Chlamydial infections can be transmitted by vaginal or anal intercourse and (less often) by oral–genital contact. Chlamydial infections, not surprisingly, are also most common in persons with multiple sex partners (Centers for Disease Control, 1985). As with gonorrhea, women seem more susceptible to chlamydial infections. About 70 percent of the female sex partners of men with documented chlamydial infections are found to be infected with chlamydia too, while 25 to 50 percent of the male sex partners of women with chlamydia have been found to be infected (Centers for Disease Control, 1985).

Symptoms

One of the difficult problems with chlamydial infections is that, much like gonorrhea, they often do not produce symptoms in infected females. According to some estimates, half of all women with chlamydial infections are symptom-free. A smaller number of men—estimated to be about 15 to 30 percent—do not have symptoms either, but since the long-term consequences for males are not as serious as for females, this is a far less serious medical problem.

In males, *C. trachomatis* most commonly causes symptoms of urethritis after one to three weeks' incubation. The two primary symptoms of urethritis are burning with urination and a whitish or clear urethral discharge. While these two symptoms typically occur together, either can occur without the other. In most cases, these symptoms are milder than in gonorrhea (Holmes et al., 1989).

Epididymitis in men under age 35 is presumed to be due to chlamydia unless proved otherwise and is marked by swelling, pain and tenderness in the scrotum (usually on one side only), and, often, fever. There may also be an associated urethritis. The pain of epididymitis can be so severe as to interfere with walking or running, but it also can be low grade, feeling more like an aching sensation than a searing pain. Epididymitis usually makes sexual activity quite unpleasant for the affected male partly because during sexual arousal the scrotum pulls up toward the body. Along with the vasocongestion in the testes, this creates pressure on the infected epididymis that is usually painful.

In females, chlamydial cervicitis does not generally produce symptoms. A cloudy mucous discharge from the cervix is sometimes seen but one study found this in only 37 percent of women who had *Chlamydia trachomatis* isolated from the cervix. In some cases there may be itchiness or mild discomfort in the genitals, but in most instances there are no symptoms, so the female has no way of knowing that she has an active chlamydial infection that requires treatment. The lack of symptoms is a problem because of the likelihood that the infection will move higher in the female reproductive tract, where it is apt to do more damage.

Females with chlamydial urethritis are in a similar situation. Only about one-third of these women develop pain, burning with urination, or frequent urination, and only a small percentage develop a urethral discharge or soreness at the opening of the urethra. Thus, few seek treatment. Although women with chlamydial endometritis may have intermittent vaginal bleeding, this occurs only in a minority; this type of chlamydial infection is also typically without any noticeable symptoms.

In contrast, chlamydial PID is more likely to be accompanied by symptoms, including the sudden onset of lower abdominal pain, vaginal bleeding, fever, and dyspareunia (painful intercourse). Another key symptom is that pressure on the lower abdomen during a pelvic exam is painful. However, as many as half of all cases of chlamydial PID may not have any symptoms, which is especially true for those cases that represent low-grade, smoldering infections that persist over time.

Chlamydial infection can occasionally spread from the Fallopian tubes to the surface of the liver (Stamm, 1988). This condition, called perihepatitis, is marked by pain in the right upper quadrant of the abdomen accompanied by nausea, vomiting, and fever. There may or may not be evidence of PID when this condition becomes symptomatic.

Diagnosis and Treatment

Because *Chlamydia trachomatis* grows only intracellularly (inside living cells), it is technically difficult and expensive to culture. In addition, because it usually takes at least three days to get the result of a culture for chlamydial infections, treatment is often started on the presumption that a chlamydial infection is present, a strategy that the U.S. Centers for Disease Control (1989) endorse. Nevertheless, a culture is the most accurate means of establishing the diagnosis.

To avoid these difficulties, several new types of antibody testing have recently become available. These tests, which can detect chlamydial infections in genital secretions with a fairly high degree of accuracy (Tam, 1984; Howard et al., 1986; Stamm, 1988), can generally be done within a few hours and are less expensive than cultures.

A number of antibiotics are very effective in treating chlamydial infections. Tetracycline or doxycycline is currently the drug of choice except in pregnant women (Centers for Disease Control, 1989). Erythromycin and sulfamethoxazole are alternative possibilities that are also highly effective. (Erythromycin is the drug of choice for pregnant women.)

It should be noted that penicillin is *not* effective against chlamydial infections. Because it is common to get chlamydial and gonorrheal infections at the same time, people are often treated for gonorrhea without realizing that they have a coexistent chlamydial infection—in part because gonorrhea has a shorter incubation time and in part because gonorrhea is easier to detect in the laboratory. This creates a situation in which the gonorrhea is cured by the penicillin, but the chlamydial infection is untouched. In some instances, this leads to a new flare-up of symptoms (chlamydial urethritis is common after gonorrhea in men), but if no symptoms occur or if they are ignored and go away spontaneously, the person remains infected and contagious to others and runs the risk of additional health complications.

It is particularly important that people who are diagnosed as having a chlamydial infection (or a suspected chlamydial infection) notify any partner with whom they had sex in the 30 days prior to the appearance of symptoms so that these individuals can be evaluated and treated (Centers for Disease Control, 1989).

CHANCROID

Chancroid is a sexually transmitted bacterial disease that until recently has been uncommon in the industrialized Western nations but is thought to be more common than syphilis on a world wide basis (Schmid et al., 1987). Caused by *Hemophilus ducreyi,* a short, compact, rod-shaped bacterium, this disease now affects an estimated 5000 to 10,000 people annually in America, a startling increase over the fewer than 1000 cases reported annually in the United States in the 1970s (Schmid et al., 1987; Leary, 1988).

Public health officials attribute the recent rise in chancroid and other previously infrequent STDs in the United States to increased prostitution tied to female drug use, as well as to the diversion of local STD personnel and funds to the fight against AIDS (Leary, 1988). Increased international travel may also play a role in this process.

Symptoms

The incubation period after exposure is short, usually between four and seven days. The hallmark lesion is a genital ulcer (sometimes called a "soft chancre," in distinction to the "hard chancre" of syphilis) that begins as a tender pimple surrounded by a reddened area. Over one to two days, it becomes filled with pus and breaks open into a sharply demarcated ulceration with ragged edges. Approximately half of those infected have more than one genital ulcer.

In males, the ulcers are most frequently on the foreskin, the frenulum, or the coronal ridge (the area separating the head of the penis from the shaft). Although the head or shaft of the penis can be affected, this is much less typical.

In females, the ulcers are usually at or near the entrance to the vagina. They may involve the labia, the clitoris, or the area just inside the vaginal opening, as well as the region between the vagina and the rectum. The cervix can also be affected, and lesions involving the breasts, the fingers, the thighs, and the mouth have also been encountered, although with far less frequency.

The other prominent clinical finding in chancroid is painful swelling of the lymph nodes on one side of the groin (the side that drains the infected region of the genitals). Although this occurs in only about half of chancroid patients, it is often a dramatic development, as the large swollen lymph nodes, called *buboes,* can rupture and exude a thick, creamy pus.

Chancroid does not appear to cause any major health complications beyond those mentioned above. *Hemophilus ducreyi* apparently does not cause disease in babies born to mothers with this infection at the time of delivery (Ronald and Albritton, 1984).

Diagnosis and Treatment

No blood test is available to diagnose chancroid, so the diagnosis is usually made on clinical grounds after a physical exam (Schmid et al., 1987).

The recommended treatment for chancroid is antibiotics—either erythromycin, taken in pill form for a week, or a single injection of ceftriaxone (Centers for Disease Control, 1989). Fortunately, these treatments are highly effective; if improvement doesn't occur promptly (within a week after therapy), it is important to consider whether the diagnosis was correct, whether the person may also be infected with another

STD—especially HIV—or whether the strain of *H. ducreyi* is antibiotic-resistant to the drug used.

Anyone who has had sexual contact with a chancroid-infected person within ten days preceding the onset of that person's infection or during the infection should be examined and treated whether there are symptoms or not (Centers for Disease Control, 1989).

GENITAL HERPES

The herpes family of viruses and the infections they cause, such as chickenpox, shingles, and cold sores, are widespread today, as they have been for thousands of years. First named by ancient Greek physicians from the word *herpein,* meaning "to creep," because of the appearance of their characteristic skin rashes, and described in some detail by Roman physicians of the first and second centuries A.D., herpes infections have recently been the subject of considerable public attention.

Genital herpes currently affects some 40 million Americans, with an additional 500,000 cases occurring annually. Viewed by some as a relatively minor skin infection with annoying but brief symptoms and by others as a life-threatening disease or even a heaven-sent directive against loose morals, the genital herpes epidemic of the 1980s had received almost as much media coverage as a presidential campaign by 1983, when it began to be outshadowed in the press by coverage of the AIDS epidemic.

Genital herpes is caused by two different but related forms of the herpes simplex virus, known as herpes virus type 1 and herpes virus type 2. In the past, herpes virus type 1 was almost exclusively a cause of cold sores and fever blisters, while genital herpes infections were almost invariably caused by the type 2 virus. Today, this distinction no longer holds true: in the United States, 10 to 20 percent of cases of genital herpes are now caused by the type 1 virus (Peter, Bryson, and Lovett, 1982), while in Japan 35 percent of first episodes are due to the type 1 virus (Corey et al., 1983). While some researchers have suggested that this crossover phenomenon may be a result of more frequent oral–genital sex in recent years than in the past, it is not clear that this explanation is correct.

A recently conducted national survey done on blood samples obtained in the late 1970s showed that 16.4 percent of the U.S. population 15 to 74 years of age was infected with herpes simplex virus type 2 (Johnson et al., 1989). The prevalence of herpes virus type 2 antibody increased from under 1 percent in the group under age 15 to 20 percent in the 30 to 44 age bracket and was significantly higher in blacks than in whites at all ages (see Figure 7–3).

Genital herpes is generally transmitted by sexual contact. Direct contact with infected genitals can cause transmission via sexual intercourse, rubbing the genitals together, oral–genital contact, anal intercourse, or oral–anal contact. In addition, normally protected areas of skin can become infected if there is a cut, rash, or sore, so that infections of the fingers, thighs, or other areas of the body are also possible.

The risk of developing genital herpes in a woman exposed to an infected, symptomatic man is estimated to be 80 to 90 percent (Straus et al., 1985). A man's risk of developing genital herpes from a single sexual encounter with an infected woman is estimated to be about 50 percent.

In some cases, genital herpes can be spread by less direct means. For example, transmission of the herpes simplex virus can occur by kissing alone, and if herpes of the mouth develops, it can then be spread by autoinoculation, that is, touching your genitals after putting your fingers in your mouth. Recently, several reports have noted that the herpes virus can live for at least several hours on toilet seats, plastic, and cloth, raising the possibility of genital herpes infection occurring by nonsexual transmission (Larson and Bryson, 1982; Turner et al., 1983; Nerurkar et al., 1983). It is unlikely, however, that this mode of transmission is very common. The herpes virus does not seem able to survive the chemical purifiers typically used in hot tubs (Nerurkar et al., 1983). Genital herpes infections can also be transmitted by artificial insemination (Moore et al., 1989), and one case report indicates that it can be transmitted by a hickey (a "love bite") as well (del Rosario, Blair, and Rickman, 1987).

Recent evidence has also shown that genital herpes can be transmitted by an asymptomatic sex partner—that is, a person who has no herpes blisters and no genital burning or itching (Rooney et al., 1986;

genital herpes (jen′ i tul her′ pēz) painful blisters of the genitals caused by infection with the herpes virus; outbreaks typically are recurrent and are highly contagious.

FIGURE 7–3

Prevalence of Herpes Simplex Virus, Type 2 Antibody in the United States in 1978, According to Age, Race, and Sex

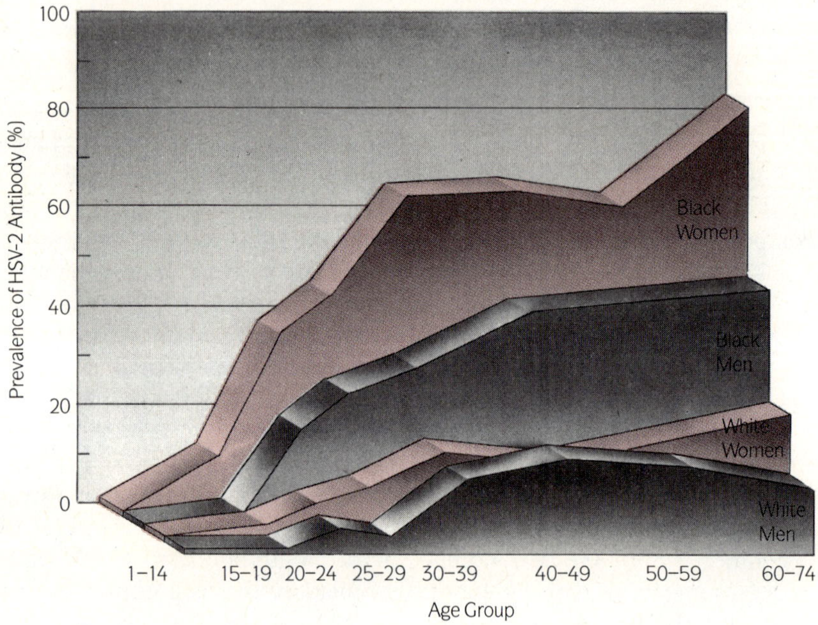

The tick marks on the x axis denote the midpoints of the age groups.

Source: From Robert Johnson, et al., NEW ENGLAND JOURNAL OF MEDICINE 321: 7–12, 1989, fig. 1, p. 10. Reprinted by permission of The New England Journal of Medicine.

Mertz et al., 1988; Brock et al., 1990). This finding is particularly troubling because it means that someone who doesn't realize that he or she is infected with the herpes simplex virus can inadvertently infect another person. While this mode of transmission is probably not too common, even if it occurs at only one-tenth the rate of symptomatic infection, asymptomatic transmission would occur in 1 out of 20 herpes victims.

The complexity of asymptomatic transmission is compounded further by the fact that someone may have large concentrations of herpes virus present in genital secretions on an episodic basis only, so that cultures of these fluids (semen, cervical mucus, vaginal secretions) that are negative for the herpes virus on one day may be positive a week later. One possibility is for persons with genital herpes to have cultures done on three occasions at least a week apart while they are totally asymptomatic: if all three cultures are negative, they can be fairly certain they won't infect a partner in their asymptomatic phase.

Symptoms

Genital herpes is marked by clusters of small, painful blisters on the genitals. After a few days, these blisters burst, leaving small ulcers in their place. In men, the blisters occur most commonly on the penis but they can also appear in the urethra or rectum. In women, blisters appear on the vaginal lips most often, but the cervix or anal area can also be affected.

The first episode of genital herpes is accompanied by fever, headache, and muscle soreness for two or more consecutive days in 39 percent of men and 68 percent of women (Corey et al., 1983). Almost all cases are marked by painful burning at the site of blister formation. Other relatively common symptoms include pain or burning during urination, discharge from the urethra or vagina, and tender, swollen lymph nodes in the groin, but these all tend to disappear within one to two weeks. More serious complications of first episodes, which occur more often in women than men, include the following: aseptic meningitis (an inflammation of the covering of the brain), estimated to occur in 8 percent of cases; eye infections, which occur in 1 percent of cases; and infection of the cervix in 88 percent of women with primary herpes type 2 infection (Peter, Bryson, and Lovett, 1982; Corey et al., 1983; Langston, 1983).

A typical first infection of genital herpes involves the appearance of 10 to 20 painful blisters on the genitals. If generalized symptoms such as fever or headache appear, they are usually most prominent within the first four days after the blisters occur, and then they diminish gradually over the first week of the infection. After the blisters burst, they may form larger reddish wet sores or ulcers, which usually heal in one or two weeks. Sores on the penis or on the mons become crusted before they heal, whereas those on the vaginal lips do not. Skin lesions last an average of 16.5 days in men and 19.7 days in women during first episodes of genital herpes (Corey et al., 1983), but if the sores become secondarily infected with bacteria, healing may be somewhat delayed.

Although the blisters disappear and the ulcers heal spontaneously within one to three weeks, the herpes simplex virus invades nerves in the pelvic region and continues to live in a dormant state near the base of the spinal cord. In about 10 percent of cases there are no further attacks, but many people have recurrent episodes of genital herpes varying in frequency from once a month to once every few years.[1] Repeat attacks are sometimes brought on by emotional stress, illness, sunburn, physical exhaustion, or extreme climates, or they may occur for no apparent reason (Glaser et al., 1985; Wyngaarden, 1988; Kemeny et al., 1989). Generally, these recurrences are less severe than the original episode because the body is able to mobilize appropriate antibodies to counteract the infecting virus. Fortunately, many who suffer from herpes find that repeat attacks tend to die out after a few years (Gillespie, 1982).

[1] If the first episode of genital herpes is caused by the type 1 virus, recurrences occur in only 55 percent of cases (Corey et al., 1983).

Recurrences are sometimes preceded by warning symptoms that occur up to 36 hours before blisters appear. These include itching or tingling sensations in or near the genitals, tenderness or aching in the groin area, and burning or pain with urination or defecation. While these symptoms are not invariably followed by active outbreaks, and while some repeat episodes of genital herpes are totally symptom-free, when such symptoms occur they deserve attention. First, they indicate the possibility that a person may be infectious *even before blisters appear.* This is possible because live herpes virus may be carried in semen or cervical or vaginal secretions even when no rashes or blisters can be seen. Second, it may be possible to prevent a flare-up of herpes by taking steps that reduce stress (e.g., getting more sleep, eating well, and avoiding substances like alcohol or drugs that might suppress the body's immunologic response system) (Gillespie, 1982; Langston, 1983).

Scientists are still puzzled by many aspects of genital herpes, and we do not understand clearly why some people never have recurrences while others have a number of repeat attacks. Certainly no one leads a completely stress-free life, nor can most people completely avoid the types of physical illnesses—like the flu—that often trigger recurrences. It is possible that there may be different strains of the herpes type 1 and 2 viruses which differ in their virulence, partly accounting for this variability, and the individual's resistance (as determined by the body's immunologic defenses) may play a role too. However, it would be a mistake to assume that people who experience recurrences of genital herpes aren't taking care of themselves properly or are being reinfected by another sexual partner, since such things usually aren't true. It is important to realize that even if no recurrences appear, a person is still infected with this virus on a life-long basis and can transmit it to a sex partner asymptomatically.

It now appears that the pattern of recurrence is strongly influenced by the type of the infecting herpes virus (Lafferty et al., 1987). Lesions affecting the mouth or lips are very common in type 1 infections but infrequent in those with type 2, while genital recurrences are six times more common than recurrences in the mouth in people infected with type 2.

One intriguing recent finding about genital herpes is that close to half of people who were previously thought to have an "asymptomatic" infection can actually be taught to recognize genital lesions that don't have the classical appearance of herpes blisters, such

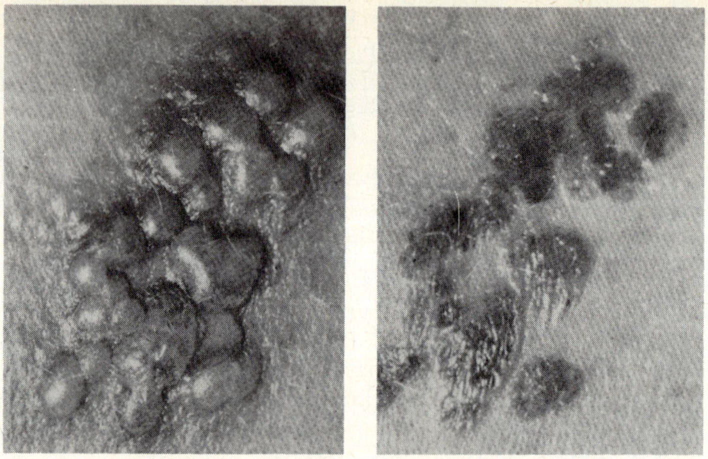

Genital herpes blisters before treatment (left) and after four days of treatment (right).

as mild external irritation or itching, or small cracks in the genital skin (Langenberg et al., 1989). Recognizing such lesions as herpes is important because it permits the person to avoid sexual contact during a time of increased transmissibility.

Genital herpes presents special problems. First, like syphilis, genital herpes in a pregnant woman can cause birth defects in the developing fetus since the virus can cross the placenta. Fortunately, this is a rare occurrence. Spontaneous abortion and premature labor were also thought to be common in pregnant women with genital herpes (Nahmias et al., 1971), but the validity of this finding has been questioned (Vontver et al., 1982). More worrisome is that the baby can be infected from the cervix or vagina during delivery, with such infections causing death or serious damage to the brain or eyes more than 50 percent of the time in those newborns who are infected (Binkin and Alexander, 1983). The rate of herpes infections in newborns has increased considerably in the last 15 years, probably mirroring the rising prevalence in the general population (Sullivan-Bolyai et al., 1983; Holmes et al., 1989). While the risk of infecting the baby may be as high as 50 percent with vaginal delivery during a first attack of genital herpes in the mother, the risk is estimated at about 5 percent during recurrent episodes (Corey et al., 1983; Prober et al., 1987). Compounding the difficulties of this situation is the fact that newborns may be infected even when the mother has no symptoms at the time of delivery. A recent study showed that cultures taken in the four weeks before delivery do not show accurately whether the infant will be exposed to the herpes simplex virus at delivery (Arvin et al., 1986). For this reason, cesarean section is often recommended to pregnant women with active genital herpes (Prober et al., 1988), but this is an individual matter that each woman should discuss with her physician. In addition, infection can occur after birth if the mother or father has oral lesions or if the virus is transmitted in breast milk.

The second serious issue regarding complications of genital herpes is that there appears to be an association between the herpes simplex type 2 virus and both cervical cancer (McDougall et al., 1980; Kessler, 1979; Graham et al., 1982) and cancer of the vulva (Schwartz et al., 1981). While only some women who have genital herpes will be so affected, because these forms of cancer are easily treated if detected early, it is advisable for all women who have had genital herpes to have a Pap smear and pelvic exam every six months.

The third source of concern is that a number of recent reports suggest genital herpes may make people more vulnerable to infection with HIV, the human immunodeficiency virus that causes AIDS (Cannon et al., 1988; Holmberg et al., 1988; Stamm et al., 1988). Current thinking holds that the genital ulcerations caused by herpes may provide HIV with an easy mode of access into the body, whereas intact genital skin surfaces may be less susceptible to attack by this virus.

The Emotional Impact of Herpes

Just as the physical severity of genital herpes varies greatly from person to person, the emotional response to the discovery of herpes varies considerably too. Most victims first experience a sense of shock, anger, and disbelief: "It can't really be happening to *me*." Their initial anger is usually (and understandably) directed at the partner who caused the infection, but it can be self-directed as well. One man told us, "I suppose this is the price I have to pay for not being more careful about who I slept with."

Not surprisingly, herpes sometimes causes conflict and suspicion in marriages or other long-term relationships. If one partner infects the other, it is taken as a sign of sexual infidelity, but this is not always true; for instance, a person may have reactivation of herpes that has been dormant for years and that preceded the relationship. Nevertheless, the discovery of herpes in a relationship can lead to so much discord and strife that the partners become combatants rather than lovers.

> *A 28-year-old woman:* When I found out I had herpes, I was scared out of my wits. I knew my husband would be outraged, but I also knew that trying to hide it was hopeless. So I told him about it, hoping that he'd understand that what was done was done. I wasn't really prepared for what happened, though. He suddenly refused to come near me. He questioned me in minute detail about everywhere I went. He was jealous and angry and rejecting, and it led us to a painful divorce. *(Authors' files)*

As might be expected, genital herpes is at least as emotionally troublesome to single people. In fact, since many single heterosexuals seem to think they have little risk of being exposed to HIV infection, it is not uncommon to find college students and other young adults who worry more about genital herpes than about AIDS. Here are some typical comments we've heard in interviews: "I couldn't stand the thought of having this infection for the rest of my life—having casual sex may be fun, but it's just not worth it." "To me, it's like playing Russian roulette, only it's my peace of mind at stake." "How could I ever find a husband if I had herpes? I'd have to marry someone else who had it too."

Some herpes sufferers have turned to dating services that provide a means of meeting others with this STD. Others feel such profound shame and depression over their affliction that they withdraw from the social scene completely. Those who continue to date face a difficult dilemma: whether and when to tell a date that they have herpes. Some people feel a moral obligation toward candor but are dismayed by how quickly their honesty scares off potential mates. (Not everyone shares this reaction, though. One woman told us: "At least I knew if they were interested in *me* if they stayed around.") Others unfortunately feel it's all right to deceive their partners, perhaps deciding to make up excuses for abstinence whenever an outbreak occurs (which will *not* always prevent transmission) or convincing themselves that there is so much herpes around that it just doesn't matter.

Cavalier attitudes about giving genital herpes to another person may be on the way out, however, in part for economic reasons. In the past few years, hundreds of civil lawsuits have successfully been brought by people whose sex partners infected them with this disease, with verdicts sometimes reaching the million dollar mark. (This type of lawsuit would not be permitted in many states where nonmarital sex is considered a felony, since personal injuries sustained while participating in a criminal act are not considered to be grounds for suing. In addition, if the person with herpes disclosed this fact to his or her partner before they had sexual contact, there would be no legal basis for a lawsuit, since the previously uninfected person would be deemed to have consented to the risk of contracting herpes.)

Those who find themselves in the throes of emotional anguish over having genital herpes—and even well-adjusted, psychologically stable people can find themselves in this position—can often obtain assistance from support groups composed of people with the same disease. Organizations such as HELP (Herpetics Engaged in Living Productively), initiated by the National Herpes Resource Center of the American Social Health Association, which has chapters in over 40 cities nationwide, provide valuable information and perspective (as well as many practical pointers) for people with herpes. In a few cases, particularly if sexual problems develop as a result of herpes or if guilt or depression becomes overwhelming, psychotherapy may be helpful. Most people, however, once past the initial anger and shock at discovering they have herpes, manage to adjust fairly easily to the disease and find that it rarely interferes with their lives. Unfortunately, media discussions of genital herpes have often presented such distorted or alarming "facts" about this disease that they have frightened many people rather than reassured or enlightened them.

Diagnosis and Treatment

The diagnosis of an active infection generally can be made with accuracy by a physician on the basis of a physical examination of the genital blisters and/or ulcers. However, other STDs can mimic genital herpes, and sometimes genital blisters or ulcers are a result of inflammation rather than infection. Thus, making a proper diagnosis is not always a simple matter. Various laboratory tests can establish the diagnosis with more certainty. These include (in increasing order of accuracy) (1) Pap smears in women, (2) blood tests to measure antibodies against herpes viruses, and (3) cultures to grow the virus in the laboratory (these are usually taken by touching a cotton swab to a blister or ulcer; the procedure is generally painless).

There is no known cure for genital herpes, although much research is being done. A new drug called acyclovir is of some usefulness in lessening the severity of symptoms, especially in first attacks. When taken by mouth within five or six days after the onset of symptoms in a first episode of genital herpes, acyclovir reduced the period of viral shedding (virus being present in body fluids such as semen or vaginal secretions) by two-thirds compared with treatment with a placebo (Bryson et al., 1983; Mertz et al., 1984). In these same studies, acyclovir shortened the healing time of genital herpes lesions by four to nine days. In addition, taken on a long-term, continuous basis, oral acyclovir seems to cut down the number and duration of recurrences: in fact, in several studies, the rate of recurrence was lowered by at least 75 percent (Douglas et al., 1984; Mindel et al., 1984; Straus et al., 1984). During genital herpes *recurrences,* however, acyclovir doesn't seem to work as well in reducing pain or viral shedding (Straus et al., 1985).

Since its safety hasn't been studied extensively in persons using this drug for more than six months, no one is certain at this time what side effects may result from long-term use of acyclovir. However, preliminary indications are that acyclovir is safe and effective for up to four years of use (Mertz et al., 1988a; Straus et al., 1988). Because there is also concern that extensive use of acyclovir will lead to the emergence of new strains of herpes simplex virus that are resistant to it (Hirsch and Schooley, 1989; Erlich et al., 1989), only people whose recurrences are particularly frequent or troublesome should consider using acyclovir on a long-term basis for suppressive therapy (Straus et al., 1985). Other antiviral medications are also being studied for treating genital herpes, and a concerted effort is being made to develop a vaccine that would prevent this infection in the first place.

General measures such as taking aspirin (or an aspirin substitute) and using cold, wet compresses to relieve pain are often helpful during an initial herpes episode or recurrent flare-ups. In addition, avoiding tight underwear or clothing can reduce irritation, and keeping the genitals clean and dry by washing with warm water and soap several times a day can also be beneficial. The skin should be dried with clean towels and a patting, rather than vigorous rubbing motion, and hand-to-eye contact should be avoided after touching the genitals. Towels and washcloths should be kept separately, since they may be contagious to others. In fact, it's wisest to use a separate towel for the face to avoid inadvertent spread of the virus from the genital region to the eyes.

Sexual contact should be completely avoided from the time symptoms of genital herpes first begin until ten days after healing is complete (for a first attack) or until two days after complete healing in recurrent episodes. Unfortunately, a few people seem to shed virus all the time—whether or not they have visible skin lesions or symptoms—so it's impossible to guarantee that there is no risk of contagion. While use of a condom can help prevent transmission of genital herpes, it is not a foolproof method (both because it doesn't cover all lesions and because it isn't always worn from the start of genital contact) and it may actually irritate the condition.

VIRAL HEPATITIS

Viral hepatitis is an infection of the liver that can vary in severity from a completely symptomless state to mild gastrointestinal symptoms (poor appetite, indigestion, diarrhea) to an acute debilitating illness with fever, jaundice (yellowish appearance of the skin), vomiting, abdominal pain, and—occasionally—more serious medical complications, including death. There are four main types of viral hepatitis: hepatitis A, hepatitis B, hepatitis C, and delta (type D) hepatitis. All four types can be sexually transmitted.

Transmission

HEPATITIS A

Hepatitis A (formerly known as infectious hepatitis) has an incubation period of 15 to 45 days. The hepatitis A virus is mainly spread by the fecal–oral route, with person-to-person transmission, food-borne epidemics (usually caused by infected food handlers), and the consumption of raw or poorly cooked shellfish from contaminated waters accounting for most cases in industrialized nations. Previous data have shown that homosexual males have a higher incidence of

Sexually Transmitted Diseases

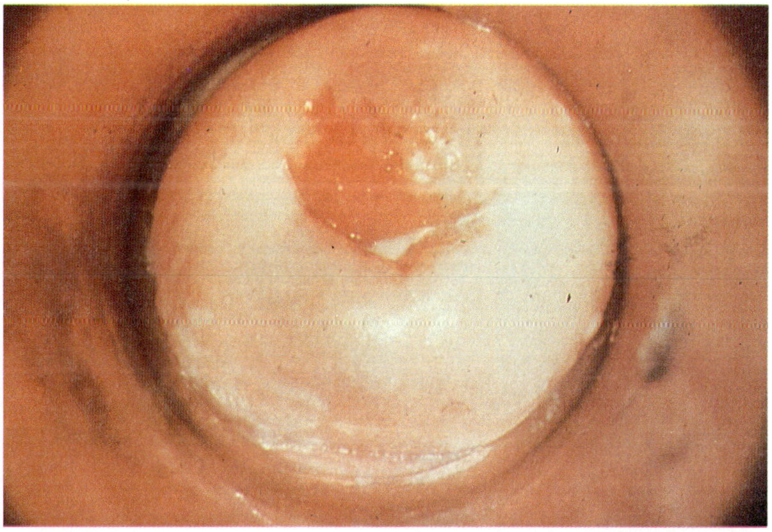

1

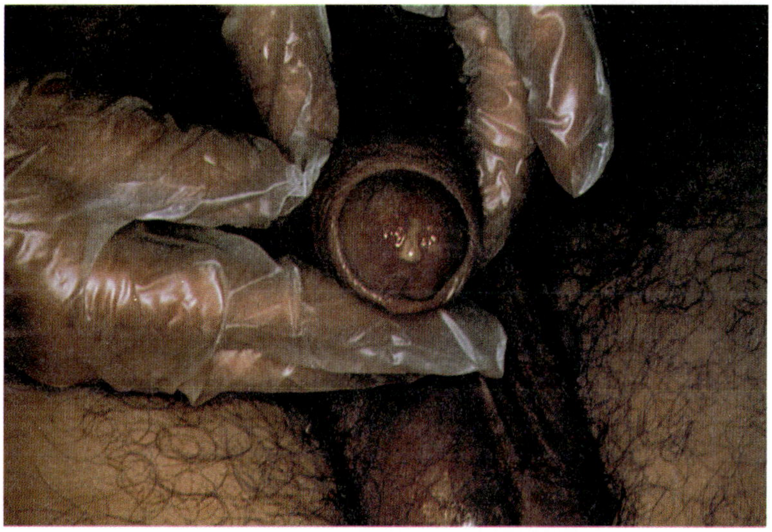

2

1 Gonorrhea causing cervicitis in the female.

2 Gonorrhea discharge from the penis.

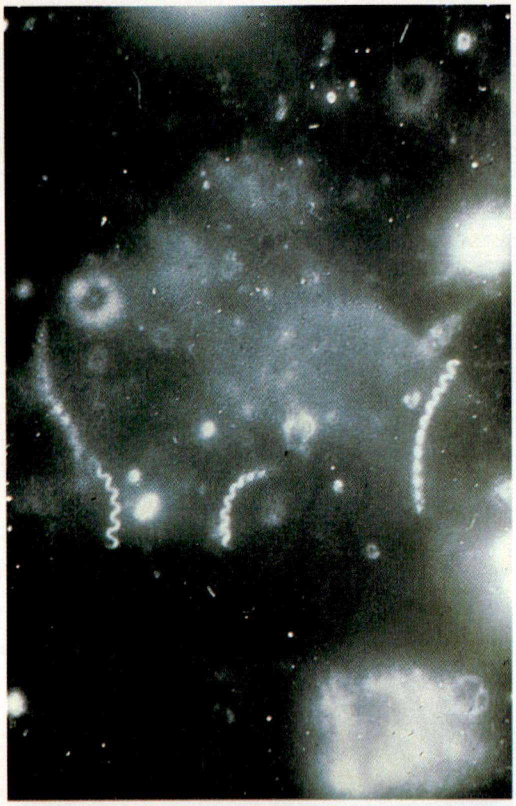

3

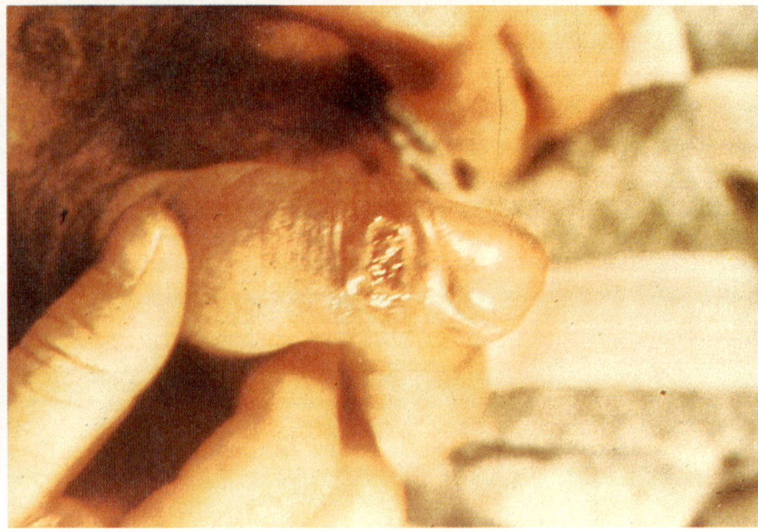

4

3 *The spiral-shaped* Treponema pallidum *is the microorganism that causes syphilis.*
4 *A typical chancre of the penis, the hallmark of primary stage syphilis.*
5 *Secondary syphilis in a female. One of the principal physical signs is a rash.*
6 *Photomicrograph of* Chlamydia trachomatis.

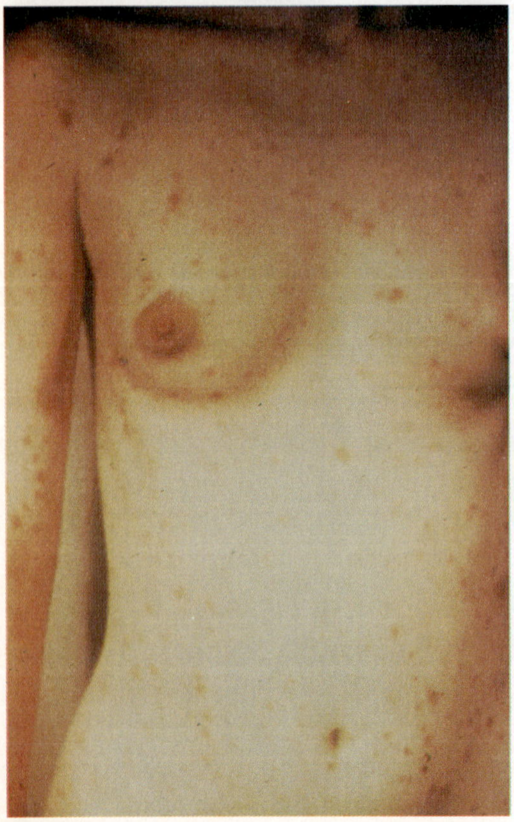

5

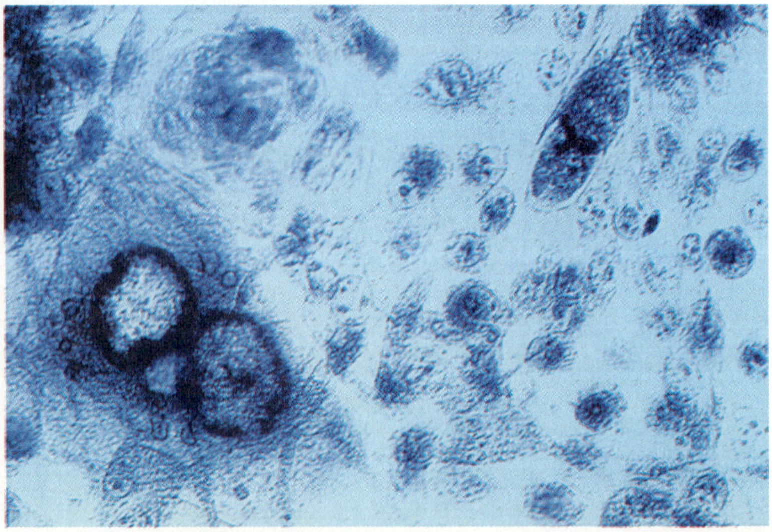

6

7
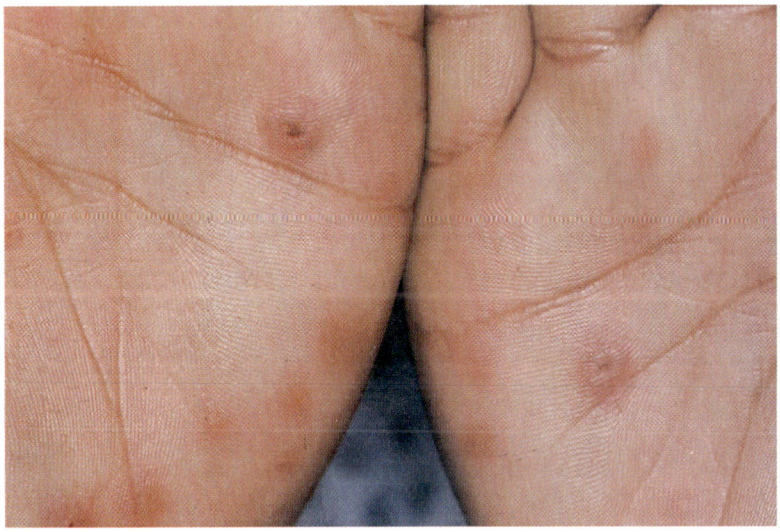

8
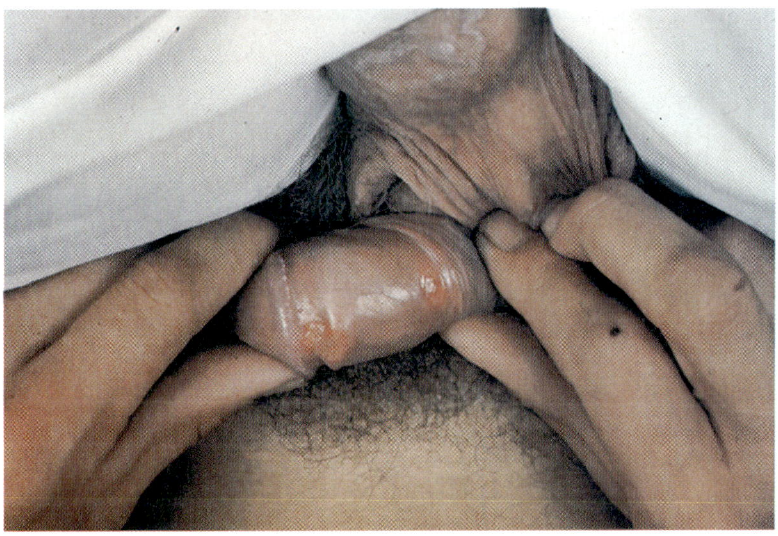

7 Typical rash on the palms in secondary syphilis.
8 Chancroid in the male.

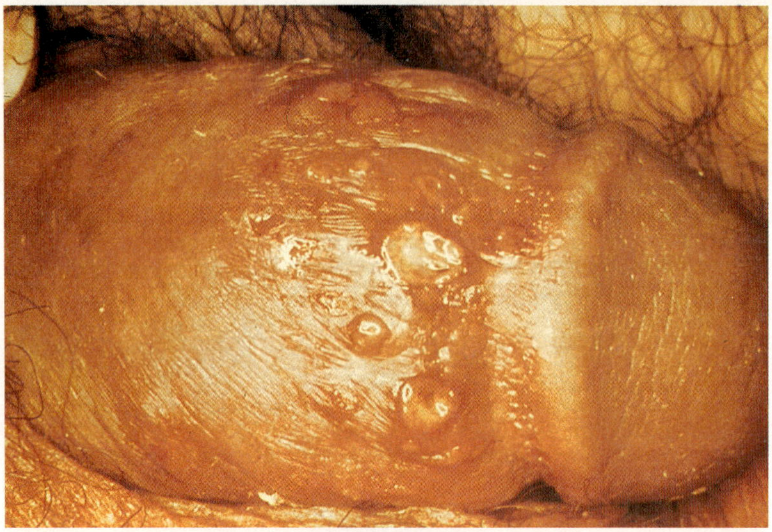

9

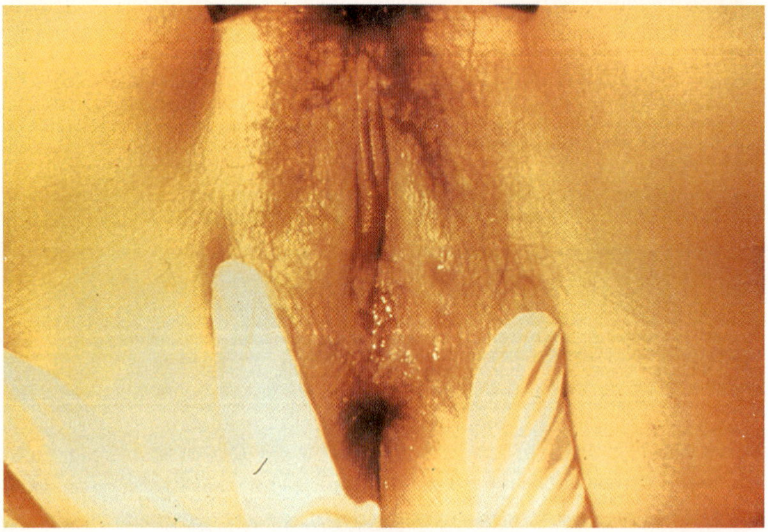

10

9 Genital herpes in the male. Characteristically, the lesions are clustered and of various sizes.
10 External genital herpes in the female. Note the involvement in the perineal region, extending toward the rectum.

hepatitis A than heterosexuals (Corey and Holmes, 1980; Fawaz and Matloff, 1981). It appears that oral–anal contact is the primary explanation for this finding, so that at least within the homosexual population hepatitis A may sometimes be sexually transmitted. (Oral–anal contact by heterosexual partners also can transmit this infection, but this is relatively uncommon.)

HEPATITIS B

Hepatitis B, previously called serum hepatitis, is usually spread by blood or blood products but it can also be transmitted by saliva, seminal fluid, vaginal secretions, and other biologic fluids (Zuckerman, 1982). Many of the approximately 200,000 annual cases of hepatitis B in the United States are sexually transmitted (Brandt, 1982; Alter et al., 1989), and evidence suggests that homosexual men have the highest rates of previous or current infection with this disorder (Reiner et al., 1982; Schreeded et al., 1982; Holmes et al., 1989). However, it is noteworthy that the proportion of hepatitis B cases accounted for by homosexual activity decreased by 62 percent between 1981 and 1988 (Alter et al., 1990). It is thought that trauma to the rectal mucosa from anal intercourse, manual stimulation of the rectum, or frequent use of enemas may predispose to the spread of this infection.

Studies of the prevalence of hepatitis B infection among various groups show that overall prevalence in homosexual males is 40 to 60 percent, whereas in heterosexual males it ranges from 4 to 18 percent (Alter et al., 1986). In this same report, it was found among heterosexual university students that students with three or more sexual partners in the four months before the study were much more likely to have been infected with hepatitis B virus than students with fewer than three partners in this same time period (14 percent versus 1.5 percent, respectively). Dan (1986) suggests that this result might mean that persons whose life-style exposes them to numerous sex partners are actually exposed to a pool of people with much higher rates of hepatitis B infection than are the group of people with few sex partners. If this view is correct, it means that a person having many sex partners has a risk of infection that is not just numerically proportional to the number of partners but is actually considerably higher since each of the partners is "riskier" from a health viewpoint—that is, more likely to be infected with the hepatitis B virus and thus more likely to be a carrier. More recently, data from a controlled study confirmed that heterosexuals with hepatitis B were more likely to have multiple sex partners than heterosexual control subjects (Alter et al., 1989).

Hepatitis B persists in an asymptomatic carrier state in approximately 5 to 10 percent of infected adults, with an estimated 400,000 to 800,000 carriers in the United States and 150 to 200 million worldwide. This condition, in which the person is still infectious although not generally ill, can persist for months, years, or a lifetime. Carriers of hepatitis B have an increased risk of developing liver cancer in their lifetime.

HEPATITIS C

Recently, scientists have finally succeeded in identifying the hepatitis C virus, solving a mystery of what caused the type of hepatitis previously called "non-A, non-B" (Alter and Sampliner, 1989; Davis et al., 1989; Di Bisceglie et al., 1989; Kuo et al., 1989). Currently, the CDC estimates that there are 150,000 cases of hepatitis C annually in the United States, with fewer than one-tenth resulting from transfusions (Alter and Sampliner, 1989). One percent of volunteer blood donors have been found to be carriers of antibody to the hepatitis C virus (Stevens et al., 1990). Furthermore, in contrast to earlier thinking on this topic, it has now been shown that heterosexual transmission plays a significant role in the spread of this form of hepatitis (Alter et al., 1989). IV drug use is another significant mode of transmission.

Hepatitis C currently accounts for more than 90 percent of the cases of hepatitis that develop after blood transfusions and is particularly devastating because at least half of those infected with it acutely eventually develop chronic hepatitis, which commonly leads to cirrhosis or cancer of the liver (Alter and Sampliner, 1989; Davis et al., 1989).

HEPATITIS D

Delta hepatitis, also called type D hepatitis, is an unusual infection in the United States that was first discovered in the late 1970s. The hepatitis D virus requires the presence of the hepatitis B virus to multiply (Hoofnagle, 1989). In a sense, it "piggybacks" onto the hepatitis B virus, either at the same time acute hepatitis B infection occurs, or later on when it infects a chronic hepatitis B carrier. In both situations,

viral hepatitis infection of the liver by a virus causing a debilitating acute illness and sometimes a chronic condition.

it is often a very severe infection, with high death rates and serious permanent liver damage in many of those who survive. Unlike other forms of hepatitis, it is most likely to occur in prolonged, severe outbreaks in isolated communities. It is especially common in the Mediterranean and the Middle East, but rare in northern Europe, the Western hemisphere, China, and southeast Asia.

Diagnosis and Treatment

Hepatitis is diagnosed on the basis of laboratory tests (e.g., blood tests that show abnormalities in liver enzymes), and the specific type of hepatitis is determined by immunologic testing of blood samples. Treatment is generally symptomatic, with hospitalization required only in the more severe cases. In 1989, a major breakthrough occurred in treating hepatitis C, with the discovery that the drug alpha interferon can often prevent the hepatitis C virus from destroying liver cells, although relapses are common when the drug is stopped (Davis et al., 1989; Di Bisceglie et al., 1989).

Persons in intimate contact with someone with hepatitis A can obtain partial immunity by getting a shot of immune serum globulin, but as a practical matter they have often been exposed for weeks before the diagnosis has been made. Viral hepatitis B vaccines are now available that are safe and effective (Hadler et al., 1986). It is currently recommended that anyone who is at high risk of acquiring hepatitis B, such as male homosexuals or bisexuals, heterosexuals with multiple sex partners, people who inject illicit drugs, all health care workers, and family members of hepatitis B carriers, be vaccinated (Hoffnagle, 1989a). There is no vaccine available for hepatitis C. Since hepatitis D depends on prior or simultaneous infection with the hepatitis B virus, it can effectively be prevented by the hepatitis B vaccine.

GENITAL WARTS

Genital warts (condylomata accuminata) are dry, usually painless warts that grow on or near the genitals and around the anus. According to one recent government estimate, there are 12 million cases of genital warts in America today, with 750,000 new cases annually (Goldsmith, 1989). They are caused by a sexually transmitted virus called the human papilloma virus (HPV) and are usually pink or grayish-white with a cauliflower-like appearance.

When epithelial cells (cells that line the outer or inner surface of the body) are infected by HPV, they undergo a transformation in which they divide continuously (Marx, 1989a), causing a buildup of abnormal tissue that eventually becomes a wart.

Although genital warts were once thought to be more of a cosmetic nuisance than a health problem, it is now clear that the virus that causes them is an important long-term cause of cancer of the cervix and other cancers of the anal and genital region, including cancer of the penis (Rando, 1988; Marx, 1989a; Reeves et al., 1989). For instance, in one large case–control study in Latin America, cervical infection with HPV types 16 or 18 was more than twice as common in cervical cancer cases as in controls (Reeves et al.,

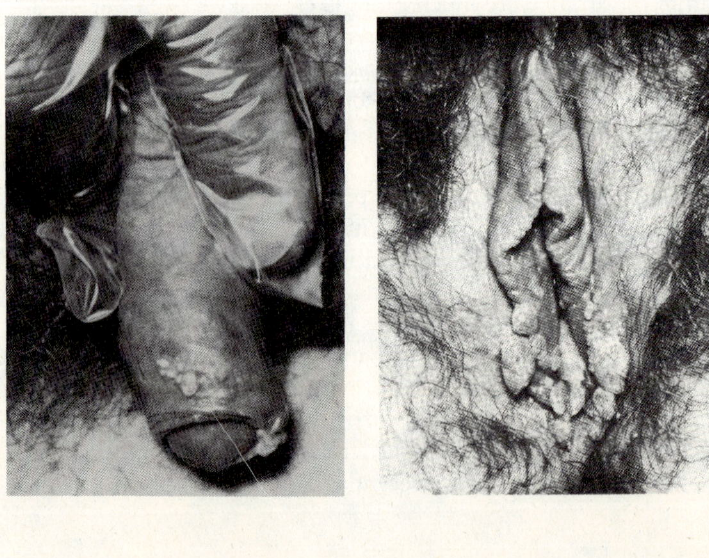

Genital warts in the male (left) and female (right).

1989). While no one believes that it is the papilloma virus alone that causes such cancers, scientists are now developing theories to explain what role these fairly common viruses may play in producing malignancies and why only some infected persons develop these cancers.

HPV was found in 29 percent of pregnant women in one study (Gissman and Schwarz, 1986); in the Latin American survey cited above, 32 percent of women in the control group had cervical infection with HPV (Reeves et al., 1989). Male sexual partners of women with HPV infection are commonly infected too; in one survey, almost three-quarters of the males were found to have HPV in genital lesions (Kennedy, 1988). In addition, since genital warts commonly coexist with other STDs, anyone with such growths should undergo thorough medical evaluation to check for the possibility of an asymptomatic case of gonorrhea, chlamydial infection, or syphilis. It is currently thought that genital warts are most likely to occur in adolescents or young adults—precisely the same age range as gonorrhea.

Symptoms

Although genital warts are, as the name implies, most often found on (or inside) the genitals, they can also be found in other locations, including the mouth, the eyelid, the lip, the nipple, and around the anus. (Genital warts, or condylomata accuminata, are not the same as ordinary skin warts, which occur on most parts of the body.)

In males, genital warts can involve any part of the penis. Common locations include just inside the opening of the urethra (where they are apt to have a bright red appearance), on the frenulum, on the head of the penis or the coronal ridge, and on the inner surface of the foreskin, as well as along the penile shaft. The appearance of the warts can range in size from tiny, solitary dotlike growths to large, irregular, rough-surfaced masses that protrude from the penis by a half-inch or more.

In females, genital warts commonly involve the labia, the opening to the vagina, the inner third of the vagina, and the cervix. In some cases, they appear as relatively isolated patches of greyish-pink tissue tags, while in other instances, the pattern of growth is distressing because extensive wart formation virtually covers the external genitals. (Rarely, genital warts can become so large as to block the birth canal at the time of labor, requiring a cesarean delivery.) As with males, genital warts in females may grow just inside the urethra.

While the primary problem with genital warts for most people is the embarrassment they cause, if they become large they may also create some mechanical discomfort (particularly during sex). In addition, large genital warts are also more likely to become secondarily infected or to become ulcerated (often because of the rubbing of underwear against them). Infrequently, genital warts may be a source of bleeding, particularly if they are quite large.

Diagnosis and Treatment

The diagnosis of genital warts is usually obvious to a medically trained examiner. Because similar lesions can be found during secondary syphilis (these are called condylomata lata), a blood test to detect syphilis is, as we mentioned above, always in order when warts appear on the genitals. Currently, tests to detect the specific type of DNA that the HPV possesses are being performed in many centers, but it is not clear what practical influence this will have on treatment decisions at present.

According to the CDC, no therapy has been shown to actually eradicate HPV (Centers for Disease Control, 1989). Thus, the goal of treatment is simply to remove visible or symptomatic warts. The available treatments include: (1) use of a liquid containing podophyllin, a caustic chemical that erodes the warts when applied repeatedly for short periods of time (this must be done by a qualified health-care professional, not self-administered, and it should not be used for pregnant women); (2) use of tricholacetic acid applied to the warts on a weekly basis; (3) use of carbon dioxide laser surgery to burn away the warts painlessly; (4) use of liquid nitrogen to freeze the warts, which usually destroys them in one or two visits; (5) use of a drug called interferon injected into the base of the warts. Unfortunately, recurrences of the warts can occur after any of these treatment methods and none of them eradicates the underlying HPV infection, which remains in tissues next to a wart that has been chemically or surgically destroyed.

Anyone with genital warts should use condoms during sexual activity with a partner to cut down the risk of transmitting HPV. (For safety's sake, this is

genital warts dry, painless warts on or near the genitals or anus that are caused by a sexually transmitted virus. Sometimes referred to as venereal warts.

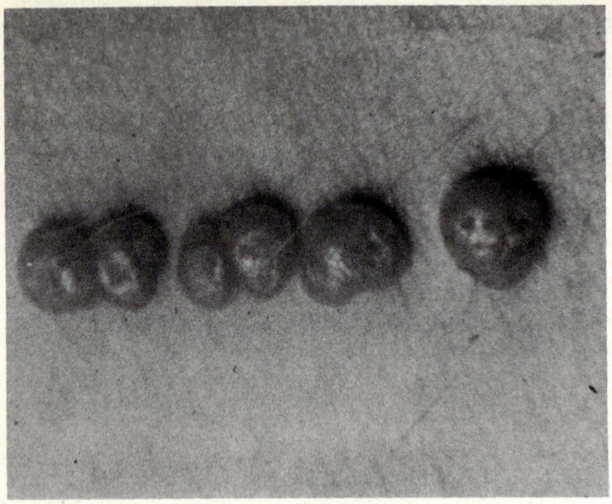

Molluscum contagiosum on the buttocks.

advisable permanently—not just when genital warts are visible.) In addition, if your partner has been exposed, it is wise to have that person get a medical checkup to see if he or she requires treatment.

MOLLUSCUM CONTAGIOSUM

Molluscum contagiosum is caused by a pox virus that typically produces raised lesions on the external genitals or on the thighs, buttocks, or lower abdomen. The painless lesions, which usually appear three to six weeks after exposure, vary from one millimeter to one centimeter in diameter and have a pinkish-orange color with a pearly top. If the lesion is squeezed, the cheesy plug of material within it can be expressed, much like a blackhead. Since the infection usually causes little trouble and often disappears spontaneously in about six months, treatment is not always necessary. Local applications of liquid nitrogen or frozen carbon dioxide have been used to remove the skin lesions.

PUBIC LICE

Pubic lice, or "crabs," are parasites that invade the pubic region (Figure 7–4). Although crabs are usually transmitted by sexual contact, they may also be inadvertently picked up from sheets, towels, or clothing used by an infested person. The lice attach themselves to pubic hair and require fresh blood at least twice a day to survive. Eggs laid by female lice are cemented onto the pubic hairs and cannot be washed off.

The crab louse (known officially as *Phthirus pubis* and called "papillon d'amour," or "butterfly of love," by the French) causes intense itching, which is mainly felt at night. A few people have no real symptoms; others develop an allergic rash that can be infected by bacteria after a lot of scratching. The lice can be killed by gamma benzene hexachloride, marketed in cream, lotion, or shampoo form under the trade name Kwell. Another highly effective treatment is a lotion called malathion (marketed under the trade name Prioderm). Neither of these drugs should be applied to the eyebrows or eyelashes, even if these areas are infested. Instead, infestations in these areas can usually be controlled by applying Vaseline or a similar petroleum jelly product twice a day for seven to ten days to suffocate the lice and their eggs. It is a myth that using brown soap to wash or that applying kerosene to the skin are the best ways to treat lice.

Although pubic lice can survive for only 24 hours once they leave the human body, eggs that fall off into sheets or onto clothing can survive for six days. For this reason, fresh bedding and clean clothing should always be used to avoid reinfestation.

FIGURE 7–4

The Crab Louse

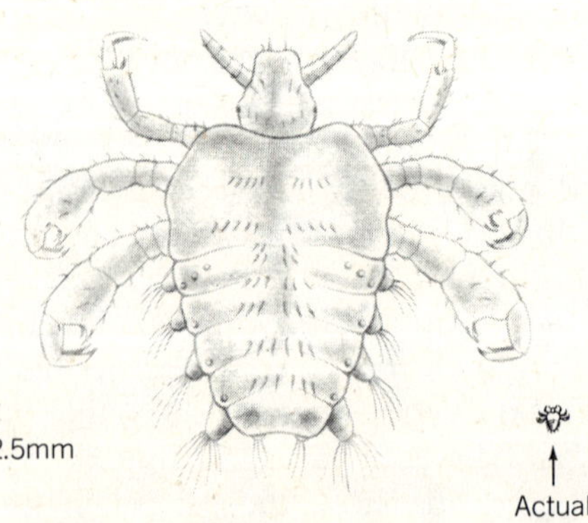

The crab louse can be transmitted by sexual or nonsexual contact and typically causes intense itching in the pubic region at night.

VAGINAL INFECTIONS

Vaginitis

Vaginitis refers to any vaginal inflammation, whether caused by infection, allergic reaction, estrogen deficiency, or chemical irritation. It is helpful to realize that while vaginitis frequently is transmitted sexually, probably 30 percent of cases arise from nonsexual causes. Vaginitis can create sexual problems by causing tenderness or pain during intercourse or by causing disagreeable odors that embarrass the woman or reduce her partner's enthusiasm for intimacy. Here we consider only the most common forms of vaginal infection.

TRICHOMONAS INFECTIONS

Trichomonas vaginitis is caused by a one-cell microorganism called *Trichomonas vaginalis,* ordinarily present in small numbers in the vagina (Holmes et al., 1989). If these organisms multiply rapidly or are transmitted by sexual contact, the resulting infection produces a frothy, thin, greenish-white or yellowish-brown, foul-smelling discharge that usually causes burning and itching of the vagina and vulva. The diagnosis is made by examining the discharge under a microscope or by cultures. The most effective treatment is a prescription drug called Flagyl (metronidazole), which should be given to the woman and her male sexual partner. Flagyl should not be used by nursing mothers because it appears in breast milk, and there is currently some concern about its safety because it has been found to produce tumors in mice.

MONILIA INFECTIONS

Monilial vaginitis is a type of fungus or yeast infection caused by an overgrowth of *Candida albicans,* a microorganism normally found in the vagina. The discharge is usually thick, white, and cheesy and is accompanied by intense itching. Diabetic women, pregnant women, and women using birth control pills or antibiotics have an increased incidence of this infection, as do women with HIV infection. Treatment involves use of special vaginal creams or suppositories, such as Monistat (miconazole) or Lotrimin or Mycelex (two different brands of clotrimazole) for one or two weeks. [Please note that Mycostatin (nystatin) is no longer recommended by the CDC because it is less effective than the drugs mentioned above (Centers for Disease Control, 1989).]

Because yeast infections can mask the presence of gonorrhea or syphilis, specific testing should be done to see if any STDs are also present. In two studies of women with STDs, more than 25 percent were found to have genital yeast infections (Oriel et al., 1972; Thin, Leighton, and Dixon, 1977)

Treatment of sex partners is not necessary with monilia infections, since the disease isn't usually transmitted sexually to begin with.

PREVENTING VAGINITIS

The vagina normally contains a number of different microorganisms. Some of these seem to play a specific role in vaginal physiology, such as maintaining the proper degree of acidity, while others can produce symptoms and infection if they multiply disproportionately. According to a review by Larsen and Galask (1982), an average of seven different species of bacteria are found in the vagina, and other microorganisms such as yeasts and viruses are also present.

Why some women develop vaginal pain or itching without having any detectable infection is unclear (Osborne, Grubin, and Pratson, 1982). It is also uncertain why many women with documented infections don't have any discharge or other symptoms. However, the fact remains that vaginitis is often an annoying condition that women and their sex partners would like to prevent if they can. Here are several suggestions for minimizing the risk of developing vaginitis:

1. Wear cotton underpants; nylon or synthetic fiber underpants or pantyhose retain heat and moisture, creating a good environment for bacteria to grow.

molluscum contagiosum a skin disease caused by a pox virus; the skin breaks out in small, bumpy lesions with a pearly top.

pubic lice parasites that invade the pubic region, often transmitted during sexual intercourse.

vaginitis (vaj in ī′ tis) vaginal inflammation from infection or chemical irritation.

trichomonas vaginitis (trick o mōn′ ess) an infection of the vagina caused by bacteria called trichomonas vaginalis. Accompanied by a frothy, thin, greenish or yellowish gray, foul-smelling discharge and burning and itching.

monilial vaginitis (mon il′ ee all vaj in eye′ tis) infection of the vagina caused by a fungus; usually accompanied by a thick, cheesy discharge with intense itching.

2. Avoid frequent douching, since this can irritate the vagina and remove important "natural" microorganisms that protect you. (Many medical authorities believe that routine douching is unnecessary and advise it only under specific conditions.)
3. After going to the bathroom, always wipe with a front-to-back motion. This way, bacteria from the rectum will not be brought forward to the vagina.
4. Avoid the long-term use of antibiotics, which can reduce the number of bacteria normally present in the vagina, allowing yeast forms to overgrow.
5. Maintain good habits of personal hygiene, including regular washing of the genital and anal regions with mild soap and water. Avoid so-called feminine hygiene sprays, which can be irritating to the skin.
6. If your partner has an infection of the genitals, avoid sexual contact. (Using a condom may be of some help in this situation.)
7. Do not put the penis in or near the vagina after anal intercourse since this can directly introduce "foreign" bacteria into the vagina.
8. Avoid forms of sexual activity that produce any vaginal discomfort.

Bacterial Vaginosis

Bacterial vaginosis is a vaginal infection that was previously known as nonspecific vaginitis or hemophilus vaginitis. The term "vaginosis" has been used in preference to vaginitis to indicate that signs of inflammation (such as redness and tenderness) are not usually present with this condition (usually in medicine, the suffix "itis" indicates inflammation). In addition, the bacterial organism *Hemophilus vaginalis,* since renamed *Gardnerella vaginalis,* is now known to be only one of several bacteria that accounts for this disorder, although it can be cultured from the vagina in about 95 percent of cases (Sobel, 1989). The primary problem seems to be one in which the normal "protective" bacterial organisms in the vagina decrease drastically in number while the infecting bacteria overgrow. The result of the overgrowth is a grayish-white discharge that usually has a foul "fishy" odor and is accompanied by burning or itching, although the latter symptoms tend to be much less intense than with many other vaginal infections.

Bacterial vaginosis is very common in sexually active women. It occurs in about 15 percent of women seen at a university student gynecology clinic, in 10 to 25 percent of pregnant women, and in close to 40 percent of women seen at STD clinics (Sobel, 1989). However, many of these infections are asymptomatic, and their long-term significance is unknown. Simultaneous infections with *G. vaginalis* are typically found in the urethras of male sex partners of women with this disorder. Treatment consists of either Flagyl (metronidazole) or an antibiotic called clindamycin, both of which are taken in pill form. The CDC states that treatment of the male sex partner is unnecessary since it has not been shown to benefit the infected female or her male partner (Centers for Disease Control, 1989).

Recent studies suggest that bacterial vaginosis may be a factor in premature rupture of the membranes and premature delivery in pregnant women (Sobel, 1989). However, since Flagyl should not be used during pregnancy, alternative treatment is indicated.

PSYCHOSOCIAL ASPECTS OF STDs

There is little question that in the 1980s our society was overwhelmed by new developments regarding STDs. First there was a tremendous amount of attention given to the still-raging genital herpes epidemic. Although the media focus on this disease was initially informative and useful, it gradually took on overtones of emotional hysteria in some quarters. This reaction may have peaked in mid-1982, but by early 1983, the public's intense fears about genital herpes were put dramatically in perspective by news coverage about AIDS.

Increased concern over AIDS has removed the spotlight from the millions of adults with genital herpes, but it has also led to a climate of fear surrounding AIDS and its contagiousness. This fear has mushroomed as it has become increasingly clear that the AIDS virus can be heterosexually transmitted.

The fear that governs many people's reactions to the AIDS epidemic is in some ways similar to the fear experienced by people when they discover that they have symptoms that *might* indicate the presence of an STD. Fear, along with a disbelief that they might have an STD, leads many people to delay a visit to a physician. They deny the reality of the situation as if pretending an infection isn't there will make it go away. This is an example of the operation of the defense mechanism called denial, in which a person simply refuses to acknowledge that a stressful or danger-

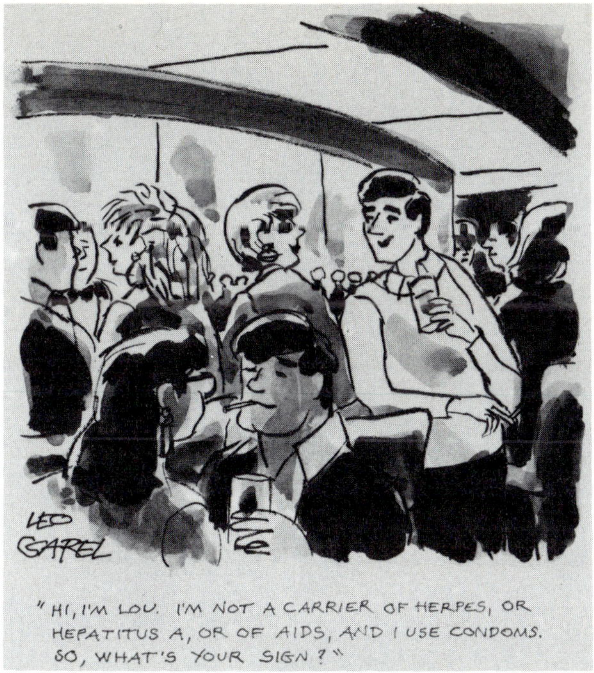
"HI, I'M LOU. I'M NOT A CARRIER OF HERPES, OR HEPATITUS A, OR OF AIDS, AND I USE CONDOMS. SO, WHAT'S YOUR SIGN?"

Reproduced by Special Permission of PLAYBOY Magazine. Copyright © 1989 by PLAYBOY.

ous situation is real. Denial is one of the most basic means people use to deal with anxiety-provoking situations.

In the case of STDs, denial is unfortunately often reinforced, because most STD symptoms disappear within a matter of a few weeks. However, infected individuals continue to harbor the infection in their bodies and expose their sex partners to the risk of infection, as well.

A better perspective on how the denial mechanism and its conscious analog avoidance come into play when people first wonder if they have been infected with an STD can be gotten from considering the following. In a recent survey of 100 consecutive first visits to a college student health clinic for the purpose of being checked for an STD, only one-fifth of the students had made their appointment within three days of the onset of their symptoms (Kolodny, 1990). More than half of the students had waited for at least two weeks before getting medical attention. Since about one-third of the overall sample did not turn out to have an STD, these students went through a lot of unnecessary worrying before being tested and given a clean bill of health. And the 40 percent of students who waited for more than two weeks before being tested not only worried during most of this time about their situation but actually contributed to endangering their own health—and the health of their sexual partner(s)—by their prolonged denial or avoidance.

The fear and denial that combine to make people delay visiting a doctor or clinic to be tested for an STD are augmented by another common defense mechanism: rationalization. Rationalization is the process of generating excuses to explain one's behavior rather than accepting the actual reason for the behavior. A clear example of rationalization was given by one of the students in the research described in the preceding paragraph when he told an interviewer: "I really didn't have time to get here any sooner. I was working on a term paper and I had a big exam coming up, and on top of that I thought I was getting the flu. Besides, I've had a discharge like this once before, and it didn't turn out to be anything" (Authors' files). The fact that this student's girlfriend had also been having symptoms of an STD apparently didn't break through his defense mechanisms. This too is a typical pattern: common sense takes a back seat to the initial refusal to believe that something is wrong.

Some people are also reluctant to go to a physician when they have symptoms of a possible STD because they're worried about getting a lecture or they're worried about the confidentiality that will be extended to them. Although physicians are legally bound to keep information they learn about their patients confidential, there are circumstances in which physicians are obligated to act differently. For example, in some states a physician's records can be subpoenaed by a court order. In all localities, a physician is supposed to report instances of certain communicable diseases to state public health departments (although as of mid-1990, most states did not require the mandatory reporting of cases of infection with chlamydia or genital herpes). Physicians' records are often accessible to insurance companies, since patients consent to having their records examined whenever they file a health insurance claim or when they apply for a new health or life policy. For this reason, anyone who is particularly concerned about this issue needs to discuss with his or her physician the limits to absolute confidentiality that might apply to his or her case.

Just a few years ago, people were dismayed if they received a lecture from their physician that advocated

bacterial vaginosis a bacterial infection of the vagina marked by a malodorous grayish-white discharge and symptoms of burning or itching; this condition is caused by an overgrowth of various bacteria, including *Gardnerella vaginalis*.

traditional sexual values and pointed out the health risks of casual sex with multiple partners. Now it is not so clear that physicians who give advice about safer sexual practices are old-fashioned or trying to impose their moral values on their patients: with what our society has learned about STD epidemics in the past decade, such physicians may simply be preaching about sensible public health practices. Nevertheless, if you encounter a physician who makes you uncomfortable by giving you unwanted moralistic-sounding advice, don't be intimidated; it will generally be in your best interests to switch to another doctor with whom you feel more at ease.

What is the impact of an STD on a person's sexuality? In most cases other than AIDS, assuming the infection is properly detected and treated, there will be little if any physical effect. During the acute phase of many STDs some people have little interest in sex because it's painful, while others continue functioning sexually without noticing that anything is wrong. Even when an STD has been untreated and has become chronic, it is not likely to depress libido or interfere with sexual functioning (genital herpes is the major exception, since sex can be quite painful during flare-ups). But even though STDs don't typically interfere with the *physical* component of sexual functioning, some people find themselves having sexual difficulties due to the psychological effects of finding out they have an STD. Often, these individuals are guilty and embarrassed about what has happened. They sometimes decide that their infection was God's way of warning or punishing them for sexual transgressions. Since they equate sex with sin, it is no wonder that such people occasionally develop subsequent sexual inhibitions.

Others develop obsessive concerns about sexual cleanliness and worry constantly about the possibility of being reinfected or catching another form of STD. Some men who fall in this category find themselves having erectile problems, while women who are exceptionally fearful about STDs may develop vaginismus as an unconscious way of protecting themselves from infection. Needless to say, such major concerns about sexual cleanliness may lead people to change their patterns of sexual behavior too—for instance, not participating in oral–genital sex.

When one partner in an intimate relationship develops an STD that the other person doesn't have, it immediately implies that the infected person has been sexually active outside the relationship. While this isn't always true, and some types of STD (such as hepatitis B) are also commonly transmitted by nonsexual means, doubt and suspicion may affect even a stable, loving relationship. If one partner infects the other with an STD, there may be even more conflict and hostility. This hostility may be expressed in sexual terms (i.e., by rejecting sexual activity with the other person) and may spill over into the entire relationship. This type of reaction can infect a relationship far more destructively than an STD. Fortunately, most people soon return to a better state of relating to their partners.

Except for AIDS, STDs are no longer as frightening as they once were, but for many people they remain somehow "different" from other infections because they are transmitted by sexual contact and generally affect the sex organs. Until people are able to think about sex as naturally as they think about breathing or eating, it is likely that this form of stigmatization will continue as a fact of life.

PREVENTING SEXUALLY TRANSMITTED DISEASES

The People's Republic of China apparently has managed to practically wipe out syphilis and many other STDs by enforcing rigid codes of sexual behavior and stopping prostitution, but most other countries must contend with the STDs as a price for social and sexual freedom. Even so, some practical guidelines can be offered to help minimize the chances of contracting an STD or spreading it once you've caught it.

1. *Be Informed.* Knowing about the symptoms of STDs can help protect you against exposing yourself to the risk of infection from a partner and help you know when to seek treatment.
2. *Be Observant.* Knowledge alone is not enough. Looking is the best way of discovering if you or your partner has a genital discharge, sore, rash, or other sign of sexual infection. (This can't be done with the lights out or in a moonlit back seat of a car.) If you see a suspicious sore or blister, don't be a hero about it: refrain from sexual contact and insist that your partner be examined. While "looking" may seem clinical and crass, you don't have to announce *why* you're looking, and often a good, close look can be obtained in the sexual preliminaries (getting undressed, giving your partner a massage). A step beyond looking is commonly used by prostitutes (and doctors) to

check for gonorrhea and NSU in men. The penis is gently but firmly "milked" from its base to its head to see if any discharge is present; the "exam" is sometimes called a "short-arm inspection."

3. *Be Selective.* Having numerous sex partners greatly increases the risk of developing an STD. Likewise, anonymous sex is risky too: you don't know if you can trust your partner or who he or she has been with in the recent past. Being selective in your choice of sex partners will improve your chances of avoiding STDs.
4. *Be Honest.* If you have (or think you *may* have) an STD, tell your partner (or partners). This can avoid spreading the infection and will alert your partner to watch for her or his own symptoms, or to be examined or tested. Similarly, if you are worried about your partner's status, don't hesitate to ask. It's foolish to jeopardize your health to protect someone else's feelings.
5. *Be Cautious.* Use of a condom will significantly lower the chances of getting or spreading STDs. Using an intravaginal chemical contraceptive (foams, jellies, creams) reduces the woman's risk of getting gonorrhea. Urinating soon after sexual activity helps flush invading organisms out of the urethra and so limits risks to a small degree. *If you think you've been exposed, promptly contact your doctor for advice.* If you *know* that you've been exposed, get medical help immediately and also abstain from sexual activity until your tests show that everything is okay.
6. *Be Promptly Tested and Treated.* A quick diagnosis and an effective course of treatment will help you prevent some of the serious complications of STDs. Treatment can be obtained from your private doctor, hospital clinics, or public health service clinics. After treatment, you must be rechecked to be certain that the disease has been eradicated. In addition, be sure to urge your partner to be tested (and treated if necessary) so as to avoid reinfection.

SUMMARY

1. Sexually transmitted diseases (STDs) is now the preferred term for what were previously called venereal diseases to minimize stigmatization and broaden the scope of infections included in this group.
2. STDs are occurring in epidemic numbers in the United States, with estimates suggesting that there are, annually, more than four million new cases of chlamydial infection, about two million new cases of gonorrhea, 750,000 new cases of genital warts, 500,000 new cases of genital herpes, 500,000 new cases of viral hepatitis, and 100,000 new cases of syphilis. Since the existence of an STD may make it more likely for a person to be infected with HIV, the AIDS virus, these statistics are particularly sobering.
3. Gonorrhea in men is usually marked by a thick discharge from the penis and burning urination. In women, gonorrhea often has no noticeable symptoms but can cause serious damage to the Fallopian tubes (PID). Because of the rapid growth in penicillin-resistant gonorrhea, the recommended treatment today is a combination of two antibiotics, ceftriaxone and doxycycline.
4. Syphilis is caused by *Treponema pallidum,* a corkscrew-shaped organism. The first symptom is a chancre two to four weeks after the infection. If untreated, syphilis goes through a secondary stage (rash, fever, aches and pains), a latent stage, and sometimes a tertiary stage where brain damage or heart problems occur. Diagnosis usually requires a blood test, and treatment is by a shot of penicillin.
5. Chlamydial infections are common STDs caused by a bacterium called *Chlamydia trachomatis.* In men, chlamydial infections generally produce a form of nongonococcal urethritis or epididymitis. In women, chlamydial infections not only cause cervicitis, endometritis, and salpingitis, but if untreated may lead to PID and subsequent infertility. In either sex, but in women particularly, chlamydial infections are frequently asymptomatic. Chlamydial infections in women are also thought to cause a number of problems during pregnancy, with eye infections and a form of chlamydial pneumonia being common in newborns of mothers who harbor chlamydial infections. Chlamydial infections are easily treated by either tetracycline, doxycycline, or erythromycin.
6. Chancroid is caused by the *Hemophilus ducreyi* bacterium and is marked by a pus-filled genital ulcer (sometimes known as a soft chancre) accompanied by painful swelling of the lymph nodes in the groin. Erythromycin is the recommended treatment.
7. Genital herpes is caused by both herpes virus type 1 and herpes virus type 2. It usually begins with painful blisters on or around the genitals that typically heal in two to three weeks in first attacks. The herpes virus remains dormant in

the body and periodically may be reactivated, causing flare-ups that are usually milder than the first episode. Although there is no cure at present for this viral infection, a drug called acyclovir is useful in lessening the symptoms of first attacks and reducing the number of recurrences.

8. Heptatitis A, B, C, and D (all caused by viruses) can be sexually transmitted, with the highest rates of infection occurring in male homosexuals and among heterosexuals with large numbers of sex partners. Hepatitis B can produce a carrier state that has a heightened risk of subsequent liver cancer, while approximately half the people infected with hepatitis C develop chronic hepatitis, with a sizable number going on to develop cirrhosis. Hepatitis D, which is infrequent in this country, only occurs in people previously or simultaneously infected with hepatitis B.
9. Genital warts, once viewed as innocuous, are now thought to be associated on a long-term basis with many forms of genital cancer. They are caused by various strains of the human papilloma virus and can be treated most effectively by laser excision.
10. Pubic lice are crablike parasites that attach themselves to pubic hair and cause intense itching. They are relatively easy to treat with a medicated shampoo or lotion called gamma benzene hexachloride (Kwell).
11. Vaginitis is most commonly caused by trichomonas or monilia. Vaginitis is not always sexually transmitted, and it is often a reflection of an overgrowth of microorganisms that normally reside in the vagina. Although preventive measures are able to minimize the chances of developing vaginitis, and most cases are easily treated, some women have long-term difficulty with this annoying but minor health problem.
12. To prevent STDs (or minimize the risk of complications), be informed, observant, selective, honest, cautious, and promptly tested and treated when symptoms appear or exposure is suspected.

Thought Questions

1. A child or teenager who has never gotten close to "having sex" can come down with a herpes infection of the genitals through auto-inoculation of oral herpes. Yet the media and most people regard genital herpes strictly as a sexually transmitted disease. What advice would you give a child with this condition for dealing with the stigma of herpes? How should parents respond to statements that automatically assume genital herpes means sexual activity?
2. How does a person with genital herpes stay safely sexually active when the infection can be transmitted asymptomatically, and a condom does not protect as well against herpes as for other STDs? What advice would you give to a person with genital herpes who is seeking a sex partner, a lover, or a mate?
3. Should the justice system deal with people who knowingly infect others with an STD? If so, should this be handled through criminal penalties or civil suits?
4. How would you respond if your partner became infected with an STD, particularly if the relationship was supposed to be monogamous? What if your partner continued to claim that he or she had not had sex outside the relationship? Should you believe your partner?
5. Regarding research priorities: Close to 30 percent of the U.S. sexually active population may have had an episode of genital warts, which is of serious concern since genital warts are associated with genital cancer. No treatment has yet been discovered which eradicates this infection, and thus infected people are advised to *always* use condoms, even in long-term, monogamous relationships. This is a huge number of people who are being adversely affected by an STD. However, relatively little funding is available to research cures and vaccines for genital warts, while AIDS, which at least currently affects far fewer people, is heavily funded for research (if not for treatment). Do you agree with these research priorities? Why or why not?

Suggested Readings

Covington, Timothy R., and McClendon, J. Frank. *Sex Care—The Complete Guide to Safe and Healthy Sex*. New York: Pocket Books, 1987. Practical, detailed information on STDs presented in an easy-to-read format, with many charts to aid the reader's grasp of material.

Holmes, King K., et al. *Sexually Transmitted Diseases,* 2nd ed. New York: McGraw-Hill, 1989. If its hefty weight (it's 1200 pages long) and technical verbiage (given that it's a highly scientific medical textbook) don't put you off, you will find this to be the definitive sourcebook on

STDs. A color insert shows numerous photos of the various skin lesions caused by STDs.

Langston, Deborah. *Living with Herpes*. Garden City, NY: Doubleday, 1983. This is an exceptionally thoughtful, scientifically accurate, detailed, yet readable book on all forms of herpes. If you have herpes, or you're close to someone who does, you should make this book number one on your reading list.

The most up-to-date material on STDs (including HIV infection and AIDS) is a weekly bulletin put out by the Centers for Disease Control called *Morbidity and Mortality Weekly Report* (it is commonly referred to by the acronym *MMWR*). Included in the wealth of data it publishes is weekly information on the numbers of cases of certain reportable communicable diseases, such as syphilis, gonorrhea, hepatitis, and AIDS.

8

HIV Infection and AIDS

The newest and most frightening STD yet discovered was first documented in 1981. Known as **AIDS**—for **acquired immune deficiency syndrome**—this devastating illness is a result of infection with the **human immunodeficiency virus (HIV).** The hallmark of AIDS is a breakdown of the immune system, the system that ordinarily protects the body against infections. Because of the collapse of the body's defenses, people with AIDS get a variety of rare infections known as opportunistic infections, usually found only in cancer or transplant patients whose resistance is lowered by medications that impair their immune responses.

Because the earliest cases of AIDS occurred primarily in gay and bisexual men and intravenous drug abusers, there was a certain amount of complacency toward the HIV/AIDS epidemic in many quarters—"This doesn't involve me" (Shilts, 1987; Presidential Commission, 1988; Kramer, 1990). As Harvard University's noted biologist Stephen Jay Gould put it, "If AIDS had first been imported from Africa into a Park Avenue apartment, we would not have dithered as the exponential march began" (Gould, 1987, p. 33). In actuality, the HIV epidemic is driven by a virus that knows no racial, sexual, or class boundaries. Today it is clear that not only are more and more heterosexuals involved in the epidemic but also that HIV infection is not restricted to certain groups of people. It occurs on college campuses, in private high schools, in small towns and wealthy suburbs, and in the famous just as in the poor, the unknown, and the homeless.

In 1988, HIV infection and AIDS was the 15th leading cause of death in the United States and ranked seventh among all causes of years of potential life lost, especially producing fatalities among people in their twenties and thirties (*MMWR* 38:561–563, 1989). In 1990, it was estimated that there were 212 cases of full-blown AIDS diagnosed each day and one death from AIDS every 12 minutes (Kramer, 1990). However, because AIDS typically develops seven to ten years after initial infection with HIV, these numbers are only the tip of the iceberg. Since the cases of AIDS being diagnosed today are largely a result of HIV infections that occurred in the early to mid-1980s, the number of AIDS fatalities will continue to grow at an alarming pace unless a scientific breakthrough occurs to help stem the tide of this epidemic. In the meantime, there are a number of measures we can each take to reduce our chances of being infected with HIV, which we will discuss in detail.

It is misleading to focus primarily on AIDS, the disease, instead of the broader spectrum of HIV infection (Presidential Commission, 1988). Thus, this chapter will emphasize the entire range of HIV infection in terms of its biology, its clinical course, its social and emotional aftermath, and the public policy issues that need to be considered to turn the tide in one of the most serious epidemics our country, and the world, has ever faced.

It is particularly important to be careful about the language we use to discuss HIV infection and AIDS because it is easy to create erroneous impressions and subtle prejudices by our choice of terminology. For example, calling AIDS a "plague" implies to some that this disease is a form of punishment for sinful behavior, whereas describing it as an "epidemic" sounds more scientific and less judgmental. Likewise, if we choose to declare war on AIDS, we must be careful to remember that the enemy is not the person infected with HIV but the virus itself.

Because new information about HIV and AIDS develops rapidly, the material presented here should not be considered the last word. Readers are urged to check with updates from other sources, especially information appearing in the U.S. Centers for Disease Control publication, *Morbidity and Mortality Weekly Report*.[1] The rapidity of new discoveries is certainly one of the brightest rays of hope for an eventual cure for this problem: In one decade, we have learned more about HIV than about any other known virus. We have also learned a great deal about how to respond humanely to this challenge, helping set the stage for eventually overcoming what now seem like formidable obstacles in bringing this epidemic under control. The message that is most important to take from this chapter, however, is that this epidemic is treatable, preventable, and predictable. Each of us can play a real part in bringing this epidemic to a close.

[1] Citations of *Morbidity and Mortality Weekly Report in this* chapter are abbreviated as *MMWR*, followed by the volume number, page numbers, and year of publication.

acquired immune deficiency syndrome (AIDS) a condition of increased susceptibility to unusual forms of cancer and infection due to disturbances of the body's immune defenses caused by infection with human immunodeficiency virus; at present, AIDS is thought to be an invariably fatal disease.

human immunodeficiency virus (HIV) the retrovirus that causes AIDS; prior to 1986, this virus was generally called HTLV-III.

EMERGING PATTERNS OF THE EPIDEMIC: AN OVERVIEW

According to the Centers for Disease Control, 160,000 cases of AIDS had been reported in the United States as of year-end 1990 (see Figure 8–1). In Western Europe, AIDS is less common, but the situation appears to be much worse in many major cities in East and Central Africa, where it is estimated that 10 to 20 percent or more of the adult population is infected with HIV (Pekkanen, 1989; Eckholm and Tierney, 1990). In addition, areas that had previously appeared to be spared from this disease are reporting increased rates of HIV infection. In Thailand, for instance, HIV infection is expanding dramatically: Among IV drug users in Bangkok the rate of HIV infection climbed from 1 percent in late 1987 to 40 percent in mid-1989, and growing numbers of female prostitutes are infected as well (Smith, 1990; Meyer, 1990).

These numbers hardly depict the full extent of the epidemic. For one thing, even in the United States, many diagnosed cases of AIDS are never reported to government centers that are tracking the disease (Hopkins and Johnston, 1988; Conway et al., 1989; Laumann et al., 1989; Masterson et al., 1989). In addition, in some countries, statistics on the extent of the HIV/AIDS epidemic appear to have been understated because of political and/or economic concerns such as wanting to avoid a drop-off in tourism, or just as a matter of national pride (Eckholm and Tier-

FIGURE 8–1

*U.S. AIDS Cases, by Six-Month Reporting Periods, 1981–1990**

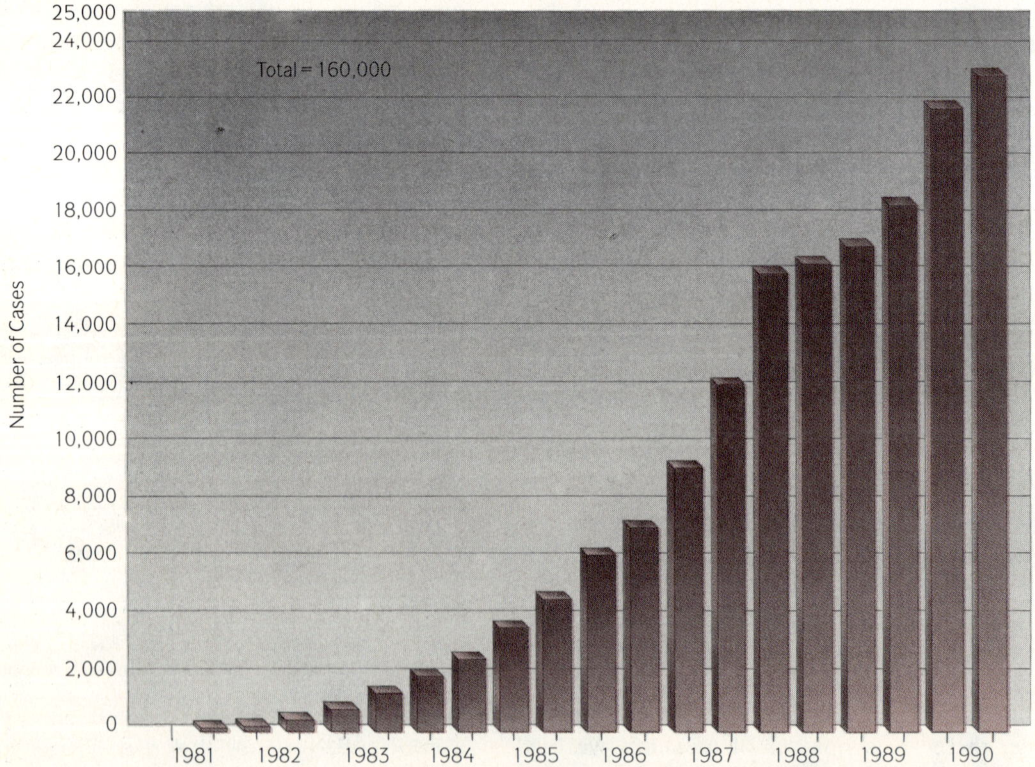

* *1990 second half data provisional.*

Sources: MMWR 37 (54): 13, 1989; *MMWR* 38 (26): 456, 1989; *MMWR* 38 (51 and 52): 892, 1990; *MMWR* 39 (26): 452, 1990; *MMWR* 39 (51 and 52): 1990.

ney, 1990). One other contributing factor to underreporting is that in some locations many cases of AIDS are never correctly identified. Thus, while "official" reports of AIDS cases worldwide totaled about 187,000 as of December 1, 1989, the World Health Organization estimated that the actual number was around 600,000 (Hilts, 1989).

Even an accurate count of AIDS cases wouldn't tell the whole story about the extent of the HIV epidemic, however, since AIDS is only the final stage of HIV infection. (Figure 8–2 provides some historical reference points.) According to the U.S. Public Health Service, 1.5 million Americans are infected with HIV and capable of transmitting it to others but have not yet developed any symptoms (Coolfont Report, 1986; *MMWR* 38: S-4, 1989); worldwide, the figure is thought to be 6 to 10 million (Mann, 1989). [Conservative projections indicate that 15 to 20 million people will be infected by the year 2000 (Pekkanen, 1989).]

Initially it was hoped that only a small proportion of people infected with HIV but without symptoms would go on to develop full-blown cases of AIDS (CDC, 1985; Liskin and Blackburn, 1986; Shilts, 1987). According to current studies, however, it appears that almost all of those infected with HIV will eventually progress to AIDS if no effective treatment becomes available (Lui, Darrow, and Rutherford, 1988; Lambert, 1990). Since AIDS is, at present, almost always fatal, the implications are staggering. The U.S. Public Health Service has predicted that by the end of 1993 there will be a cumulative total of 450,000 cases of AIDS in America, with one million cases by 1998 (Altman, 1989a). Other projections suggest that between one and two million Americans will have been diagnosed with AIDS by the turn of the century (*The New York Times,* March 4, 1987, p. A20; Hopkins and Johnston, 1988; Masters, Johnson, and Kolodny, 1988).

Two different patterns of AIDS and HIV infection have been recognized around the world. In North America, parts of South America, Australia, New Zealand, and many Western European countries, most AIDS cases have occurred as a result of homosexual transmission or as a result of IV drug abuse. In contrast, in most of Africa and in the Caribbean, the vast majority of cases appears to be due to heterosexual transmission (Institute of Medicine, 1988; Mann, 1989). Whether these two patterns will continue, or whether eventually most cases of AIDS will be as a result of heterosexual transmission, is an unanswered question at the present time.

FIGURE 8–2

The History of the HIV/AIDS Epidemic: A Timeline

1981 ► Five cases of *Pneumocystis carinii* pneumonia in young homosexual men in Los Angeles and 26 cases of Kaposi's sarcoma in young homosexual men in New York and California are reported to the CDC, arousing attention.

1982 ► New disease is named acquired immune deficiency syndrome (AIDS); first cases of AIDS detected in patients with hemophilia and in recipients of blood transfusions.

1983 ► U.S. Public Health Service issues guidelines for the prevention of AIDS; first cases of heterosexual transmission reported.

1984 ► A retrovirus, first called HTLV-III, is identified as the cause of AIDS; later, it is renamed the human immunodeficiency virus, HIV.

1985 ► Blood tests to identify antibodies to the AIDS virus become widely available and are first used routinely to screen the nation's blood supply; AZT (zidovudine) is first used in clinical trials; the news that Rock Hudson has AIDS mobilizes world-wide media attention.

1986 ► Surgeon General's Report on AIDS is issued by Dr. C. Everett Koop; clinical testing shows that AZT can improve survival and quality of life for people with AIDS; cumulative total of AIDS cases crosses 25,000.

1987 ► FDA approves AZT for severe HIV infection; President Reagan orders that all immigrants and federal prisoners be tested for HIV; the AIDS Quilt Project begins.

1988 ► President's Commission on the HIV Epidemic issues broad report urging focus on HIV infection rather than just AIDS, early diagnosis, and antidiscrimination measures; aerosol pentamidine found to be effective in preventing PCP pneumonia.

1989 ► National HIV prevalence study blocked by political pressures; FDA licenses aerosol pentamidine; cumulative total of AIDS cases crosses 100,000 in U.S.

1990 ► Recommended dose of AZT halved by FDA; first report of a dentist who may have transmitted HIV to patients published by CDC.

As shown in Figure 8–3, of the first 100,000 cases of AIDS in the United States, 63 percent involved homosexual or bisexual men who were not intravenous drug users, 19 percent occurred in heterosexual IV drug users, 7 percent occurred in homosexual or bisexual drug users, 7 percent occurred in heterosexual partners of people with AIDS or of people in high-risk groups, and 3 percent involved people who had received transfusions of contaminated blood products (*MMWR* 38:561–563, 1989). In Africa cases are divided almost equally between men and women (Peterman and Curran, 1986). Elsewhere in the world, as the HIV epidemic has grown, there has been a notable shift in statistics: For example, in Central and South America, where earlier reports showed 3 to 10 times as many men with AIDS as women, this ratio has now changed substantially, and in some regions men and women are affected equally (Hilts, 1989). In fact, while AIDS was initially regarded as a problem primarily affecting homosexual and bisexual men, it is now clear that heterosexual transmission is common and that no single group can be singled out as "at risk" for developing this disease.

FIGURE 8–3

*A Profile of the First 100,000 Cases of AIDS in the United States**

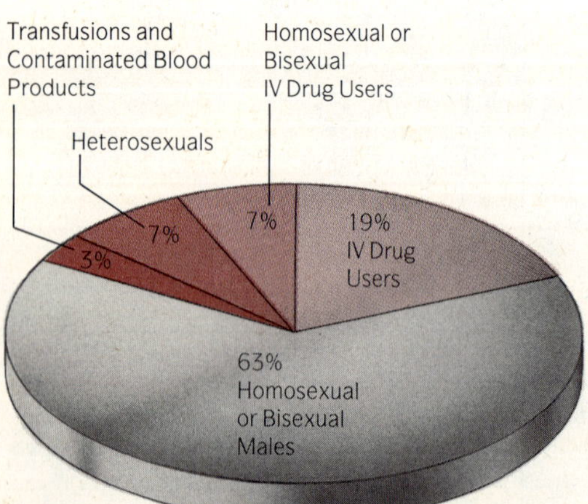

* *Note: The 100,000th case was reported to the CDC in July, 1989.*

Source: CDC AIDS Surveillance Reports, AMA/NET AIDS Information Service, September 1989.

In the United States it has become apparent that the nature of the HIV epidemic is shifting significantly from its early days, when the overwhelming number of AIDS patients were gay and bisexual men. In the past few years, AIDS has had a disproportionate impact on the poor, on blacks, and on Hispanics in inner-city populations, where the primary impetus for its spread has been needle sharing by drug addicts, followed by the transmission of HIV infection to sex partners of infected individuals (Altman, 1989; *MMWR* 38: 229–236, 1989; *MMWR* 39: SS-3, 22–30, 1990). Notably, AIDS is particularly affecting women in these populations (Figure 8–4). In addition, the geographic nature of the epidemic is changing. What had initially been a problem of New York and California has now become a problem that affects every state and territory and is not limited to large metropolitan areas alone.

This evolving view of the epidemic is buttressed by newly emerging data showing that HIV is spreading rapidly among some groups of teenagers and that among adolescents, equal numbers of males and females are infected (Kolata, 1989; Vermund et al., 1989; Burke et al., 1990). A 1989 study by the Centers for Disease Control found that 1 percent of teenagers in cities like New York and Miami, where the HIV epidemic has been pronounced, are already infected with the AIDS virus. And among teenage runaways in New York City, an alarming 7 percent of 1,800 surveyed were found to be infected. Little wonder, then, that many experts agree with Dr. Gary Strokash, a specialist in adolescent medicine, who believes that HIV infection among teenagers is "dreadful and it's going to be devastating"; in fact, he states, it "is going to be the next crisis" (*The New York Times,* October 8, 1989, Section 1, p. 1).

THE ORIGINS OF HIV

Although there is no certainty at present about how the AIDS virus originated, many scientists believe that it began in central Africa (Norman,, 1986; Cohen, Sande, and Volberding, 1990). One possibility is that a slightly different strain of the AIDS virus first infected monkey colonies there (Breo, 1986; Kanki et al., 1986; Essex and Kanki, 1988; Smith et al., 1988) and subsequently spread to humans. Viruses frequently cross over from animal species to humans; this is a natural part of the process of evolution that

FIGURE 8–4

Annual Incidence (adjusted for reporting delays) of AIDS Among Women 15–44 Years of Age, by Race/Ethnicity and Year of Diagnosis, United States, 1982–1988

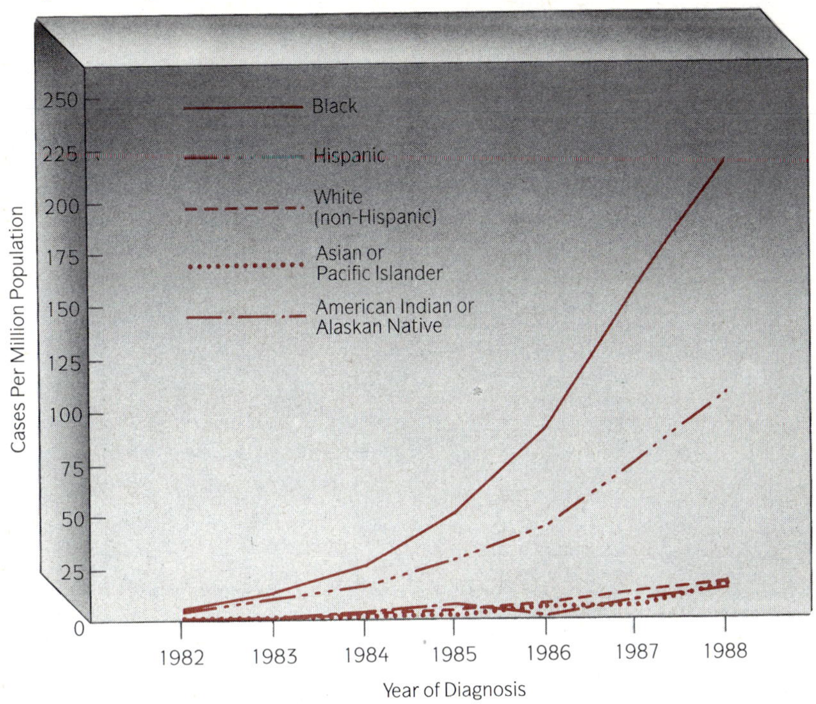

Source: MMWR 39 (55-3): 26, 1990.

has been going on for tens of thousands of years. Today, in fact, our world offers many possibilities for exotic or previously undetected viruses to spread to new locales because of the efficiency and wide availability of modern transportation systems. It is likely that both the various types of HIV and the strains of the AIDS virus that infect monkeys arose from a common viral ancestor (Cohen, Sande, and Volberding, 1990).

Whatever the beginning may have been, one research study using long-stored frozen blood samples found evidence for the existence of HIV in central Africa in 1959 (Nahmias et al., 1986). From there, AIDS may have been carried across the Atlantic Ocean by Haitians who once lived in or visited central Africa. From Haiti, AIDS may have spread to the United States by two routes: Haitian immigrants and vacationing American homosexual males, who often traveled to Haiti. If this explanation is correct, the early clustering of AIDS cases in the United States in gay males may have been largely accidental. If this scenario is true, it is likely that in the future far more AIDS cases in the United States will arise from heterosexual transmission.

The earliest known case of AIDS in the United States (not recognized as such at the time), based on the laboratory analysis of long-frozen blood and tissue samples, appears to have been in a teenage boy in 1968 in St. Louis (Garry et al., 1988). There have also been recent retrospective reports of cases of AIDS in a Norwegian family during the 1960s (Froland et al., 1988) and a fatal HIV infection in a 25-year-old British sailor in 1959 (Corbitt, Bailey, and Williams, 1990).

PERSONAL PERSPECTIVES

"We Are All At Risk"

The following is excerpted from a letter to the editor of *The New York Times* that was published on June 16, 1990:

I am a 36-year-old happily married, white female, who has never had syphilis, gonorrhea or chlamydia, has never used crack, never been an intravenous drug user, never had a blood transfusion. I test positive for the human immunodeficiency virus.

Clearly I contracted the acquired immune deficiency syndrome virus through heterosexual contact. Whoever he is (or was), he was either a recipient of a tainted blood transfusion or bisexual or an intravenous drug user. Equally clearly, that man would today be classified as a risky sexual partner, but it was not apparent to me at the time.

I think many women got infected as I did, but for the following reasons we are not getting counted:

(1) White, middle-class women just don't know they might have HIV. I never would have known it—I feel fine and I never looked better—except my husband and I applied for life insurance a year and a half ago. He tested negative; I tested positive. Because I haven't had sex with anyone other than my husband since we were married, this means I have been positive for at least five years with no symptoms. I know of at least a score of women from my support groups of similar socioeconomic background with a similar story.

(2) White-middle-class women know they have HIV, but (as with me) they are terrified their medical condition will leak out of their doctors' offices. If they die, the diagnosis is more easily hidden for a middle-class woman with a private physician than for the impoverished or homosexual population. So white middle-class women don't get counted.

(3) If a white, middle-class woman is sick and getting worse, her doctor might very well not think to test for HIV. Should death occur, it's essentially classified as death from uncertain causes.

I think it is very incorrect to depend on reporting systems that attribute AIDS cases to any other conceivable risk category before allowing that transmission was through heterosexual contact (the Centers for Disease Control and the New York City Health Department use such systems). It gives white middle-class society a false sense of security. The information systems appear to be structured so as not to generate information that would at first terrify, although it could eventually benefit, white middle-class society.

I think it is incorrect to discuss heterosexual transmission of AIDS as if it will, most probably, continue to affect just minorities (sexual, racial, socioeconomic or any other). That is the way heroin addiction was first perceived, and look how widespread the drug problem is today. We are all our brother's keeper. Problems do not remain isolated in the ghettos. AIDS will emerge into the population at large if we continue to think in terms of risk groups, to think in terms of the other getting it, not me.

We are all at risk. If I could become HIV positive, any woman (or man) can too.

Source: Letter to the Editor "If I Could Be HIV Positive, Any Woman Can." from the *New York Times*, June 16, 1990.

THE BIOLOGY OF HIV

The Virus

AIDS is caused by the human immunodeficiency virus (HIV), a virus discovered in the mid-1980s. HIV is so small that 16,000 could fit on the head of a pin. Typically, HIV gains entry to the body by sexual contact or by intravenous drug use with a contaminated needle. (It is believed that in most cases the virus must enter through a break in the skin or other tissue, such as with a cut, a sore, or a tear. This is one reason that drug addicts are at particularly heightened risk of infection.) Once inside, the virus selectively attacks two types of white blood cells, T-helper cells and macrophages. T-helper cells are the key coordinators of the immune system. They send out chemical signals that stimulate the production of antibodies and largely control the development of several other types of cells that make up the immune system (see Understanding the Immune System on pages 216–217). Macrophages, on the other hand, roam the bloodstream as scouts with two primary missions: to detect invading substances and to capture them, removing them from the circulation. Because they literally devour intruders, macrophages are classified in a group of cells known as **phagocytes,** from the Greek *phagein,* to eat. Macrophages not only search for invading microbes and engulf them, they also send an alarm to the rest of the immune system by secreting messenger proteins, called **lymphokines.**

After attaching itself to the outer surface of the T-helper cell by a biochemical process that is very much like a key fitting in a lock, HIV injects its core inside the cell, establishing a permanent infection. (The HIV core consists of two strands of RNA as well as a group of structural proteins and enzymes that are important for later steps in the life cycle of the virus.) Once this occurs, the virus copies its genetic information into the DNA of the host cell, actually becoming part of that cell's genetic structure.[2] In this form, it can remain inactive and hidden for years (Redfield and Burke, 1988). However, if the immune system is activated in response to another invader, infected helper T-cells proliferate, producing large quantities of new HIV particles that are then released from the host T-cell. These new viruses not only attack other T-cells but also other cells of the immune system and the brain. The entire process is summarized graphically in the figure accompanying the boxed item on pages 216–217.

HOW HIV IS TRANSMITTED

Sexual Transmission

In more than 78 percent of all AIDS cases the virus has been sexually transmitted (Peterman and Curran, 1986). It is not, however, as highly contagious as some other STDs such as syphilis, gonorrhea, and hepatitis B (see Chapter 7). Current estimates suggest that the risk of being infected with HIV from a single act of heterosexual vaginal intercourse with an infected person is 1 in 500 for a woman and 1 in 700 for a man (Turner, Miller, and Moses, 1989). The risk from a single episode of anal intercourse with an infected partner is considerably higher—probably on the order of 1 in 50 to 100 (Voeller, 1986). This risk with anal intercourse is higher because the lining of the rectum is very delicate and tears easily during anal sex, allowing infected white blood cells and HIV in the ejaculate to enter the tissue and bloodstream of the receptive partner easily (whether male or female).

Since the risk of catching gonorrhea from a single heterosexual exposure to an infected partner is 50 percent for women and 25 percent for men, and the risk of sexual transmission of hepatitis B appears to be more than 8 times greater than the risk of transmitting HIV (Kingsley et al., 1990), it is clear that HIV is far less contagious. Nevertheless, anyone who engages in risky sexual activity has a small but definite chance, each time, of becoming infected with HIV—and the more chances taken and the more exposures, the greater the likelihood of infection. What's more, there have been numerous instances documented in which infection occurred with a single episode of heterosexual intercourse (Peterman et al., 1988; Haverkos and Edelman, 1988; Glaser, Strange, and Rosati, 1989), which means that even though the *average* risk may be only 1 in 500 per sexual encounter, there is still a chance that HIV can be transmitted with only one sexual contact.

While it is certain that vaginal and anal sexual intercourse are the primary means by which HIV is transmitted, it is also clear that it can be transmitted by other forms of sexual activity (see Table 8–1).

Oral–genital sex, which is known to transmit every other form of STD, has now been shown conclusively to be a means of transmitting HIV (Perry, Jacobsberg, and Fogel, 1989; Spitzer and Weiner, 1989; Staver, 1990; *The New York Times,* October 7, 1990, p. 37). Earlier difficulties in proving that oral–genital sex could transmit HIV infection primarily reflected the problem of finding people who had engaged exclusively in oral–genital contact and never in coitus or intravenous drug use (Masters, Johnson, and Kolodny, 1988). Thus, one study of 45 married couples

[2] This is where the name retrovirus originated. Usually, the genetic material in cells is DNA, and when genes are expressed, the DNA is initially copied into messenger RNA, which then functions as the model for the production of proteins. In a retrovirus, this process is essentially reversed: The RNA is converted into DNA before it can be expressed or duplicated. In other words, retroviruses reverse what had seemed to be the normal flow of genetic coding (Haseltine and Wong-Staal, 1988).

phagocytes white blood cells that engulf invading microorganisms.

lymphokines messenger proteins secreted by macrophages that activate the immune response.

TABLE 8–1

Risk Estimates of HIV Transmission from Various Sexual Practices

Safer—Probably No Risk for HIV Transmission
Abstention from sexual contact
Monogamous relationship, both partners uninfected
Self-masturbation
Touching, massaging, hugging, stroking
Dry kissing (social kissing)
Low but Real Risk for HIV Transmission
Anal or vaginal intercourse with proper use of intact condom
French kissing
Fellatio without ejaculation in the mouth
Genital–genital contact without penetration
Contact with urine (exclusive of contact with mouth, rectum, or cuts or breaks in the skin)
Unsafe—Moderate Risk for Transmitting HIV
Fellatio with ejaculation in the mouth
Cunnilingus (risk may be greater during menstruation when blood is present or if there are sores in the mouth)
Sharing sex toys and implements
Sex play (such as S/M activities) that causes bleeding
Unsafe—High Risk for Transmitting HIV
Numerous sexual partners
Unprotected anal receptive sex with infected partner
Unprotected anal penetration with the hand (fisting)
Anal douching in combination with anal sex
Oral–anal contact (rimming)
Vaginal intercourse with an infected partner without a condom

Source: Modified from AIDS KNOWLEDGE BASE: A TEXTBOOK ON HIV DISEASE FROM THE UNIVERSITY OF CALIFORNIA, SAN FRANCISCO AND SAN FRANCISCO GENERAL HOSPITAL, ed. by Cohen, Sande, and Volberding, 1990, Chapter 11.1.4. Reprinted by permission of the Massachusetts Medical Society.

in which one spouse had AIDS found that the frequency of oral–genital sex correlated with the previously uninfected partner's becoming infected with HIV (Fischl et al., 1987), but this was not proof of a cause-effect relationship. While it does not appear at present that the risk of transmitting HIV via oral–genital sex is as high as the risk during coitus, there has been no way to quantify the risk based on current knowledge. It would certainly seem sensible in an individual set of circumstances to assume that the risk is higher if you or your partner has cuts or sores on the genitals, on the lips, or inside the mouth, but this doesn't help in determining the magnitude of risk for oral–genital sex when such conditions are not present. However, it is important to remember that oral–genital sex cannot "create" the AIDS virus if one person isn't already infected: If you are certain that both you and your partner are uninfected, there is no reason to abstain from oral sex.

There has been a great deal of skepticism about whether French kissing, or soul kissing (which involves exchanging saliva with your partner), can transmit HIV. While some reports claiming to document such transmission have appeared (Rozenbaum et al., 1988; Piazza et al., 1989), there is also evidence that saliva inactivates HIV (at least in the laboratory setting). Furthermore, the concentration of HIV is much lower in saliva than in blood or semen. On the other hand, since it is very common to have minor cuts or abrasions of the gums, lips, or inner mouth that may provide a place for the virus to enter, it is a biological possibility. That it may be an actuality, under some circumstances, is suggested by one recent report that described the transmission of HIV infection from a 70-year-old woman who had been infected by a blood transfusion to her 72-year-old husband, who had had no sexual activity other than passionate kissing for many years (Illa, 1989).

Absolute, incontrovertible proof that HIV can or cannot be transmitted by French kissing is not yet available and may be extremely difficult to obtain. Nevertheless, it is clearly possible that this type of transmission could occur. While this doesn't mean you should demand a medical certificate from your partner before embarking on a first kiss, or that kissing should be reserved only for long-term relationships, it would certainly be wisest to avoid French kissing a person you know to be infected with HIV.

Substantial evidence has accumulated showing that having another STD is an important risk factor for becoming infected with HIV via sexual contacts. (Such a risk factor is often referred to as a co-factor, a condition that plays a causative role, although it is not the sole cause of the infection.) This observation was first made in Africa, where the high rate of coexistent STDs (especially those causing genital sores or ulcers) is thought to be particularly important in the large proportion of heterosexually transmitted cases of HIV infection (Institute of Medicine, 1988; Mann, 1989). The association between other STDs and HIV infection has been noted in the United States as well. For example, a small study done at King's County Hospital in New York found that more than a quarter of women with pelvic inflammatory disease had HIV infection. Researchers in Baltimore found an association between syphilis and HIV infection in men and a similar association with a history of genital warts in women (Quinn et al., 1988). Others have found that the risk of HIV infection is substantially higher in people with genital herpes than in others (*JAMA* 259: 1048, 1988). However, heterosexual transmission is possible even when there are no other STDs present (Turner, Miller, and Moses, 1989; Cohen, Sande, and Volberding, 1990).

Nonsexual Transmission

Aside from sexual transmission, the major route by which HIV is transmitted is by intravenous drug users sharing needles or syringes that are contaminated by small amounts of infected blood. Once infected in this way, someone can then pass on the infection by sexual contact as well as by further sharing of needles.

Intravenous drug users may have a higher susceptibility than others to infection with HIV because their general health and nutritional status are often poor and their immune defenses may already be partly broken down by other illnesses.

The AIDS virus can also be transmitted by the transfusion of contaminated blood or blood products. As of 1989, about 3 percent of AIDS cases in the United States have fallen into this category. The routine use since 1985 of screening tests to detect HIV antibodies in donated blood and blood products (see (page 220) has substantially lessened the risk of using contaminated blood for transfusions. However, the blood supply is not completely safe because the screening tests are not foolproof, as we will discuss shortly. As a result, it is estimated that there are still about 1,000 cases a year in which the recipient of a blood transfusion is infected with HIV because of receiving a contaminated unit of blood (Ward et al., 1988). To put this in perspective, although the risk of HIV infection with a single unit of transfused blood is approximately 1 in 40,000, this is much safer than the risk of dying from general anesthesia (about 1 in 10,000).

Because of this small but real risk, some people having elective, nonemergency surgery have donated their own blood months or weeks before their surgery and have had it frozen and stored so it can be used if needed in a transfusion. This procedure has received strong endorsements from the medical community in the last few years (Presidential Commission, 1988; Silver, 1989). In addition to preventing any chance of inadvertently transmitting HIV, it also has the benefit of completely eliminating the risk of other transfusion-linked infections, such as hepatitis.

It is important to recognize that there is absolutely no risk to *giving* blood as long as a sterile needle is used, which is standard and mandatory procedure throughout the United States and Canada.

HIV can also be transmitted from an infected mother to her developing child during pregnancy or childbirth. Current research suggests that 20 to 50 percent of infants born to infected mothers will be infected (European Collaborative Study, 1988; Cohen, Sande, and Volberding, 1990), although how many of these children will develop AIDS is not known at present. Because of the high risk that the baby will be born HIV-infected, women infected with HIV should not become pregnant if they can help it.

UNDERSTANDING THE IMMUNE SYSTEM

The primary strike force of our immune system consists of one trillion white blood cells that attack and repel our microbial enemies. Although the immune process is complex and multidimensional, here is a basic summary of the system's operations. Keep in mind that the same principles apply to how our bodies fight off any type of infection, from the common cold to serious, life-threatening conditions.

When a foreign invader manages to evade the body's first lines of defense—the skin and mucous membranes—it is quickly detected by macrophages, a type of white blood cell that acts like an armed scout roaming the bloodstream to clean up debris and sound the alarm when an enemy is encountered. One of the key duties of the macrophage is to search for antigens—chains of unique proteins attached to the surface of invaders that serve as identifiers, allowing the body to recognize what is "foreign" compared to what is "self." In addition to detecting suspicious intruders and engulfing them, macrophages also activate the main portion of the immune system by secreting messenger proteins called lymphokines. In addition, some macrophages carry a fragment of what they've ingested as a type of biochemical flag to signal another element of the immune system, the helper T-cell. (This surface fragment is known as an antigen because it becomes an *anti*body *gen*erator.)

T-cells are manufactured in the bone marrow, as are all white blood cells. They are programmed for their work in the thymus, a butterfly-shaped gland in the upper chest. Here, one type of T-cell, the helper T-cell, is prepared to respond to specific "foreign" antigens and to recognize a string of molecules on every cell of the body that identifies it as self. A separate class of T-cells, called killer T-cells, is special troops that attack infected cells.

When macrophages engulf invaders, such as HIV, the antigen they attach to their surface acts like a distress flag that summons help. This immunologic assistance comes first in the form of a back-up army made up of the helper T-cells. These T-cells travel through the circulation in specialized groups. Each group recognizes only a certain type of antigen. When the antigen displayed on the surface of the macrophage fits into the receptor on the T-cell's surface, the two stick together. This "key-in-the-lock" phenomenon causes the macrophage to release a chemical that activates the T-cells and sounds a general alarm to the immune system as a whole, particularly mobilizing the killer T-cells, which multiply and concentrate their attack on the invader, following their chemical programming.

Another part of the immune system is also activated in this process. These are a separate class of white blood cells, called B-cells, that ordinarily are stockpiled in the spleen and lymph nodes. B-cells have the primary task of manufacturing antibodies, protein substances that seek out and bind tightly to specific invader antigens, marking the enemy for elimination. Many varieties of antibody are produced by B-cells. Each one binds to a specific antigen. Unless you have previously been exposed to an invading microbe, the body typically requires a number of weeks to generate a measurable antibody response. But if you've been previously exposed, either through a vaccination or by fighting off the actual microbe in question, the antibody response is much quicker because the body "remembers" the invader and is biochemically programmed to manufacture antibodies with greater rapidity. When antibodies stick to the antigen surface of invading microbes, they usually prevent them from attacking other cells and make them easier targets for macrophages to capture.

With HIV infection, something in this immune process goes wrong. Although antibody production is stimulated quickly in

Schematic Depiction of the Immune Response

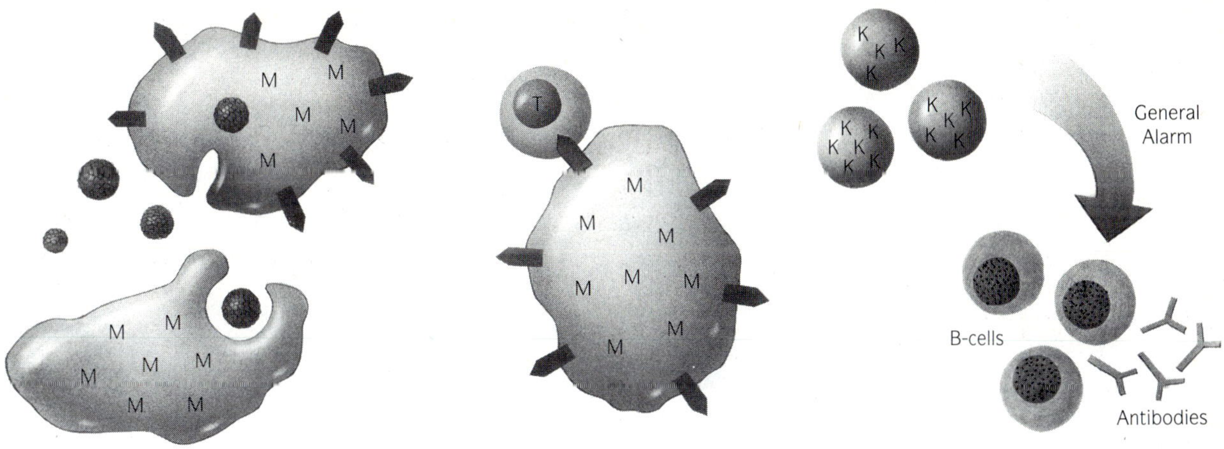

1. *When infectious microbes gain entry to the body, macrophages [M] attack and engulf them. Fragments of the ingested microbes (antigens) are carried like flags on the surface of some macrophages to signal T-cells.*

2. *A helper T-cell [T] locks on to the surface antigen and is activated by chemical messages from the macrophage.*

3. *Once activated, the helper T-cell sounds a general alarm, mobilizing killer T-cells [K] and leading B-cells [B] to produce antibodies.*

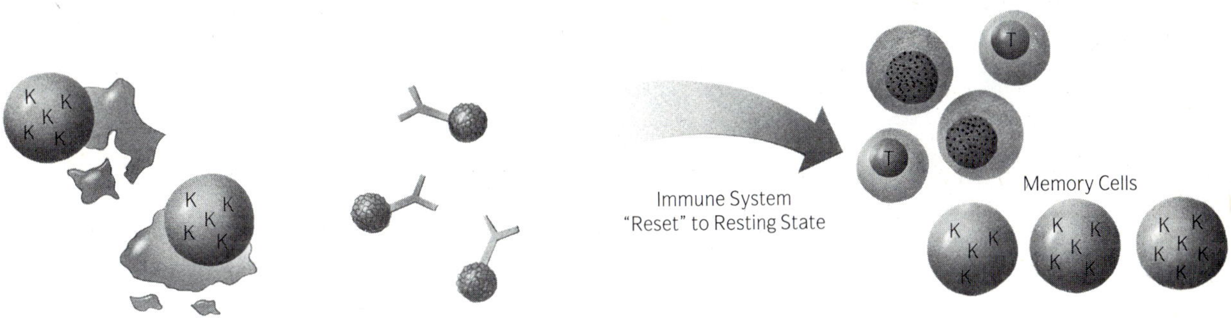

4. *Infected cells are sought out and destroyed by killer T-cells, interrupting the disease-causing replication cycle.*

5. *Antibodies manufactured by B-cells bind to the invading microbes, inhibiting their infectiousness and targeting them for attack and destruction.*

6. *When the infection is controlled, an "all clear" is sent to the entire immune system via chemical signals. Specialized antigen-specific memory cells remain permanently to provide a swift response against another invasion by the same microbe.*

most cases, the HIV antibodies that are manufactured seem to be unable to work effectively. This may be partly because HIV manages to get inside T-cells and macrophages, where it copies its own genetic code into the host cell's DNA, so that it actually becomes part of the host cell's genetic structure. In this situation, any activation of the immune system actually stimulates production of the invading virus—the exact opposite of what should be happening. Over time—in fact, usually over a period of years—this insidious invasion wreaks havoc by destroying helper T-cells, so that the body's front line of defense is seriously depleted. This is the primary reason that as the T-cell count drops drastically, the body is unable to respond appropriately to fend off the opportunistic infections and cancers that typically make AIDS a fatal disease.

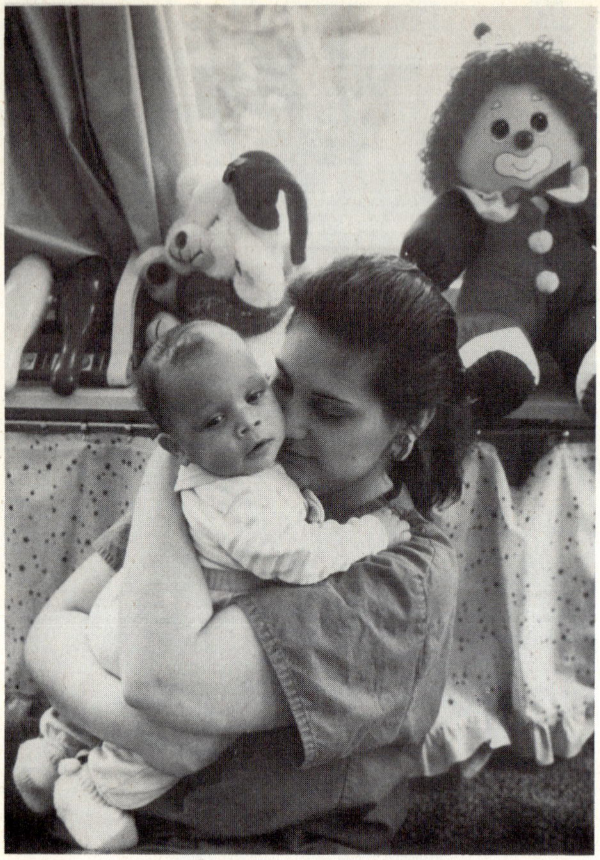

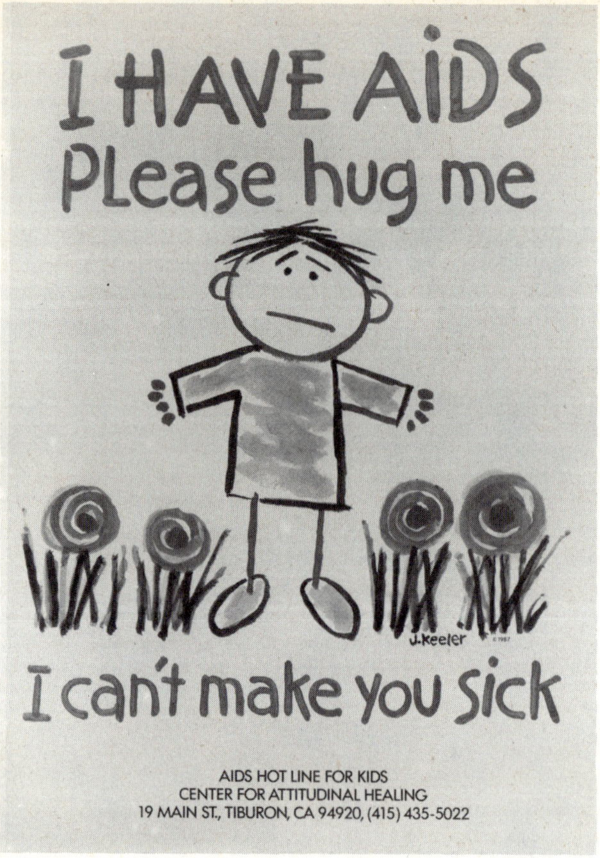
I HAVE AIDS
Please hug me
J.Keeler
I can't make you sick
AIDS HOT LINE FOR KIDS
CENTER FOR ATTITUDINAL HEALING
19 MAIN ST., TIBURON, CA 94920, (415) 435-5022

A volunteer holds a 10-month-old baby with AIDS in the playroom of the Farrano Children's Center in Albany, New York.

Most experts also feel that a woman infected with HIV who becomes pregnant should consider having an abortion, although of course this is a complicated personal decision. The best solution is for women infected with HIV to avoid pregnancy completely.

HIV can also be transmitted from a sperm donor or an organ transplant donor to an uninfected person, although instances of this sort are rare (Chiasson, Stoneburner, and Joseph, 1990; *MMWR* 39: 249–256, 1990). Nevertheless, the possibility of transmission in this fashion has led several states to pass legislation requiring that all sperm donors be screened for HIV.

Another rare type of transmission is during breast feeding. Since HIV appears in breast milk (Levy, 1989), it can be passed from a mother to her nursing infant (Ziegler et al., 1985). Furthermore, several cases have been reported from a Russian hospital where babies who had been infected by a contaminated syringe infected their mothers during nursing. Presumably, blood from sores in the baby's mouth entered the mother's body through cracks in the mother's nipples (Pokrovsky and Eramova, 1989; *American Medical News,* July 20, 1990, p. 36).

HIV can also be transmitted by needlestick injuries, which occur when doctors or nurses giving someone an injection accidentally stick themselves with the needle after it has been used. It is currently thought that HIV transmission occurs in less than one-half of 1 percent of such injuries (*MMWR* 38: S-6, 1989), and so far less than 30 such cases have been confirmed in health-care workers over the last decade (Herman, 1990). (In contrast, the risk of infection with hepatitis B virus after such an exposure is estimated to be 23 to 43 percent, and the CDC estimates that more than 10,000 cases of occupationally acquired hepatitis B occur annually in the United States [Fahey and Henderson, 1990].) At least one instance of HIV infection due to contaminated acupuncture needles has also been reported (Vittecoq et al., 1989).

How HIV Is *Not* Transmitted

Despite the finding of a low degree of infectiousness, many people have been so frightened by the AIDS epidemic that they worry that HIV infection might be transmitted by casual contact such as shaking hands with an infected person or coming in contact with the virus on a doorknob, toilet seat, or water fountain. Researchers agree that such fears are unfounded: There is no evidence at all that the AIDS virus is transmitted by casual contact of this sort (Tanne, 1985; Liskin and Blackburn, 1986; Heywood and Curran, 1988). While HIV has been identified in blood, tears, urine, saliva, semen, and vaginal secretions (Liskin and Blackburn, 1986; Wofsy et al., 1986; Levy, 1989), many studies have shown that people in close daily contact with persons with AIDS—such as a parent caring for a child with AIDS and nurses, doctors, and dentists working closely with AIDS patients—do not develop HIV infections from these contacts (Friedland et al., 1986; Jason et al., 1986; Fischl et al., 1987; Heywood and Curran, 1988). In many instances, of course, family members share drinking glasses or eating utensils with a person with AIDS, yet transmission of HIV by such acts has never been demonstrated.

Earlier concerns that the AIDS virus might be transmitted by insects such as mosquitoes now have been put to rest. Although HIV can survive for 48 hours in mosquitoes fed on infected blood (Booth, 1987), there is no indication that the virus reproduces inside mosquitoes or any other type of insect. Furthermore, if HIV were transmitted by insect bites, there would likely be a high rate of infection in preadolescent children in Africa and other tropical areas, but there is no evidence that this has occurred (Heywood and Curran, 1988).

PROTECTING AGAINST HIV INFECTION: SAFER SEX GUIDELINES

Experts are somewhat divided on exactly what constitutes "safe" sex. Complete abstinence is one solution, but this option isn't appealing to most people. Another possibility is a mutually monogamous relationship with an uninfected partner. While there is no way to tell by someone's appearance if he or she is free of HIV, a blood test can be done to detect whether or not HIV infection is present (see page 220). If you and your partner are both tested and are found to be uninfected and you each remain sexually faithful to each other, you are effectively assured that you won't get AIDS (making allowances for the slim chance of becoming infected by nonsexual means such as a blood transfusion). If such an approach is either impractical or unrealistic in your circumstances, the following guidelines may be of some help:

1. *Completely safe sex is possible if there is no exchange of body fluids.* While this means cutting out oral sex and intercourse as options—because even without ejaculation there is a danger of transmitting HIV in pre-ejaculatory fluid and vaginal secretions—techniques such as massage, use of vibrators, and mutual masturbation can be used. In addition, any sexual practices that can cause injury or rips in tissue should be avoided.
2. *Proper and consistent use of condoms will greatly reduce the risk of transmission of HIV as a result of sexual contact.* Studies have found that the pores of latex ("synthetic") condoms are so small that even viruses cannot pass through, and thus latex condoms, used properly, can prevent the transmission of HIV (Kish et al., 1983; Conant et al., 1986; Minuk, Bohme, and Bowen, 1986). (So-called natural membrane or animal skin condoms do occasionally leak virus particles, and thus are

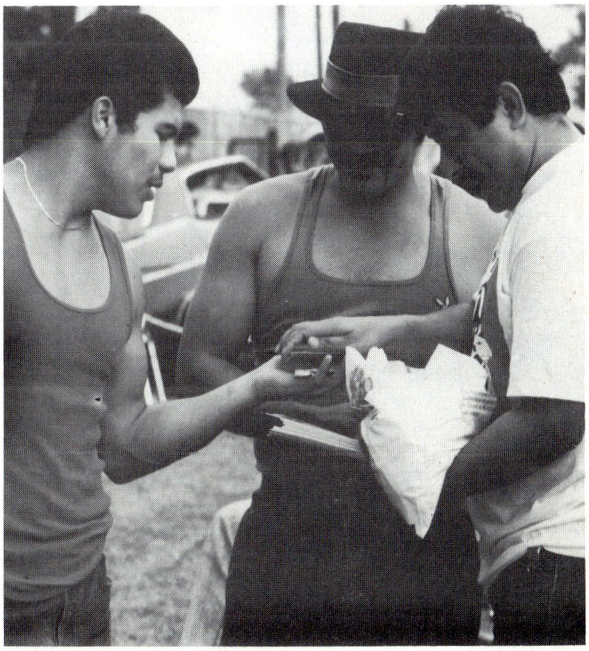

In Austin, Texas, a health department worker hands out condoms at a community festival.

not recommended [Goldsmith, 1987].) However, since improper use of condoms or a tear in the condom can certainly lead to leakage, this method is *not* a foolproof means of preventing infection (see Chapter 5). In fact, condoms fail more often than you might think. One survey found that 22 percent of heterosexuals and 31 percent of homosexuals had experienced condom failure in the preceding three months (Miller, Downer, and Kreuger, 1988). Remember, condoms are not perfect contraceptives, and they're not perfect barriers to HIV or other STDs, either.

3. *Use of spermicides containing nonoxynol-9 may offer additional protection.* Nonoxynol-9 kills HIV under laboratory conditions (Hicks et al., 1985), although it is uncertain whether under real-life conditions it provides as much protection as a condom. The best solution seems to be to use *both* a condom and a spermicide with nonoxynol-9 during intercourse.

4. *Be selective in choosing your sex partners.* As we've already noted, it isn't possible to judge who is infected with HIV by any symptoms, since it can take years after becoming infected for symptoms to develop. Furthermore, the great majority of people who are infected with HIV don't realize they're infected, so don't rely on a potential sex partner to warn you that there may be a danger of transmission. Under current conditions, it is prudent to realize that people who have had a large number of sex partners and people who inject drugs are statistically more likely to have been exposed to and infected by HIV. Similarly, males who have had same-sex experiences in the past decade are statistically more likely to be infected with HIV. Selectivity regarding a prospective sex partner can be life saving.

5. *Learn as much as you can about someone BEFORE you have sex together, but don't blindly trust whatever you are told.* Research such as that summarized in the Focus in Brief shows that people often lie about how many sex partners they have had. *The Kinsey Institute New Report on Sex* notes, "Researchers suspect people are even more likely to lie about homosexual activity, sex with prostitutes, or the use of illegal drugs" (Reinisch, 1990, p. 465).

6. *Stay away from high-risk sexual activity with a new partner until you have developed enough trust and rapport in your relationship to know each other fairly well.* While this doesn't mean that you should refrain from all sexual contact with a new partner for a period of months, it is perfectly sensible to start out slowly and to be forthright about which types of sex you'd prefer to leave until later in the relationship.

These guidelines need to be applied with a certain amount of common sense in order to be most useful to you. For example, we don't think it is advisable to have sexual intercourse knowingly (gay or straight) with a partner you know is infected with HIV even if you use a condom. (We are sensitive to the problems this poses in long-term, committed relationships, including marriages, when one partner becomes infected and the other partner is not. Still, we stand by this position: Condoms may reduce the risk of transmitting HIV, but they are far from fail-safe.) Likewise, if you suspect (but can't prove) that a prospective sexual partner has been an intravenous drug user, it may be most prudent to evaluate the situation cautiously, and refuse to have any sexual contact without first having blood tests done.

DETECTING HIV INFECTION

Several different blood tests can be used to detect HIV antibodies. The most widely used test is called **ELISA** (for **enzyme-linked immunoabsorbent assay**), which was developed to screen blood used for transfusions. Like all biomedical tests, ELISA is not infallible, although the accuracy of current versions of ELISA, which is very high, is improved substantially from five years ago. ELISA tests fail to detect HIV antibodies in about 0.3 percent of samples known to be positive (a mistake known as a "false negative"). In addition, this test incorrectly "finds" HIV antibodies in about 1 percent of samples (in other words, using the ELISA test alone, 1 out of 100 tests will be mistakenly called positive when it actually is not—a situation known as a "false positive") (*MMWR* 39:380–383, 1990).

Because of these inaccuracies, which may seem minor from a statistical viewpoint but which are certainly anything *but* minor if they involve *your* test, it is important to verify any positive result found by ELISA by using a different, more complicated (and expensive) test after repeating the ELISA test. This confirmatory test is called the **Western blot test.** When used together (ELISA test first, repeated if positive, and then confirmed by the Western blot test), the accuracy of testing for HIV antibodies is much better than most other medical screening tests, al-

FOCUS IN BRIEF

Dishonesty in Dating

Much of the advice about protecting yourself against exposure to HIV hinges on establishing possible risk factors of your sex partner. However, as the data from 18- to 25-year-old college students summarized here shows, sizable percentages of men and women lie about sex to their partners.

Actual Experiences	Men (N = 196)	Women (N = 226)
Has told a lie in order to have sex	34%	10%
Lied about ejaculatory control	38	—
Lied about likelihood of pregnancy	—	14
Sexually involved with more than one person	32	23
Partner did not know	68	59
Has been lied to for purposes of sex	47	60
Partner lied about ejaculatory control or likelihood of pregnancy	—	46
	34	—

Hypothetical Willingness to Lie	Men	Women
Would lie about having negative HIV-antibody test	20	4
Would understate number of previous sex partners	47	42
Would disclose existence of other partner to new partner		
Never	22	10
After a while, when safe to do so	34	28
Only if asked	31	33
Yes	13	29
Would disclose a single episode of sexual infidelity		
Never	43	34
After a while, when safe to do so	21	20
Only if asked	14	11
Yes	22	35

Source: From "Sex, Lies and HIV" by Cochran and Mays, THE NEW ENGLAND JOURNAL OF MEDICINE, vol. 322, pp. 774–775, 1990. Reprinted by permission of The New England Journal of Medicine.

though even this method of screening is not perfect. In fact, several laboratories have reported false positive rates of less than 1 in 100,000 tests using these two tests combined (Burke et al., 1988; MacDonald et al., 1989).

A false positive test can be the result of technical error in performing the test or a clerical error in identifying the blood sample. A false positive test can also occur if some of the chemicals used in the test react to a substance in the blood so that a mistaken reading

enzyme-linked immunoabsorbent assay (ELISA) the screening test used to detect HIV antibodies in blood samples; positive ELISA results must always be confirmed with a second, more specific test, such as the Western blot.

Western blot test a confirmatory test used to supplement ELISA testing. Western blot tests are more accurate than ELISA tests, but their complexity and expense preclude their use as the primary screening method in testing for HIV.

is given. (False positives are more common in women than in men and may also be related to previous pregnancy.)

Testing is complicated somewhat by the fact that infrequently, a person may be infected with HIV for more than two years before antibodies become detectable by either ELISA or Western blot testing (Loche and Mach, 1988; Imagawa et al., 1989). In addition, in rare cases a person who was initially seropositive (that is, had detectable HIV antibodies) may become seronegative (have no detectable HIV antibodies in the bloodstream), even though they are still infected with HIV (Farzadegan et al., 1988). In such cases, it appears that HIV "hides" in macrophages and monocytes, where it is somehow camouflaged from the usual testing. Fortunately, the incidence of disappearing HIV antibodies is low—0.4 percent (4 out of 1,000 persons tested)—and the phenomenon is still of uncertain significance.

Despite these various possibilities and problems with testing, we should stress that a confirmed positive test *is* cause for concern and should be followed up by careful, long-term medical evaluation. In addition, as noted emphatically by a panel of experts, "All persons who are antibody positive for HIV, whether they are symptom free or ill, must be considered to be potentially infectious to others by sexual transmission, by sharing of drug injection equipment, by childbearing, or by donation of blood, semen, or organs" (Consensus Conference, 1986).

It is important to realize that finding HIV antibodies in someone's blood does not, by itself, mean that the person has AIDS. The diagnosis of AIDS is made when a major disease such as *Pneumocystis carinii* pneumonia or Kaposi's sarcoma that signals an underlying deficiency in the immune system occurs in the absence of other conditions known to be risk factors for these illnesses. AIDS can also be diagnosed if a person has a positive HIV antibody test, evidence of a suppressed immune system (for instance, a low T cell count), and at least one disease from a list of some of the lesser infections associated with AIDS.

THE STAGES OF HIV INFECTION

As we have already noted, it is important to look at the entire spectrum of HIV disease instead of simply looking at AIDS, because HIV is a slow-acting virus. People who become infected today may not have any symptoms of their infection for 10 years or more, although sometimes they become ill at a much more rapid pace. Despite such variability, it is clear that HIV infection is a chronic, progressive disease (Cohen, Sande, and Volberding, 1990). Full-blown AIDS is the end stage of an infection that begins long before we can recognize that people are physically ill. Understanding the stages of this progression can help our understanding both of people who are infected with HIV and of what we can do to avoid this infection.

Initial Infection

No matter how someone is infected with HIV, when this virus enters the bloodstream the person's immune system typically responds by producing antibodies to the invading organism. Most people have no symptoms that accompany the initial infection or the production of antibodies, but 10 to 25 percent may have a brief illness that occurs two to five weeks after the virus enters the body (Cooper et al., 1985; Tucker et al., 1985). Symptoms include fever, chills, aches, swollen lymph glands, and itchy rashes (similar to the symptoms of infectious mononucleosis, or mono). Because of the nonspecific nature of these symptoms, which are frequent accompaniments to many types of viral infections—including the common cold—do *not* assume that a two-day bout of swollen glands, a runny nose, and fever means you've been infected with HIV! Antibodies to HIV can usually be detected within two months after the initial infection, but there are some cases in which antibodies do not appear for a year or longer (Francis and Chin, 1987; Ranki et al., 1987; Imagawa et al., 1989).

The Asymptomatic Carrier State

The infected person then passes into a phase called the **asymptomatic carrier state.** (Asymptomatic means no symptoms.) In this phase, a person looks and feels perfectly healthy, but the infection is present and antibodies persist. Many asymptomatic carriers also have a reduced number of T-helper cells in their blood. *The presence of the live virus in the asymptomatic carrier state means that such a person can infect others without realizing that he or she is infected.* It is important to realize that asymptomatic carriers do not have AIDS (the illness), although they are infected with the virus that causes AIDS.

Here are some personal reactions that illustrate the surprise and anguish many people who are asymptomatic HIV carriers express on learning of a positive test result (Authors' files):

> *A twenty-three-year-old married woman:* I was tested for HIV when I applied for an overseas job. When the results came back, I was absolutely sure they were wrong. There was no way I could have been infected, I thought. I never messed around, I never did drugs, and I never had a blood transfusion. Plus, I had never felt better in my life. But it turned out that my husband was positive, too, and that he had a bisexual affair when he was a sophomore in college. I was devastated, let me tell you.
>
> *A twenty-eight-year-old male rock musician:* I found out I was infected when I went to donate blood for a friend who was having surgery. It sounds so simple now, but I was stunned when I heard the news. The counselor at the blood bank told me, "How can you be surprised? You've got about every risk factor in the book." Now that I've come to terms with it, I guess I had led a pretty wild life, but it's tough to think that I'll be dead in a few years unless they find some cure.
>
> *A twenty-six-year-old gay man:* When someone from the public health department called to tell me that one of my sex partners from a few years back had come down with AIDS, I had nightmares every night. I kept putting off the time to go get tested, because I didn't want to get the news. And I kept saying to myself, "Relax—you feel so good; you couldn't possibly be sick." But I finally went for testing and found out just what I didn't want to hear. What do I do now about my sex life? Do I tell someone "I've got it" just before we get it on? And what do I tell the people I've been with the past few years? "Oh, hey, I got it from Larry and now I've passed it on to you?"

It is uncertain how long infected people can remain asymptomatic and not develop any signs of illness. Many individuals remain in the asymptomatic carrier state for periods of five years or longer before developing AIDS or related symptoms. Current evidence suggests that about 20 percent of asymptomatic carriers will develop full-blown cases of AIDS within six years (Bachetti and Moss, 1989; Cohen, Sande, and Volberding, 1990), and some data suggest that with the passage of additional time, as many as 99 percent may eventually develop AIDS (Lui, Darrow, and Rutherford, 1988). The best long-term data now available, based on blood samples frozen and stored as part of a hepatitis study conducted in San Francisco in the late 1970s, show that 11 years after infection with HIV, 53 percent of subjects had progressed to full-blown AIDS, and under a quarter of the subjects were still symptom-free (Bachetti and Moss, 1989; Lambert, 1990).

Much remains to be done to clarify how and when HIV infection progresses to AIDS. Different groups may have different rates of progression. For instance, homosexual men seem to develop full-scale AIDS more rapidly than hemophiliacs (Goedert et al., 1986). Similarly, adults over age 35 who are infected with HIV have been reported to progress more rapidly to AIDS than younger adults and adolescents (Moss et al., 1988; Goedert et al., 1989). Such differences may be a result of various factors. For example, repeated infections with HIV may reactivate the virus when it has been relatively dormant in the body. It is also possible that persons who have current or past infections with various other viruses (for instance, the hepatitis B virus) may be most at risk for developing AIDS. Another theory is that use of certain illicit drugs—most particularly, volatile nitrites like amyl nitrate ("poppers")—may somehow set the stage for developing AIDS more easily by lowering natural resistance to HIV. Whether any of these theories will prove correct is uncertain at present.

It is also important to realize that there have been only relatively brief follow-up studies done on people infected with HIV, which is understandable since this infection was first identified in the early 1980s. It is possible that 15 or 20 years after infection, unless a cure or other form of treatment is found, most people will progress to full-blown AIDS or will have died from other complications of HIV infection. On the other hand, since data from the 1980s are based primarily on HIV infection in homosexual males and in IV drug users, it is possible that this pattern may not accurately predict the experience that will be found in heterosexual, non–drug-abusing populations.

Symptomatic HIV Infection

In some people, HIV infection leads to symptoms that are less serious than AIDS itself. This stage was previously known as **AIDS-related complex (ARC),** but this term has now been generally discarded after the recognition that it was not a specific disease entity and had no special significance for treatment or outcome (President's Commission, 1988; Cohen, Sande, and Volberding, 1990). Symptomatic HIV infection

asymptomatic carrier state the phase of HIV infection in which a person is symptom-free (although able to infect others); this period may last for years.

AIDS-related complex (ARC) a constellation of signs and symptoms of infection with HIV, including such features as swollen lymph nodes and fevers or nightsweats, that falls short of a full-blown case of AIDS. This term has now generally been discarded in favor of the term "symptomatic HIV infection."

should be understood as part of a continuum of effects. As HIV multiplies within the body over time, it slowly destroys immune defenses. As these defenses deteriorate, susceptibility increases to a variety of infections that the immune system normally holds in check. These include non–life-threatening infections such as **shingles** or **thrush** (a fungus infection of the mouth), as well as more dangerous infections such as tuberculosis.

Symptomatic HIV infection is also commonly marked by persistently swollen lymph nodes in several locations in the body (for example, the neck, the armpits, just above the collarbones), which can occur alone or with other symptoms. The most common symptoms are diarrhea, weight loss, fatigue, and fever, but these tend to be episodic, not constant. In addition, neurologic problems are frequently encountered (Koralnik et al., 1990). However, it should be emphasized that many people with symptomatic HIV infection are well enough to lead relatively normal lives much of the time, continuing to work productively, to participate in sports and other recreational activities, and to appear quite healthy. Here is how one person described it:

> *A 32-year-old male architect:* I've been infected with HIV for more than six years now. Until last year I was completely free of any symptoms, but this year I've lost 12 pounds and have started to have occasional bouts of night sweats and fevers. But I still manage to jog three miles each day, play tennis on most week-ends, and keep an active social calendar. My doctor tells me that staying in good physical condition will help my fight against this killer—and so far it has. (Authors' files)

Unfortunately, people with symptomatic HIV infection do not always realize they are infected, either because their condition has been misdiagnosed, because they haven't gone to a doctor, or because they minimize the significance of the physical problems they are having. People in this situation may unknowingly and unintentionally expose their sex partners to HIV infection.

It is virtually inevitable that all people with symptomatic HIV infection will go on eventually to develop AIDS (Brachetti and Moss, 1989; Goedert et al., 1989; Cohen, Sande, and Volberding, 1990).

AIDS and Its Symptoms

While no single pattern of signs and symptoms fits all cases of AIDS, some of the most common are progressive, unexplained weight loss, persistent fever (sometimes accompanied by night sweats), swollen lymph nodes, and slightly raised reddish-purple coin-sized spots on the skin. These skin spots often turn out to be a form of cancer of the small blood vessels, a condition called **Kaposi's sarcoma** (pronounced kah-poh′-sees, often abbreviated as KS). Kaposi's sarcoma was rare in the United States before the start of the HIV epidemic. About one-quarter of homosexual males with AIDS in the United States have been found to have Kaposi's sarcoma, although KS is relatively infrequent in heterosexual IV drug users and hemophiliacs with AIDS (Beral, 1989).

When symptoms of AIDS first appear they may remain unchanged for many months or they may be quickly followed by one or more opportunistic infections, that is, infections that occur when immunity is broken down. One of the most common of these infections is an unusual, often-fatal form of pneumonia caused by ***Pneumocystis carinii,*** the presence of which establishes the diagnosis of AIDS in almost two-thirds of the cases seen in the United States.

Among other common infections in people with AIDS are severe fungal infections (including a form that spreads to the covering of the brain, causing meningitis), tuberculosis, and various forms of herpes

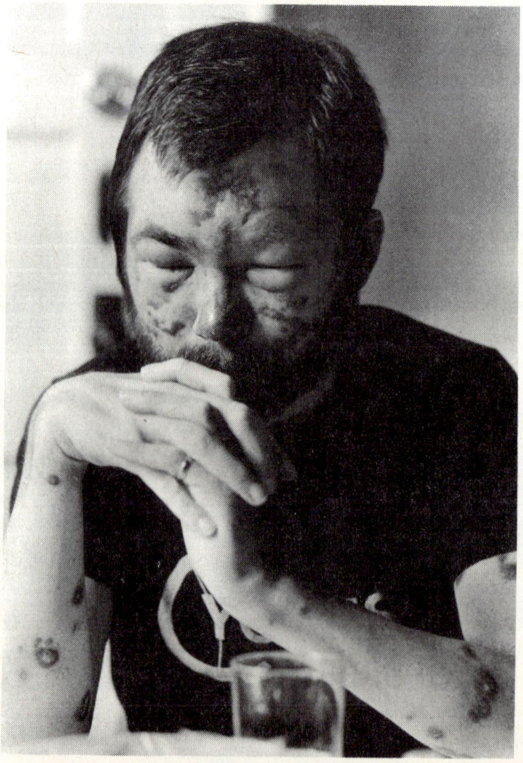

An AIDS patient with typical skin lesions of Kaposi's sarcoma.

that are more severe and recur more often than usual. **Encephalitis** (inflammation of the brain) is another life-threatening condition that occurs with greatly increased frequency in people with AIDS. In fact, because HIV can directly infect brain cells, a variety of neurological disturbances is seen in an estimated 30 to 65 percent of AIDS patients (Liskin and Blackburn, 1986; Gabuzda and Hirsch, 1987; Ho et al., 1989). These conditions include memory disturbances, psychiatric symptoms, severe mental confusion (dementia), difficulty walking, seizures, and coma. Although treatment can often fend off these infections temporarily, the typical course is for one after another overwhelming infection to occur until the victim finally dies because the depressed condition of the immune system becomes progressively worse, leading eventually to one final infection that cannot be overcome.

The human side of these symptoms is difficult to grasp unless you have been involved personally in caring for someone with AIDS. Here is a description offered by one man who took care of his brother for the last year of his life, as they both dealt with this devastating disease:

> Tom was determined to handle his affairs with dignity. While he was a realist until the very end, he was also able to look at the cards life had dealt him without bitterness or a sense of defeat. "Everyone's got to die sometime," was a phrase he used over and over again, mostly to cheer his visitors out of their dismay at his appearance. Still, once he became so weak that he was unable to walk more than a few steps at a time, we both realized things were going downhill rapidly. What worried him most of all was that he might develop AIDS dementia. Fortunately, even through three hospitalizations and a ferocious bout of shingles, Tom's mind stayed sharp until he was done living. While this was an emotionally trying time for us all, it gave me a chance to get to know my brother on a level I never would have known him before. (Authors' files)

At present, AIDS is almost always fatal within a matter of two to four years after it is first diagnosed. (The median survival for AIDS patients in San Francisco is 12.5 months, with less than 9 percent of patients surviving for 3 years [Payne et al., 1989].) Despite this, many people with AIDS are able to lead relatively normal lives early in the course of their disease, although coping with the social, economic, and emotional aspects of their illness is especially difficult for many, as we will discuss shortly. As more treatments are developed and become available for AIDS and for the severe infections associated with it, both the quality and quantity of life for people with AIDS will improve substantially.

While some people with AIDS continue their employment and usual activities for six months or more after the diagnosis is established, eventually the weight loss, constant fatigue, and multiple infections take such a toll that even ordinary movement becomes a major effort and the person becomes an invalid. (In Africa, AIDS is often called "slim" because in its late stages its victims look like they have been starving.)

TREATMENT OF HIV INFECTION AND AIDS

Medical Aspects

Although as of late 1990 no successful cure for AIDS or HIV infection has been found, there are some definite signs of progress against this disease. Most notable has been the identification of a drug called **AZT** (**azidothymidine,** marketed in the United States under the trade name **zidovudine**), which has proved to be an effective life-prolonging treatment. AZT was initially found to slow the progression of disease in patients with full-blown AIDS. Subsequent studies not only confirmed that AZT delayed the progression of disease in AIDS patients (Fischl et al., 1987a; Curran, 1989) and patients with asymptomatic HIV infection (Volberding et al., 1990) but also showed that it could be effective in lower doses than were used initially (Friedland, 1990; Volberding et al., 1990). By using lower doses, it is possible to minimize the serious side effects many people experience with this drug (Collier et al., 1990; Fischl et al., 1990), the most common of which is suppression of bone marrow function. Since the bone marrow serves as the

shingles a painful, blistering skin rash caused by the herpes zoster virus.

thrush an infection of the mouth and throat caused by monilia; this type of infection is more bothersome than life-threatening.

Kaposi's sarcoma a previously rare form of cancer of the small blood vessels, causing purplish spots on the skin or in the mouth; a common sign of AIDS in homosexual men.

Pneumocystis carinii a microorganism that causes life-threatening pneumonia in persons with AIDS; one of the leading causes of death in AIDS patients.

encephalitis a viral infection of the brain that is among the most serious opportunistic infections persons with AIDS face.

azidothymidine (AZT) (or **zidovudine**) a medication that has been shown to prolong life in HIV-infected persons and to slow the progression to symptomatic AIDS.

body's factory for producing new blood cells, suppression of this function causes severe anemia (low red blood cell count, which cause severe fatigue) and lowering of the white blood cell count (further reducing the body's ability to fight infections).

Clearly, AZT can prolong life for people with HIV infection. This is the major reason that AIDS experts are now calling for early detection and treatment (Cohen, Sande, and Volberding, 1990; Friedland, 1990). On the down side, however, there is evidence that some strains of HIV develop resistance to AZT when they are exposed to the drug over long time periods (Larder, Draby, and Richman, 1989). If this resistance becomes widespread, the overall utility of using AZT would be reduced considerably.

Progress has also been made in treating some of the infections that are the actual causes of death in people with AIDS. For example, a drug called **pentamidine** helps to prevent *Pneumocystis carinii* pneumonia; other drugs are available for fighting encephalitis and other life-threatening complications of AIDS.

Additional interest is focused on a variety of now-experimental drugs that are being rapidly developed to assist in the fight against the HIV epidemic. Among the dozens of approaches that appear most promising at this time are:

1. *Synthetic CD4*. CD4 is the receptor on the surface of T-helper cells that is unlocked by gp 120, a surface protein on HIV (see color insert, plate 11). By creating synthetic forms of CD4, which are infused into the bloodstream, HIV is lured to these "decoy" molecules and is thus prevented from attaching to as many healthy T-helper cells. While this approach has been found to work in the laboratory, it is not yet ready for full-scale testing in humans. The problem is partly that the synthetic CD4 doesn't live very long in the body.
2. *Compound Q*. This extract of the root of a Chinese cucumber has been used successfully in China to treat certain types of malignancies. It is currently being tested by the FDA for its effectiveness in treating AIDS under an accelerated drug-testing program that allows promising but unproven therapies to be tested rapidly, with a minimum of red tape. In laboratory studies already completed, it has been shown to destroy HIV-infected macrophages, while leaving healthy macrophages unharmed. However, it has not yet been tested extensively in humans, so that while it appears promising, it is still far from certain whether it will eventually prove to be effective in combatting AIDS.
3. *Enzyme blockers*. A number of scientists are searching for ways to block the key enzymes HIV needs to replicate. One of these is an enzyme called protease; if it could be blocked effectively, HIV would be unable to multiply within T cells or macrophages, and thus would be unlikely to harm the immune system seriously. While progress with this approach is still in its early stages, many experts feel this offers the best possibility for effective treatment.
4. *Vaccines*. Vaccines can be used either to *prevent* infection from occurring or *treat* an infection after it has occurred. Dr. Jonas Salk, famed developer of the first polio vaccine, has tried the latter approach with some preliminary signs of success. First, he and his colleague, Dr. Clarence Gibbs, Jr., a virologist, developed an AIDS vaccine that contained killed HIV cells. Then they administered the vaccine to two chimpanzees that had already been infected with HIV. Both chimps had a sharp rise in HIV antibodies. A third chimpanzee, who was not infected with HIV, also had a sharp rise in anti-HIV antibodies after two immunizations (Gibbs et al., 1989). Finally, Salk and Gibbs gave the vaccine to 19 people who were infected with HIV, all of whom had low T cell counts and other evidence of badly damaged immune systems. Although the vaccine did not eliminate the virus, only one of them had developed symptoms of AIDS within a year, and eight had a notable improvement in their immune systems (Levine et al., 1989).

Progress has also been made in the search for a preventive vaccine, which if successfully developed would be a key element in actually halting the worldwide spread of HIV infection. Researchers have recently succeeded in producing a vaccine that protected 8 out of 9 monkeys against simian AIDS (an AIDS-like disease caused by a retrovirus closely related to HIV) (Murphy-Corb et al., 1989). On the basis of this finding, many experts now believe that eventually it will be possible to develop a safe and effective AIDS vaccine for human use, although most expect that it will take 5 to 10 years to accomplish this task (Hilts, 1989).

One of the technical difficulties in devising a workable vaccine is that there are several different strains of HIV that the vaccine must protect against simultaneously. Another practical problem is that in order to be effective, a vaccine must have long-lasting protective effects—measured in years, not weeks or months. Whether such long-lasting immunity against HIV can be devised is uncertain at present.

HIV and AIDS

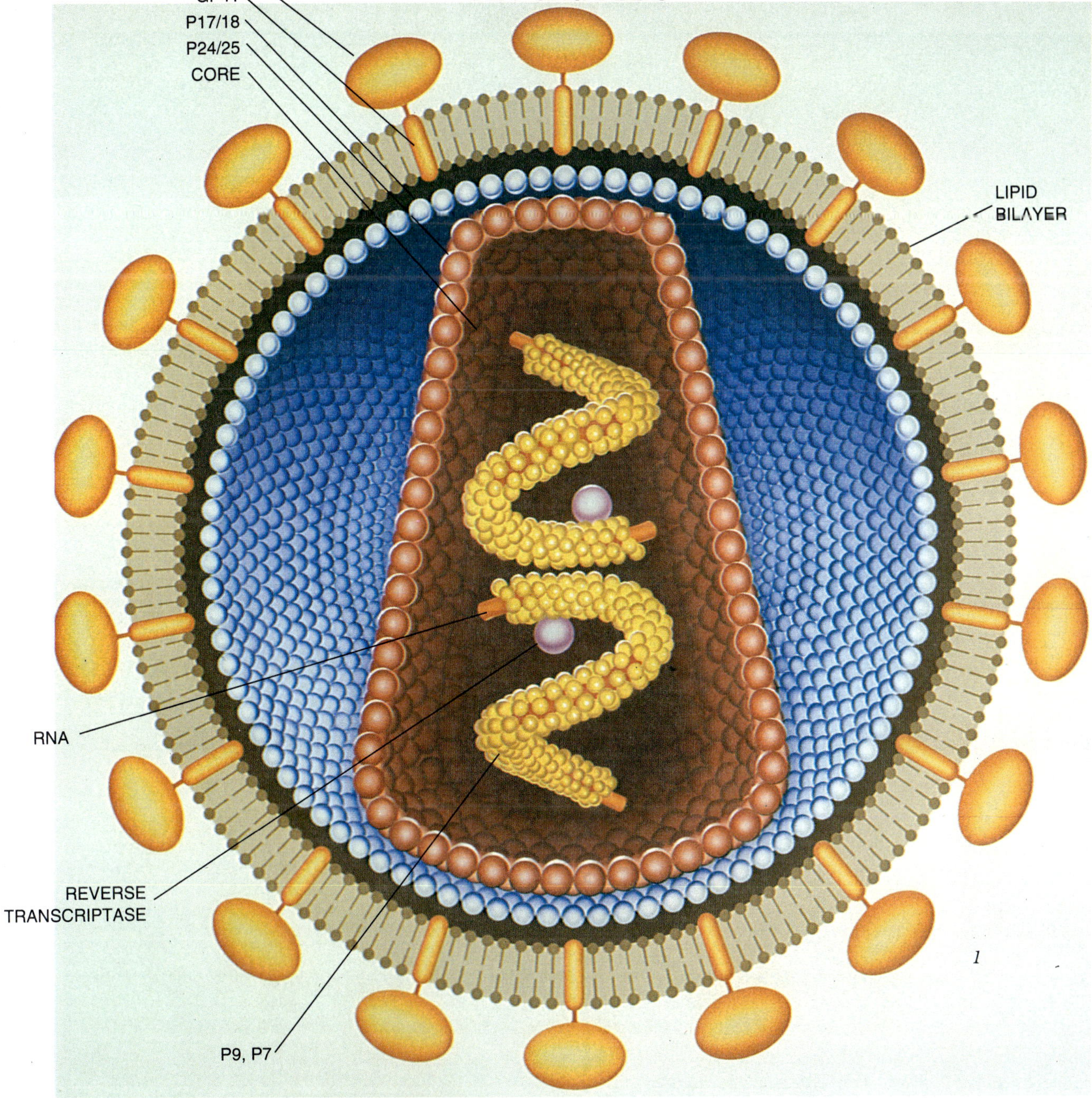

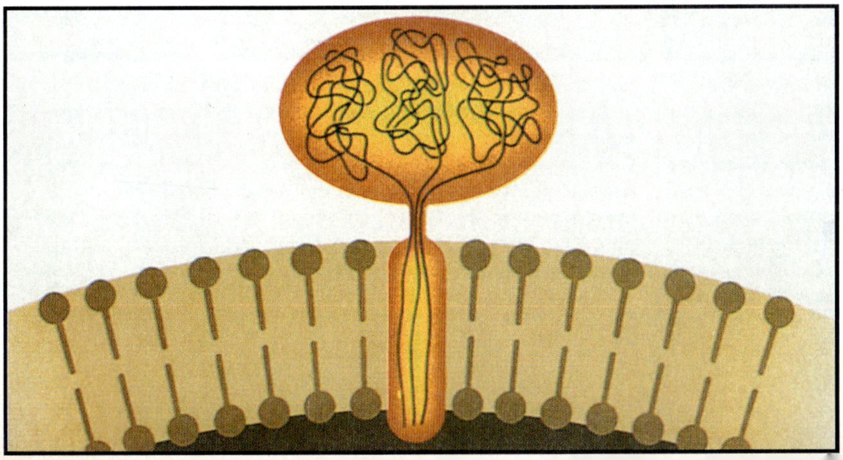

*1 VIRION STRUCTURE is shown in cross section. The knobs consist of a protein called gp120, which is anchored to another protein called gp41. Each knob includes three sets of protein molecules (*box at left*). The virus's core includes a protein called p25 or p24. In the core, along with the RNA that carries the virus's genetic information, is an enzyme known as reverse transcriptase. Reverse transcriptase enables the virus to make DNA corresponding to the viral RNA. The DNA inserts itself into the host cell's chromosomes and remains latent until it is activated to make new virus particles.*

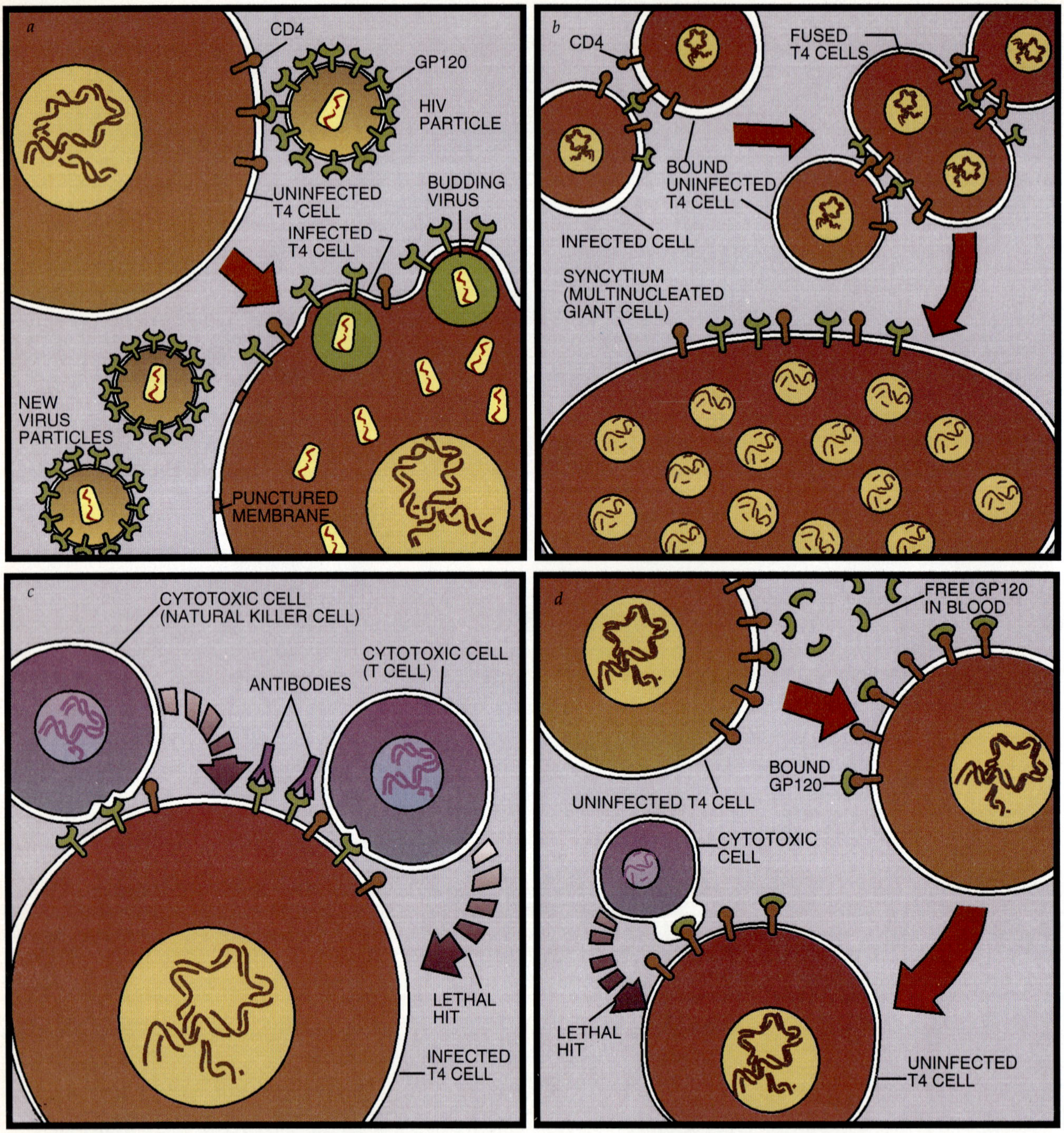

2

*2 Destruction of T4 Cells, which are critical to immune defense, is the major cause of the progressive immune dysfunction that is the hallmark of HIV infection. The virus is known to kill cells by replicating, budding from them and damaging the cell membrane (*a*). HIV might also kill T4 cells indirectly, by means of a viral protein, gp120, that is displayed on an infected cell's surface. A molecule on T4 cells—the CD4 receptor—has a strong affinity for gp120, and healthy T4 cells can bind to the gp120 and merge with the infected cell (*b*). The end result, called a syncytium, cannot survive, and all the once healthy cells it contains are destroyed along with the infected cell. HIV can also elicit normal cellular immune defenses against infected cells (*c*). With or without the help of antibodies, cytotoxic defensive cells can destroy an infected cell that displays viral proteins on its surface. Finally, free gp120 may circulate in the blood of people with HIV (*d*). The free protein may bind to the CD4 receptor of uninfected cells, making them appear to be infected and evoking an immune response.*

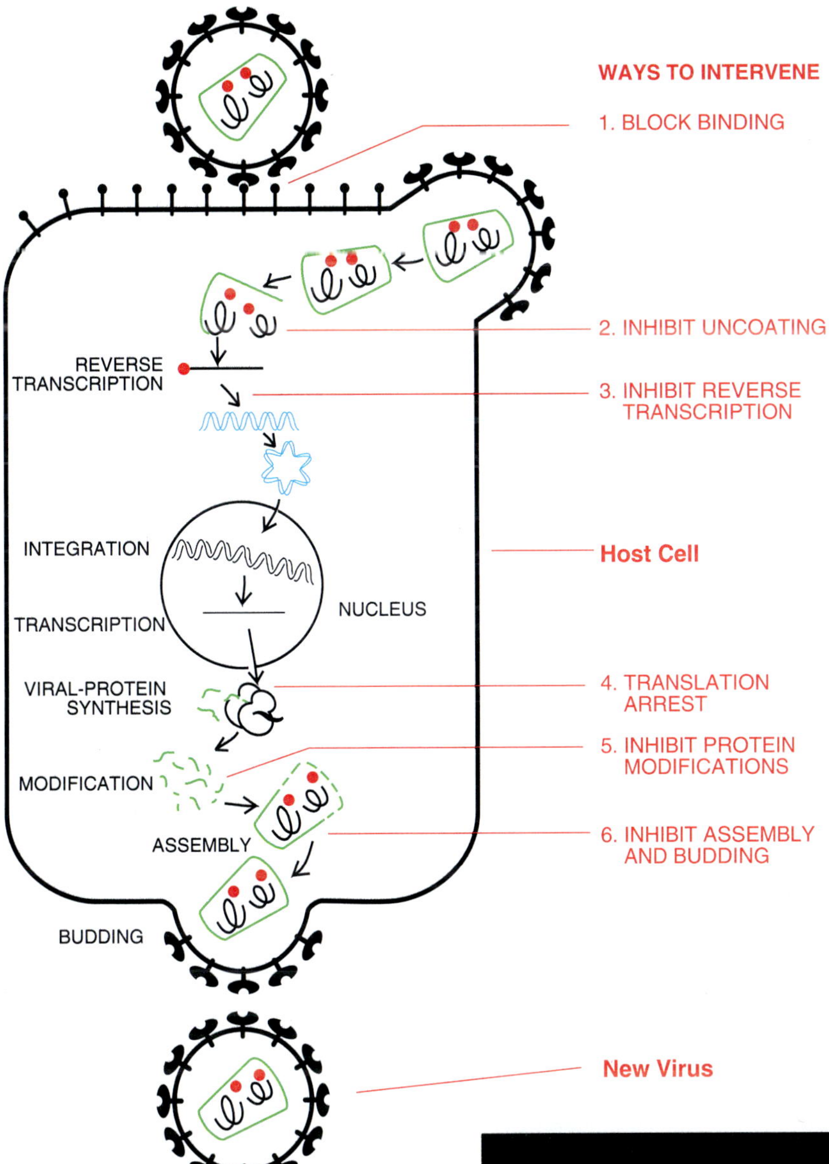

3

3 HIV LIFE CYCLE is subject to attack by drugs at several stages. Antibodies or chemicals could block the binding of HIV to CD4 receptors on the surface of helper T cells (1). Other agents might keep viral RNA and reverse transcriptase from escaping their protein coat (2). AZT and similar drugs work by blocking the reverse transcription of viral RNA into viral DNA (3). Drugs are also being sought to block the translation of messenger RNA into viral proteins (4). Since the newly produced viral proteins must undergo chemical and structural modifications before they can be assembled into new infectious virus, it may be possible to interfere successfully with this modification process (5). Finally, antiviral substances such as interferon may be able to keep the new virus particles from assembling themselves and budding out of the cell (6).

4 Photomicrograph of a T-cell infected by HIV.

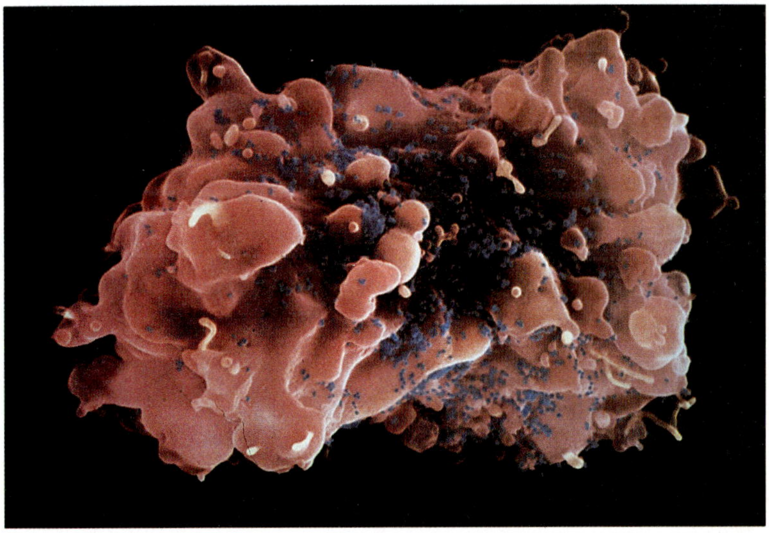

4

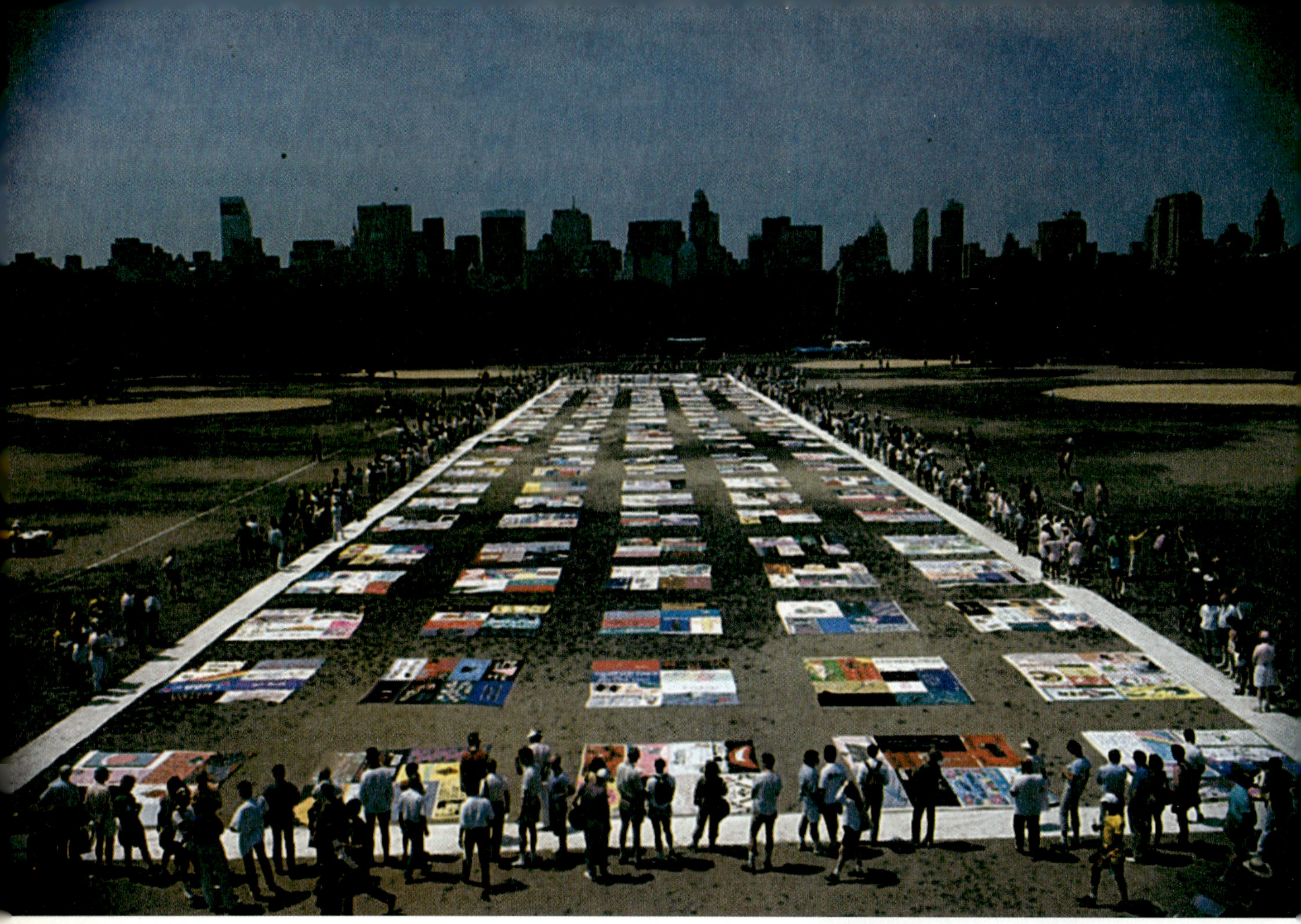

5

5 An aerial view of the AIDS Quilt.
6 and 7 Close-up views of panels from the AIDS Quilt Project.

6

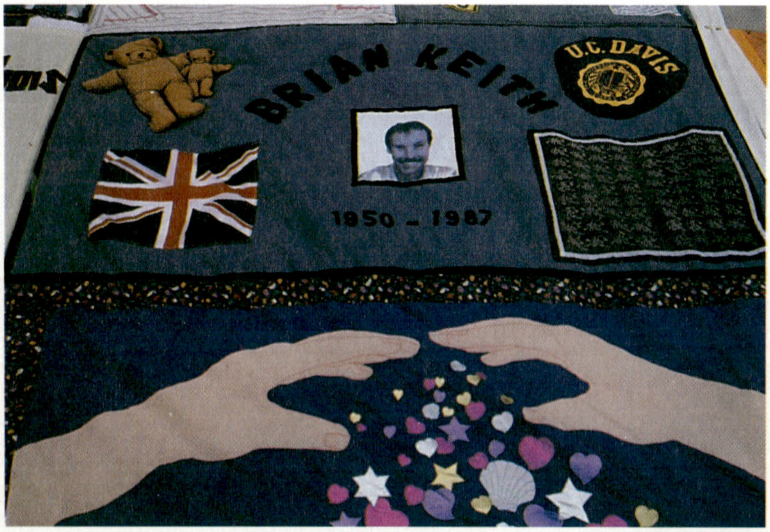

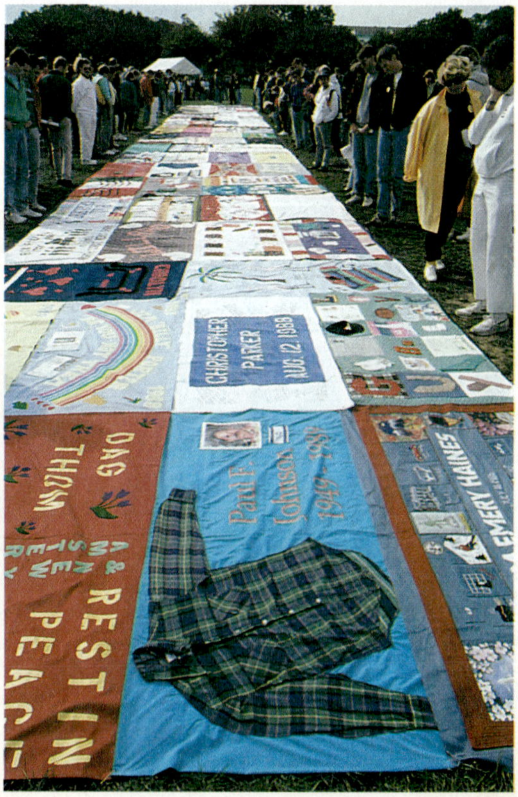

7

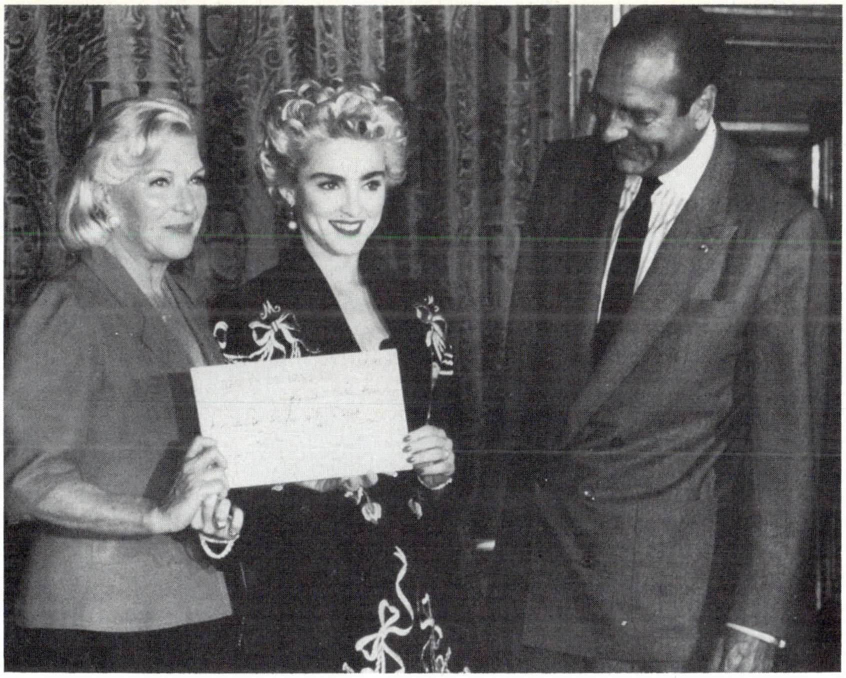

Madonna, shown here in Paris handing over a check to be used for AIDS research, has been among many entertainers who have become actively involved in fundraising to combat the HIV/AIDS epidemic.

Another difficulty is that vaccines work by triggering a person's immune system to produce antibodies that help to kill a virus. In HIV infection, however, the antibodies that are usually produced seem to be unable to kill the virus, which is why people with HIV antibodies eventually go on to develop AIDS. Overcoming this hurdle may be the primary stumbling block in developing an effective vaccine.

Finally, the matter of safety is also of paramount importance: In any vaccine containing killed virus, there is always a slight risk that some viral particles survive or get reactivated so that once injected into an individual, they can cause the very disease they are intended to prevent. Despite such obstacles, development of the monkey vaccine is a major step forward in the fight against the HIV epidemic.

Caring for People with AIDS

Because people with AIDS may have only minimal symptoms of their disease, may be struggling against acute, life-threatening infections, or may be anywhere on the spectrum between these two extremes, special care and support systems have been devised in many cities to provide a broad range of necessary services to those who need help. In San Francisco, for example, the following components exist (Cohen, Sande, and Volberding, 1990):

1. A walk-in clinic for everyone from the "worried well" to those who are dying.
2. A specialized AIDS inpatient unit for those requiring hospitalization.
3. An extensive array of community-based care, including the following services that are provided at the residence of the person with AIDS: assistance with shopping, housecleaning, meal preparation, special nursing services, legal assistance, and obtaining necessary medications.
4. Volunteer organizations providing a variety of forms of support. The best-known of these groups in San Francisco is the Shanti Project, which assigns a trained volunteer counselor to every newly diagnosed person with AIDS and provides a wide range of services, from ongoing support groups to low-cost housing for those who need it.
5. A hospice program for those in the terminal stage of illness. Hospices aim to make the last weeks or months of a dying person more comfortable, both physically and psychologically, by providing a broad range of services. In addition to providing care aimed at minimizing a dying person's distress when no cure is realistically possible, hospices generally try to deal with many

pentamidine a medication used to prevent *Pneumocystis carinii* pneumonia.

WHEN SOMEONE YOU KNOW HAS AIDS

When a devastating illness like AIDS strikes a family member or friend, it is natural to feel unable to offer much help or hope and to think you can't do anything that would make a difference. Instead of giving in to these feelings, here are some concrete suggestions for what you *can* do to make a difference.

- Simply being there as often as you've been in the past (or maybe even a little more often) is one of the best ways to convey your concern and caring. But be sure to call first. Let your friend decide if he or she wants a visitor right at that time.
- Offer to help out in various ways. Washing dishes, doing the grocery shopping, or picking up the cleaning may seem like small tasks to you, but providing such help is likely to be greatly appreciated. Your effort is tangible proof that you care, so it is much more than "just" cooking dinner or doing a few chores.
- You should realize that dealing with a fatal disease is not simple. You can get many helpful hints from AIDS groups in your area, but recognize that this doesn't make you an expert on the subject. So don't try to be one—it can only serve to create conflicts with your friend's health-care providers.
- Be aware that holidays are a time when loneliness can be particularly hard to deal with. (This is especially true if your friend is in the hospital.) A special visit that helps your friend feel included in the holiday spirit is a thoughtful act. And creative use of decorations, snacks, or gifts with the holiday theme—like a Christmas stocking stuffed with hard candies, paperbacks, and toiletries—are a concrete way of leaving a reminder of your feelings even after your visit is over.
- While it isn't useful to dwell on all the details of your friend or relative's medical condition and treatment, don't pretend the illness doesn't exist. Questions like "How are you feeling" are certainly appropriate (just as they would be for someone with any other type of illness).
- Include news of the outside world in your conversations to help your friend avoid feeling completely isolated and uninvolved. Tell him or her about mutual friends and what's going on at work, discuss your favorite sports teams, and bring up current

aspects of the lives of their patients, including spiritual needs, family matters, and legal and financial concerns. Hospices also help family members and friends deal with bereavement and loss.

Across the country, both families and friends of people with AIDS and community volunteers are learning new ways of relating and communicating: of bringing caring, compassion, and dignity as powerful tools to deal with this epidemic. While it would be a mistake to believe that this completely counterbalances the prejudices against people with HIV infection and AIDS that exist in many segments of our society, it is certainly a much-needed step in the right direction. For some specific suggestions about what you can do to help if you know someone with HIV infection or AIDS, see When Someone You Know Has Aids, above.

event items from the national and international scene.

- Reach out and touch your friend. A hug, a kiss, or an arm around a shoulder means more than you probably realize.
- Don't lie to your friend about how he or she looks or how he or she is doing. You don't have to blurt out everything you're thinking—there is a place for tactful gentleness in all human relations. If you try, you can probably find something optimistic to focus on, even if the optimism has to be put in terms of hope for the future: "I bet things will be better by the weekend."
- Don't give your friend lectures if he or she isn't dealing with the illness in the way you think is best. You don't know what medical, legal, or other advice he or she has been given, and you can't know exactly what his or her feelings are.
- Realize that from time to time, your friend or relative may get angry with you even though you've tried to be helpful. When this happens, don't take it personally. Anger may be a way of venting feelings of inadequacy and helplessness when dealing with illness. In a way, it's a compliment that your friend knows you care enough to get angry with you, knowing deep inside that such feelings won't be misunderstood.
- Try to be in touch with significant others in your friend or relative's life. This helps you stay informed about progress (or complications) on the medical front, and allows you to offer help when needed—help your friend may be embarrassed to ask for. For example, your friend's spouse or lover may need a break from nursing duties. You can offer to spell them for a Saturday afternoon, so they can get out and attend to their own needs for awhile.
- Do not confuse acceptance of AIDS with resignation from living. Accepting the reality of this disease may free your friend or relative from a sense of turmoil and uncertainty. Acceptance can also provide your friend with a sense of his or her own power.
- If you have been particularly close to your friend or relative, recognize your own needs for support or counseling. Many AIDS organizations have support groups you can join for just this purpose.

PATTERNS OF THE EPIDEMIC: A LOOK AT THE NUMBERS

Regrettably, ten years after the first recognition of AIDS and six years after the development of tests to detect antibodies to HIV, no national prevalence survey has been done to establish definitively the exact dimensions of the HIV epidemic in the United States. (Prevalence denotes the proportion of a population that is currently infected.) In fact, former Surgeon General C. Everett Koop acknowledged this problem when he said, "How many are infected? That's our whole problem—we don't know that number. We use the number of a million or a million and a half, but it could be 400,000 or it could be 4 million. We just don't know" (*The New York Times,* July 22, 1988, p. B4). Nevertheless, a substantial number of prevalence studies have been done in various segments of the population. By studying the range of results found in such studies, it is possible to form a preliminary picture of the HIV epidemic as it currently exists.

Before considering these surveys, it is useful to look back at the evolution of the HIV epidemic from several different viewpoints. First, it is helpful to keep in mind that the early years of the HIV epidemic hit hardest in New York, New Jersey, and California. In fact, many scientists and politicians in the Midwest and in the South (outside of Florida) voiced doubts that AIDS would ever take much of a toll in their locales. While it is obvious today that this attitude of denial was incorrect, denial occurred in other ways as well. For example, as recently as the mid-1980s many scientists considered it unlikely that HIV could be transmitted by heterosexual intercourse, giving detailed explanations as to why the pattern in Africa and the Caribbean was somehow "different" from the United States (Kant, 1985; Schultz et al., 1986; Stibbe, 1986; Shilts, 1987; Langone, 1988). The AIDS epidemic was considered rather simplistically to be a problem of the gay community and of people who abused drugs. As Figure 8–5 shows, this is far from correct. Even more recently, there have been many observers who contend that the epidemic is mainly a problem for minority communities—inner-city populations that are heavily black and Hispanic. This "ghettoization" of the problem also reflects a signal misunderstanding: HIV doesn't recognize skin color or social class when it invades a host.

Patterns and Trends of HIV Infection

Counting cases of AIDS only tells us what happened 7 to 10 years ago, because that is the average length of time from initial infection with HIV to the point where AIDS is diagnosed. Thus, to identify current trends in the epidemic, it is useful to examine information about the prevalence of HIV infection in various segments of the broader population. Here is a rundown on what is known.

FIGURE 8–5

Heterosexually Acquired AIDS Cases, by Half-Year of Report—United States, 1983–1988

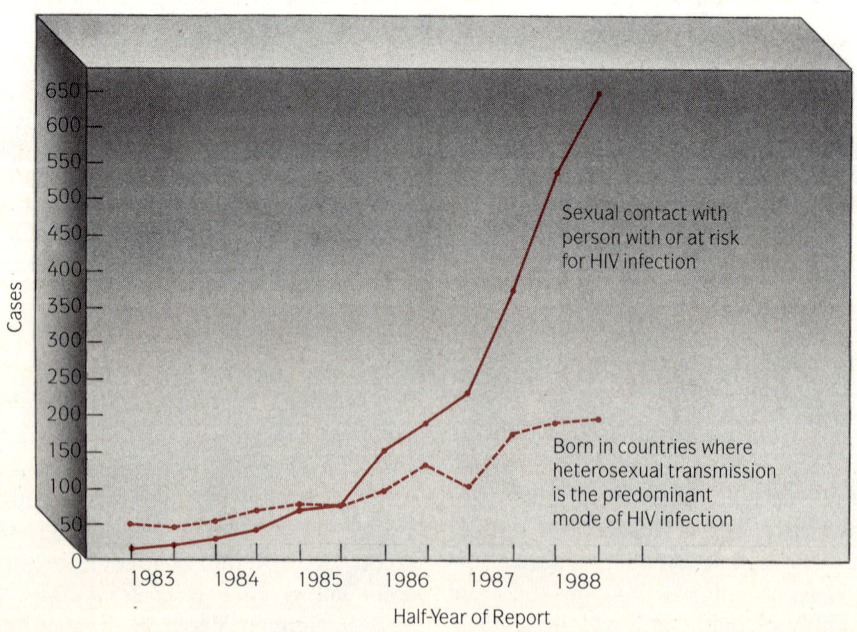

Source: MMWR 38: 430, 1989.

HOMOSEXUAL AND BISEXUAL MALES

In San Francisco and New York City, HIV infection among gay and bisexual men hovers around the 50 percent mark. Although it had previously been thought that no new cases of HIV infection were occurring in these groups because of effective community-wide education resulting in their careful adherence to safer sex guidelines, several recent studies have shown that there has been some slippage in this (Siegel et al., 1988; Ekstrand et al., 1989; *American Medical News,* June 29, 1990, p. 3), so that a modest number of new infections are occurring in these groups annually. Elsewhere in the United States, prevalence rates among homosexual and bisexual males are somewhat lower. For instance, in Milwaukee the figure recently stood at 24 percent, whereas in Albuquerque, New Mexico, it was 14 percent (*MMWR,* S-4, 1989).

INTRAVENOUS DRUG USERS

Among IV drug users surveyed through treatment programs, hospitals, and drug treatment centers, HIV infection rates are considerably higher on the East Coast than on the West Coast. For instance, in New York City and northern New Jersey, rates are in the 50–60 percent range (*MMWR* 36: S-6, 1987; Hahn et al., 1989), and in Washington, D.C., one study reported a seroprevalence rate of 28 percent, which is similar to the rate reported from Baltimore. In contrast, in Los Angeles only a 3 percent seroprevalence rate was found (*MMWR,* S-4, 1989, Table 6), and in Sacramento the seroprevalence rate in IV drug users participating in a drug treatment program was 2 percent (*MMWR* 38: 370, 1989).

HETEROSEXUALS

There have been relatively few studies of HIV infection in the general heterosexual population. One of the first studies (done in 1987) tested 800 heterosexual men and women in four locations (New York, Los Angeles, Atlanta, and St. Louis) and found that 5 percent of the men and 7 percent of the women with at least 6 sex partners a year for the preceding 5 years were seropositive (Masters, Johnson, and Kolodny, 1988). (Having at least 6 sex partners a year would be considered by many to be an operational definition for promiscuity; we should also point out that only a small portion of the general heterosexual population would meet this criterion.) In contrast, none of the women and only 1 of 200 men in strictly monogamous relationships were seropositive.

A similar study of sexually active heterosexuals with no known risk factors for HIV infection was conducted by Margaret Fischl and her co-workers in Miami. Of 346 people they studied, 5 percent were seropositive, with the only potential risk factor identified being multiple sexual partners (Fischl et al., 1988a). (This result was remarkably similar to our own study, described in the preceding paragraph, but Fischl's study has not been widely publicized.)

The appearance of HIV infection in middle-class heterosexuals mainly as a result of sexual contact with IV drug users is now being documented with increasing frequency (Glaser, Strange, and Rosati, 1989).

One interesting point to keep in mind is that in women, HIV infection appears to be linked increasingly to heterosexual transmission. For example, in New Jersey, the percentage of women who gave birth to HIV-infected babies whose only apparent risk factor was heterosexual intercourse rose from 14 percent in 1982–1985 to 43 percent in the time period from 1986 to 1988 (Weiss, 1989).

AIDS Surveillance

AIDS cases have been reported in all 50 states, but the geographic distribution of cases—which has shifted over time—varies considerably from one region to another. In 1988, the annual incidence of reported cases of AIDS ranged from a high of 81.2 cases per 100,000 persons in Washington, D.C., and 38.9 per 100,000 persons in New York to a low of 0.6 per 100,000 persons in North Dakota (*MMWR,* S-4, 1989). Updated statistics are shown in Figure 8–6. Whereas before 1983, 63 percent of all AIDS cases in the United States were reported from New York, New Jersey, and Pennsylvania, this proportion gradually dropped to 32 percent of cases in 1988.

The U.S. Centers for Disease Control has noted that the reported cases of AIDS are underestimates because of incompleteness of reporting, delays in reporting, and the fact that not all persons with AIDS have access to adequate medical or diagnostic care, so that "reported AIDS cases may represent fewer than 80% of all cases of recognized or unrecognized severe morbidity associated with HIV infection" (*MMWR,* S-4, 1989, p. 4).

FIGURE 8–6

Acquired Immunodeficiency Syndrome (AIDS)—Cases per 100,000 Population, Reported to the CDC by State, United States, 1989

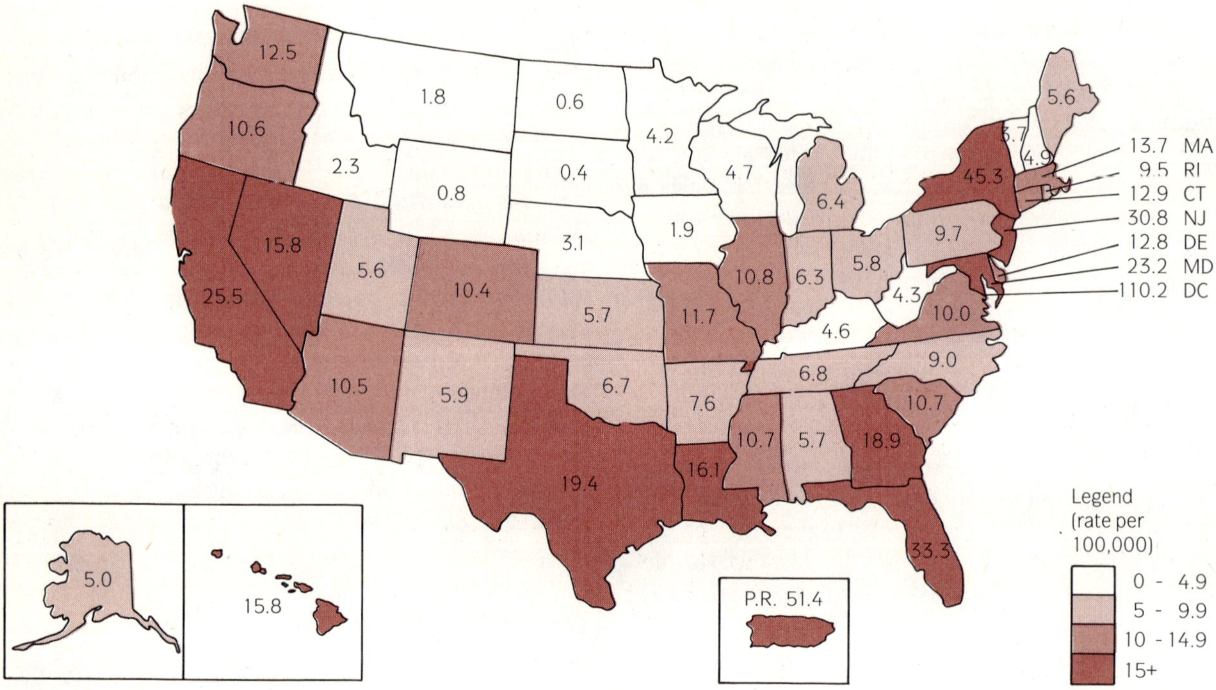

Source: MMWR 37 (54): 15, 1989.

PERSONAL ASPECTS OF THE HIV EPIDEMIC

The HIV/AIDS epidemic has many faces. Thus far in this chapter, we have primarily examined its biologic side. But the epidemic also has intensely personal aspects. Now we will turn to a discussion of the social, emotional, and behavioral facets of the HIV epidemic.

Social and Emotional Reactions

The impact of the HIV epidemic on our society has already been divisive and emotional. For many, the epidemic is a ready-made excuse for intensified prejudice against homosexuals, particularly among the misinformed, who think that shaking hands with a gay person or being served by a homosexual waiter could transmit a fatal infection. Some people have even suggested that everyone infected with HIV should be quarantined—a concept that is not only inhumane but also economically unfeasible since it would involve the enforced isolation for a period of many years of an estimated 1.5 million Americans now infected with HIV. Others are complacent about this major public health crisis because they mistakenly see AIDS as a problem confined to homosexuals, bisexuals, and drug users rather than a problem for American society as a whole.

Fortunately, our society's awareness of and sensitivity to the HIV/AIDS epidemic have been heightened considerably in the past few years by a number of small steps that have succeeded in humanizing and demystifying the epidemic. One particularly noteworthy step in this direction was the creation of the AIDS Quilt Project, begun in 1987 by Cleve Jones. This project was started as a way of memorializing a friend who had died of AIDS. It has now grown to a giant quilt containing more than 11,000 panels sewn by friends and families of persons who have died and has been viewed by millions. (A photograph of a portion of the Quilt Project is shown in the color insert, plate 12.)

Other signs of increased awareness of the HIV/AIDS epidemic crop up in diverse places. In many cities, obituaries now routinely mention AIDS as a cause of death, in contrast to the situation just 5 or 6 years ago, when the topic seemed taboo. AIDS fund-raisers hosted by well-known entertainers such as Elizabeth Taylor and Madonna are frequent and successful in raising funds for research. Even television soap operas have woven AIDS-related story lines into their scripts, although the same national television networks still refuse to air condom advertisements because of worries about the sensitivities of some of their viewers.

In the gay community, which has clearly been most directly affected in the first decade of the HIV epidemic, the initial fear and dismay quickly gave way to highly organized educational efforts combined with compassionate caring for people with AIDS and active lobbying for more government funding, antidiscrimination legislation, and streamlined guidelines for approving new treatment methods. Recognition of the realities of sexual transmission of HIV has generally led to widespread changes in the sexual behavior of this group: Most gay men now avoid the bathhouse scene entirely and a large number have cut back to having sex with only a small number of partners who are well-known to them (*The New York Times,* October 13, 1985, p. L41; Riesenberg, 1986; Winkelstein et al., 1987). In addition, a large majority of gay men have adopted safer sex practices, either by avoiding anal sex entirely or by carefully using condoms for anal intercourse (Becker and Joseph, 1988; Turner, Miller, and Moses, 1989). As a result of these patterns, particularly the cut-back in number of sexual partners, the incidence of other STDs such as gonorrhea and syphilis in gay men has also declined noticeably.

There are also some homosexual males who are so overwhelmed by fear of AIDS that they decide to be completely abstinent sexually until a vaccine or cure is found. In an occasional variation on this theme, a small number of male homosexuals and bisexuals have switched to heterosexual partners, at least temporarily. And, for reasons that are more than understandable, it is not unusual to find homosexual men who have developed such a degree of AIDS anxiety that they have become preoccupied with every minor physical ailment they experience. To these gay men, a sore throat, a skin rash, or a fever is a sign of impending doom, and they may even mistakenly tell their partners that they have AIDS before it is diagnosed. Among the very fearful it is common to see a sharp drop in sexual interest and sexual activity.

Anyone who discovers that one of his or her previous sex partners has AIDS or tests positive for HIV infection has definite reason for concern. So far in the epidemic, this situation has primarily affected gays and IV drug users, but heterosexuals are increasingly

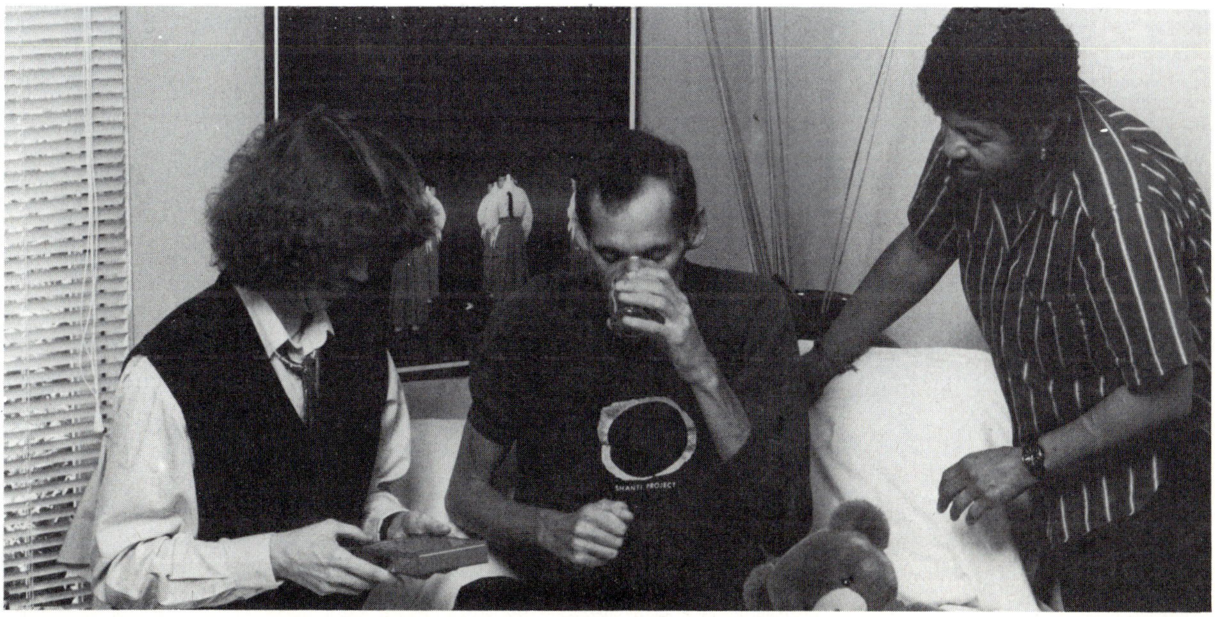

Two women help an AIDS patient at a hospice take his medicine.

AIDS

We are stretched
to meet a new dimension
Of love, a more demanding range
Where despair and hope must intertwine.
How grow to meet it? Intention
Here can neither move nor change
The raw truth. Death is on the line.
It comes to separate and estrange
Lover from lover in some reckless design.
Where do we go from here?

Fear. Fear. Fear. Fear.

Our world has never been more stark
Or more in peril.
It is very lonely now in the dark.
Lonely and sterile.

And yet in the simple turn of a head
Mercy lives. I heard it when someone said
"I must go now to a dying friend.
Every night at nine I tuck him into bed,
And give him a shot of morphine,"
And added, "I go where I have never been."
I saw he meant into a new discipline
He had not imagined before, and a new grace.
Every day now we meet it face to face.
Every day now devotion is the test.
Through the long hours, the hard, caring nights
We are forging a new union. We are blest.

As closed hands open to each other
Closed lives open to strange tenderness.
We are learning the hard way how to mother.

Who says it is easy? But we have the power.
I watch the faces deepen all around me.
It is the time of change, the saving hour.
The word is not fear, the word we live,
But an old word suddenly made new,
As we learn it again, as we bring it alive:

Love. Love. Love. Love.

Source: "AIDS" is reprinted from THE SILENCE NOW, New and Uncollected Earlier Poems by May Sarton, by permission of W.W. Norton & Company, Inc. Copyright © 1988 by May Sarton.

---

going to have to confront the same possibility as the HIV epidemic spreads into the broad population. Just how does it feel to be in such a situation?

> *A 28-year-old heterosexual man:* I heard from a friend that a girl I used to date had come down with AIDS. At first I thought it was just a crazy story, something to try to scare me with, but when I checked it out I was horrified to discover it was true. God, I thought, we had sex together a couple of dozen times, and we never used a condom because she was on the pill. My doctor sent me for a blood test, which much to my relief came back okay, but in the 24 hours before I got that report I can only say that I had visions of a slow, agonizing death right before my eyes, and I was plenty worried. You can be sure that I'll remember this episode for a long time.

> *A 33-year-old divorced woman:* I had been divorced for about three years when I found out my "ex" was in the hospital with AIDS. I knew he had messed around with drugs from time to time, but I never thought of him as addicted or anything like that. So this news shook me up pretty badly. When I was tested myself and the doctor told me I was positive, I broke down on the spot and cried. I have two kids, and I'm not ready to die. So far I've been lucky. My T cell count is pretty good and I haven't had any major problems, just some minor infections and stuff. But I am still furious that he did this to me, even though I know he didn't mean to. (Authors' files)

For some heterosexuals, concern about AIDS is mounting as people become aware that AIDS is not just a homosexual disease. For instance, it is not unusual now for a person to ask a potential partner to have a blood test for HIV antibody before beginning sexual relations. As one college-age woman told us, "It's not that I'm totally nervous about AIDS, but considering the stakes are so high, what's the purpose in pretending that everyone you'll meet will be honest? If someone doesn't care enough about me to have the test, the relationship isn't going to go anywhere anyway" (Authors' files). But as we will discuss shortly, many heterosexuals continue to demonstrate complacency about their personal risks of encountering HIV or becoming infected with it.

Immediately after learning that they are infected with HIV or that they have AIDS, most people react with shock, anger, and denial. Here is how it is described by a counselor at one HIV testing center in New York:

> Typical responses have included crying hysterically, going blank and numb, ranting and shouting—"I'm going to die now!"—and questioning—"Did the test tell how long I have to live?" Some clients try to bolt out of the office. . . . Some clients report that they were prepared for this and have a plan of action/treatment. Most clients, however, are "freaked out." (James, 1990, p. 280.)

These are perfectly normal defense mechanisms that can initially cushion the blow of receiving such a diagnosis. In the weeks or months after the diagnosis, this initial reaction typically undergoes a transition to guilt, sadness, and resignation to one's fate—a sort of unhappy acceptance of the situation. Of course, different people react in very different ways.

People who are diagnosed as being HIV infected or having AIDS are usually young adults who have generally been healthy, so they have relatively little preparation for facing a life-threatening disease with a very bleak prognosis. As if this was not difficult enough, those who are infected, whether gay or straight, must also face a hostile and fearful society. Many are ostracized at work, rejected by their family and friends, and put in a situation of social isolation (Volberding, 1985). It is emotionally difficult to find that your landlord wants to evict you, that your dentist refuses to take care of you any longer, or that your employer wants to fire you—all of which are uncalled for discriminatory actions. Fortunately, federal legislation that prohibits discrimination against the disabled has been extended to apply to people with AIDS and people infected with HIV, but such legislation doesn't change people's attitudes quickly.

The scope of the emotional anguish people with AIDS must face is often even broader than the discriminatory problems just listed. Consider, for instance, the situation of a woman who knows she is dying from AIDS and has just discovered that her six-month-old baby is also infected with HIV. Who will care for her baby after her death? How can she resolve the guilt she probably feels over transmitting this infection to her child? And who will care for her four year-old child who *isn't* HIV-infected? As another example, what about the personal turmoil in the life of a woman infected from a blood transfusion who has unwittingly transmitted her HIV infection to her husband?

As another problem you might expect, people infected with HIV also are apt to have sexual difficulties. In a study of 120 gay men who were infected with HIV, Meyer-Bahlburg and co-workers (1989) found that two-fifths of their sample reported decreased sexual satisfaction, two-fifths had some degree of difficulty with erectile failure, and more than half had some degree of negative feelings during sex. A similar interview-survey of a group of 50 HIV-infected heterosexuals noted that a drop in sexual desire is common and that more than 40 percent have had the appearance of symptoms of sexual dysfunction (Kolodny and Kolodny, 1990).

In addition to the emotional anguish caused by dealing with all of these issues, people with AIDS must face the prospect of numerous medical complications and hospitalizations, must deal with concerns about the economic cost of their illness, and must come to terms with their own identities and emotions as part of the ultimate task of preparing for death.

Behavioral Aspects

Although it is clear that in the absence of an effective vaccine or cure it will require massive changes in patterns of sexual and drug-related behavior to stem the tide of the HIV epidemic, there is little evidence that such changes are occurring in the general population.

The gay community has been a major exception. It has been notably successful in implementing risk-reducing behavior since the exact nature of the AIDS epidemic became clear. While widespread changes have occurred, these changes have been "expectably incomplete" (Becker and Joseph, 1988), and concerns are now mounting that a "second wave" of HIV infections in younger gay men may be occurring (Linn et al., 1989; Staver, 1990). Part of the reason for this is that widespread use of drugs and alcohol by young

PERSONAL PERSPECTIVES

Dealing with the Realities of AIDS

The following letter, which has been edited only to remove identifying information, was written by a 31-year-old man who had been found to have AIDS approximately three months earlier.

> My first reaction to the news, as you might imagine, was one of absolute shock and disbelief. I had been all too aware of the mysterious plague that was haunting us all, yet I hardly imagined it could affect me, of all people. After all, I generally was rather fastidious in my choice of sexual partners. After a few bleak, disheartening visits to the baths years ago, I had sworn off the faceless, nameless, passionless groping that others have only given up recently out of fear. My choice was made for aesthetic reasons, not because of the danger of lurking microbes, yet apparently I should have thought more about those evil microbial beings, for it seems they were searching for me, looking for a moment of weakness to spring and seize my soul.
>
> I spent weeks trying to decide who had betrayed me. In my mind, I had decided on three likely candidates, but eventually I realized the futility of this cerebral detective game. Instead, I became more concerned with practical matters. I wrote a will, spoke to my best friends, and tried to come to grips with the knowledge that I probably had—at best—two years to live.
>
> I must be honest with you and tell you that the thought of suicide crossed my mind. I told my parents that I had an unusual form of leukemia, since news of the true diagnosis would have probably killed them both. . . .
>
> When I was in the hospital, I began to notice that people avoided me in a variety of ways. Not only did the nurses and orderlies and people delivering food rush in and out of my room as though pausing to talk might infect them, too, even my doctor kept a determined distance between us. This distance, which I've now come to accept, was perhaps most apparent in the fact that very few people, including my friends, could bear to have eye contact with me. When I looked directly at them, they diverted their gaze, as though ashamed or afraid.
>
> I'm not a religious person, as you know, but I've been praying a lot lately. There's little else to do except hope for a medical miracle, because right now it looks like the odds are a million to one against my making it. If that honesty is too brutal for you to bear, think how it makes me feel. Now I know how a prisoner on death row must feel as he awaits his execution date.
>
> I suppose that my brothers in the gay world are rightfully distraught because this gruesome epidemic is turning back the clock. But it's hard for me now to think about equal rights and the movement. For me, equal rights would mean being able to live. If that's selfishness, I suppose I have a terminal case.

The author of this letter died in late 1983, less than a year after the original diagnosis was made.

gay men may be altering their judgment and their planning for using safer sex practices. Another reason is that some people tire of following safer sex guidelines and relapse to risky behavior patterns (Miller, Turner, and Moses, 1990).

For example, in a longitudinal study done in San Francisco, it was noted that between 1985 and 1986 the average number of sex partners decreased by 20 percent for those men not in a monogamous relationship, but 37 percent of the men continued to engage in sexual activities that were "probably risky" (such as ingesting semen during oral–genital sex) and 38 percent still engaged in high risk activities such as anal sex without a condom (Stall et al., 1986). Through the end of 1987, while almost a third of the subjects changed to and maintained low-risk behaviors, 16 percent relapsed to risky sex after an initial short-term behavior change (Ekstrand et al., 1989). A similar longitudinal study done in New York showed that 48 percent of the gay men studied continued to engage in risky sex, including sex with multiple anonymous partners, and that for every two men who shifted to safer sex practices over time, one slipped back from safer sex to riskier sex (Siegel et al., 1988).

A number of other studies also show, collectively, that positive behavioral changes have occurred among gay and bisexual males, but that these risk-reducing changes are far from complete (Martin, 1986, Joseph et al., 1987; Becker and Joseph, 1988; Doel et al., 1989). One review of 24 separate studies of changes in sexual behavior by gay men in response to AIDS found that overall, approximately 20 percent had not altered their unsafe sex practices and that a portion of this resistance to change was probably due to frequent use of recreational drugs (Stempel and Moss, 1988). For example, substantial numbers of gay men continue to engage in anal sex with multiple partners—even though these men know that they are infected with HIV (van Griensven et al., 1989). About half of these men either do not use condoms at all or use them very erratically (Masters, Johnson, and Kolodny, 1988, van Griensven et al., 1989; Linn et al., 1989).

Among heterosexuals there seems to be considerably less concern for safe sex in terms of changed behavior, although the matter has not been studied in much detail. One recent study in San Francisco found that among patrons of bars, single heterosexual women were less likely to engage in safe sex practices than single homosexual men (McKusick and Hoff, 1989). In another study, it was found that only 6 of 200 heterosexual women who had at least 6 sex partners a year routinely asked their partners to use condoms during vaginal intercourse (Masters, Johnson, and Kolodny, 1988). Likewise, a survey of Canadian college students reported that among those with more than 10 sex partners, only 21 percent of the men and 7.5 percent of the women used condoms regularly (MacDonald et al., 1990). And a recent study of women in the military found that a growing number are becoming infected with HIV "through unprotected sex with bisexual or IV [intravenous] drug-using men" even though most of them reported having only one or two sexual partners (Staver, 1990).

Although condom sales jumped dramatically in the late 1980s as a result of the public's awareness of AIDS, regular condom use has not become very common among heterosexuals, nor have heterosexuals in general shifted to strictly monogamous sex. One indication of this is that from 1986 to 1987, rates of syphilis in the United States jumped by more than 80 percent (*MMWR* 38, 39), with the rise attributable entirely to more cases in the heterosexual population. The incidence of syphilis continued to increase in 1988 and 1989, confirming that there has been little behavioral change in spite of a growing number of

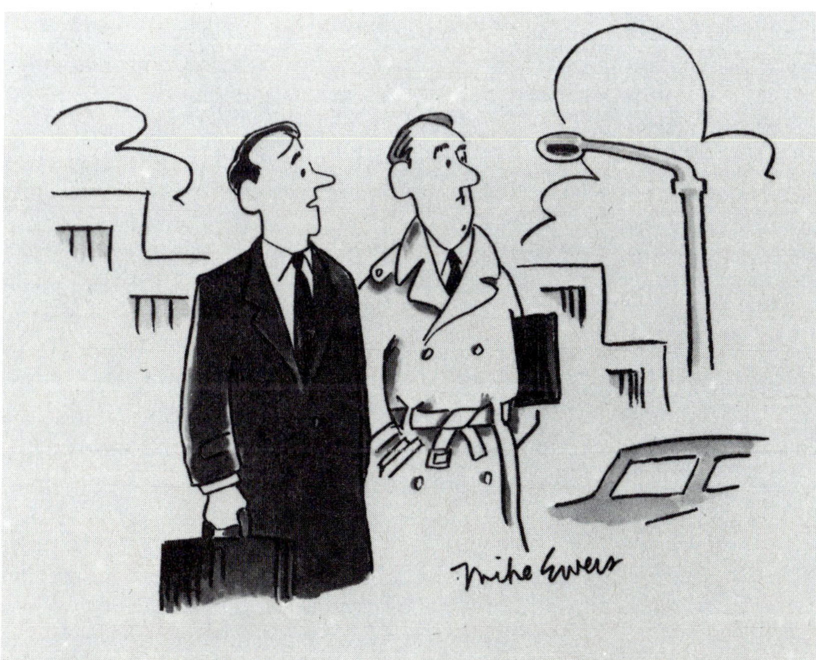

"REMEMBER WHEN 'SAFE SEX' MEANT HER HUSBAND WAS OUT OF TOWN?"

AIDS cases due to heterosexual transmission. In fact, even among persons attending STD clinics, condom use is sporadic at best (*MMWR* 39: 685–689, 1990). And only a minority of sexually active adolescents uses condoms at all (Goodwin, 1990).

Other signs of a general lack of concern in most heterosexuals about the HIV epidemic are apparent, although no one has thoroughly studied them as yet. For instance, in most urban areas prostitution continues to thrive, despite considerable publicity about the possible transmission of HIV. (Since a majority of prostitutes are also IV drug users, there is an obvious danger of HIV infection with such sexual activity [Turner, Miller, and Moses, 1989].) Furthermore, most male customers of prostitutes prefer not to use condoms; although few data are available on this point, one recent study showed that about half of the men who patronized prostitutes never used condoms, and many others used condoms erratically (Wallace et al., 1988).

Condom use is also very low in black and Hispanic groups who are at heightened risk of exposure to HIV infection because of widespread drug use in their communities (Altman, 1989; Miller, Turner, and Moses, 1990; *MMWR* 39: 685–689, 1990). In addition to this cultural bias, there is another relatively recent development contributing to the spread of HIV: The use of cocaine in a particularly powerful form known as crack. The use of crack cocaine, which is highly addictive, is often done in binges of almost continual use over several days. In order to support their drug habits, many female crack addicts resort to prostitution (often with as many as 10 or more clients per day); since many of their clients have a history of IV drug abuse, and thus have a heightened likelihood of HIV infection, many observers believe this has become an important factor in the heterosexual transmission of HIV (Goldsmith, 1988; Weiss, 1989; Miller, Turner, and Moses, 1990).

Even in more "traditional" settings, there are many indications that inadvertent HIV transmission is not unusual in the heterosexual world at large. Walk through a singles bar on a weekend evening, or browse through the classified personal ads in many newspapers and magazines, and you will quickly realize that heterosexuals have hardly given up on the sexual revolution. Despite lip service to the notion of safe sex, many heterosexuals continue to behave sexually much as they did in the days before AIDS, which is certainly understandable since many have been led to believe that AIDS is "just" a gay disease. This was borne out in a national poll conducted by the *Los Angeles Times* in mid-1989 that showed concern about AIDS among the general public declining, as well as a drop in people who say they have made substantial changes in their life-styles because of the epidemic (*Stamford Advocate,* July 16, 1989, p. B1).

The following comments from interviews with single heterosexuals in late 1990 reflect this overall sense of complacency (Authors' files):

> *A twenty-six-year-old woman:* I don't want to sound like a fool, but I don't know anyone with AIDS, and I doubt that the guys I would date are shooting up drugs or anything like that. Maybe if I lived in New York or San Francisco I'd be more worried, but I don't want to live my life in fear.
>
> *A twenty-nine-year-old man:* I think the papers made too big a thing out of the whole AIDS business. Last year I heard a government report that said the epidemic was leveling off. And even though I've had sex with five or six partners every year, I've never had a problem.

The same lack of concern is all too apparent on college campuses today, where despite well-intended attempts at preventive AIDS education, sexual behavior patterns are not much different from a decade ago. Several surveys of college students bear this out, showing that relatively few students are worried about personal exposure to HIV or are consistently using safer sex practices (Baldwin and Baldwin, 1988; DeBuono et al., 1990; MacDonald et al., 1990). One of these studies, done in Southern California with a sample of 851 students, found that 66 percent had not used condoms at all in the preceding three months despite being sexually active. In addition, students with four or more sex partners annually were not using condoms more than students with fewer partners per year (Baldwin and Baldwin, 1988). Similarly, a survey of 350 students at a large East Coast university showed that most felt they had little or no risk of exposure to HIV, and also felt that they could somehow intuitively sense when a prospective sexual partner wasn't "safe." Many said that they did not use condoms at all, and "In general, students equated 'safer sex' with 'not-for-fun' sex" (Caron and McMullen, 1987).

These attitudes are commonplace on campuses across the country. The medical director of the student health service at a large midwestern university recently described it this way, requesting anonymity so he could avoid getting embroiled in political problems from the administration:

Students here seem almost oblivious to the AIDS epidemic, as though it doesn't travel to this part of the country. We can see this from the soaring chlamydial epidemic we have going on, which is sort of a marker for sexual behavior. What no one realizes is that we had five HIV-infected students diagnosed here last year—but the president of the university has put a tight lid on the news, because he's afraid of the reaction from alumni donors and prospective freshmen if news leaked out about this problem. (Authors' files)

The situation on college campuses is not unusual; in many ways, it mirrors the broader picture fairly accurately. We have not, as yet, succeeded very well in implementing widespread behavioral change to fight the HIV epidemic because the American public has received mixed messages, watered-down messages, and often no messages at all about what needs to be done to turn the tide (Shilts, 1987; Masters, Johnson, and Kolodny, 1988; Turner, Miller, and Moses, 1989). Politicians and religious leaders have blocked many efforts at developing educational materials about AIDS with public funding because of concerns that they would be too sexually explicit; school-based AIDS education programs have frequently foundered because of arguments over the "moral" way to teach about AIDS and HIV (for instance, some people claim it is only permissible to teach that abstinence is the only way to avoid AIDS); on some college campuses, condom dispensers have been removed to avoid offending certain alumni groups. Until more effective HIV/AIDS education messages are sent to the public, this epidemic will probably continue to grow at a frightening rate.

PUBLIC POLICY ISSUES

The history of the early years of the HIV epidemic, thoroughly chronicled in Randy Shilt's book, *And the Band Played On* (1987), is in many ways a story of tragic dimensions. Lives were wasted and precious time was lost in combatting a deadly disease because of homophobia, complacency, and the federal government's relative inaction. For instance, in 1983, *Time* quoted Donald Currie, then manager of the San Francisco Kaposi's sarcoma hotline, as saying, "If the same number of Boy Scouts had been dying of this, there would have been a hell of a lot more money for research" (*Time,* March 28, 1983, p. 55). Yet it was still almost five years before the government approved adequate funds for AIDS research (Winkenwerder, Kessler, and Stolec, 1989). Even as recently as 1990, Larry Kramer, founder of Gay Men's Health Crisis, has said, "I am so frightened that the war against AIDS has already been lost. It is beyond comprehension why, in a presumably civilized country, in the modern era, such a continuing, extraordinary destruc-

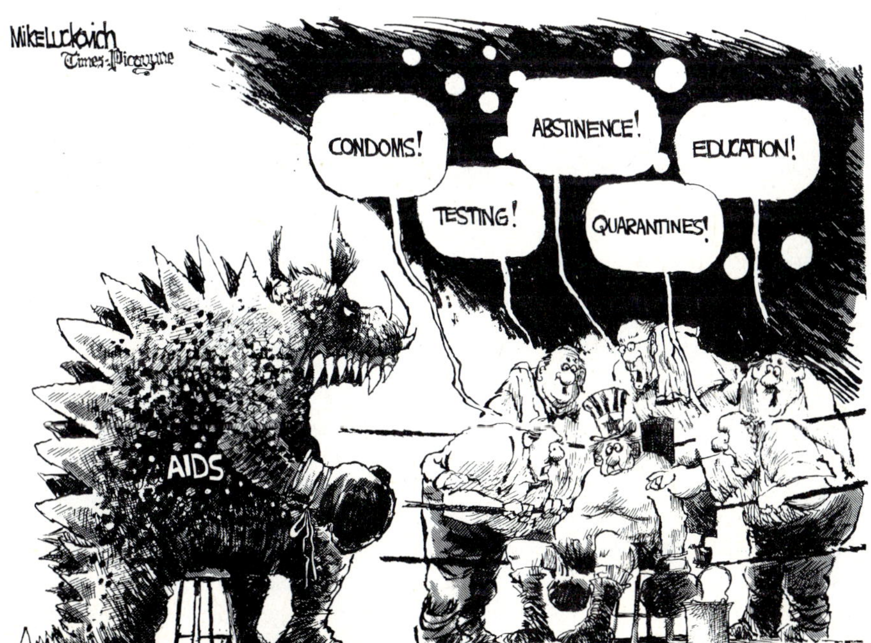

By permission of Mike Kovitch and Creators Syndicate.

tion of life is being attended to so tentatively, so meekly and in such a cowardly fashion" (Kramer, 1990).

Today there is still considerable complacency about the epidemic. Homophobia continues to play a major role in how people view questions about HIV infection and AIDS. There is another side to our ineffectiveness in dealing with the epidemic, however. For years, more emphasis was put on protecting individual rights to privacy than protecting public health. Furthermore, much-needed research on sexual behavior and other aspects of the HIV epidemic has been stalled or killed for strictly political reasons. Implementation of a federally funded national sex research survey—a study that many believe is essential to fighting successfully against the further spread of HIV (Turner, Miller, and Moses, 1989)—was blocked because a handful of politicians objected to asking explicit questions about private sexual behavior (*USA Today,* March 31, 1989, p. D1).

Given this hodge-podge situation with different groups arguing for and against certain policy choices for their own self-interested reasons, it can be difficult to sort out the issues. The following discussion of a number of pivotal policy issues draws on the recommendations of the National Research Council, the Institute of Medicine of the National Academy of Sciences, and the Presidential Commission on the HIV Epidemic (as well as other authoritative sources) to present consensus opinions emerging at the beginning of the 1990s on how to proceed in our efforts to control the HIV/AIDS epidemic.

Education and Research

Since it is clear that science, by itself, cannot stop the spread of this epidemic (even if a vaccine were discovered tomorrow, it would take years of testing before it would receive approval and become widely available), it is important that every effort be made to implement widespread behavioral changes in our society to control the spread of HIV. To be effective, this type of education must go beyond simply informing people about facts—it must also motivate them to modify their behavior.

We have previously recommended the following steps for development of broad educational programs in this country (Masters, Johnson, and Kolodny, 1988):

1. A comprehensive AIDS curriculum must be developed for widespread use in public schools. In order to be effective, such a program must begin well before young people begin to engage in sexual activity and drug use, which means such programs must begin no later than fourth or fifth grade.
2. Special education programs must be targeted at specific groups whose behaviors or situations place them at high risk of being exposed to HIV. These include intravenous drug abusers and their sex partners, homosexual and bisexual men, prostitutes and their customers, and heterosexuals who have multiple sex partners. Furthermore, special programs must be developed for groups that may have unique requirements in program design, including minority populations, the blind and the deaf, and people who cannot read.
3. A broad-based, multimedia general education campaign that encourages responsible behavior should be undertaken as soon as possible. This campaign should encompass the television and movie community (where scriptwriters can incorporate warnings about HIV into their prime-time shows or movies), celebrities from the world of rock, sports stars, and other high visibility spokespersons who have particular credibility with adolescents and young adults.
4. All colleges and universities should provide their students with extensive educational and counseling services related to prevention of HIV infection.
5. To coordinate and implement the entire educational effort, a special office should be created in the U.S. Department of Health and Human Services and it should be given enough budgetary support and administrative power to accomplish its mission.

In addition, it is imperative that the progress that has been made in the last decade in fighting the HIV epidemic be built on and expanded by promptly and intensively increasing behavioral and biomedical research (Institute of Medicine, 1988; Presidential Commission, 1988; Turner, Miller, and Moses, 1989).

Testing

Earlier in the course of the HIV epidemic, there was considerable resistance to the idea of widespread testing for the presence of infection because of concerns about the accuracy of the blood tests that were available, concerns about privacy and confidentiality, and a sense of futility: What good did it do to know that you're infected with the AIDS virus if there was no treatment available to prolong your life? Today, there is a vastly different perspective on this issue: Most experts agree that virtually anyone at risk should undergo confidential testing on a voluntary basis (Lo et al., 1989; Francis et al., 1989; Cohen, Sande, and Volberding, 1990).

The reasons for this change are relatively straightforward. First, the accuracy of tests for HIV infection have improved significantly. Second, worries about lack of confidentiality of test results have been lessened considerably as many states have passed legislation specifically addressing this issue and as many states provide anonymous testing sites. Most important, however, early detection of HIV infection is the only way to ensure early medical treatment, and it is clear that early medical treatment can prolong life and prevent (or at least postpone) some of the serious complications of AIDS (Arno et al., 1989; Francis et al., 1989; Friedland, 1990.)

Widespread voluntary testing also leads to many personal benefits. For example, in many cases, persons who have been tested will discover that they are *not* infected, which will not only be psychologically reassuring, but may also help them make important personal decisions about marriage, pregnancy, or other issues. On the other hand, people who discover that they are infected can (1) protect their sexual partners from infection; (2) make arrangements for appropriate medical care; (3) avoid situations where they would have additional exposures to HIV; and (4) make informed plans concerning careers, insurance, finances, and other related matters.

There are certainly some personal drawbacks to widespread testing. For one thing, positive test results may cause profound anxiety or depression. A second problem is the small chance of having a false positive result, which could certainly have a serious impact on a person's life. Another difficulty is that unless your test results are absolutely confidential (not all tests done in hospitals or doctors' offices are, especially if you sign a form authorizing the release of your medical records to an insurance company), you may find that you encounter problems. For example, military applicants who turn out to be HIV positive are denied jobs in the military. And someone who tests positive may have difficulty obtaining certain types of insurance coverage in the future.

Widespread voluntary testing also benefits the general public as well as individuals. For example, public health authorities would gain a better picture of trends in the HIV epidemic and would be better able to address broad policy issues such as educational campaigns and other prevention programs targeted at special population groups. Furthermore, this sort of information is essential to the economic planning that will be needed to deal with the epidemic in the future, as well as the planning for the delivery of health-care services.

While mandatory testing of blood, organ, and tissue donors and the military population is currently in place in the United States, attempts at mandatory premarital testing for HIV proved ineffective in Illinois and Louisiana and have now been discontinued. Routine (but not mandatory) prenatal HIV screening has been advocated by some experts but has not yet been implemented in most locales (Minkoff et al., 1988).

Public Health Measures

Contact tracing and notification—tracking down the sex partners of people with a reportable STD and informing them that they may have been exposed, without revealing the identity of the "index case"—has been one of the most time-tested public health strategies (Gostin, 1989). In fact, public health statutes usually authorize contact tracing for STDs, but in an odd quirk, most states today do not classify HIV infection as an STD. (The reason for this is that these states wish to avoid the automatic contact tracing programs that would be triggered by existing laws if HIV infection was classified as an STD.) Nevertheless, a number of states, such as Colorado, and cities have implemented contact tracing and notification programs, with generally good results. A few other states, such as California, have a voluntary contact tracing program.

By focusing on people with a high probability of exposure to HIV, contact tracing is efficient in detecting those with previously unidentified infection. This detection has important implications for prevention in two ways: (1) uninfected sex partners of an already infected person are warned that they have been exposed, which may lead them to behavioral changes that would reduce their risk of subsequent infection and (2) identifying persons with a previously undetected HIV infection should allow them to take steps to protect their own sex partners, minimizing the risk of spreading HIV further.

There has been some controversy about the physician's role in contact tracing and partner notification. Concerns about protecting the confidentiality of HIV-infected persons have created conflicting opinions on this issue, but in many states, including New York and California, while protecting patient confidential-

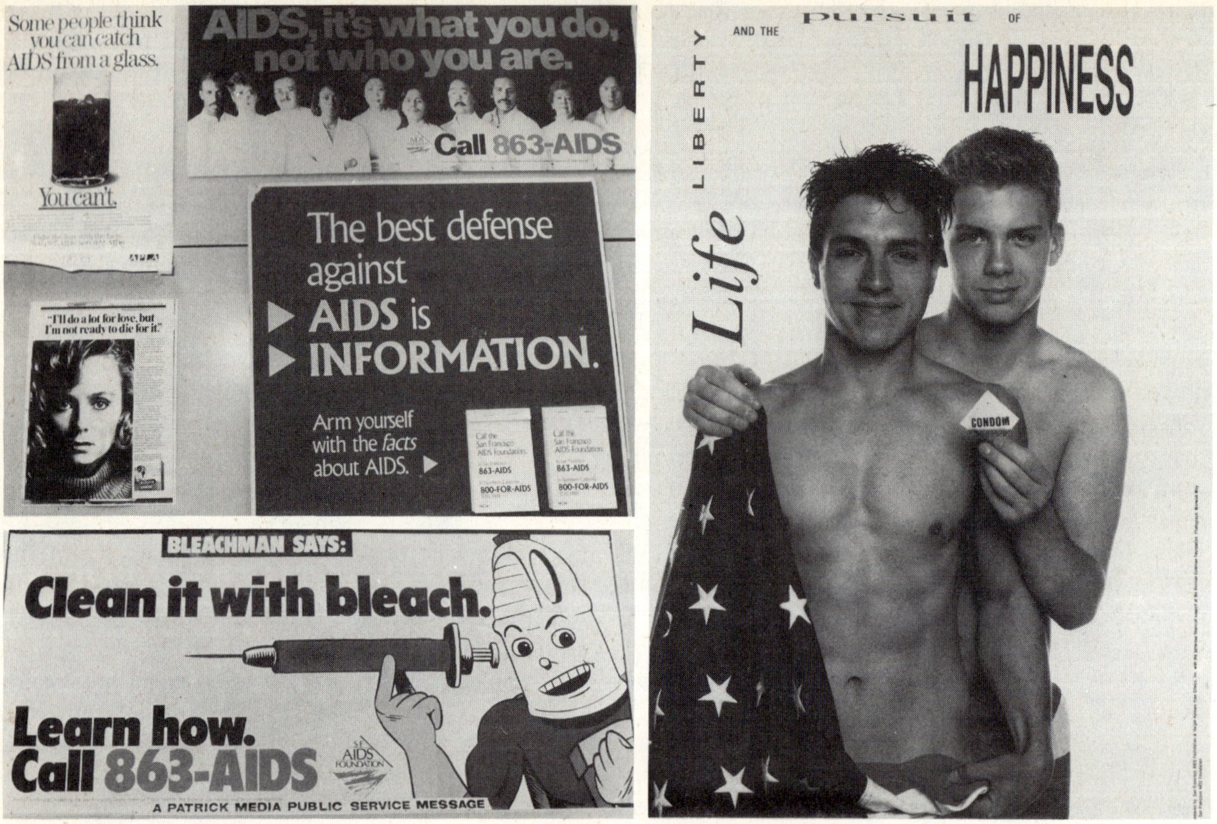
Some people think you can catch AIDS from a glass.
You can't.
AIDS, it's what you do, not who you are.
Call 863-AIDS
"I'll do a lot for love, but I'm not ready to die for it."
The best defense against AIDS is INFORMATION.
Arm yourself with the facts about AIDS.
863-AIDS
800-FOR-AIDS
BLEACHMAN SAYS:
Clean it with bleach.
Learn how.
Call 863-AIDS
A PATRICK MEDIA PUBLIC SERVICE MESSAGE
Life
LIBERTY
AND THE
pursuit
OF
HAPPINESS
CONDOM

A wide variety of educational posters have been used to reach different target populations. The poster showing two naked young men wrapped in a U.S. flag was funded by the San Francisco AIDS Foundation in 1990 after research showed that many young gay men were having sex without using condoms.

ity is a legal obligation, there is also a responsibility to warn anyone who is in clear and imminent danger of becoming infected. This means that if an HIV-infected man refuses to inform his sex partners of his infection, a physician is authorized to disclose this information to the partners in order to protect their health and well-being (Dalton, Burris, and the Yale AIDS Law Project, 1987).

Although public health laws in all jurisdictions in this country carry provisions for quarantine of persons with communicable diseases, and a few states have laws authorizing the compulsory isolation of persons with AIDS or HIV infection who are aware of this but continue to engage in high-risk behaviors (Gostin, 1989), there is virtual unanimity among public health authorities that quarantine is unnecessary—and inhumane—in the HIV epidemic (Cohen, Sande, and Volberding, 1990).

Another possible public health measure that has stirred considerable controversy is the use of *sterile needle and syringe exchange programs* as a means of reducing the spread of HIV among intravenous drug abusers. While such programs have been operating successfully in Europe for years, in the United States they have been primarily restricted to small-scale pilot projects in a few cities such as New York, Seattle, and Portland, Oregon. The main obstacle in America is concern that providing sterile needles and syringes to drug abusers is condoning an illegal act and might lead to more widespread drug abuse (Stryker, 1989). The available evidence suggests that this isn't happening in Europe, but needle-exchange programs do not eliminate HIV risk behavior, either (Miller, Turner, and Moses, 1990).

Antidiscrimination Issues

Because AIDS first appeared in this country in groups that were already stigmatized—homosexuals and IV drug abusers—society's response has been strongly shaped by bias, assignments of blame, and a disregard for the needs of those most directly affected by the epidemic. In addition, fears about casual transmission of HIV that were widespread in the early days of the epidemic (fears that have now been effectively proven to be unfounded) fueled many examples of discriminatory responses to people with AIDS or HIV infection. For instance, office workers sometimes shunned a colleague with AIDS because of worries that they might become infected by indirect physical contact with him. Landlords tried to evict tenants with AIDS on the grounds that they had an easily communicable disease that might affect other building occupants. In some particularly sad cases, infected children have been banned from attending school on the grounds that they posed a health hazard to their classmates.

Today we have made a good deal of progress in moving beyond these discriminatory practices, but fear of discrimination is still a major stumbling block to the acceptance of potentially effective public health strategies by gay rights groups and other AIDS activists. The federal Rehabilitation Act of 1973, section 504, prohibits discrimination against "otherwise qualified" handicapped persons, and the courts have consistently found that HIV-related conditions are covered by this—but the coverage only applies to federally funded programs (Gostin, 1989). To address this issue, legislative attempts to counter HIV-related discrimination have already been passed in many states. It will probably take a growing realization that HIV infects people from all walks of life (not just gay and bisexual men and IV drug abusers) to change attitudes toward the epidemic enough so that HIV-infected persons are regarded no differently than people with cancer, heart disease, or high blood pressure.

Additional Considerations

Society must face a large number of challenging issues as part of addressing the HIV epidemic. What can be done about the problem of HIV infection in the homeless? Who will care for HIV-infected babies whose parents have died of AIDS? How can we put an end to the patterns of drug abuse that contribute in major ways to the spread of HIV infection? How will we finance the health-care requirements of the hundreds of thousands of people who are already HIV infected? Unfortunately, it is clear that the answers to these challenges are not always easy or affordable, so choices have to be made in terms of budgets and allocation of human resources and other means in this epic fight. One set of such recommendations is described in the section that follows.

THE PRESIDENT'S AIDS COMMISSION

In 1987, President Reagan created a special commission to investigate the HIV epidemic and to make recommendations that could be used to protect the public health, assist in finding a cure for AIDS, and provide care for those already infected. (As a historical note, it should be pointed out that many observers felt that the commission should have been created years earlier; furthermore, there was initially considerable controversy over the make-up of the commission, with many groups dismayed that the gay community was not adequately represented and others worried that the commission was lacking in medical and scientific expertise.) At the end of a year of hearing expert testimony from some 600 witnesses, the commission issued a widely acclaimed final report. Among its key recommendations were the following:

- Early diagnosis of HIV infection is essential both for obtaining optimal medical care and counseling and for protecting others. This requires encouragement of extensive voluntary testing.
- "HIV infection is a disability and should be treated as such under federal and state law. . . . Infected persons should be encouraged to continue normal activities, such as work or school, and live in their own home as long as they are able" (Presidential Commission, 1988, p. xviii)
- Strong measures should be implemented for protecting the confidentiality of persons who are infected with HIV. At the same time, public health authorities should immediately begin a system of confidential partner notification so that all partners who have been exposed to an HIV-infected person can be counseled, tested, and followed up.
- States should begin to require the reporting of all HIV-positive tests, not just cases of AIDS, to better track the course of the epidemic.
- Prevention and treatment of intravenous drug abuse should be made a top national priority. A new policy of "treatment on demand" should be implemented (at a cost to the government of about $1.5 billion annually), since the ability to control the course of the HIV epidemic depends to a large extent on being able to curtail IV drug abuse.

The commission also called for new federal and state funding to reverse the national nursing shortage, emphasized the need for developing comprehensive drug and alcohol education programs and "age appropriate, comprehensive health education programs" from kindergarten through grade twelve, and suggested that there is a responsibility for all citizens to treat HIV-infected persons with respect and compassion.

A CONCLUDING NOTE

The HIV epidemic can be stopped in its tracks if people take personal responsibility over their behavior by abstaining from IV drug use and consistently following safer sex guidelines.

Medical science today is technologically equipped to solve the puzzles of HIV infection—although how long it will take to accomplish this is not entirely clear.

But what is clear is this: Within the next few years, every single person in the United States will know someone who is infected with HIV. How we will respond to this challenge, both as individuals and as a society, cannot be known as yet. Yet one thing is certain: We are all in this together. As well-known author James Carroll puts it:

> Now no one is immune. Those things that have always cut us off from one another—sexism, homophobia, racism, hatred of addicts—have the additional effect of making this disease more powerful. However understandable the common impulse to blame is, however "human" it is, the fact now is that we indulge it at our common peril.
>
> The climate in which prevention thrives is marked not by blaming, but by caring. It is marked by the frank and open exchange of real information, even information that we once regarded as inappropriate for exchange. It is marked by willingness to consider, in the name of prevention, ideas and strategies that at first may offend us. We have to work constantly, in other words, at changing those attitudes that feed the infection, at keeping open minds as well as open hearts. (Carroll, 1990, pp. 20–21)

SUMMARY

1. Acquired immune deficiency syndrome (AIDS) is an illness resulting from infection with HIV, the human immunodeficiency virus. AIDS, which was first recognized as a clinical entity in 1981, is characterized by a breakdown of the body's immune defenses, ultimately leading to susceptibility to opportunistic infections and death.
2. Although the earliest cases of AIDS were detected primarily in homosexual and bisexual men and intravenous drug users, the pattern of the HIV/AIDS epidemic is changing today, with increasing numbers of people infected by heterosexual transmission and an increasing number of infections among women. Similarly, although the epidemic began heavily concentrated in New York and California, it has now expanded to involve the entire country.
3. As of the end of 1990, there had been a cumulative total of 160,000 cases of AIDS reported in the United States. This was only a small fraction of the estimated number of cases around the world, with Africa being the most heavily affected region.
4. HIV, a retrovirus believed to have evolved from a virus that infects monkeys in Africa, selectively attacks T-helper cells and macrophages once it gains entry to the body. Once HIV invades these white blood cells, it turns them into factories for manufacturing its own genetic information, in effect duplicating itself many times over. HIV particles actively attack other cells in the immune system and other parts of the body, including the brain, causing considerable damage.
5. HIV is transmitted by three primary routes: sexual contact, blood-to-blood transmission (as with needle sharing among intravenous drug users or with contaminated blood transfusions), and perinatally, from an infected mother to her infant. Anal intercourse—whether homosexual or heterosexual—is the riskiest form of sexual contact, but vaginal intercourse and oral–genital sex are also capable of transmitting HIV. HIV is *not* transmitted by casual contact (such as a handshake) or by mosquitoes.
6. Completely safe sex is only possible under a few sets of circumstances, including abstinence, restricting sexual contact only to activities that do not involve the exchange of body fluids, or sex in a mutually monogamous relationship between two uninfected partners. However, proper and consistent use of condoms reduces the risk of HIV transmission during sex. Limiting the number of sex partners also materially reduces the risk of exposure.
7. HIV infection can be detected by a number of different blood tests. The most commonly used screening test, the ELISA test, is only accepta-

ble if a positive result (indicating infection) is confirmed by another more sophisticated test. The Western blot test is usually used for this purpose. Using the two tests in combination, false positives are now very unusual—according to some studies, less than 1 in 100,000.

8. HIV infection proceeds through several distinct stages. The *initial infection* is often completely unrecognized, although 10 to 25 percent of people who are infected have a brief illness several weeks after the infection occurs. This is typically followed by an *asymptomatic carrier state* in which the person feels healthy but is a carrier of live HIV and is capable of infecting others. It is now known that this asymptomatic period can last for 7 to 10 years or longer. The next stage of illness is *symptomatic HIV infection,* in which destruction of the immune system begins to manifest by annoying but non–life-threatening infections such as shingles or thrush. Weight loss, swollen lymph nodes, and fatigue are other common symptoms. The last stage of HIV infection is full-blown *AIDS,* which may be accompanied by Kaposi's sarcoma (a form of skin cancer), *Pneumocystis carinii* pneumonia (a previously rare, often fatal lung infection), and a variety of neurological disorders and other opportunistic infections.

9. While HIV infection and AIDS are not curable, they are treatable. AZT (also known as zidovudine) prolongs life for AIDS patients and slows the progression to AIDS for those infected with HIV. Other drugs are effective in treating the opportunistic infections that occur commonly in AIDS, and currently a number of drugs are being studied as a means of combatting HIV infection. Vaccines that may be useful in treatment as well as prevention are currently being avidly pursued.

10. Counting cases of AIDS doesn't say a great deal about the dynamics of HIV infection today because it generally takes 7 to 10 years for AIDS to develop after the initial infection. Thus the focus is changing to emphasize tracking patterns of HIV infection. While infection rates are around 50 percent in homosexual and bisexual men in large cities in New York and California, elsewhere in the country they are generally in the range of 20 to 25 percent. Among intravenous drug users, infection rates also vary according to geography, with cities in the Northeast having rates in the 40 to 50 percent range, but relatively low rates (less than 10 percent) in the rest of the country. In the second decade of the HIV epidemic, there may be a shift of infections involving more women and more adolescents.

11. Although social reactions to the HIV/AIDS epidemic have been distorted by a combination of homophobia and complacency, along with fear about the possibility of casual contagiousness, there are signs that such prejudices (and the discrimination they cause) are lessening and awareness is improving.

12. The gay community has been remarkably successful in its campaigns to promote risk-reducing behavior and safer sex practices, resulting in a marked decline in the rate of new HIV infections in many areas. However, there are now signs that a "second wave" of HIV infections may be occurring in gay and bisexual men partly as a result of drug and alcohol use and partly because people are getting tired of being careful. Among heterosexuals, there is much less concern about the risk of contracting HIV. This is shown particularly by infrequent patterns of condom use, little (if any) reduction in number of sex partners, and participation in sexually risky acts. The link between crack cocaine and heterosexual transmission of HIV has also been recognized.

13. There are serious gaps in our nation's current approach to public policy issues related to this epidemic. For one thing, there is no national leadership for comprehensive HIV/AIDS educational efforts. For another, in spite of the availability of effective treatments for people with asymptomatic HIV infection, we have not succeeded in getting across the message that anyone at risk for this infection should voluntarily undergo testing. Lingering concerns about the frequency of false positive test results (which are now uncommon) and about possible breaches of confidentiality seem to be a part of the problem. In addition, standard practices used in combatting STDs have not been brought into play in the HIV/AIDS epidemic in most locations because of political pressures, although measures such as contact tracing and notification appear to be efficient and effective.

Thought Questions

1. Many cities and states have refused to initiate contact tracing and notification programs to locate and test the sexual partners of persons found to be infected with HIV. Do you think this is a good policy? Why or why not? If someone you had sex with several years ago was found to be

infected with HIV, would you want to be informed about it?

2. If you were pregnant and discovered you were infected with HIV, with a 20 to 50 percent chance of transmitting this infection to your baby, what would you do?
3. If you were a marriage counselor treating a couple and discovered that one of the partners was infected with HIV but refused to tell the other person despite the fact that they were having sex together, how would you proceed?
4. The press often publishes stories in which famous people are identified as being infected with HIV. The media contend that this is a legitimate function of a free press and that the public has a right to know such information, especially since it reminds them of the realities of the HIV/AIDS epidemic. But such disclosures violate the famous person's right to privacy and may pose problems for their families or their careers, as well. How do you feel on this issue?
5. In some cases, people who have been infected with HIV from sexual contact have sued the person who gave them the infection. Do you think this type of legal action is right or wrong? What if the person who transmitted the infection didn't realize he or she was infected? Would this change your thinking at all?

Suggested Readings

Bayer, Ronald. *Private Acts, Social Consequences.* New York: Free Press, 1989. A thoughtful analysis of the tensions between public health principles and individuals' rights in the context of the HIV epidemic.

Dalton, Harlon L., Burris, Scott, and the Yale AIDS Law Project. *AIDS and the Law.* New Haven, CT: Yale University Press, 1987. A detailed, comprehensive guide for the general public on ethical and legal questions posed by the HIV epidemic.

Institute of Medicine/National Academy of Sciences. *Confronting AIDS: Directions for Public Health, Health Care, and Research.* Washington, DC: National Academy Press, 1986; and *Confronting AIDS: Update 1988.* Washington, DC: National Academy Press, 1988. A well-balanced sourcebook, and its update, on policy issues; not highly technical in most regards, this well-referenced, balanced discussion examines the complex medical, social, ethical, and financial problems arising from the HIV/AIDS epidemic.

Miller, H. G., Turner, C. F., and Moses, L. E., eds. *AIDS—The Second Decade.* Washington, DC: National Academy Press, 1990. Emphasizing trends in the HIV/AIDS epidemic expected to emerge in the decade of the 1990s, this scholarly volume emphasizes the increasing risks to females and adolescents as the epidemic evolves. There is also a detailed examination of prevention strategies and methodological issues in AIDS surveys.

Shilts, Randy. *And the Band Played On: Politics, People, and the AIDS Epidemic.* New York: St. Martin's Press, 1987. An impressive history of the early years of the AIDS epidemic that is told in vivid detail. This book is must reading for anyone who wants to understand the background of our country's early response to AIDS.

Turner, Charles F., Miller, Heather G., and Moses, Lincoln E., eds. *AIDS: Sexual Behavior and Intravenous Drug Use.* Washington, DC: National Academy Press, 1989. A thorough discussion of various aspects of sexual behavior and IV drug use as they affect the transmission of HIV, with particular emphasis on implementing social strategies to reduce risky behavior.

9

Sexual Dysfunctions and Sex Therapy

Like many other body processes, when sexual function goes along smoothly, it is usually taken for granted and given little thought. But if sexual function is a problem in one way or another, it can be a source of anxiety, anguish, and frustration that often leads to general unhappiness and distress in personal relationships.

This chapter begins with a description of sexual dysfunction—conditions in which the ordinary physical responses of sexual function are impaired. Our attention then turns to the causes of these dysfunctions. The concluding portion of the chapter discusses the methods and effectiveness of sex therapy in dealing with these problems.

MALE SEXUAL DYSFUNCTION

For most men in most societies, sexual adequacy is considered a yardstick for measuring personal adequacy. The man who does not "measure up" sexually is often embarrassed, confused, or depressed over his plight, which he regards as reflecting poorly on his manhood. The sexually dysfunctional male may change his behavior to avoid sexual situations (fearing in advance that he will fail); he may cope with his dilemma by inventing excuses (blaming the dysfunction on his partner, for example); or he may try to overcome his problem by diligently "working" at sex, which usually makes the situation worse instead of better.

Erectile Dysfunction (Impotence)

Erectile dysfunction, or **impotence,** is the inability to have or maintain an erection that is firm enough for coitus. Erectile dysfunction is classified as either primary or secondary: the male with **primary erectile dysfunction** has never been able to have intercourse, whereas the male with **secondary erectile dysfunction** has succeeded in having intercourse once, twice, or a thousand times before his dysfunction began. Secondary erectile dysfunction is about ten times more common than primary erectile dysfunction (Kolodny, Masters, and Johnson, 1979).

Erectile dysfunction can occur at any age and can assume many different forms. Total absence of erection is infrequent except in certain medical conditions. More typically, the male with erectile dysfunction has partial erections that are too weak for vaginal insertion (or anal intercourse). Sometimes firm erections quickly disappear if intercourse is attempted. In other instances, a man with erectile dysfunction may be able to have normal erections under some circumstances but not others. For example, some men with erectile dysfunction have no problem during masturbation but cannot get erections during sexual activity with a partner. Other men have solid erections during extramarital sex but only feeble erections with their spouses. The reverse of this pattern is also common: some men who have no sexual difficulty with their wives are unable to function during attempts at extramarital sex.

Isolated episodes of not having erections (or losing an erection at an inopportune time) are so common that they are nearly a universal occurrence among men. [For this reason, Masters and Johnson (1970) classified a man as secondarily impotent only if his erection problems occurred in at least 25 percent of his sexual encounters.] Such isolated episodes do *not* mean that a man has a sexual dysfunction; they may reflect a temporary form of physical stress (having the flu, being tired, having overindulged in food or drink) or may relate to other problems like tension, lack of privacy, or adjusting to a new sexual partner. If the man does not take such incidents in stride and becomes deeply upset by his "failure" to respond the "right" way physically, he may set the stage for difficulties in later sexual situations because he is worried about his ability (or inability) to perform.

One aspect of erectile dysfunction that is not widely recognized is that this problem sometimes disappears spontaneously. In one survey, it was found that 30 percent of men with erectile problems not caused by physical conditions were functioning normally six months later without receiving any treatment (Segraves et al., 1985). While such spontaneous "cures" are most likely in males who have had erectile difficulties for relatively short periods of time—typically less than three years—we have also seen instances of an abrupt return to normal sexual functioning after ten years or more of erectile dysfunction. Although there is no simple explanation for why these instances occur, it often seems to be linked to reduction in stress levels in a man's life.

Fears of sexual performance—"Will I lose my erection?" "Will I satisfy my partner?"—are likely to dampen sexual arousal and cause loss of erection. The stronger and more insistent such fears become, the greater is the likelihood that they will become self-fulfilling prophecies, and the man will experience an actual inability to get and keep an erection. On a long-term basis, performance fears may lead to lowered interest in sex (avoidance), loss of self-esteem, and attempts to control the anxiety by working hard to overcome it (which usually reduces sexual spontaneity and causes sex to be even more of a "performance" instead of just being *fun*). In addition, fears of performance often cause one or both partners to become spectators during their sexual interaction, observing and evaluating their own or their partner's sexual response. By becoming a spectator, a person usually becomes less involved in the sexual activity because of the distraction of watching and evaluating what is going on.

The spectator role, which can affect men and women, is found not only in cases of erectile dysfunction. When a person slips into the spectator role because of performance fears, the reduced intimacy and spontaneity of the situation combined with preexisting fears usually stifle the capacity for physical response. This cycle tends to feed on itself: erectile failure leads to performance fears, which lead to the spectator role, which results in distraction and loss of erection, which heightens the fears of performance. Unless this cycle is broken, there is a strong possibility that sexual dysfunction will be firmly established.

Men react to erectile dysfunction in various ways, ranging from great dismay (probably the most typical response) to studied nonchalance (the least typical). While there are some men and women who see sex as more than a throbbing, erect penis and do not judge the satisfaction of a sexual encounter on the basis of having intercourse alone, for most people the practical limitations of erectile dysfunction are bothersome. One 34-year-old man relates his personal feelings in dealing with it:

> After a while, the problem becomes so predictable that you start to make excuses in advance. It's as though you lose any chance of having sexual pleasure because you become preoccupied with the notion of failure. And the failure hits you right in the gut—you don't feel like much of a man. *(Authors' files)*

The partner of a man with erectile dysfunction may blame herself for not being attractive enough to turn him on or not being skilled enough to arouse his passion, or she may fear that she is pressuring him and causing his difficulties. On the other hand, the partner may blame the man in various ways for his sexual problems. We have encountered women who accused their husbands of extramarital sex, being homosexual, or not being in love with them as explanations of erectile dysfunction. Sometimes the impact of erectile dysfunction can alter the fabric of a close relationship by introducing strain, doubt, irritability, and frustration, all of which have effects outside the bedroom.

Premature Ejaculation

Premature ejaculation, or rapid ejaculation, is a common sexual dysfunction but is difficult to define precisely. Older definitions that used a specific duration of intercourse as the dividing line ("less than two minutes," for example) or that specified a minimum number of penile thrusts before ejaculation have now been discarded. This is fortunate because some men actually tried to time themselves with a stopwatch to determine if they were normal, and others tried to hurry their thrusting ("just four more thrusts, dear") although this usually speeds up ejaculation instead of delaying it.

In *Human Sexual Inadequacy*, an attempt was made to define premature ejaculation in terms of the interaction between sexual partners, not just the male alone. (Prior to 1970, premature ejaculation had frequently been classified as a form of impotence, a belief that reflected a poor understanding of the underlying physiology.) A man was considered to ejaculate prematurely if his partner wasn't orgasmic in at least 50 percent of their coital episodes, but it was acknowledged that this definition was still lacking (Masters and Johnson, 1970). Specifically, it couldn't be applied to situations in which a woman was infrequently orgasmic or never had orgasms during intercourse, and it was an arbitrary way of estimating normality at best. Later, Helen Kaplan (1974) suggested that premature ejaculation occurred if the male didn't have voluntary control over when he ejaculated—although most sex therapists agree that total voluntary control over the timing of ejaculation is the exception rather than the rule.

The American Psychiatric Association has recently sidestepped this issue neatly by defining premature ejaculation in terms of "reasonable voluntary control."

erectile dysfunction (impotence) the inability to have or maintain an erection firm enough for coitus. Can be classified as **primary** (always existing) or **secondary** (having functioned in the past).

premature ejaculation unintentional ejaculation during noncoital play, while the male is trying to enter his partner, or soon after intercourse begins.

"The judgment of 'reasonable control' is made by . . . taking into account factors that affect duration of the excitement phase, such as age, novelty of the sexual partner, and frequency and duration of coitus" (American Psychiatric Association, 1980, p. 280). Another view suggests that premature ejaculation does *not* exist if both partners "agree that the quality of their sexual encounters is not influenced by efforts to delay ejaculation" (LoPiccolo, 1977, p. 1234).

Despite the shortcomings of these definitions (or the definitions of this shortcoming), it is usually not too difficult to decide when rapid ejaculation is problematic in a sexual relationship. Although Kinsey and his co-workers suggested that rapid ejaculation was a sign of biological competence, noting that "it would be difficult to find another situation in which an individual who was quick and intense in his responses was labeled anything but superior . . . however inconvenient and unfortunate . . . from the standpoint of [the] wife" (Kinsey, Pomeroy, and Martin, 1948, p. 580), today most sexologists disagree with this idea. Kinsey's belief may have influenced his finding that 75 percent of men ejaculated within two minutes of vaginal entry, but it now seems unlikely that this figure is accurate (Hunt, 1975). While it is certainly true that some people see sex as primarily for the male's pleasure—and some females may actually be grateful to "get it over with" quickly—these ideas, which were once widespread, seem to have been replaced today by a more egalitarian view of sexual interaction except among the least educated and lowest socioeconomic levels.

Clearly, the male who persistently ejaculates unintentionally during noncoital sexual play or while trying to enter his partner has a problem. While this extreme situation is found in fewer than 10 percent of cases, it is likely to be particularly distressing. More typically, the premature ejaculator is able to participate in a variety of sexual activities and only loses his ejaculatory control soon after intercourse begins. Premature ejaculation may occur in some situations and not in others. For example, a man may have this problem only during extramarital sex.

Some men are not bothered at all by ejaculating rapidly. Many others question their masculinity and have low self-esteem (Perelman, 1980; Kaplan, 1989). Fears of performance often heighten the lack of ejaculatory control and can lead to erectile dysfunction by the "fears–spectator–failure–greater fears" cycle described earlier (Kolodny, Masters, and Johnson, 1979). Erectile difficulties can also occur if a premature ejaculator struggles to control his sexual arousal by using distraction (thinking about the office or counting backwards from 1000): if he succeeds too well in distracting himself from involvement in the sexual interaction, he may lose his erection as well as the urgency to ejaculate.

While many of the female partners of men with premature ejaculation are understanding and accepting of the involuntary nature of the problem, others "feel angry and 'used,' leading them to seek professional guidance, to seek another lover, or to avoid sex" (Perelman, 1980, p. 201). Because most males have a tendency to ejaculate more quickly if it has been a long time between sexual opportunities, avoidance is likely to worsen the problem and may worsen the relationship too. Similarly, if the man tries to reduce his arousal by shortening the time of noncoital play, his tactic not only is ineffective but also may backfire by further convincing the woman of her partner's selfishness (Kolodny, Masters, and Johnson, 1979).

Although premature ejaculation is less frequent than erectile dysfunction among male patients at the Masters & Johnson Institute (Masters and Johnson, 1970; Kolodny, Masters, and Johnson, 1979), we believe it is probably the most common sexual dysfunction in the general population. We estimate that 15 to 20 percent of American men have at least a moderate degree of difficulty controlling rapid ejaculation, but less than one-fifth of this group consider it to be enough of a problem to seek help. Some men find that they can overcome premature ejaculation on their own by using a condom to cut down on genital sensations; others discover that a glass or two of an alcoholic beverage may reduce their ejaculatory quickness; and others find that controlling ejaculation is no problem "the second time around"—that is, once they have already had one orgasm and attempt intercourse within the next two or three hours. Over-the-counter creams and ointments that "desensitize" the penis deaden sensations. If they help control rapid ejaculation at all, they do so at the cost of not feeling very much or by the power of suggestion.

Ejaculatory Incompetence and Retarded Ejaculation

Ejaculatory incompetence is the inability to ejaculate within the vagina despite a firm erection and relatively high levels of sexual arousal. It must be distinguished from **retrograde ejaculation,** which is a condition where the bladder neck does not close off properly during orgasm so that the semen spurts backward into the bladder, where it is mixed with urine. **Retarded ejaculation** can be thought of as the opposite of premature ejaculation; here, although intravaginal ejaculation eventually occurs, it requires a long time and strenuous efforts at coital stimulation, and sexual arousal may be sluggish.

Ejaculatory incompetence is an infrequent disorder mainly seen in men under age 35. The most common pattern (about two-thirds of patients) is **primary ejaculatory incompetence** or never having been able to ejaculate in the vagina. **Secondary ejaculatory incompetence** refers to men who have lost the ability to ejaculate intravaginally or who do so infrequently after a prior history of normal coital ejaculation. In either the primary or secondary version of this dysfunction, ejaculation is usually possible by masturbation (about 85 percent of patients in our series) or by noncoital partner stimulation (about 50 percent of patients in our series). In about 15 percent of our cases, men with ejaculatory incompetence had never experienced ejaculation except through nocturnal emissions. Rarely, ejaculatory incompetence can be situational, occurring with one partner but not another (Munjack and Kanno, 1979).

Ejaculatory incompetence can be a source of sexual pleasure because it permits prolonged periods of coitus. A few of our patients have told us that they were regularly able to sustain an erection for one or two hours of intercourse—much to the delight of their partners, many of whom marveled at this staying power. However, once the woman discovers that her partner is unable to ejaculate intravaginally, a new reaction most likely sets in. She may assume that the man does not find her attractive, is not enjoying the experience, or is "withholding" orgasm as a sign of selfishness (Munjack and Oziel, 1980). If reproduction is a goal of the sexual partners, ejaculatory incompetence can be even more frustrating and may lead to accusations and arguments that can threaten even the best of relationships, as this example from our files shows:

> *A 27-year-old married man:* I'm sick and tired of being psychoanalyzed by my wife because of this problem we're having. I want a baby just as much as she does, but my penis doesn't seem to understand. But that's no reason to accuse me of being homosexual.

Retarded ejaculation is seen in all age groups from adolescence on and is probably two or three times more common than ejaculatory incompetence. Although it may also be a source of sexual enjoyment, sometimes the prolonged periods of coital thrusting required to bring about ejaculation are uncomfortable both physically and psychologically for the female, whose own sexual needs may have been amply met in a briefer time frame. The woman may become resentful of the sexual demands placed on her by her partner. Her feeling corresponds to the male whose female partner needs to be stimulated coitally for a long time to reach orgasm.

Here again, it is important to distinguish between the fairly consistent pattern of sexual dysfunction and the occasional episodes when a man cannot ejaculate intravaginally or requires a long period of vaginal containment and thrusting to ejaculate. Occasional difficulty with ejaculation is *not* a sign of sexual disturbance and is often related to fatigue, tension, illness, too much sex in too short a time, or the effects of alcohol or other drugs (see Chapter 10). In addition, a male may be unable to ejaculate with a partner he's not very emotionally involved with (e.g., when he's just having sex because he feels it's expected of him).

Painful Intercourse

Painful intercourse, or **dyspareunia,** is generally thought of as a female dysfunction but it also affects males. Most typically, the pain is felt in the penis but it can be felt in the testes or internally, where it is often associated with a problem of the prostate or seminal vesicles. Causes of painful intercourse in males are discussed later in this chapter.

FEMALE SEXUAL DYSFUNCTION

Until fairly recently, it was presumed that women were less sexual than men. Females with a sexual dysfunction were therefore not seen as incomplete or "unable to measure up" as men with sexual problems were. In the past two decades, traditional views of female sexuality were all but demolished, and women's

ejaculatory incompetence the inability to ejaculate within the vagina. Can be classified as **primary** (always existing) or **secondary** (having been able to ejaculate in the past).

retrograde ejaculation condition in which the semen spurts backward into the bladder during orgasm because the bladder neck does not close off properly. It occurs in men with multiple sclerosis and diabetes and following some types of prostate surgery.

retarded ejaculation condition in which ejaculation in the vagina occurs only after a lengthy time period and strenuous efforts.

dyspareunia (dis′ puh roo′ nē uh) painful intercourse.

sexual needs became accepted as legitimate in their own right. But as part of this process, female sexual responsivity became something of an expected accomplishment, with women—helped along by numerous magazine articles, how-to books, and TV talk shows—suddenly put on the spot with performance pressures of their own.

As a result, females began to develop more awareness of the existence of sexual dysfunctions. The woman who sees herself as "unresponsive" in one way or another often becomes embarrassed, confused, or depressed just as men do. She too may try to cope by avoidance, inventing excuses, or studiously "working" at sex to find the "right" technique to unlock her sexual potential.

Vaginismus

Vaginismus is a condition in which the muscles around the outer third of the vagina have involuntary spasms in response to attempts at vaginal penetration (Figure 9–1). Females of any age can be affected, and the severity of the reflex is highly variable. At one extreme, vaginismus can be so dramatic that the vaginal opening is tightly clamped shut, preventing not only intercourse but even insertion of a finger. Less severe, but still considerably distressing, is when any attempts at coitus—no matter how gentle, relaxed, and loving—result in pelvic pain. In its milder versions, vaginismus may allow a woman to have intercourse, but only with some discomfort. The frequency of vaginismus in the general population is unknown, but judging from our patients, it accounts for less than 10 percent of cases of female sexual dysfunction. We estimate that 2 to 3 percent of all postadolescent women have vaginismus.

Although some women with vaginismus are very fearful of sexual activity, which may impair their sexual responsiveness, most women with this dysfunction have little or no difficulty with sexual arousal. Vaginal lubrication occurs normally, noncoital sexual play may be pleasurable and satisfying, and orgasm is often

FIGURE 9–1

Vaginismus

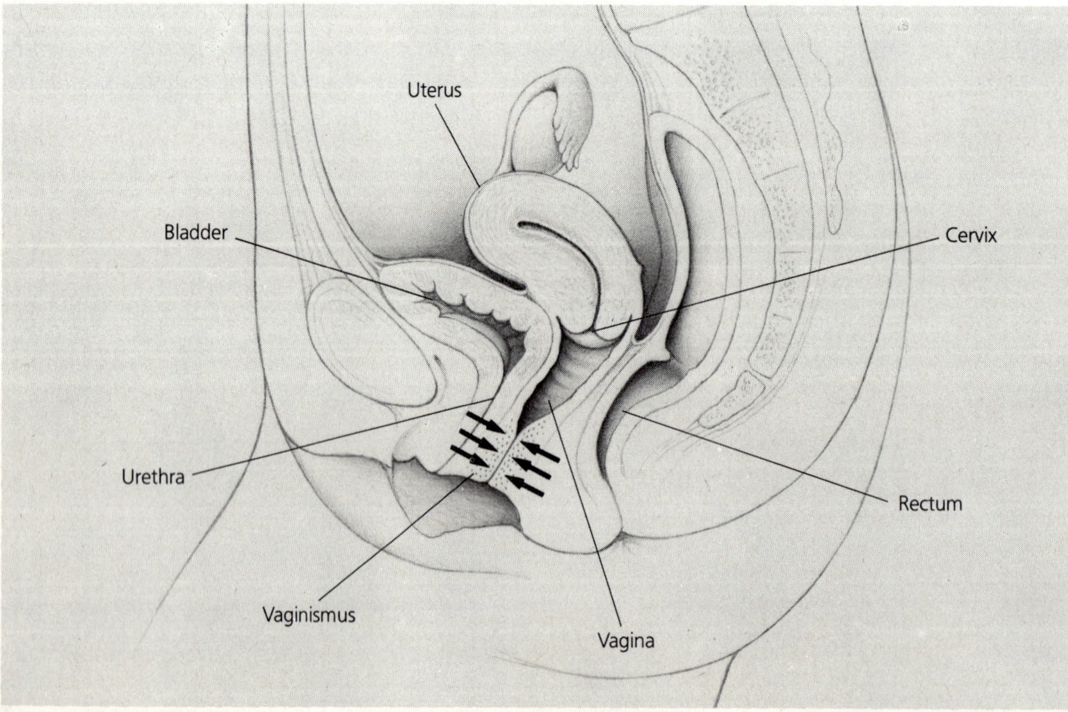

The involuntary muscular spasms of vaginismus at the outer third of the vagina are shown by the arrows.

unaffected (Kolodny, Masters, and Johnson, 1979). Women with vaginismus usually have normal sexual desire and are upset by their inability to enjoy intercourse. Vaginismus can be particularly troubling to a couple who want to have children, and it is often this consideration that pushes the couple to seek help.

The male partner of the woman with vaginismus may be completely baffled about why sexual difficulties arise. Often, he has no specific knowledge of the involuntary muscle spasms involved and either thinks that he is doing something that hurts his partner or sees her as deliberately avoiding intercourse by "tensing up." If he thinks he is hurting her, he may become more and more passive in sexual situations. Erectile dysfunction may develop, especially if he assumes the blame for the situation. If, instead, he blames the woman, he may lose patience after a while and become resentful or openly hostile or may simply seek other sexual partners.

Vaginismus may be suspected from a woman's history (e.g., the woman may have had difficulty using a tampon or a diaphragm), but identification of this dysfunction can be made with certainty only by a careful pelvic examination. Unfortunately, not all physicians are well versed in detecting sexual problems, and women are sometimes mistakenly told "everything's normal" when vaginismus is unquestionably present.

Anorgasmia

Before the publication of *Human Sexual Inadequacy* in 1970, the term **frigidity** was generally used to describe a number of female sexual difficulties ranging from not having orgasms to not being interested in sex to not becoming sexually aroused. As this term lacked diagnostic precision and was increasingly used in a negative, disparaging way, portraying women as "cold" or "rejecting," many sexologists abandoned its use. Masters and Johnson (1970) and Kaplan (1974) substituted the term **orgasmic dysfunction** to describe women who have difficulty reaching orgasm; **anorgasmia** is currently used as a synonym.

As with many sexual dysfunctions, there are several categories of anorgasmia. **Primary anorgasmia** refers to women who have never had an orgasm. **Secondary anorgasmia** refers to women who were regularly orgasmic at one time but no longer are. **Situational anorgasmia** refers to women who have had orgasms on one or more occasions but only under certain circumstances—for example, women who are orgasmic when masturbating but not when being stimulated by their partner. Women who are orgasmic by a variety of means but do not have orgasms during intercourse are described in a subcategory of situational anorgasmia called **coital anorgasmia.** Finally, **random anorgasmia** refers to women who have experienced orgasm in different types of sexual activity, but only on an infrequent basis.

As indicated by these definitions, there are many forms of anorgasmia. Within these classifications, the diversity is even greater. Some anorgasmic women get little pleasure out of sex and see it as an obligation of marriage or a means of maintaining a relationship. Other anorgasmic women find that sex is stimulating and satisfying. One woman told us: "Since I've never had an orgasm, I don't really know what I'm missing; but I certainly know when I'm having fun." Many women with orgasmic difficulties voice opinions somewhere between these extremes, as shown by these comments from our files:

> *A 22-year-old single woman:* I enjoy sex, but I keep pushing to reach for an orgasm, and the worry that it won't be there keeps gnawing away inside me. I'd feel a lot better if I knew I could come every time.
>
> *A 31-year-old married woman:* I've always been able to have orgasms when I masturbate, but it's never happened with my husband. After eight years of marriage this has really become a strain on our relationship—for him, because he feels he's inadequate; for me, because I'm missing a special kind of sharing.
>
> *A 19-year-old college student:* There's so much talk about orgasms that I've been wondering what's wrong with me, that I don't have them. I used to enjoy sex a lot, but lately it's a bad scene because I just get reminded of my own problems.

Not having orgasms can create fears of performance that propel a woman into the spectator role, dampening her overall sexual responsiveness, just as is true for a man. Anorgasmia can also lead to less self-esteem, depression, and a sense of futility.

vaginismus (vaj in iz′ mus) involuntary spasms of the muscles around the vagina in response to attempts at penetration.

frigidity (frı jıd′ ı tē) an outdated term formerly used to describe female sexual difficulties.

orgasmic dysfunction (or gaz′ mik) the inability of a female to reach orgasm.

anorgasmia (an′ or gaz′ mē uh) the inability of a woman to reach orgasm. Can be classified as **primary** (always existing), **secondary** (having been orgasmic in the past), **situational** (existing only in certain situations), **coital** (existing only during coitus), or **random** (existing on a frequent basis during different types of sexual activity).

It must be stressed that the stimulation of intercourse *alone* is not always sufficient for female orgasm to occur. Many women usually require additional stimulation (e.g., stroking the clitoris) during intercourse to have coital orgasms. Unfortunately, some people believe that "genuine" coital orgasms are only the result of penis–vagina contact, which is simply not the case.

There is some controversy today about the number of women who are anorgasmic during intercourse. A number of studies, viewed as a group, suggest that about 10 percent have never experienced coital orgasm (Kinsey et al., 1953; Chesser, 1956; Fisher, 1973; Hunt, 1975; Levin and Levin, 1975). Perhaps another 10 percent have coital orgasms on an infrequent basis. Kaplan (1974) suggests that these women should not necessarily be thought of as having a problem, since she believes that not having orgasms during intercourse is within the normal range of female sexual response. Hite (1977) voices a similar opinion, pointing out that many of the women she surveyed preferred noncoital orgasms to those occurring during intercourse. To us, their approaches are flawed for several reasons: (1) If the same line of reasoning were applied to males, premature ejaculation would be viewed as "within the normal range," since it appears to affect a similar number of men. (2) Many coitally anorgasmic women are easily able to begin having orgasms during intercourse with the aid of short-term sex therapy. (3) There is no reliable research evidence that a sizable fraction of women are incapable of coital orgasm. Furthermore, since many women who have coital anorgasmia are distressed by their situation, what is gained by telling them that everything is normal and it's no cause for concern?

We would like to make it clear that we believe that people should seek sex therapy with attainable goals and a genuine sense of need. A woman who is content not to have orgasms or who is unconcerned about how she reaches her orgasms should not be pushed into sex therapy. We also believe that it is usually a mistake to undertake sex therapy for female anorgasmia when the primary motivation is to satisfy the male partner.

Anorgasmia in its different forms is far and away the largest category of female sexual dysfunction, accounting for about 90 percent of cases in most large studies. Many women, however, are not orgasmic during every sexual encounter yet do *not* have a sexual dysfunction. Lack of orgasm must be viewed in terms of the individual's desires, the skill and sensitivity of her partner (as well as his attractiveness, cooperation, etc.), the circumstances of sexual activity (privacy, timing, comfort, and so on), and other factors too numerous to mention here. A woman who sometimes has orgasms should be classified as having orgasmic dysfunction only if her orgasmic frequency is so low that it is a source of distress or dissatisfaction.

The male partner of an anorgasmic woman may feel sympathetic while also feeling threatened, since many men assume it's their responsibility to make their partner orgasmic. If he sees his role as "tutor" or "coach," he may become impatient or angry if his partner doesn't reach orgasm in response to his attentions. If he concentrates on romance and carefully orchestrated sexual technique, he may become resentful if the female does not achieve orgasm. Some men give up trying and become resigned to the situation, while others are convinced that their partners are deliberately withholding orgasm. If a man discovers that his partner has been faking orgasm, he is particularly likely to be upset or angered.

Rapid Orgasm

Although premature ejaculation in men has been widely discussed, its female counterpart—**rapid orgasm**—has been almost completely ignored by sexologists. This is probably because the condition is relatively rare. In more than three decades of our research, we have encountered only a handful of women who complained of reaching orgasm too quickly. The primary problem for these women is that once orgasm occurs they have little interest in further sexual activity and often find that it is physically uncomfortable. In contrast, most women who have rapid orgasms remain sexually interested and aroused (often going on to additional orgasms) and thus consider it an asset, not a liability. The male partner of a woman who reaches orgasm rapidly is also likely to view it in a positive light, either seeing it as a sign of a very responsive partner or giving himself a pat on the back for his lovemaking skills.

Painful Intercourse

Dyspareunia, or painful intercourse, in women can present a major stumbling block to sexual satisfaction. In this condition, which can occur at any age, pain can appear at the start of intercourse, midway through coital activities, at the time of orgasm, or after intercourse is completed. The pain can be felt as burning, sharp, searing, or cramping; it can be external, within the vagina, or deep in the pelvic region or abdomen.

The incidence of dyspareunia is unknown. We have found that about 15 percent of adult women experience coital discomfort on a few occasions per year. We estimate that 1 to 2 percent of adult women have painful intercourse on more than an occasional basis.

Dyspareunia detracts from a person's sexual enjoyment and can interfere with sexual arousal and orgasm. The fear of pain may make the woman tense and decrease her sexual pleasure; in many cases, the woman may avoid coital activity or abstain from all forms of sexual contact. The partner of a woman with dyspareunia may either be very understanding and sensitive to her feelings or resentful and demanding in spite of her discomfort.

CAUSES OF SEXUAL DYSFUNCTION

It is customary to classify the causes of **sexual dysfunction** as either **organic** (physical or medical factors such as illness, injury, or drug effects) or **psychosocial** (including psychological, interpersonal, environmental, and cultural factors). The precise cause of a specific dysfunction in a given person cannot always be identified, and in some instances it may be a combination of several different factors.

Organic Factors

It is generally estimated that 10 to 20 percent of sexual dysfunction cases are caused primarily by organic factors (Kolodny, Masters, and Johnson, 1979; Munjack and Oziel, 1980; Kaplan, 1983). In another 15 percent of cases, organic factors may contribute to the sexual difficulty, although they may not be the direct or sole cause of the disorder. Given these facts, it is important for a person seeking treatment for a sexual dysfunction to have a thorough physical examination as well as appropriate laboratory testing of blood and urine samples to identify or rule out organic conditions that might be affecting sexual function. We now review each sexual dysfunction to examine organic factors that may be important. Many of these disorders are discussed more fully in the next chapter.

MALE SEXUAL DYSFUNCTION

Erectile dysfunction can result from many medical conditions. Diabetes (a condition in which the body improperly handles blood sugar regulation) and alcoholism are the two most prominent organic causes of erectile dysfunction. Together, they probably account for several million cases in the United States alone. Other organic causes of erectile dysfunction include spinal cord injury, multiple sclerosis, or other neurological disorders; infections or injuries of the penis, testes, urethra, or prostate gland; hormone deficiencies; and circulatory problems. Both prescription medications (such as drugs for high blood pressure) and street drugs like uppers (amphetamines), downers (barbiturates), and narcotics sometimes cause difficulty with erection.

Premature ejaculation rarely results from organic causes. In over 500 cases of premature ejaculation seen at the Masters & Johnson Institute, we have found only one instance where an organic condition proved to be of importance.

With *ejaculatory incompetence,* organic causes can be eliminated as a possibility if ejaculation occurs in noncoital situations. In cases of complete inability to ejaculate, drug use and neurological disorders are sometimes found, accounting for about 1 out of 20 cases. Drug use and alcoholism account for about 10 percent of cases of retarded ejaculation. Some prescription medicines, such as guanethidine (trade name Ismelin, used to treat high blood pressure) and monoamine oxidase inhibitors (used to treat depression) can also cause retarded ejaculation.

Painful intercourse in males can be due to several different organic problems, although psychosocial factors appear to cause at least half of such cases. Inflammation or infection of the penis, the foreskin, the testes, the urethra, or the prostate are the most likely organic causes of male dyspareunia. A few men experience pain if the tip of the penis is scratched or irritated by the tail of an IUD (the stringlike portion that protrudes through the cervix into the vagina).

rapid orgasm the female counterpart of premature ejaculation, marked by characteristically having orgasm so quickly in a sexual encounter that it is distressful. This is a very rare complaint.

sexual dysfunction conditions in which the ordinary physical responses of sexual excitement or orgasm are impaired. Can be classified as **psychosocial** (caused by psychological, interpersonal, environmental, and cultural factors) or **organic** (caused by physical or medical factors such as illness, injury, or drugs).

Other men develop painful penile irritation when exposed to a vaginal contraceptive foam or cream.

FEMALE SEXUAL DYSFUNCTION

Vaginismus is most frequently a psychosocial problem rather than an organic one. However, any of the organic causes of female dyspareunia can condition a woman into vaginismus as a natural protective reflex (Kolodny, Masters, and Johnson, 1979). Even when the underlying organic problem is detected and successfully treated, the vaginismus may remain, particularly if it has been present for a long time.

Anorgasmia is linked to organic causes in less than 5 percent of cases. Severe chronic illness of almost any variety can impair female orgasmic response. Specific disorders that sometimes block orgasm include diabetes, alcoholism, neurological disturbances, hormone deficiencies, and pelvic disorders such as infections, trauma, or scarring from surgery. Drugs such as narcotics, tranquilizers, and blood pressure medications can also impair female orgasm. *Rapid orgasm* in women has no known physical causes.

Female dyspareunia can be caused by dozens of physical conditions, although psychosocial factors may be as frequent as organic ones (Lazarus, 1980). Any condition that results in poor vaginal lubrication can produce discomfort during intercourse. The chief culprits here seem to be drugs that have a drying effect (e.g., antihistamines, used to treat allergies, colds, or sinus conditions; certain tranquilizers; and marijuana) and disorders such as diabetes, vaginal infections, and estrogen deficiencies. Other causes of female dyspareunia include the following:

1. Skin problems (blisters, rashes, inflammation) around the vaginal opening or affecting the vulva.
2. Irritation or infection of the clitoris.
3. Disorders of the vaginal opening, such as scarring from an episiotomy, intact hymen or chronically infected remnants of the hymen that are stretched during intercourse, or infection of the Bartholin's glands.
4. Disorders of the urethra or anus.
5. Disorders of the vagina, such as infections, surgical scarring, thinning of the walls of the vagina (whether due to aging or estrogen deficiency), and irritation due to chemicals that are found in contraceptive materials or douches.
6. Pelvic disorders such as infection, tumors, abnormalities of the cervix or uterus, and torn ligaments that support the uterus.

Psychosocial Factors

It has been much more difficult to develop a clear understanding of how psychosocial factors "cause" sexual dysfunction. Much of the research to date has found *associations* between factors such as developmental traumas, psychological traits, behavior patterns, and relationship difficulties and the existence of a sexual dysfunction, but research of this sort cannot prove what *causes* sexual dysfunctions. Furthermore, many people whose histories are loaded with potentially devastating psychosexual events have completely normal sexual function, while others who have unremarkable histories turn up with sexual dysfunctions.

Despite these problems, we can identify some psychosocial factors that are currently thought to contribute to the origins of sexual dysfunction. Since many of these are nonspecific—that is, they may lead to a number of dysfunctions in either men or women—we consider them in terms of several broad categories.

DEVELOPMENTAL FACTORS

Many authorities have suggested that troubled parent–child relationships, negative family attitudes toward sex, traumatic childhood or adolescent sexual experiences, and gender identity conflicts may all predispose one toward developing later sexual dysfunctions, either singly or in combination (Masters and Johnson, 1970; Kaplan, 1974; Leiblum and Pervin, 1980). For example, a child who is brought up believing that sex is sinful and shameful may be handicapped in later sexual enjoyment. Children who have been repeatedly and severely punished for touching their genitals or for innocent sex play with other boys or girls are also liable to become fearful about sex in any form and may have difficulty developing a positive view of sex as an intimate, pleasurable, desirable activity.

A traumatic first coital experience—either physically or psychologically painful—is another common problem found in the backgrounds of many people with sexual dysfunctions. Such an experience can raise fear about sexual encounters, lead to avoidance, or cause considerable guilt. Another variation is shown in this comment from one of our patients:

> *A 48-year-old coitally anorgasmic woman:* When I was 21 and still a virgin I had been looking forward to my wedding night in a romantic, idealized way. But the wedding day was exhausting, my husband and I both had too much to drink, and when we tried to make

> love for the first time, instead of being blissful and tender, it was hurried and disastrous. It seems as though we were never able to catch the spark of loving sex after that—it's always been disappointing and unpleasant for me. *(Authors' files)*

One other developmental factor will be mentioned briefly. In *Human Sexual Inadequacy* (Masters and Johnson, 1970), it was noted that a rigid religious background during childhood seemed to be associated with many sexual dysfunctions. What was striking about these cases was not the specific set of religious teachings (since these did not always condemn sexuality) but that sex was strongly regarded as evil and dirty in these rigidly religious families. Since 1970, when these findings were published, we have gathered more information in this area. We can now say that a rigid religious upbringing seems to be a common factor only in certain dysfunctions: vaginismus and primary anorgasmia in women and ejaculatory incompetence and primary impotence in men. Furthermore, by interviewing many individuals from similar backgrounds who did *not* have sexual dysfunctions, we have become even more confident that it is generally *not* the religious beliefs that are troublesome but the severely antisexual attitudes that are forced on the child.

PERSONAL FACTORS

People's feelings obviously have a lot to do with how they function sexually. We have already noted that fears of performance often suppress sexual function. Other types of anxiety, including fears of pregnancy, venereal disease, rejection, loss of control, pain, intimacy, and even success, can also block the pathways of sexual response.

Other feelings can also affect sexual responsiveness. Guilt, depression, and poor self-esteem are encountered frequently in association with sexual dysfunction. Sometimes, though, it is difficult to know which came first, the feeling or the dysfunction. It is natural for people who have sexual problems to become depressed about them or to feel less good about themselves. Thus, identifying such a feeling does not always mean it caused the dysfunction.

Other personal factors that can play a part in sexual dysfunction are lack of sexual information and blind acceptance of cultural myths. Uncertainty about the location of the clitoris or lack of awareness of its importance in female sexual response are prime examples of lack of sexual information. Believing that the capacity for sexual function disappears with aging or that the pace of sexual activity must be set by the male are examples of how cultural myths can translate into personal attitudes and behavior.

Although a number of different studies have attempted to correlate sexual dysfunctions with particular types of personalities, no solid evidence exists documenting such a relationship.

INTERPERSONAL FACTORS

Interpersonal factors are of tremendous importance in most sexual dysfunctions. The most common problem is poor communication, in both sexual and nonsexual areas of the relationship. Communication problems either can lead directly to a sexual dysfunction (through misunderstandings or defensiveness) or can play a key role in perpetuating a dysfunction. As we have stressed throughout this book, sex is a form of communication, and effective communication is extremely important in sexual relationships. Other interpersonal factors frequently involved in sexual dysfunctions include power struggles within a relationship, hostility toward a partner or spouse, preference for another partner, distrust or deceit, lack of physical attraction to a partner, and gender-role conflicts (which often become power struggles). Conflicts in the sex value systems of partners or widely different sexual preferences in terms of timing, frequency, or type of sexual activity may also contribute to dysfunctions.

It must be recognized, however, that such problems do not *always* lead to sexual difficulties. Some couples find that sex is most enjoyable when they are angry at each other. Other couples with terrible communication have fantastic sexual relationships. As always, we must be careful not to oversimplify.

ADDITIONAL CONSIDERATIONS

Until the detailed studies of Masters and Johnson were released, it was generally thought that sexual dysfunctions were invariably due to deep-seated personality problems that originated in childhood (Kaplan, 1974; LoPiccolo and Heiman, 1978; Apfelbaum, 1980a). Today, most sexologists recognize that many people with sexual dysfunctions have completely normal personalities, no signs of emotional illness, and simple, straightforward explanations for their problems.

Yet there are still some major differences between how psychoanalysts and behaviorists explain sexual dysfunction. The traditional psychoanalytic viewpoint

SEXUAL FAKERY

A 28-year-old married woman tells her husband that for six years of marriage she's been "faking" orgasms. He gets so angry at her that he kicks her off the end of their bed. Later, with professional counseling, he admits that his anger was self-directed—he couldn't believe he didn't see through her act.

A 24-year-old man who's been having problems with erections finds himself with an intimate invitation from a girl he's just begun dating. "Look," he tells her, "I'm not feeling so good tonight, so don't expect too much." *(Authors' files)*

No one knows how many people lie to their partners by faking sexual responsivity or personal satisfaction. When one partner tenderly asks another, "How was that for you?" the usual answer ("terrific!") may be more a matter of tact than truth. Although there are certainly times when sexual deception may seem the better part of valor by allowing a person to save face or by protecting a partner's feelings, many problems may arise if it becomes habitual. This can be illustrated by considering what seems to be the most common form of sexual fakery: a woman who fakes orgasms.

The woman who "fakes" is sabotaging communication rather than doing her partner a favor. Although she may succeed in temporarily massaging his ego by making him feel like a great lover, her pretense convinces him that he's doing everything "just right." As a result, he will probably continue doing what he thinks she enjoys, having no reason to change his style and being unaware of her need for anything different.

While men have an impossible time trying to fake erections and while male orgasm usually produces unmistakable external evidence, "faking" can still occur. This usually takes the form of trying to hide an inability to achieve erection, using fatigue or illness as an excuse. In other instances, a man may try to hide his own difficulties by convincing his partner that he wants only to please her—that *he* is satisfied when *she* is satisfied—although this pretense works only with noncoital acts. In a few cases of ejaculatory incompetence, men have faked intravaginal ejaculation successfully for years without their partner's detection. Whatever the particular deception, the result is very similar to the female version of sexual fakery. By undermining effective communication, the man cuts off an opportunity to gain his partner's understanding and thus lessens his chances of being able to change the situation.

Sexual fakery has no long-lasting advantages. It may save a partner's feelings temporarily, but this is usually at the cost of the other person's pleasure. The sexual lie is all too likely to become a barrier between partners. If the barrier becomes thick enough, it can dissolve the relationship.

---

has been that the dysfunction is not the primary problem but is instead a symptom of a deeper psychological disturbance. Analysts have suggested that ejaculatory incompetence, erectile dysfunction, and premature ejaculation result from castration anxiety and unresolved Oedipal wishes that are usually present at the unconscious level. Similarly, the analytic viewpoint generally suggests that vaginismus and anorgasmia also reflect unresolved Electra conflicts as well as unconscious hostility toward men because of penis envy. In essence, old fears of being punished for sexual play that were supposedly learned in early childhood are reawakened (in the unconscious) by adult sexual encounters and cause psychological conflict, anxiety, and dysfunction.

In sharp distinction, the learning theory viewpoint sees sexual dysfunction as a conditioned, or learned, response. A man may develop erectile dysfunction if his partner constantly criticizes his performance or if he feels guilty after every sexual encounter. A woman may be anorgasmic because she was conditioned to believe that sex was "wrong" or shameful or because she was taught that "nice" girls don't enjoy sex. Premature ejaculation may originate from early sexual experiences in which ejaculating quickly was desirable. Such experiences might include situations with a risk of being discovered by someone else, as in sex in a parked car; sex with a prostitute who typically encourages speed so she can see more customers; or group masturbation, where ejaculatory speed was seen as a sign of virility. If the conditioning is powerful enough, it cannot be easily "unlearned" even when circumstances change.

The learning theory model also points out that some dysfunctions are maintained by positive reinforcement. That is, the dysfunction may result in increased tenderness or attention from a partner, or it may give a person the upper hand in a power struggle. Furthermore, behaviorists generally believe that a precise understanding of causation is less important in treating a sexual dysfunction than recognizing the conditions that *maintain* the difficulty, since these are the ones that need to be changed.

Perhaps as sex research becomes more sophisticated it will be possible to approach the question of causation with more certainty. At present, the understanding of this area remains limited.

DISORDERS OF SEXUAL DESIRE

Since the mid-1970s, sex therapists have become increasingly aware of a new category of sexual problems that are not, strictly speaking, sexual dysfunctions. In these conditions, which are collectively referred to as disorders of sexual desire, the capacity for physical sexual response is usually preserved, and the problem is one of lack of willingness to participate in sexual relations due to either disinterest or fear. If lack of interest in sex is the predominant problem, it is classified as **inhibited sexual desire (ISD).** If lack of participation in sex is mainly due to overwhelming fear, it is classified as **sexual aversion.**

In deciding when a disorder of sexual desire is present, it is necessary to remember that while some people seem to be interested in sex at almost any time, others have low or seemingly nonexistent levels of sexual interest. Only when lack of sexual interest is a source of personal or relationship distress, instead of voluntary choice, is it classified as ISD. Schover and co-workers (1982) suggest that ISD is present if there is both a low rate of sexual activity and "a subjective lack of desire for sexual activity; desire here includes sexual dreams and fantasies, attention to erotic materials, awareness of wishes for sexual activity, noticing attractive potential partners, and feelings of frustration if deprived of sex."

People with ISD characteristically have low interest in initiating sexual behavior and are generally unreceptive to a partner's sexual advances, although they may reluctantly "give in" to their partner's wishes from time to time to preserve peace in the relationship. Generally, people with ISD are sexually functional (in physiological terms), but this disorder can also coexist with one or more sexual dysfunctions. ISD can be primary (lifelong) or secondary, and it can be either generalized (occurring all the time) or situational. Although the exact incidence of this problem is unknown, it has been appearing frequently in sex therapy clinics around the country in the recent past, accounting for as many as three out of ten cases in some clinics (Lief, 1977; Schover and LoPiccolo, 1982; Leiblum and Rosen, 1988).

The causes of inhibited sexual desire include both organic and psychosocial conditions. Hormone deficiencies, alcoholism, kidney failure, drug abuse, and severe chronic illness may each play a role. Ten to 20 percent of men with this disorder have pituitary tumors that produce excessive amounts of prolactin; the prolactin suppresses testosterone production and sometimes causes impotence as well as ISD (Schwartz and Bauman, 1981). A majority of cases of ISD appear to be psychosocial in origin, reflecting problems such as depression, prior sexual trauma, poor body image or self-esteem, interpersonal hostility, and re-

inhibited sexual desire (ISD) a condition marked by very low interest in sexual behavior.

sexual aversion a severe phobia (irrational fear) of sexual activity or the thought of sexual activity, which generally leads to avoidance of sexual situations.

lationship power struggles. In some cases, ISD seems to develop as a means of coping with a preexisting sexual dysfunction. For instance, a man with erectile dysfunction who develops a low interest in sex finds that this allows him to avoid the unpleasant consequences of sexual failure such as embarrassment, anxiety, loss of self-esteem, and frustration.

Women or men with ISD may be sexually functional or may have difficulties with sexual arousal and orgasm. In many cases, they seem not to be able to recognize early signs of sexual arousal in themselves and use a limited set of cues to define a situation as sexual (LoPiccolo, 1980). For example, such persons may ignore warmth and tenderness as possible signs of sexual feelings while waiting to be swept off their feet by a tidal wave of sexual passion. In addition, many people with ISD believe their initial desire is a good predictor of their ultimate response to a sexual situation, so if they are not feeling "turned on" at the first touch or kiss, they give up all hope of enjoying themselves.

ISD is not a source of difficulty in all marriages or relationships where it occurs. Sometimes a couple reaches an acceptable accommodation to the situation: for example, a person with ISD may agree to participate in sex when his or her partner requests it, regardless of personal interest. Alternatively, some couples reach a workable solution by allowing—or even encouraging—the partner with an intact sex drive to seek sexual activity outside the relationship. Most frequently, however, when only one person in the relationship has low sexual desire, it poses a major strain.

Sexual aversion is a severe phobia (irrational fear) to sexual activity or the thought of sexual activity which leads to avoidance of sexual situations. It too affects both males and females. The intense fear or dread found in sexual aversion is sometimes expressed in physiological symptoms such as profound sweating, nausea, diarrhea, or a racing, pounding heartbeat (Crenshaw, 1985). But in many cases, the phobia expresses itself in purely psychological terms: simply put, the person is terrified of sexual contact.

Perhaps surprisingly, people with sexual aversion are likely to be able to respond fairly naturally to sexual encounters—if they can get past the initial dread. Some patients with this disorder have told us they have more difficulty with undressing and touching in a sexual context than they do with participation in intercourse.

Between 1972 and 1985, we have seen 164 cases of sexual aversion at the Masters & Johnson Institute. The primary causes seem to be (1) severely negative parental sex attitudes, (2) a history of sexual trauma (e.g., rape, incest), (3) a pattern of constant sexual pressuring by a partner in a long-term relationship, and (4) gender identity confusion in men. In the typical case of sexual aversion, the frequency of sexual activity drops to only once or twice a year—if that often. This can obviously become a major source of relationship stress, and the partner of the person with sexual aversion often becomes angry and considers leaving the relationship. Fortunately, the success rate for treating sexual aversion is over 90 percent even in cases of long duration (Kolodny, Masters, and Johnson, 1979). Schover and LoPiccolo (1982) have also reported that cases of ISD and sexual aversion usually have successful treatment outcomes.

SEX THERAPY

Prior to 1970 the treatment of sexual dysfunctions and problems was generally the province of psychiatry (Levine, 1976). Treatment usually took a long time, and successful reversal of the sexual distress was very uncertain. The traditional psychiatric model of individual treatment (one therapist working with one patient) was almost always used.

Today, sex therapy is a field that includes practitioners of many different backgrounds—psychology, medicine (both psychiatry and other specialties), social work, nursing, counseling, and theology to name just a few. There are also many approaches to sex therapy, some of which are described below.

The Masters and Johnson Model

Beginning in 1959, Masters and Johnson began their innovative program for treating sexual dysfunctions. It is considerably different from prior approaches in a number of ways. For example, they primarily work only with couples (instead of individuals) because they feel that there is no such thing as an uninvolved partner in a committed relationship in which there is any form of sexual distress. This does not mean that the partner always *causes* the problem but points out that he or she is *affected* by it, as the relationship is affected. This strategy shifts the therapeutic focus to the relationship instead of the individual. Furthermore, it provides a more effective means of identifying the full dimensions of a problem. Masters and Johnson found that the input of both partners usually proved more useful than the one-sided view that an individual provided. Finally, this strategy provides an opportunity to gain the cooperation and understanding of both partners in overcoming the distress.

A logical extension of this approach is the use of *two* therapists—a man and woman working together as a *cotherapy team*. This team increases therapeutic objectivity and balance by adequately representing male and female viewpoints and gives each partner a same-sex therapist to whom he or she can (theoretically) relate more easily. The cotherapy team also provides a model for the patient couple in important ways: for example, they can easily demonstrate effective communication skills.

Another important element of the Masters and Johnson approach is the integration of physiologic and psychosocial data in assessment and treatment. In the past, many psychiatrists never examined their patients because they feared that this might trigger unwanted sexual feelings that could complicate the treatment relationship. Masters and Johnson recognized that it was important to identify organic conditions that might require medical or surgical treatment instead of sex therapy. They also found that explaining the anatomy and physiology of sexual response to patients often had important therapeutic benefits of its own.

Finally, the Masters and Johnson model involves a rapid, intensive approach to treating sexual problems. Couples are seen daily for a two-week period (the average duration of therapy is actually just under 12 days). This format permits a day-to-day continuity that appears to be beneficial in certain aspects of sex therapy, such as reducing anxiety or helping patients overcome mistakes. Couples are also urged to free themselves whenever possible from their ordinary work, family, and social activities during the two weeks of therapy to be able to devote their attention to their own relationship without outside distractions.

It became apparent during the pilot phase of this clinical model that the therapy process was much more effective when couples were seen on a daily basis than in cases where couples were seen in the prevailing format of the 50-minute hour once or twice a week.

Against this general background, some additional treatment concepts of the Masters and Johnson approach are important:

1. *Therapy is individualized to meet the specific needs of each couple*. The couple's values and objectives are the primary determinants of exactly what is done. Therapists must avoid imposing their own values on their patients.
2. *Sex is assumed to be a natural function, controlled largely by reflex responses of the body*. Although many different factors can interfere with sexual function by disrupting these natural reflexes, sex therapy does not generally involve "teaching" the desired sexual response. Masters and Johnson focus instead on identifying obstacles that block effective sexual function and on helping people remove or overcome these obstacles. When this happens, natural function usually takes over promptly.[1]
3. *Because fears of performance and "spectatoring" are often central to cases of sexual dysfunction, therapy is approached at several levels*. Pressures to perform are removed initially by banning direct sexual contact. Couples are then helped to rediscover the sensual pleasures of touching and being touched without the goal of a particular sexual response (the "sensate focus" exercises). The therapists also help couples relabel their expectations so they do not judge everything they do as "success" or "failure." They also give people "permission" to be anxious, which helps them to talk about their anxiety more openly. This open communication often reduces the severity of the anxiety.
4. *Determining who's "to blame" for a sexual problem is discouraged as counterproductive*. Instead, couples are assisted in finding out what makes them feel comfortable and relaxed as opposed to tense or nervous. In this approach, each person is urged to take responsibility for himself or herself rather than waiting for his or her partner to provide the "right" mood, the "right" touch, or the "right" style of making love.
5. *Helping couples see that sex is just one component of their relationship is stressed*. Often, when a sexual problem occurs in people's lives, it causes them to worry about sex so much that they devote a disproportionate amount of time to thinking and talking about this topic. One typical objective of therapy is to help couples achieve a balanced perspective toward sex in which it is neither the totality of their relationship nor the most neglected part of their relationship. In fact, a general truism of sex therapy is that

[1] Sometimes removing the obstacles to natural function is not enough, particularly for people who have a life-long pattern of sexual dysfunction. They may also need specific therapeutic attention to facilitate arousal or to improve sexual techniques. In this situation, there is some "teaching" going on.

when a couple's relationship improves outside the bedroom, it is apt to have positive results inside the bedroom too.

THE MASTERS AND JOHNSON THERAPY FORMAT

On the first day of therapy, the couple begins by briefly meeting with their cotherapists, who introduce themselves and explain the events of the next few days. Following this overview, the patients are separated and a detailed history is taken from each partner by the same-sex therapist. After a break for lunch, when the cotherapists get together to discuss what they have learned, a second history is taken, but this time on a cross-sex basis: that is, the male therapist interviews the female patient and the female therapist interviews the male patient. Rounding out a busy day, each patient has a complete physical examination. Blood samples are obtained the following morning for laboratory evaluation of general health.

The second day of therapy is the time of the "roundtable session" in which the couple and both cotherapists meet together. Here, the therapists present their assessment of the sexual *and* nonsexual problems that the couple is facing and give an honest opinion of the chances of successful treatment. The patients are encouraged to comment on the therapists' impressions and to correct any factual errors that have been made. The therapists try to explain the most plausible causes of the sexual dysfunction(s) or problem(s) and begin to outline the approach for treatment. Generally, there is some discussion of sex as a natural function, how fears of performance originate, the effect of spectatoring, and the importance of communication skills. The roundtable usually concludes with suggestions to try the "sensate focus" exercises (described in the next section) in the privacy of their own home or hotel room.

Each initial history-taking session usually lasts one and one-half to two hours, and the cross-sex histories average about 45 minutes apiece. The roundtable generally lasts about 90 minutes, although any of these times are quite variable, depending in part on how talkative the couple is. Daily sessions after the roundtable average about an hour in length.

From the third day, the patient couple and the cotherapists continue to meet in a four-way interaction, although occasionally the therapists may see each patient separately to discover if there are any individual concerns that one partner is hesitant to discuss in the presence of the other. Each partner is asked to describe the events of the previous 24 hours, with particular attention to communication patterns and interaction during the sensate focus assignments.

Interestingly, a majority of time in the therapy sessions is usually spent on nonsexual issues (such as dealing with anger, self-esteem, and power struggles), although there is a direct attempt to provide information about sexual anatomy and physiology while attending to the couple's other needs. Couples who have negative sexual attitudes are encouraged to adopt new viewpoints.

SENSATE FOCUS

At the beginning of therapy, each couple is asked to refrain from direct sexual interaction involving genital contact. This approach helps to remove performance pressures and provides a framework for breaking the fear–spectatoring–failure–fear cycle that is often deeply ingrained. To learn more effective ways of sexual interaction, the idea of sensate focus is introduced.

In the first stage of sensate focus exercises, the couple is told to have two sessions in which they will each have a turn touching their partner's body—with the breasts and genitals "off limits." The purpose of the touching is *not* to be sexual but to establish an awareness of touch sensations by noticing textures, contours, temperatures, and contrasts (while doing the touching) or to simply be aware of the sensations of being touched by their partner. The person doing the touching is told to do so on the basis of what interests him or her, *not* on any guesses about what his or her partner likes or doesn't like. It is emphasized that the touching should not be a massage or an attempt to arouse the partner sexually.

The initial sensate focus periods should be as silent as possible, since words can detract from the awareness of physical sensations. However, the person being touched must let his or her partner know—either nonverbally (by body language) or in words—if any touch is uncomfortable.

Although many people say, "Oh, we've touched lots of times before—can't we just skip this and go on to a more advanced level?" this first stage of sensate focus is critical in several ways. It allows the therapists to find out additional information about how a couple interacts that supplements their histories in important ways. This stage also has a specific treatment value of its own, as shown by the fact that many men who

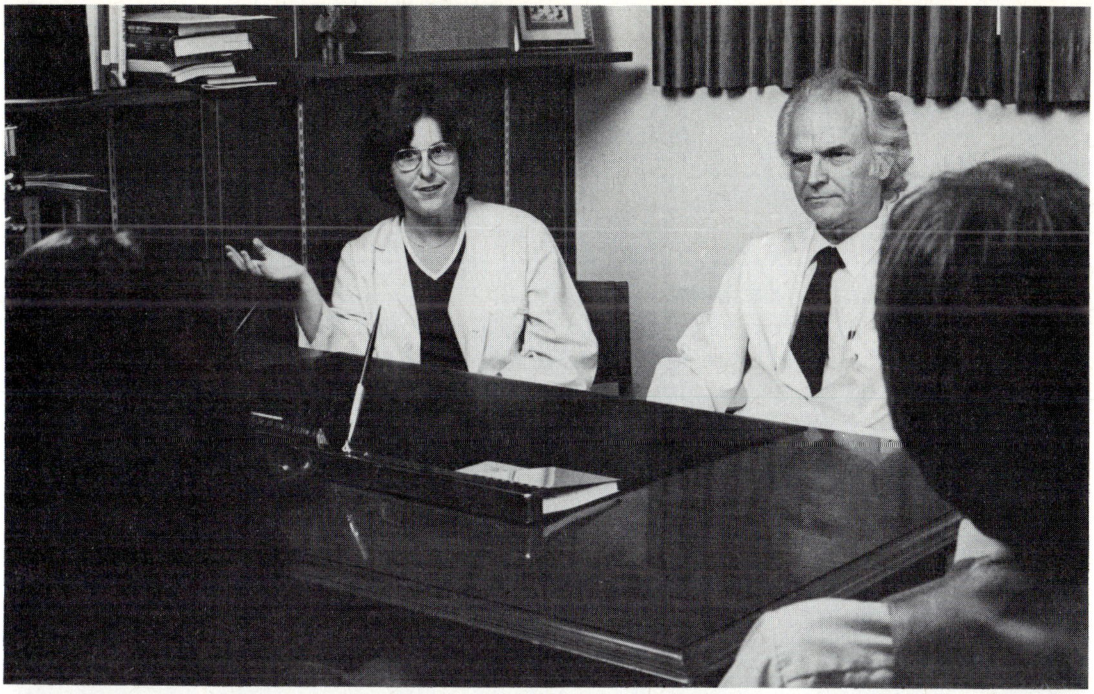

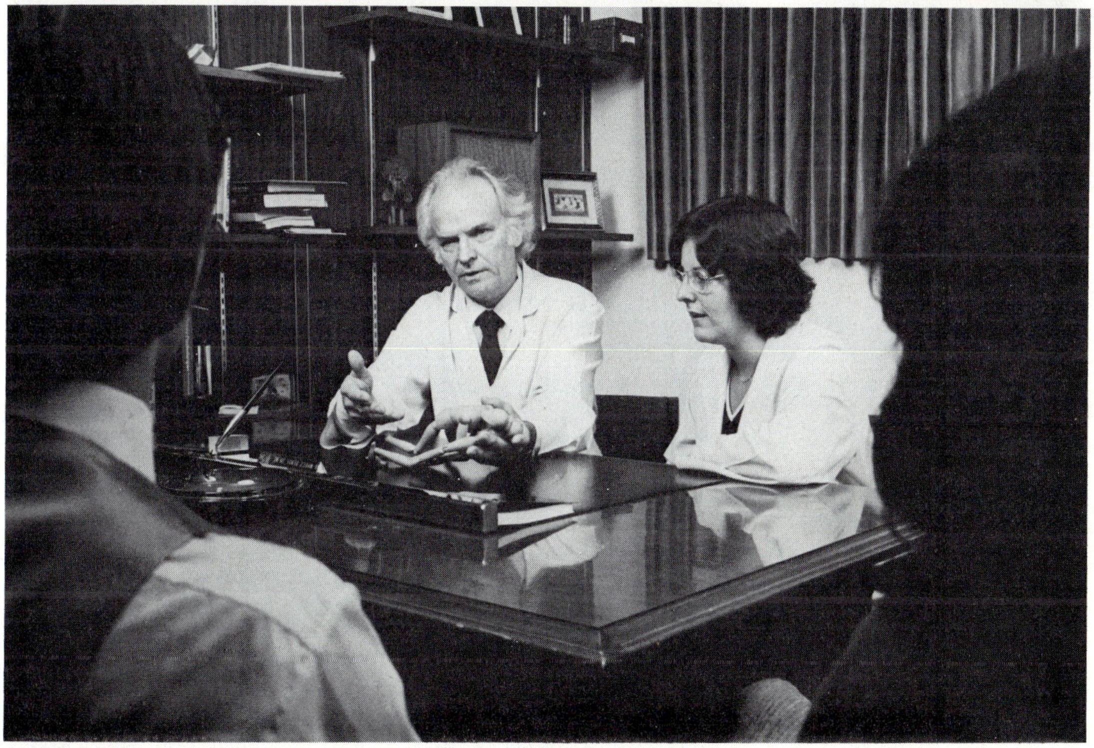

In therapy sessions at the Masters & Johnson Institute, wide-ranging discussions cover much more than sexual issues. In some cases, questions about sexual positions are answered using wooden artist's dolls for "demonstration" purposes.

have not had erections for years in attempts at sex suddenly discover a king-size erection probably because the performance demand was removed. After all, they were told that sexual arousal was not expected but even if it occurred, it was not to be put into action. Finally, it provides an excellent means for reducing anxiety and teaching nonverbal communication skills.

In the next stage of sensate focus, touching is expanded to include the breasts and genitals. The positions shown in the drawings are recommended but not required. The person doing the touching is instructed to begin with general body touching and to not "dive" for the genitals. Again, the emphasis is on awareness of physical sensations and not on the expectation of a particular sexual response.

At this stage, the couple is usually asked to try a "hand-riding" technique as a more direct means of nonverbal communication. The couple takes turns with this exercise. By placing one hand on top of her partner's hand while he touches her, the woman can indicate if she would like more pressure, a lighter touch, a faster or slower type of stroking, or a change to a different spot. The male indicates his preferences when the situation is reversed. The trick is to integrate these nonverbal messages in such a way that the person being touched doesn't become a "traffic cop" but simply adds some additional input to the touching, which is still primarily done based on what interests the "toucher."

In the next phase of sensate focus, instead of taking turns touching each other, the couple is asked to try some mutual touching. The purpose of this is twofold: first, it provides a more natural form of physical interaction (in "real-life" situations, people don't usually take turns touching and being touched); and second, it doubles the potential sources of sensual input. This is a very important step in overcoming spectatoring, since one thing the spectator can try is to shift attention to a portion of his or her partner's body (getting "lost" in the touch) and away from watching his or her own response. Couples are reminded that no matter how sexually aroused they may feel, intercourse is still "off limits."

The next stages of sensate focus are to continue the same activities but at some point to shift into the female-on-top position without attempting insertion. In this position, the woman can play with the penis, rubbing it against her clitoris, vulva, and vaginal opening regardless of whether there is an erection or not. If there is an erection, and she feels like it, she can simply slip the tip of the penis a bit inside the vagina, all the while focusing on the physical sensations and stopping the action or moving back to simple nongenital touching or cuddling if she or her partner becomes goal-oriented or anxious. When comfort is developed at this level, full intercourse can usually occur without difficulty.

As simple as these techniques may sound, it is important to realize that they are used as part of a de-

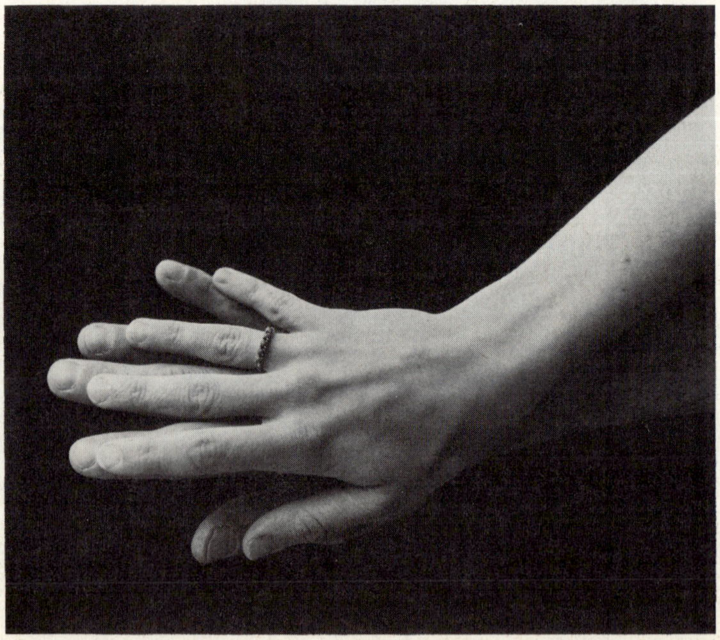

The "hand-riding" technique for conveniently giving nonverbal messages.

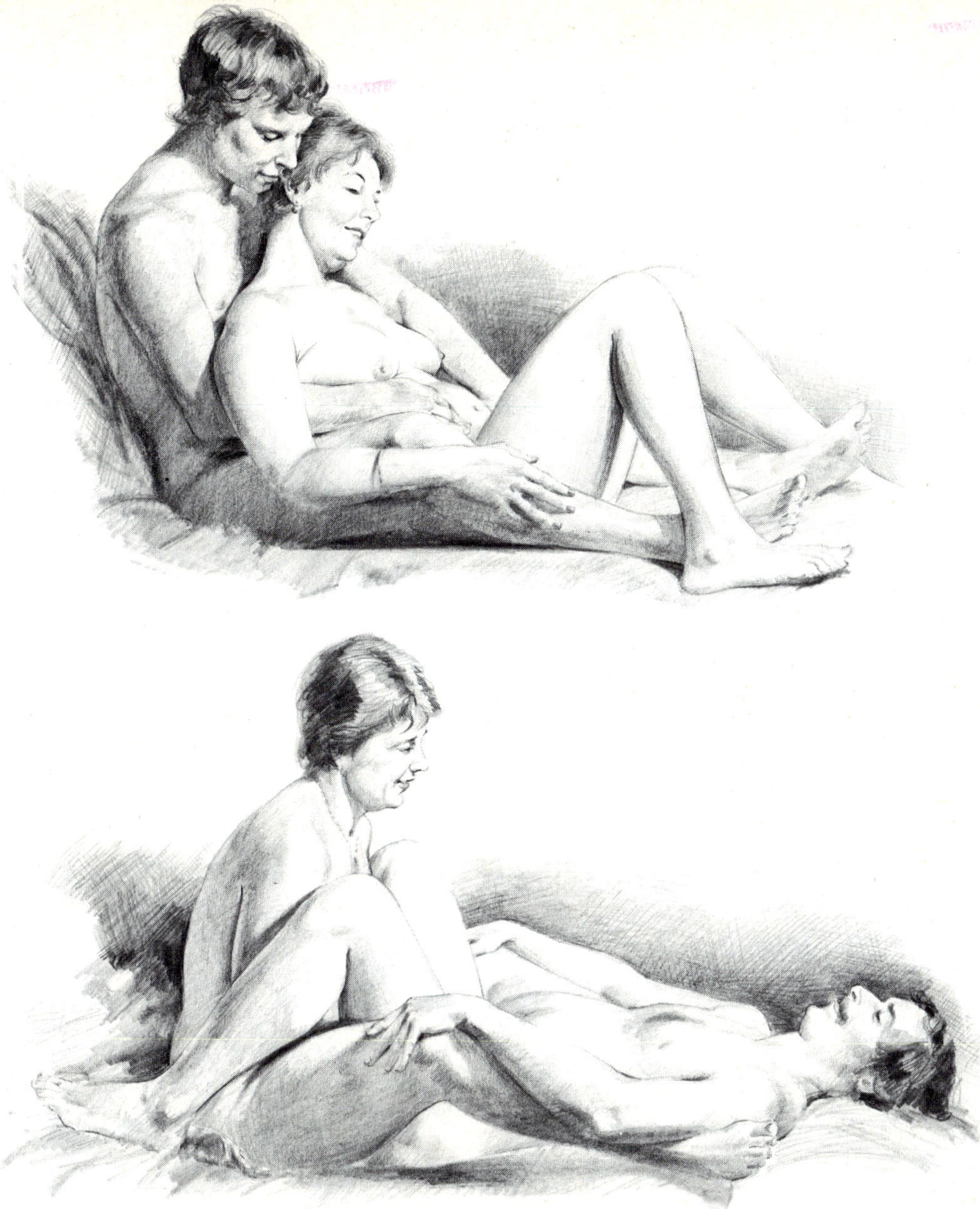

These positions are suggested to couples for the sensate focus exercises at the stage that includes genital exploration. When the man is touching his partner, the position in the top drawing is used; when the woman is touching her partner, the position in the bottom drawing is used. Couples are urged to modify these positions to whatever they find comfortable and to experiment with other positions, too.

tailed program of psychotherapy, not just as a grab-bag of "gimmicks." The remarkable thing is how dramatically and effectively these techniques work, even in cases where severe sexual dysfunctions have been present for 10, 20, or 30 years.

SOME SPECIFIC TREATMENT STRATEGIES

The general features of the Masters and Johnson treatment model just described are supplemented by some additional methods used in the treatment of various dysfunctions.

In *erectile dysfunction*, it is important to help the man understand that he cannot "will" an erection to occur on demand any more than he can "will" his blood pressure to drop or his heart rate to increase. He *can* set the stage for his own natural reflexes to take over by not trying to have erections and by moving out of his performance fears. Not surprisingly, the man with erectile dysfunction often finds himself having firm erections during the early stages of sensate focus experience. While this can be reassuring to him, it is also important for the man (and his partner) to realize that losing an erection is *not* a sign of failure; it simply shows that erections come and go naturally. For this reason, the woman may be instructed to stop stroking or fondling the penis when an erection occurs, so the man has an opportunity to see that it will return with further touching. A related problem is that many men with erectile dysfunction try to rush their sexual performance once they get an erection out of fear that they will promptly lose it. The "rushing" adds one more performance pressure, and the usual result is a rapid loss of erection.

When intercourse is attempted (only after the man has gained considerable confidence in his erectile capacity *and* has been able to reduce his spectatoring behavior), the woman is advised to insert the penis. This reduces pressures on the man to decide when it is time to insert and removes the potential distraction of his fumbling to "find" the vagina.

In treating *premature ejaculation*, the couple approach is particularly important since the condition may actually be more distressing to the woman than the man. In addition to discussing the physiology of ejaculation, the therapists introduce a specific method called the "squeeze technique" that helps recondition the ejaculatory reflex. When genital touching is begun, the woman uses the "squeeze" periodically. As shown in Figure 9–2, the woman puts her thumb on the frenulum of the penis and places her first and second finger just above and below the coronal ridge on the opposite side of the penis. A firm, grasping pressure is applied for about four seconds and then abruptly released. The pressure is always applied front to back, never from side to side. It is important that the woman use the pads of her fingers and thumb and avoids pinching the penis or scratching it with her fingernails. For unknown reasons, the squeeze technique reduces the urgency to ejaculate (it also may cause a temporary, partial loss of erection). It should not be used, however, at the moment of ejaculatory inevitability: instead, it must begin at the early stages of genital play and continue periodically, every few minutes. The "squeeze" can be used whether the penis is erect or flaccid, but the firmness of the

FIGURE 9–2

The Squeeze Technique Used in Treating Premature Ejaculation

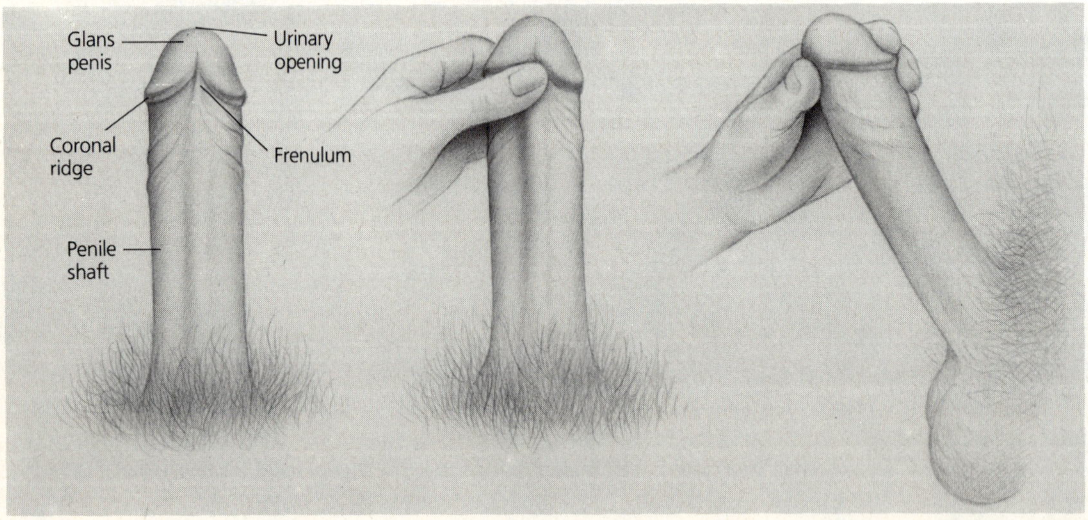

FIGURE 9–3

The Basilar Squeeze Technique Used in Treating Premature Ejaculation

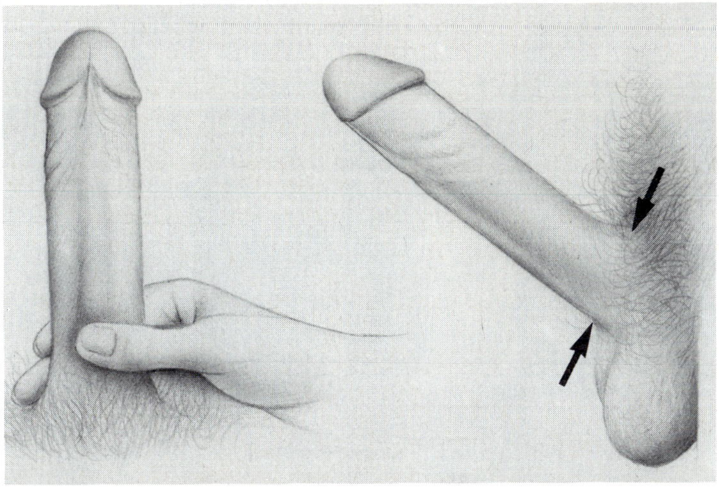

Unlike the squeeze at the coronal ridge, the basilar squeeze can be applied by the man during vaginal containment of the penis. Firm pressure is applied for about four seconds and then released; the pressure should always be from front to back (as shown by the arrows), never from side to side.

pressure should be proportionate to the degree of erection.

When the couple begins to have intercourse, the woman is asked to use the squeeze three to six times before attempting insertion. Once the penis is fully inside her, she should hold still for 15 to 30 seconds, with neither partner thrusting, and then move off the penis, apply the squeeze again, and reinsert. This time a slow thrusting pattern can begin. Once the man improves his ejaculatory control, both partners are taught the "basilar squeeze," another version of the squeeze technique (Figure 9–3), so that intercourse need not be interrupted by repeated dismounting to apply a squeeze.

The basilar squeeze should only be employed during coitus. The male partner should initiate the basilar squeeze because, once fully mounted, he has the easier anatomical access to the base of the penis, and he obviously is far more subjectively aware of his level of sexual excitation than is his female partner. For the first six months after introduction of the squeeze technique, the male partner is encouraged to avoid any attempts at "brinksmanship," that is, seeing how close he can come to the state of ejaculatory inevitability before initiating the appropriate squeeze technique. The squeeze techniques are far more effective if initiated before the plateau phase of the sexual response cycle has been attained.

Ejaculatory incompetence is treated by in-depth attention to the underlying psychological components combined with sensate focus experiences that seek to lead the man through a sequence of (1) ejaculating by masturbation while alone, (2) ejaculating by masturbation in the presence of his partner, (3) ejaculating by manual stimulation received from his partner, and (4) having the partner stimulate the penis vigorously to the point of ejaculatory inevitability and then quickly inserting it in the vagina. In most cases, when the man has ejaculated in the vagina once or twice, the fears or inhibitions about this act disappear completely. In some cases where the treatment sequence has not worked, it may be helpful to have the man ejaculate (via manual stimulation) externally onto the woman's genitals. After he becomes used to seeing his semen in genital contact with his partner, intravaginal ejaculation may occur more easily.

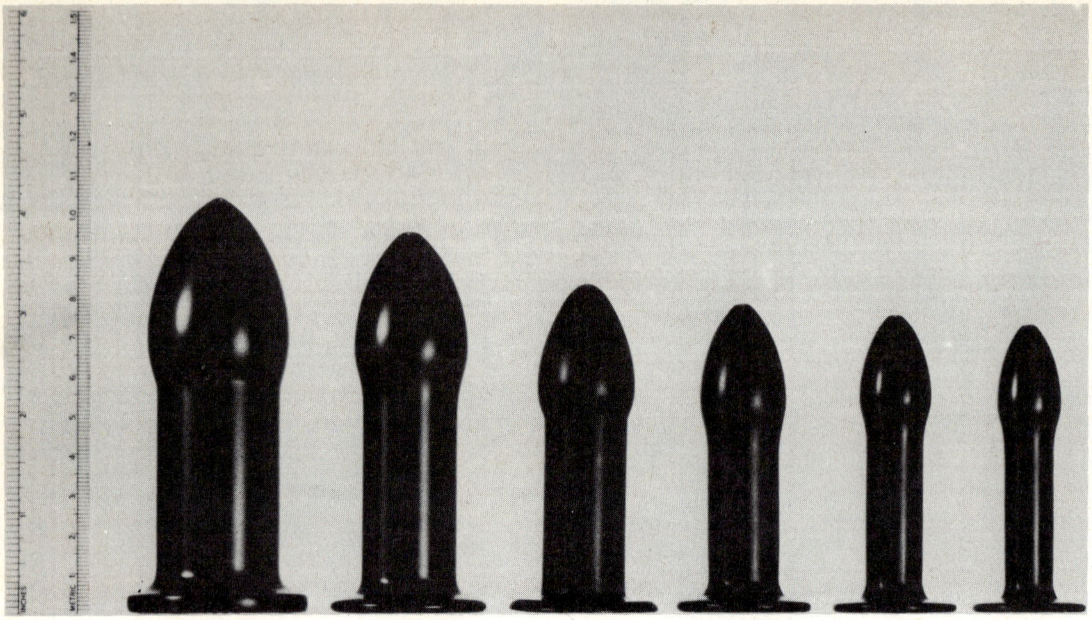

Plastic dilators used to treat vaginismus to allow the woman to learn how to recondition the reflex response of the muscles surrounding her vagina. Treatment begins with the smallest dilator and progresses gradually to the larger sizes.

Vaginismus is treated by explaining the nature of the involuntary reflex spasm to the couple and demonstrating the reflex in a carefully conducted pelvic examination with the male partner present and the woman urged to watch by use of a mirror. After this is done, the physician teaches the woman some techniques for relaxing the muscles around the vagina. The most effective method seems to be having her first deliberately tighten these muscles and then simply let go. It is much more difficult to relax on command. Next, the woman is given a set of various-sized plastic dilators. The smallest of these, slightly thinner than a finger, is gently inserted in the vagina by the physician—often to the amazement of the woman, who may have never been able to insert *anything* in her vagina. She is then shown how to insert the dilator herself, using plenty of sterile lubricating jelly, and is asked to practice this at home several times a day, keeping the dilators in place for 10 to 15 minutes at a time. Most women with vaginismus find that within five or six days they are able to use the largest dilator in the set, which is similar in thickness to an erect penis. If relationship issues have been dealt with adequately (often a key part of the therapy), the transition to successful intercourse is usually easy at this point. At this time, it is particularly important for the woman to insert the penis so she feels in control.

The strategies used in treating *anorgasmia* depend greatly on the nature of the dysfunction. Different approaches are needed for a woman who has never had an orgasm than for a woman who is easily orgasmic with masturbation, manual stimulation, or oral–genital sex. Similarly, depending on the cause(s) of the anorgasmia, treatment strategies will vary widely from case to case. For example, a woman with a poor body image may be helped to find various ways of regarding her body more positively. A woman who is distracted from high levels of arousal by disturbing fantasies might be taught thought-blocking techniques, while another woman who cannot get beyond plateau may be encouraged to experiment with fantasies as an aid to boosting her into orgasm.

Common techniques used in treating anorgasmia include (1) encouraging a woman to explore her own body, especially focusing on genital exploration and stimulation in a relaxed, undemanding fashion; (2) dealing with performance anxieties and spectatoring, with particular attention to reducing performance pressures from her partner; (3) fostering sexual communications so that the woman is able to let her partner know what type of touch or stimulation she prefers at a given moment; and (4) reducing inhibitions that limit the woman's capacity for arousal or that block orgasm. A woman helped by this last technique is often given "permission" to have sexual feelings and learns to overcome fears that orgasm involves losing consciousness or losing control of her bladder. In most cases, these strategies make it fairly simple for the woman to reach orgasm via masturbation or stimulation by her partner. To make the transition to having orgasms during intercourse, a "bridging" technique is used in which either partner stimulates the clitoris manually during coitus with active thrusting.

These methods have now been used for more than 30 years in the treatment of sexual dysfunctions, with approximately four out of five patients successfully treated. Between 1959 and 1973, patients were followed for five years after therapy to evaluate the permanence of treatment results. More recently, a two-year follow-up has been used. About 1 couple in 20 returns to the Masters & Johnson Institute for additional therapy sometime after their two-week course of treatment. Statistics describing the Masters & Johnson Institute's experience for the various categories of dysfunction are shown in Table 9–1.

Other Approaches to Sex Therapy

Important contributions to sex therapy have been made by a number of other workers using treatment methods that differ from the Masters and Johnson model. Most therapists, for example, see patients once a week rather than daily (Schmidt and Lucas, 1976; Caird and Wincze, 1977; Schiller, 1981). Many therapists believe that a single therapist can work as effectively as a cotherapy team (H. Kaplan, 1974, 1979; Annon, 1976; Ellis, 1980; Schiller, 1981; Arentewicz and Schmidt, 1983; LoPiccolo et al., 1985), which reduces the expense of sex therapy. Others have experimented successfully with group therapy formats or individual therapy (Kaplan, 1974; Barbach, 1980; Zilbergeld, 1980; Cotten-Huston and Wheeler, 1983). Hypnosis has also been reported to be useful in treating sexual difficulties (Alexander, 1974; Fuchs et al., 1975; Fabbri, 1976; Brown and Chaves, 1980). Here, we consider some of the most common approaches used by other therapists.

HELEN KAPLAN: THE NEW SEX THERAPY

Psychiatrist Helen Kaplan (1974, 1979, 1989) has written extensively on the treatment of sexual dysfunctions, integrating many methods of Masters and Johnson with principles of psychoanalytic therapy. In her view, human sexual response is best seen as *triphasic*, or consisting of three separate but interlocking phases: desire, arousal, and orgasm. She believes that desire phase disorders are most difficult to treat because they tend to be associated with deep-seated psychological difficulties (1979). She also states that "the standard sex therapy methods seem to be effective

TABLE 9–1

Results of Sex Therapy at the Masters & Johnson Institute

	N[a]	Failures	Successes[b]	Success Rate
Primary impotence	65	21	44	67.7%
Secondary impotence	674	134	540	80.1
Premature ejaculation	543	35	508	93.6
Ejaculatory incompetence	113	27	86	76.1
Male totals	1395	217	1178	84.4
Anorgasmia	811	207	604	74.5
Vaginismus	130	2	128	98.5
Female totals	941	209	732	77.8
Combined totals	2336	426	1910	81.8

[a] Cases seen between 1959 and 1985.

[b] A case was categorized as successful only if the change in sexual function was unequivocal and lasting. For all patients seen before 1973, follow-up lasted five years. From 1973, the follow-up period was reduced to two years. If a patient were successful during the two-week sex therapy program but then slipped back into dysfunction, the case was listed as a failure.

primarily for those sexual problems which have their roots in mild and easily diminished anxieties and conflicts" (1979, p. xviii). To deal with more complex cases, she uses a lengthened form of sex therapy that seeks a deeper level of insight and addresses unconscious conflicts. One of her underlying theories is that a sexual disorder usually results from multiple levels of causes—some more immediate and accessible, some more remote and hidden.

The details of Kaplan's treatment methods differ considerably in some ways from the Masters and Johnson methods. In the treatment of premature ejaculation, for example, she advocates use of the "stop–start" technique instead of the squeeze. In the "stop–start" method, introduced by James Semans in 1956, the female partner stimulates the penis manually until the man feels that he is rapidly approaching ejaculation, at which time she stops all stimulation until the sense of ejaculatory urgency disappears. Stimulation then begins again, and the stop–start cycle is repeated several times before the man is allowed to ejaculate (Kaplan, 1974, 1989).

BEHAVIORAL THERAPY

Modern behavioral methods for treating sexual difficulties are generally traced back to Joseph Wolpe (1958) and enjoy widespread acceptance today (Bancroft, 1977; LoPiccolo, 1977; Leiblum and Pervin, 1980; Leiblum and Rosen, 1989). While many methods used by Masters and Johnson are very similar to behavioral techniques, there are some theoretical and practical differences in approach.

The operant approach to behavioral therapy is to carefully analyze the problematic behavior (e.g., the sexual dysfunction) and to use positive and negative reinforcers best suited to the individual case. Gradual exposure to imaginary scenes of sexual activity may be used before exposure to real-life sexual situations in sensate focus exercises. These techniques are both forms of *desensitization*, in which the controlled exposure to limited amounts of anxiety helps to eliminate the anxiety. *Relaxation training* (learning specific breathing and muscle exercises to reduce tension) and *assertiveness training* (learning how to say what you feel and what you need) are other methods used to reduce anxiety. *Directed masturbation* (LoPiccolo and Lobitz, 1972), which is used in the treatment of anorgasmia, is a nine-step program for helping a woman learn to masturbate to orgasm and then include her partner in her orgasmic response, first in manual stimulation and then during intercourse.

An interesting and logical way of approaching sexual problems has been suggested by behavioral psychologist Jack Annon (1976). He uses a four-level model, represented by the acronym PLISSIT, to go from the simplest to more advanced levels of treatment. The four levels are P = permission, LI = limited information, SS = specific suggestions, and IT = intensive therapy. This model makes use of the fact that in simple cases of sexual difficulties, reassurance and education are sometimes enough to solve the problem. Specific suggestions might include instruction in the squeeze technique or in sensate focus, without dealing with major psychosocial issues. Intensive therapy goes beyond these steps to deal with relationship conflicts, psychological problems, and other complex issues that may be present.

ADDITIONAL PSYCHOTHERAPY METHODS

There are now so many different approaches to sex therapy that it is practically impossible to describe them all. Only brief mention of a few other notable methods can be made here due to space limitations. Lonnie Barbach (1975, 1980) has pioneered in the use of women's groups for treating anorgasmia. These groups have the particular advantages of being relatively inexpensive and quite successful. Psychologist Albert Ellis has developed Rational-Emotive Therapy (RET) as a useful approach to sexual and nonsexual problems. RET helps people overcome irrational beliefs and unrealistic expectations that feed into their sexual dysfunction. Blending behavioral methods with unique strategies for dealing with emotional discomfort (such as shame-attacking exercises, risk-taking exercises), RET principles can be applied in individual, couple, or group therapy.

Some sex therapists follow the controversial practice of "body work therapy" in which the therapist has sexual activity with the patient (Apfelbaum, 1980a). Many ethical objections have been raised to this practice (Marmor, 1980a).

A different approach, still controversial but more widely accepted, is the use of a "surrogate partner" in sex therapy. The surrogate is usually a trained woman who is paid to participate in therapy and sexual activity with a single male to improve his chances of success; there are also a few male surrogates who work with female partners. The surrogate does not function as a cotherapist but usually makes periodic reports to the therapist on the patient's progress and follows their instructions closely (Masters and Johnson, 1970). Although some people have criticized this practice as being only a thinly veiled form of prostitution, others see it as an important means of helping people who are unable to find a partner who will accompany them in sex therapy.

BIOMEDICAL METHODS

In the last decade, a number of significant advances have been made in treating organic forms of male sexual dysfunction by techniques other than "talking" therapies. The most dramatic example of this approach is the use of surgery to implant a device in the penis that makes intercourse possible when the physical capacity to have an erection has been lost due to illness or injury. This form of treatment, called a penile prosthesis, is discussed in more detail in Chapter 10.

An even newer method that is currently being studied in many centers involves the use of a drug called papaverine hydrochloride, which is injected into the body of the penis. This drug causes engorgement of the penis with blood, with the resulting erection typically lasting for several hours, thus permitting sexual intercourse to take place. Men can be taught to administer these injections themselves, and thus far the reports of success using this approach have been heartening (Zorgniotti et al., 1985; Sidi et al., 1986). However, one unwanted side effect of this treatment is that in 5 to 10 percent of users there has been at least one episode of priapism (persistent, painful erection), which requires emergency medical care.

Inhibited male sexual desire that is caused by excessive levels of prolactin in the blood can often be treated successfully with the use of a drug called bromocriptine. In addition, men with erectile dysfunction and/or low sex drive due to a deficiency of testosterone can usually be treated successfully with injections of testosterone on a monthly or bimonthly basis.

Unfortunately, there have not been corresponding treatment advances in dealing with female sexual dysfunction by using biomedical approaches.

THE EFFECTIVENESS OF SEX THERAPY

Because there are many different models of sex therapy and the specialty is still fairly young, evaluating the effectiveness of these approaches is difficult. Most studies to date have not had control groups, and many reports are based on a small number of cases. Other problems are (1) lack of uniform definitions of the dysfunctions, (2) differences in selection of patients, (3) differences in defining success or failure, and (4) lack of adequate follow-up (checking the results periodically after therapy is over). Additional methodological issues have been raised in several detailed reviews (Schumacher, 1977; Hogan, 1978; Kilmann, 1978; Kilmann and Auerbach, 1979).

Psychologists Bernie Zilbergeld and Michael Evans (1980) have criticized the Masters and Johnson data on the effectiveness of sex therapy on a variety of methodological grounds. Specifically, they have questioned the criteria Masters and Johnson used to rate treatment outcomes, suggesting that the results obtained may have reflected undue leniency in deciding how to classify cases. In addition, they suggested that the Masters and Johnson results may have been artificially inflated by selecting only the best candidates for treatment (and rejecting fairly large numbers of cases that appeared "difficult"). In actuality, however, fewer than 1 out of 50 couples who apply to the Masters & Johnson Institute are turned down for therapy, and the criteria used to evaluate the outcome of sex therapy at the Masters & Johnson Institute are relatively stringent (Kolodny, 1981a; Masters et al., 1983). These criticisms also seem to lose sight of the fact that other sex therapy programs are reporting rates of success that are similar to those of the Masters and Johnson program (Rachman and Wilson, 1980; Schover and LoPiccolo, 1982; Apfelbaum, 1983; Arentewicz and Schmidt, 1983).

Some critics of sex therapy have suggested that it is a dehumanizing, mechanistic process. Psychiatrist Natalie Shainess (1973), for example, argues that sex therapy "debases" sex and that Masters and Johnson "have tended to detach the sex act from the moods, feelings, and emotions of desire and love." In her view, sex therapy is a kind of "coaching that reduces one partner to a push-button operator" (Cadden, 1978, p. 487). Psychiatrist Thomas Szasz (1980, p. xvi) sees sex therapists as "determined to conceal moral values and social policies as medical diagnoses and treatment."

As most sex therapists agree, success or failure is a subjective commodity. Some sex therapy patients who are classified as "failures" may see their treatment as very beneficial. Others, who attained enough change in their sexual function to be called a "success" by their therapists, may continue to feel unhappy or anxious. Sometimes two partners disagree about whether therapy was helpful. In all these situations, it is impossible to say that one viewpoint is right or wrong.

Although sex therapy offers no instant, magical cures, a variety of studies show that it can be of significant help to many people. Furthermore, the gains made in sex therapy tend to be long-lasting rather than short-lived (Leiblum and Pervin, 1980). Thus, while sex therapy is no cure-all and some people admittedly require a different type of professional help, sex therapy has managed to improve the lives of thousands of people with sexual distress.

CHOOSING A SEX THERAPIST

Unfortunately, sex therapy is an unregulated profession today. People can call themselves sex therapists even if their "training" consists only of attending a few workshops or reading a book. Judging from letters received at the Masters & Johnson Institute and from situations we have encountered with our patients, there are many fraudulent sex therapists who are deliberately bilking the public, and there are hundreds of well-meaning persons who try to do sex therapy but simply are not qualified. Worse yet, emotional problems may be created by improper therapy, sexual problems may worsen, and the lack of success may discourage a person from seeking further care.

To minimize the risk of falling prey to unqualified sex therapists, the following guidelines may be of assistance:

1. Turn first to sex therapy centers that are affiliated with universities, medical schools, or hospitals. Alternately, your local medical society, psychological association, or your family physician may be able to provide a list of qualified therapists. Two professional organizations, the Society for Sex Therapy and Research (New York, NY) and the American Association of Sex Educators, Counselors, and Therapists (Washington, DC), publish national directories. AASECT has a sex therapist certification program; SSTAR has tougher membership requirements that it believes are equivalent to certification.
2. Ask about the education and training of the sex therapist. Unless he or she is willing to discuss this with you, do not continue any further. In addition to a genuine graduate degree from a recognized university, be sure to verify that the therapist has received postgraduate training in sex therapy that included personal supervision. Attendance at a weekend seminar isn't the same as in-depth training.
3. Avoid therapists who make unrealistic promises or guarantees of cure and therapists who tell you that part of your "treatment" includes having sexual relations with them.
4. Be sure the therapist is willing to discuss treatment costs, schedules, and plans in an open, straightforward fashion. (Many sex therapy clinics have a sliding scale fee arrangement where charges are adjusted to the client's ability to pay.)

PREVENTING SEXUAL DYSFUNCTION

The prevention of sexual dysfunctions probably begins in the parenting role by providing children with sex information appropriate for their age and by permitting them to discuss sexuality in an open, honest fashion. Severely negative family attitudes about sex may predispose a child to later sexual difficulties. After childhood, the following pointers apply:

1. Approach sex as an opportunity for exploration and intimacy instead of as a job to be done. Goal-oriented sex creates performance demands, which can lead to spectatoring and impaired responsivity. Remember that there's no "right" way of having sex; it's a matter of personal interest and comfort.
2. Try to develop open, effective lines of communication with your partner. Guessing about what your partner wants is difficult at best; making your partner guess about your needs is equally problematic. Effective communication includes being able to say no just as well as yes: if you never say no, your partner can't be sure if your yes is genuine or not.
3. Don't believe everything you read or hear about sex. Many books and articles about how people "should" respond are oversimplified at best and may be inaccurate and misleading. It's easy to talk yourself into a problem by comparing yourself to what "others" say.
4. If you're having a sexual problem of any sort, discuss it with your partner instead of pretending it doesn't exist. Often, by using some of the sensate focus methods or the self-help readings listed at the end of this chapter, a solution can be found. *However, if the problem doesn't go away fairly quickly, seek professional help*. It's usually

much easier to treat recent problems than problems that have solidified over a long time.

SUMMARY

1. Sexual dysfunctions are conditions in which the physical responses of sexual function are impaired. In males, the principal sexual dysfunctions are erectile dysfunction, premature ejaculation, ejaculatory incompetence, and retarded ejaculation; in women, they are anorgasmia, vaginismus, and dyspareunia.
2. Overall, about 10 to 20 percent of cases of sexual dysfunction have organic causes such as diabetes, alcoholism, infection, neurologic disease, and drugs. Psychosocial causes can be classified as developmental (e.g., negative sex attitudes, sexual trauma), personal (e.g., anxiety, depression, guilt), or interpersonal (e.g., poor communication, relationship conflicts, hostility).
3. Inhibited sexual desire and sexual aversion are examples of sexual problems that do not necessarily cause dysfunction but can lead to considerable emotional distress.
4. Sex therapy as a distinct specialty originated with the work of Masters and Johnson. Their approach involves a cotherapy team working with couples on a daily basis over a two-week period emphasizing integration of physiologic and psychosocial information. Sex is seen as a natural function; sensate focus exercises are used to reduce anxiety and improve spontaneity; and methods such as the "squeeze" technique (for premature ejaculation) and use of vaginal dilators (for vaginismus) are sometimes employed along with careful attention to relationship dynamics.
5. Other approaches to therapy include Helen Kaplan's work (integrating sex therapy and psychoanalytic methods), behavioral models, Rational-Emotive therapy, and group therapy.
6. Although sex therapy is not foolproof, it has been shown to be highly effective in most studies. Many so-called sex therapists, however, have little or no formal training in the field, so it is important to choose a sex therapist carefully.

Thought Questions

1. Researchers have concluded that about 10 percent of women have never experienced coital orgasm. Do you think this finding is correct? Why or why not?
2. The text states that ejaculatory incompetence may be a potential source of sexual pleasure due to the man's ability to prolong coitus. Do you agree or disagree with this idea? Explain.
3. Psychological, familial, cultural, and biological factors can all contribute to the development of sexual dysfunction. How should these factors be changed to reduce the number of people who are sexually dysfunctional in our population?
4. Why do women fake orgasms? What are their motives? Is it always wrong for a woman to fake an orgasm? Can men accurately discriminate fake from real orgasms? *Should* men wonder whether their partners are faking? How should a man deal with these suspicions? How should a woman who has not had an orgasm but whose partner thinks she has respond to the situation? How should a woman who has been habitually faking orgasms and wants to change handle the situation?
5. Should a sex therapist *ever* engage in sexual activities with a client? How often do you think this happens? What if the client is attracted to the therapist and wants to engage in sex with him or her?
6. What should a couple who are committed to their relationship do if they find that they have very different levels of sexual needs? What if one member experiences sexual aversion or inhibited sexual desire? How should the partner best respond?
7. For most men who develop erectile dysfunctions, do you think they would prefer to learn that the cause was physiological or psychological in nature? Assuming the cause was psychological, how should the partner act so that she demonstrates sexual desire but at the same time avoids making what could be interpreted as a demand for performance?

Suggested Readings

Belliveau, Fred, and Richter, Lin. *Understanding Human Sexual Inadequacy*. New York: Bantam, 1970. A translation into nontechnical language of *Human Sexual Inadequacy*, accurately summarizing the content in easily readable form.

Castleman, M. *Sexual Solutions*. New York: Touchstone, 1989. An updated revision of a comprehensive guide to dealing with sexual problems, this book covers a lot of territory concerning sexual dysfunctions and sex therapy.

Heiman, Julia; LoPiccolo, Leslie; and LoPiccolo, Joseph. *Becoming Orgasmic: A Sexual Growth Program for Women*. Englewood Cliffs, N.J.: Prentice-Hall, 1976. A personal sensitively written book designed to help women overcome sexual difficulties.

Kaplan, Helen. *The Illustrated Manual of Sex Therapy*. New York: Quadrangle/New York Times, 1975. A beautifully produced book with tasteful illustrations and clear, concise explanations of Kaplan's approach to sex therapy.

Kaplan, Helen S. *How to Overcome Premature Ejaculation*. New York: Brunner/Mazel, 1989. This slim book (only 118 pages with large type) describes the causes and treatment of premature ejaculation in easy-to-understand terms.

Leiblum, S. R., and Rosen, R. C. *Sexual Desire Disorders*. New York: Guilford Press, 1988. An outstanding collection of thoughtful and carefully documented papers summarizing the various treatment approaches to disorders of sexual desire.

Ambitious students who are willing to wade through more technical terminology might also be interested in Helen Kaplan's *Disorders of Sexual Desire* (Brunner/Mazel, 1979), Lonnie Barbach's *Women Discover Orgasm* (Free Press, 1980), Leiblum's and Rosen's *Principles and Practices of Sex Therapy* (Guilford Press, 1989), and the original *Human Sexual Inadequacy* (Little, Brown, 1970) by Masters and Johnson.

10

Sexual Disorders and Sexual Health

Sexual health is tightly interwoven with total health: both depend on freedom from physical and emotional limitations. The preceding chapter emphasized emotional causes of sexual distress and ways of dealing with these problems. In this chapter, we consider the physical conditions that affect sexuality. Our discussion covers four major topics: sex and disability, the impact of illness on sexuality, drugs and sex, and infections involving the sex organs. Learning about these problems is important because it increases our understanding of the physiology of sex and helps us better grasp the emotional dimension of such situations.

SEX AND DISABILITY

A number of common myths and stereotypes about sexuality of disabled people have been identified by the Sex & Disability Project of George Washington University. These myths, which "can drastically and unnecessarily curtail the sexual expression of disabled people" (Chipouras et al., 1979), are as follows:

1. Disabled people are asexual.
2. Disabled people are dependent and childlike, so they need to be protected.
3. Disability breeds disability.
4. Disabled people should stay with and marry their own kind.
5. Parents of handicapped children don't want sex education for their children.
6. Sexual intercourse culminating in orgasm is essential for sexual satisfaction.
7. If a disabled person has a sexual problem, it's almost always the result of the disability.
8. If a nondisabled person has a sexual relationship with a disabled individual, it's because he or she can't attract anyone else.

These myths collectively show how uncomfortable our society is with the idea of disabled persons as sexual beings. Somehow, many people seem to think, the disabled should worry about more important things in their lives and not concern themselves with an area that is obviously intended for healthy, "normal" people to enjoy. Fortunately, many of those who are disabled have refused to be intimidated by this line of reasoning and have joined forces with a number of workers in the health-care professions as activists in seeking more attention to the sexual needs and feelings of people who have one form of disability or another. In fact, this movement has led to the development of a sexual bill of rights for the disabled (Chipouras et al., 1979) that covers the following items:

1. The right to sexual expression.
2. The right to privacy.
3. The right to be informed.
4. The right to have access to needed services such as contraceptive counseling, medical care, genetic counseling, and sex counseling.
5. The right to choose one's marital status.
6. The right to have or not have children.
7. The right to make decisions that affect one's life.
8. The right to develop to one's fullest potential.

Although we are not yet in an era when the disabled are totally free to exercise these rights, we have made considerable progress in this direction in the last decade. As attitudes toward the disabled continue to change and as our society accepts sexuality as a positive, enhancing aspect of all of our lives, we may finally see the disappearance of myths and stereotypes and a more tolerant, open, and informed attitude taking their place.

Spinal Cord Injuries

A dramatic example of the impact of a disability on sexuality can be seen in people who have had injuries of the spinal cord. These injuries occur in a variety of circumstances, such as auto or motorcycle accidents, stab or bullet wounds, crushing industrial accidents, diving accidents, and serious falls. The injury usually results in **paraplegia** (paralysis of the legs) or **quadriplegia** (paralysis of all four limbs) and loss of all sensations in the body below the level of the injury. Normal bowel and bladder control is usually lost, and persons with spinal cord injuries are apt to have a significant loss of sexual function as well.

Most spinal-cord-injured (SCI) men lose the ability to have normal erections in response to psychological arousal, although they may be able to have brief reflex erections (which they cannot feel) in response to mechanical stimulation such as pinching or rubbing close to the genitals. In some cases, SCI males have partial erections in response to psychological stimuli such as watching erotic movies or listening to erotic tapes but

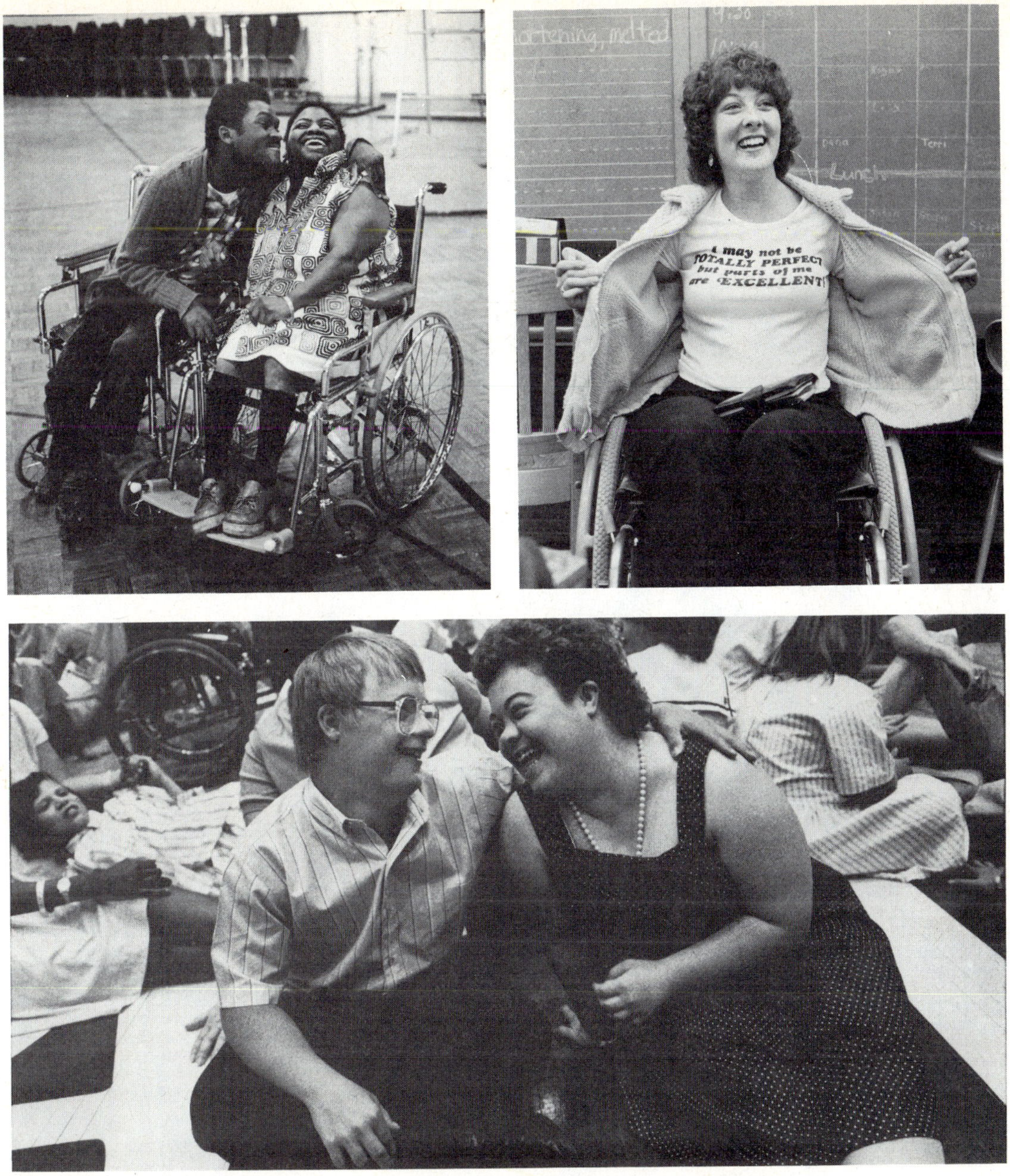

The joy of loving and being loved is shared by disabled people. Despite popular misconceptions, the disabled also have sexual feelings and needs, which can be expressed in a multiplicity of ways.

don't realize that they're responding in this manner (Kennedy and Over, 1990). Most (but not all) SCI males also become infertile and lose the ability to ejaculate. [Szasz and Carpenter (1989) state that under 10 percent of men with complete spinal cord injuries experience ejaculation with intercourse.] Those who are still able to ejaculate do so with no pelvic sensations of orgasm, and in many of the cases retrograde ejaculation (a backflow of semen into the bladder) occurs. On the other hand, intercourse may

paraplegia paralysis of both lower extremities.
quadriplegia (kwahd ruh pleej' ee ah) paralysis of all limbs.

PERSONAL PERSPECTIVES

Sex and Disability

Understanding the impact of a major disability on a person's sexuality is not simply a matter of understanding sexual physiology or even the medical side of the disability. The following candid observations explain, in their own ways, other aspects of the disability that may be eye-opening.

First, Don Smith talks about his reactions after a spinal cord injury at age 19:

> I felt asexual for a long time because a man's sex was supposed to be in his penis, and I couldn't feel my penis. So that contributed to my feeling of being asexual; it didn't occur to me that it felt good to have the back of my neck licked, or that it felt good to have my arms stroked lightly. Stroking the wrists, then to the arms, then up the arms is a sequence that I've since learned can be very exciting.
>
> A lot of my first sexual contacts were just to gain experience. I wanted to find out what was going on and what I liked. With the help of two really excellent lovers, I learned about my body.

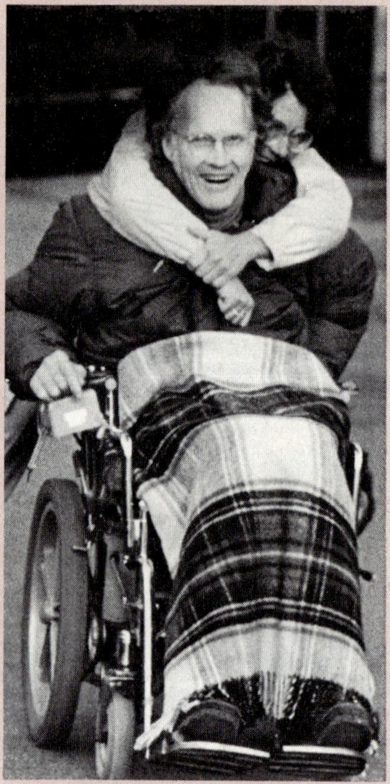

> I learned to take goals out of my lovemaking; I don't have to have intercourse or any kind of penetration if I'm going to have sex. I don't even have to do anything with the genitals if I'm going to have sex. I can take my time; I feel less pressure and less performance anxiety. That's not to say it's all gone, because it's there; I want to be there for my partner. *(Bullard and Knight, 1981, p. 16)*

A spinal-cord-injured woman discusses some aspects of her relationships with men:

> I find that I am often suspicious of the motives of men who are attracted to me sexually. That is, some men want to be caretakers; some men can't find able-bodied partners (and assume that disabled women are also unable to find partners). Other men are sexually intrigued with disabled women, believing they will have a "kinky" experience; some men want a "strong mother confessor" figure they can depend on or want a woman who will be totally dependent on them. I don't intend to do a general indictment of the whole male race, but I do believe disabled women must be very selective in choosing partners.
>
> Many of my relationships have matured into strong relationships with sexual dimensions, some of my partners have been "affairs," flings, one-night stands, etc. During my sexually active years, I have had several different partners; among them three long-term relationships. I have had one sexual experience

be possible for about four out of five men with incomplete spinal cord injuries. Even when erections do not occur, a technique called "stuffing" can be used. This involves tucking the soft or semifirm penis into the vagina, with the woman thrusting her hips, taking care not to move so the penis falls out.

Women with spinal cord injuries generally have normal fertility and can have children. While they usually retain their interest in sex, they typically lose their genital sensations and orgasmic responsiveness, and their vaginal lubrication is greatly reduced. Some SCI women—as well as SCI men—report experiencing "phantom" (nongenital) orgasms which include both psychological feelings of orgasm (e.g., intense with a gay woman. *(Becker, 1978)*

A 25-year-old woman with cerebral palsy talks about her sexual feelings:

> When I was a teenager, I was intensely jealous of the beautiful, able-bodied women I saw on television and in the movies. I thought that sex was for them, not me, and I was angry because I knew I'd never have a baby. In fact, I was pretty much resigned to never finding a husband and being celibate all my life.
>
> Fortunately, I learned how to masturbate at age 12 or 13. I figured out a way of getting a rubber hose attachment from the faucet near my genitals while I was bathing, and I quickly found myself looking forward to baths for reasons quite apart from cleanliness. The almost electric, tingly feeings of sexual excitement began to build up for me slowly for hours before bath time, and the sudden surge of a climax was sheer joy. Even now, years later, I still get excited thinking about this wonderful way of stimulating myself or having a partner do it for me. But what was most important was that my discovery of the joys of masturbating let me know that I was a sexual being, that it was legitimate to have these feelings. *(Authors' files)*

Finally, consider the comments of a man remembering his reactions after a spinal cord injury resulting in quadriplegia at age 16:

> At home I felt like the town eunuch for a few years. I saw a lot of the women I had been dating before I broke my neck, but now there was nothing sexual going on between us. I kept secretly blaming them for not giving me a chance, not treating me as needing or wanting or even being capable of having a sexual relationship. Now I realize that I wasn't *acting* like I needed or wanted or was capable of having a sexual relationship. The simple truth was that I was just plain scared. I didn't know what I could do, how I could pleasure or be pleasured, and I sure didn't want to look like a jerk while trying to find out, or worse yet, find out I was a failure and face the eventual rejection.
>
> My eunuch years also included a lot of martyrdom. I remember deciding that if I ever really fell in love with someone, I would end the relationship because I thought, being in a wheelchair, I could never really make anyone happy. *(Bullard and Knight, 1981, pp. 65–66)*

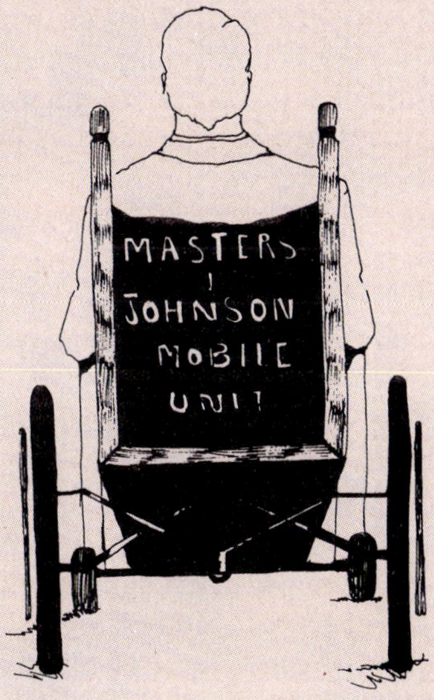

As these heartfelt recollections show, the disabled are very much interested in and able to have sexual feelings and relationships. It is the mistaken assumption of an able-bodied society that impose an asexual image on these individuals, which is equivalent to denying the very core of their humanity.

pleasure) and physical sensations in some unaffected areas of the body that resemble prior patterns of orgasmic response.

Many people cannot understand why a spinal-cord-injured person who has no genital sensations would want to have intercourse. While the motivations of all cord-injured people are not the same, the following reasons are commonly given by people in this situation:

1. Having intercourse is a special act of sharing and intimacy quite apart from genital feelings.
2. Having intercourse can be intensely *psychologically* arousing.

3. Being able to engage in intercourse can provide a boost to a person's self-concept.

In addition, many cord-injured males mention that being able to have intercourse makes them feel more like a man, while some cord-injured females note that having intercourse enhances their sense of femininity. There are also some cord-injured persons who have intercourse primarily to please their partner (just as some people *without* cord injuries do, too).

While a number of people have pointed out that the SCI woman is less handicapped sexually than the SCI man because she is still able to have intercourse, this is an oversimplification of a complex issue and perpetuates a view of females as sexually passive. Many cord-injured women are distressed by their sexual limitations and require counseling to help them reaffirm their sexuality (Thornton, 1979). Unfortunately, as Zwerner (1982) points out, sexuality counseling is not included in many rehabilitation programs for SCI women, forcing many to seek out such services on their own or to do without their potential benefits.

The sexual abilities of the spinal-cord-injured and their ways of coping with their situation vary greatly. While some adopt a completely defeatist attitude and avoid all sexual opportunities, others have a continuing interest in sex which they express through active involvement with a partner. What must be stressed is that there are many methods of sexual interaction besides intercourse (Mooney, Cole, and Chilgren, 1975). Oral–genital sex, kissing, use of a vibrator (which a quadriplegic can sometimes apply by holding the base with his or her teeth), massage, and cuddling are only a few of the available options for having intimacy and sexual pleasure. In fact, recent research has shown that applying a vibrator directly to the penis of a cord-injured man produces a predictable series of body reactions that are quite similar to the nongenital physical changes found in the sexual response cycle of non-SCI men (Szasz and Carpenter, 1989). (Note: This type of stimulation should only be used in SCI males with medical consultation because there is a high risk of a dangerous reaction of soaring blood pressure and severe headache unless the proper medication is used in advance.) In addition, many SCI people find that unaffected regions of their body become extraordinarily sensitive and erotic, so that stimulation above the region of sensory loss can produce arousal and sometimes orgasm.

It is also possible for the SCI man with permanently impaired erections to have a device implanted surgically that will permit him to have erections and to participate in intercourse. (This topic is discussed in more detail on page 291.)

An experimental procedure called electroejaculation now offers some hope for fathering children to the nation's 145,000 spinal-cord-injured men who had previously been considered infertile (Raymond, 1987). The procedure, which is based on a method widely used in animal husbandry, involves inserting a probe into the rectum and then passing an electric current into the instrument until ejaculation is electrically induced. While this method is far from foolproof, and has a small but definite risk of injury to the rectum, success rates of about 45 percent have been attained so far (Bennett et al., 1988).

Blindness and Deafness

If a person is blind or deaf from birth (or from a very young age), the sexual learning that occurs during childhood and adolescence can be seriously hindered. The person who has been blind since birth, for instance, is deprived of the ability to see the various shapes of human bodies both clothed and undressed that most of us silently notice and learn from. As a result, the person with lifelong blindness may be quite uncertain about the anatomic relation of one part of the body to another. (One 15-year-old boy was quite surprised to learn that the female breasts weren't located just above the waist, where he imagined them to be.) The person who has been deaf since birth often has difficulty understanding abstract concepts like maleness, parenting, and intimacy (FitzGerald and FitzGerald, 1977). Since very few parents of deaf children can communicate with them effectively with sign language, sex education in the home is often difficult.

Neither blindness nor deafness produces any physical limitations on the body's sexual responsivity in and of itself. However, the sexual ignorance of many deaf or blind persons may create a predisposition toward sexual and relationship problems. In addition, the distorted body image and poor self-esteem that many deaf or blind persons experience can also contribute to later sexual difficulties. Since blind persons do not have the visual cues surrounding sexual behavior that most of us depend on, and deaf people are apt to have significant problems in communicating with others, it's not surprising that such difficulties might occur.

Fortunately, sex education curricula have been de-

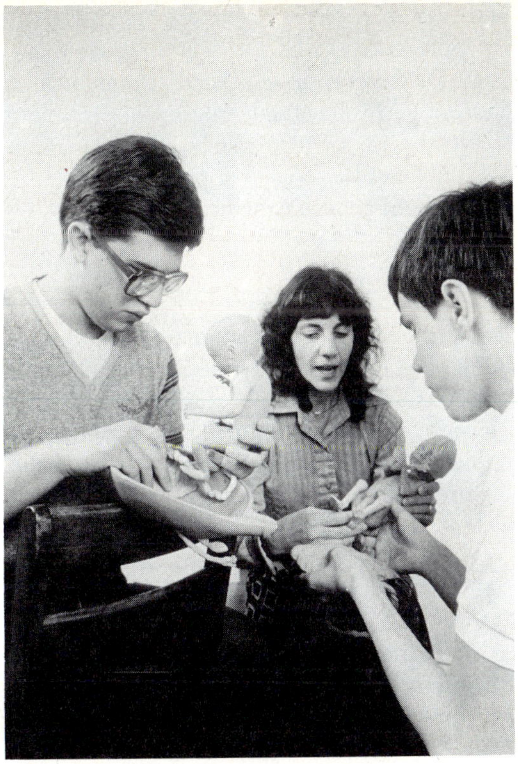

Two blind students are being educated about pregnancy by an instructor using lifelike plastic models. This type of sexual education is invaluable to persons with sensory disabilities.

vised for the deaf and blind. Most of these programs emphasize both social and biological aspects of sexuality and make good use of innovative methods of teaching as well. For instance, blind students may be given sex-related articles like condoms, tampons, birth control pill packages, and vibrators to handle, so they develop familiarity with these products by touch. In fact, in Europe the touch method is sometimes used for anatomy lessons with live nude models (Helsinga, 1974). Many deaf students are now being taught by sex educators trained in sign language, and special visual materials have been prepared to make sex education easier despite the existence of hearing impairment.

Mental Retardation

Until very recently, people who are mentally retarded have been viewed as either asexual (in a state of childlike innocence) or as totally impulse-ridden and unable to control their primitive sexual urges. These myths, along with the general public's distaste for seeing the retarded as persons in their own right, have combined to make the topic of sexuality and the retarded a threatening one that arouses indignation and sometimes anger. One reflection of this attitude that has recently been changed was the involuntary sterilization that was often performed on young retarded adults or even adolescents to ensure that they couldn't reproduce (even though there is no evidence that most forms of retardation are genetically transmitted).

It is important to recognize that not all mentally retarded people are alike in their learning capacity, emotional stability, social skills, or capacity for independent living. The mildly retarded, for example, are educable and often lead productive lives, holding jobs, marrying, and raising families. Their lives are often indistinguishable from the lives of "normal" people, and they are usually capable of learning responsible sexual behavior without difficulty (Monat, 1982). The moderately retarded do not fit into our society so easily and are more apt to behave in a childlike manner both sexually and in other areas of living. They may alarm people by masturbating or disrobing in public or acting in a fashion that appears to be reckless or aggressive when showing affection for others, and they often require a protected or restricted environment to live their lives as comfortably and safely as possible. Yet they too are capable of learning much about sexuality and reproduction; for example, they can be taught how babies are conceived, what menstruation is (and how to deal with it), and how to channel their sexual impulses into appropriate (i.e., nonpublic) masturbation. They also can learn how to avoid taking advantage of others and how to avoid sexual abuse. The severely or profoundly retarded, who must generally be institutionalized for their own safety, present a different range of problems since they are much more difficult to teach and are often capable of only the most rudimentary forms of communication.

The primary way of helping retarded people learn to handle their sexual feelings and express their sexual desires is through appropriate sex education. Kempton (1978) notes: "The retarded need sex education more than anyone else because they cannot readily learn about sexuality from friends, books, or from observing the behavior of others, and they have more than usual difficulty with sorting out reality from unreality" (p. 138). In addition, cause-and-effect relationships are not always clear to the retarded; for instance, they may not realize that having intercourse can cause pregnancy. While some parents of retarded children have worried that sex education simply puts ideas into their children's heads, the available evidence suggests that withholding sex information does not deter sexual behavior and providing sex education does not lead to irresponsible sexual acts: in fact, just the opposite is likely to happen (Kempton, 1978; Monat, 1982).

A number of specific issues regarding sex and the mentally retarded are too complex to discuss meaningfully here. These issues include the following:

1. Providing privacy for the institutionalized retarded.
2. Providing appropriate contraceptive protection for the retarded. (In general, the IUD seems to be the best option for retarded women who are sexually active. Birth control pills are appropriate for use by the mildly retarded, but condoms, diaphragms, and foams are usually not practical since they are too easily forgotten and too difficult for many to use.)
3. Providing opportunities for long-term relationships and marriage, if desired.

Further information about these and related topics can be found in several books listed at the end of this chapter.

SEX AND MEDICAL ILLNESS

A wide variety of medical illnesses cause sexual problems. Until fairly recently, these situations were generally overlooked by health-care professionals, who were often uncomfortable discussing sexuality, uninformed about sexual aspects of illness, and untrained in providing useful ways of dealing with these problems. Fortunately, this situation is rapidly changing today because fundamental research in this area is increasing and most health-care schools include specific education about sexuality in their curricula.

Illnesses affect sexuality in direct and indirect ways. Physically, an illness can disrupt the normal reflexes of sexual response, as seen in persons with multiple sclerosis. Sometimes the treatment of an illness creates a sexual problem: medications that cause sexual side effects or surgery that results in sexual impairment are common examples. In other instances, sexual problems arise from the general effects of illness such as weakness, fatigue, or pain. There is an emotional side too: people with an illness may assume that it is "wrong" for them to have sexual feelings or may believe erroneously that their illness will prevent them from enjoying sex or from functioning sexually.

Now we describe the sexual problems encountered in some specific types of medical disorders.

Neurologic Conditions

Sexual behavior and sexual function are both controlled in important ways by the nervous system. The brain itself is the ultimate synthesizer of sensory input (touch, sight, sound, taste, smell) and transforms electric impulses sent to it by nerve fibers into perceptions of pleasure, pain, and human emotion. Similarly, impulses sent from the brain to other organs, including the genitals, translate sexual desire into sexual response. For these reasons, it is easy to see why many diseases or injuries of the nervous system can lead to sexual difficulties.

Multiple sclerosis (MS) is a disease that typically affects young adults and involves patchy damage to the protective covering of nerves throughout the body. Loss of erections and ejaculation eventually affects more than half of men with MS (Schover et al., 1988), while difficulty reaching orgasm (or complete anorgasmia) affects a similar fraction of women (Lilius, Valtonen, and Wikström, 1976). Early in the disease there may be a partial numbness in the genitals, and sometimes any type of touch to the affected body region produces irritating, unpleasant sensations (Lundberg, 1977). For this reason, painful intercourse is another common problem. The sexual effects of MS tend to vary over time, so a person may have difficulties for several weeks or months and then go through a period of relatively normal sexual function.

People with **brain tumors** are somewhat less likely to encounter sexual difficulties. Although pituitary or hypothalamic tumors commonly cause erectile dysfunction and decreased sexual desire (Lundberg and Wide, 1978), tumors in other regions of the brain do not usually lead to sexual problems. **Epilepsy** is another neurologic disorder with little physical effect on sexual function (Jensen et al., 1990). Some people with epilepsy, however, feel inferior because of their condition and may avoid sexual opportunities in the mistaken fear that arousal will cause a seizure. Although **polio** can cause spinal cord damage, it affects muscular function, not sensations. For this reason, most people with paralysis from polio are not impaired in their sexual function, although their inability to move may create problems in coital thrusting.

Another common neurologic condition is **Alzheimer's disease**, which affects an estimated 2 to 4 percent of people over age 65 (American Psychiatric Association, 1987). Alzheimer's disease is a progressive form of degenerative brain disease of unknown cause that produces dementia, usually resulting in death after five to seven years. People with Alzheimer's disease usually have a loss of brain functions, including difficulties with memory, judgment, and abstract thought. There is usually speech impairment and deterioration in mental alertness, along with personality changes, but these features may be minimal early in the disease. According to Shapira and Cummings (1989), the most typical pattern of sexual behavior shown by male Alzheimer victims is a loss of interest in sex. However, there was marked variability in their sample, with a small number of Alzheimer patients showing a heightened interest in sex. These researchers also noted that it was common for the wife of the Alzheimer's patient to stop having sex with her husband as he became increasingly dependent and childlike, and as caring for him became more and more of a drain on her time. This sometimes caused considerable guilt on the wife's part, however.

Endocrine Conditions

The most common type of endocrine disorder is **diabetes,** which affects approximately 4 percent of the U.S. population. About 50 percent of diabetic men have erectile dysfunction, which either can be an early symptom of this disorder or may not occur for many years after the diagnosis (Podolsky, 1983; Pfeifer, 1988). Retrograde ejaculation occurs in about 1 percent of diabetic men, but sex drive is usually unaffected. Although the sexual difficulties of diabetic men had been well known for at least two centuries, sexual problems in diabetic women were not identified until the 1970s. Although one study found that about one-third of diabetic women have secondary anorgasmia, which usually occurs four to six years after the disease is discovered (Kolodny, 1971), other studies have not completely confirmed this finding. A report by Jensen (1986), for instance, found that 14 percent of diabetic females had orgasmic dysfunction and 20 percent had reduced sexual desire. In addition, some diabetic women have problems with vaginal lubrication. Prather (1988) provides a recent review of previous research in this area.

FOCUS IN BRIEF

Sexual Dysfunction in Diabetic Males

- Erectile dysfunction affects approximately 50 percent of men with diabetes.
- In more than 90 percent of the cases, the erectile difficulties have a gradual onset, typically progressing from occasional episodes of erectile failure to complete impotence over a period of 6 to 12 months.
- Characteristically, the male's sex drive remains normal and ejaculation is undisturbed.
- The primary causes of erectile dysfunction due to diabetes are diabetic nerve damage and abnormalities in the small blood vessels supplying the penis.
- Approximately 1 percent of diabetic men develop retrograde ejeculation, a condition in which semen spurts backward into the bladder at the time of ejaculation.
- The erectile dysfunction caused by diabetes does not usually lessen genital sensations.
- Penile implants can be used to permit the diabetic male to have intercourse successfully.

multiple sclerosis (MS) a chronic neurological disorder affecting both motor and sensory function in an episodic but progressive fashion.

brain tumors abnormal growths in the brain which can either be malignant (cancerous) or nonmalignant.

epilepsy a disease of unkown origin marked by the periodic occurrence of seizures (convulsions).

polio an infection caused by a virus that can, in severe forms, cause paralysis.

Alzheimer's disease a progressive form of degenerative brain disease that causes dementia (deterioration of mental abilities).

diabetes a chronic disorder of how the body handles sugar because of an insulin deficiency. Complications of this disease include circulatory and neurological problems.

The primary cause of these sexual problems in both diabetic men and women is a form of nerve damage that is a complication of diabetes (Rowland et al., 1989; Tejada et al., 1989). In a smaller fraction of cases, these dysfunctions are due to circulatory problems. Unfortunately, both types of problems tend to be permanent and untreatable (except for the possibility of using penile implants to overcome erectile dysfunction). In cases where diabetics have sexual difficulties for other reasons, such as anxiety or poor communication, sex therapy can be beneficial (Kolodny, Masters, and Johnson, 1979; Clarke, 1988).

Disorders of the pituitary, thyroid, or adrenal glands are also commonly associated with sexual difficulties. In each of these conditions, sex drive is likely to be altered along with sexual function. About 40 percent of women with an underactive thyroid or adrenal glands have orgasmic difficulties, and a similar percentage of men have problems with erections (Kolodny, Masters, and Johnson, 1979). Sexual dysfunction is even higher in people with underactive pituitary glands. Fortunately, these conditions are easily treatable by giving the proper amount of the "missing" hormone in pill form.

Heart Disease

In severe forms of chronic heart disease, the capacity for sexual activity is likely to be greatly limited. In milder types of heart problems, however, there may be no physical limitation on sexual activity. Nevertheless, several studies of men who had heart attacks have shown that six months to a year after recovery, sexual difficulties are common (Singh et al., 1970; Green, 1975; Mehta and Krop, 1979). The primary factor here is not a physical one but a mental one: anxiety, misconception, and avoidance conspire to create sexual difficulties. The man may be worried that his heart attack will cause sexual problems or that sexual excitement will cause another heart attack. This worry is also expressed in stories about men dying from a massive heart attack in the midst of a passionate sexual episode. There is no solid evidence to support this as a meaningful risk for most heart patients, and the cardiac cost of sexual activity—including intercourse and orgasm—seems to be about the same as the cost incurred in walking up two flights of steps (Masur, 1979; McLane, Krop, and Mehta, 1980). Women who have had heart attacks seem to be less likely to develop subsequent sexual problems than men (Kolodny, Masters, and Johnson, 1979; Schover and Jensen, 1988).

Cancer

Until the last decade, most people have automatically assumed that a person with cancer could not possibly have sexual feelings or sexual needs. Now it is clear that this view is incorrect, and increasing attention is being paid to the sexuality of people with cancer (Derogatis and Kourlesis, 1981). Several types of cancer and their impact on sexuality will be briefly examined.

BREAST CANCER

An American woman has about a 1 in 11 chance of developing breast cancer, the most frequent female cancer and the second leading cause of cancer death in women after lung cancer (Council on Scientific Affairs, 1989). More than 130,000 new cases of breast cancer are discovered each year, and early detection significantly increases the chances of survival and even cure.

Unfortunately, recent research shows that more than one-third of women with breast cancer only discover this condition accidentally (Lund, 1988). Most don't routinely examine their own breasts or have mammography (x-rays of the breasts), even though the medical evidence is strong that such procedures can be life-saving (Tabar et al., 1985; Brody, 1988; Eddy et al., 1988). (Self-examination of the breasts is discussed in the boxed item on page 36.) In fact, for the first time ever, 11 major medical organizations such as the American Cancer Society, the National Cancer Institute, and the American Medical Association have finally agreed that all women age 40 or over should undergo mammography.

A mammogram, which costs about $100, can detect tumors as small as the point of a pencil—tumors that are far too small to be detected by a woman during a breast self-exam. The actual procedure involves x-raying each breast separately while it is placed in a compression device that exerts gentle pressure on the breast, flattening it so that an accurate x-ray picture can be taken. A side view and a front-to-back view of each breast are usually taken, for a total of four x-rays. The great majority of women (88 percent) undergoing mammography report no discomfort with the procedure or only mild discomfort; only 2 percent

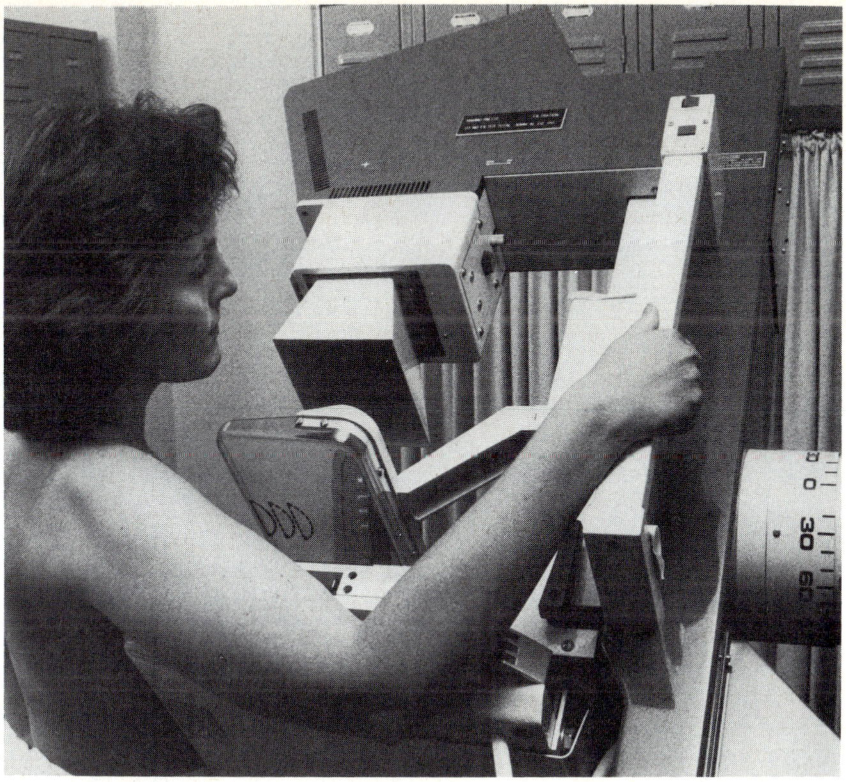

A machine used for mammography. Today, two mammograms are taken of each breast. This is the diagonal view; the other is horizontal. The shield will press slightly down on the breast to get the best results.

report severe discomfort or actual pain (Stomper et al., 1988).

While experts agree that there is no need for women under age 35 to have a mammogram because breast cancer is unusual in this age range, many suggest that women between the ages of 35 and 39 should have one mammogram done to serve as a baseline to be compared to future screenings. Current recommendations are that women in their 40s should have a mammogram every two years unless they have a family history of breast cancer, in which case they should be screened annually. From age 50 on, women should ideally have a mammogram every year.

In addition, recent studies by the Breast Cancer Detection Demonstration Project (Gail et al., 1989) provide a way of calculating a woman's risk for developing breast cancer. The calculation involves an equation with four factors: age when menstruation began, whether her mother or sisters have had breast cancer, her age at the birth of her first live-born child, and the number of negative breast biopsies a woman has had.

It is hoped that by identifying women at particularly high risk for breast cancer, they can be encouraged to take steps geared toward both prevention and early detection. Possible preventive actions include, for example, losing weight if the woman is overweight, lowering fat consumption, and stopping the use of alcohol, since each of these factors has been tied to an increased risk of breast cancer (Kelsey et al., 1981; Helmrich et al., 1983; Graham, 1987; Schatzkin et al., 1987; LaVecchia et al., 1987). Early detection can be improved by regular monthly breast self-exams and by regular mammograms from age 40 on. The value of early detection is quite clear from this statistic: when found at a localized stage, five-year cancer survival rates usually exceed 85 percent (King, 1989).

Breast cancer is usually treated by **mastectomy,** surgical removal of the affected breast. This operation typically creates psychological conflicts for the woman, with concerns about physical attractiveness and possible rejection by her husband or sexual partner ranking high on the list (Witkin, 1975; Notman, 1978). Perhaps this response is not surprising in light

mastectomy (mas tek′ tuh mē) surgical removal of the breast.

of the degree to which our society emphasizes the breast as a symbol of sexuality and femininity. As a result, the woman who has a mastectomy is likely to feel "incomplete" and unfeminine.

Although surgical removal of a breast does not "cause" sexual problems in a direct, physical sense, the psychological impact of mastectomy can be profound. Women react in a variety of ways ranging from relatively easy adjustment to depression, loss of sexual desire, or sexual dysfunction. Following mastectomy, a few women avoid all forms of sexual activity. More typically, the frequency of sexual activity declines and women initiate sexual activity less often than they did before (Frank et al., 1978).

Nudity may be a matter of self-consciousness for the woman or discomfort for her partner. The couple may shift away from intercourse in the female-on-top position, since the male looks directly at the area of the surgical scar. Women who are without a partner at the time of the mastectomy may be particularly worried about dating and what to tell a prospective sexual partner; they may also be afraid that no man could possibly fall in love with a woman with one breast. The following comment is typical of the reactions many women have:

> After having a mastectomy at age 45, I was absolutely convinced my love life was over. After all, I thought, it was bad enough being single, but now with an ugly scar and a disfigured body, I could hardly be the target of anyone's ardent desires. For two years I moped around in this semidepressed state, feeling sorry for myself and feeling lonely, too. So when a neighbor asked me to his company's Christmas party, I was reluctant to accept at first. You can imagine my surprise when our date led to more invitations and the kindling of a romantic spark between us. Although I was acutely uncomfortable with the situation, I finally convinced myself to tell him about my "condition"—and was absolutely flabbergasted when it didn't scare him away, or even bother him. While we didn't wind up getting married, it wasn't because of any sexual problems we had—in fact, sex turned out to be the best part of our relationship, and it gave me confidence in myself to know that I could still be an attractive sex partner. *(Authors' files)*

For women in ongoing relationships, how their partner responds is an important ingredient of their overall adjustment (Wellisch, Jamison, and Pasnau, 1978). In many cases, it is possible to use plastic surgery techniques for breast reconstruction as a way of helping a woman adjust to mastectomy most comfortably. However, it is notable that fewer than 1 percent of women who have had a mastectomy undergo such a procedure, which may suggest that this option is often not discussed with them (Winder and Winder, 1985). Currently, some physicians favor removal of the tumor without removing the entire breast (a procedure called "lumpectomy" or "segmental mastectomy") and radiation therapy as treatment options for the breast cancer patient (Fisher et al., 1989). These alternative treatments results in less disfigurement and less profound psychological effects, and in many cases they are just as effective as a total mastectomy.

CANCER OF THE CERVIX AND UTERUS

Cancer of the cervix accounts for slightly more than 60,000 new cases of cancer annually, and cancer of the lining of the uterus is found in another 38,000 women (Silverberg, 1981). Risk factors include infection with herpes simplex virus type 2 or human papilloma virus (Raymond, 1987; Layde, 1989) and may also include cigarette smoking (Slattery et al., 1989). There are two forms of cervical cancer: carcinoma in situ (CIS) and invasive cancer of the cervix (ICC). Although neither form is likely to cause symptoms, both can be detected by Pap smears during routine pelvic exams. CIS is really a precancerous condition involving cells on the surface of the cervix that do not invade other tissues. On average, it takes eight years or more for CIS to progress to true cancer, or ICC (Eddy, 1980; Richart and Barron, 1980). Treatment of CIS while it is still precancerous results in virtually 100 percent long-term survival. Treatment of ICC depends on whether the cancer cells have spread beyond the cervix: either surgical techniques or radiation therapy can be used. Sexual difficulties are common but depend on the amount of pelvic scarring that occurs (Abitbol and Davenport, 1974; Lamberti, 1979). One report suggests that surgery is less disruptive to sexual function than radiation therapy (Seibel, Freeman, and Graves, 1980).

Cancer of the lining of the uterus is rare before age 40 and is usually marked by abnormal bleeding early in its course. Later symptoms include cramping, pelvic discomfort, bleeding after intercourse, or lumps in the groin. Pap smears are *not* a foolproof way of detecting this form of cancer; usually a D&C (dilatation and curettage, scraping the inside of the uterus) is done to establish the diagnosis. Depending on the findings, treatment ranges from surgery (removal of the uterus and ovaries) to radiation therapy, drug therapy, or hormone therapy. If the cancer has not spread beyond the uterus, the patient has an 83 percent chance of being cured—that is, of not having the cancer recur within the next five years (Silverberg, 1981). Surgical removal of the uterus, called **hysterectomy,** does not usually have any negative effects on female sexual function. It may actually be beneficial since physical problems such as bleeding or cramping are corrected. However, some women have impaired sexual responsiveness and/or decreased sexual interest after a hysterectomy because they see the operation as a lessening of their femininity (Utian, 1975; Dennerstein, Wood, and Burrows, 1977; Roeske, 1978).

CANCER OF THE PROSTATE

Prostate cancer accounts for 17 percent of cancers in men, or about 70,000 new cases annually (Silverberg, 1981). The disease is rare in men under 40 and is generally diagnosed by a rectal examination. Treatment consists of surgical removal of the prostate **(prostatectomy),** radiation therapy, or hormone therapy. Prostatectomy for prostate cancer frequently causes erectile dysfunction because nerves that supply the penis are damaged. When the prostate is removed for reasons other than cancer, erectile dysfunction is a less frequent complication, although a high percentage of men develop retrograde ejaculation.

CANCER OF THE TESTIS

Cancer of the testis is a relatively rare condition that is most common in the twenties and thirties. Since only about half of these cancers are accompanied by pain, it is important for males to learn a method of testicular self-examination (see the boxed item on page 44) and to seek prompt medical attention if a testicular lump or swelling is noticed.

Treatment of testicular cancer (surgery, drugs, radiation) is sometimes a cause of sexual dysfunction and generally results in infertility. It is common to find that men with this form of cancer develop considerable guilt over their previous sexual practices, often blaming the problem incorrectly on masturbation, sexually transmitted disease, or an "overactive" sex life. Other men with this problem feel that the surgical removal of one testis makes them "less than a man." They may also develop fears of sexual performance and spectatoring, leading to difficulty with erection for strictly psychological reasons.

DES DAUGHTERS AND SONS

Approximately six million people—pregnant women and their daughters and sons—were exposed to the synthetic estrogen DES (diethylstilbestrol) and other DES-like drugs from 1940 to 1971, when it was widely used to treat so-called high-risk pregnancies—those with a threatened miscarriage or those complicated by a medical problem such as diabetes. In 1971, physicians found evidence of a rare form of cancer of the vagina or cervix (technically called clear cell adenocarcinoma) in daughters whose mothers had taken DES and related drugs during pregnancy (Herbst, Ulfelder, and Poskanzer, 1971). Subsequently, a number of reproductive abnormalities were found in some of the sons of women given DES during pregnancy, including incomplete development of the testes, undescended testes (cryptorchidism), anatomical abnormalities of the penis, and preliminary evidence of infertility (Gill, Schumacher, and Bibbo, 1977). Still more recently, there is some preliminary concern about cancer of the testis in DES-exposed sons, although this finding requires further substantiation.

While the cancer found in DES daughters is relatively infrequent (it is estimated to occur in about one of every 800 exposed women), noncancerous abnormalities are found in the vagina in one-third of these individuals and abnormalities of the cervix are present in almost every case (Robboy et al., 1981). It is not certain if a higher rate of vaginal/cervical cancer (or other forms of cancer, such as cancer of the breast or uterus) will emerge as this population of women ages, so that long-term medical follow-up is important. In fact, evidence suggests that there is an increased risk of cancer—including breast cancer—in the mothers who took the drug during pregnancy (Hoover, Gray, and Fraumeni, 1977; Meyers, 1983). It also appears that there is a higher rate of ectopic pregnancies and miscarriages in DES daughters.

If you were born after 1940, you should ask your mother whether she had any drugs prescribed for her during pregnancy—especially to prevent miscarriage or to treat a problem pregnancy associated with diabetes. If she did (or thinks she might have), go to your physician for evaluation. While it would be help-

hysterectomy (his′ tur ek′ tuh mē) partial or total removal of the uterus.

prostatectomy (pros′ tuh tek′ tuh mē) surgical removal of the prostate gland.

PELVIC EXAMS AND PAP SMEARS

One aspect of sexual and reproductive health care that often seems shrouded in mystery is the pelvic exam, sometimes called a vaginal or internal exam. Many women are embarrassed or anxious about having a "female check-up" done, yet the information gained from such an exam is important in many ways. For instance, the pelvic exam can be used to diagnose such diverse conditions as pregnancy, vaginal infections, cancer of the cervix, certain causes of infertility, and tumors of the uterus. It is also needed to fit a diaphragm or to insert an IUD.

The pelvic exam is done with the woman lying flat on her back on an examination table with her knees bent, legs apart, and heels in special footrests called stirrups. The physician or nurse conducting the exam begins by inspecting the outer genital structures, checking the labia, clitoris, and vaginal opening for signs of infection, irritation, rashes, swellings, sores, or other problems. Next, wearing thin rubber gloves, the examiner gently inserts a finger just inside the vagina to check for vaginismus or other abnormalities. Following this, an instrument called a speculum is slipped into the vagina to spread the vaginal walls apart. (If the speculum is metal, it should be warmed first so it won't be shockingly cold.) Although some women find that insertion of the speculum may be a bit uncomfortable, it is generally not painful if properly positioned. Since this instrument comes in different sizes, a woman who has a lot of discomfort should ask the examiner to try a narrower or shorter instrument.

With the speculum in place, the cervix is visually inspected and a Pap smear is taken. The Pap smear (or, officially, the Papanicolaou smear, named for its inventor) is done by gently scraping the area around the mouth of the cervix with a thin wooden spatula. Contrary to what many people believe, this is a painless procedure—most women don't even realize when it's been done (it takes only about two seconds). The scraping is then smeared on a glass microscope slide for later evaluation. The Pap smear shows early changes in cervical cancer or other abnormalities of the cervix. Generally, a second smear is also taken to examine vaginal secretions for microscopic signs of infection.

The speculum is then withdrawn slowly and gently from the vagina while the examiner carefully looks at the lining of the vagina for any unusual signs. Next, a bimanual exam is done. This involves inserting two gloved fingers into the vagina and pressing downward on the lower abdomen with the other hand. By this maneuver, the examiner can feel the size, shape, and position of the ovaries, uterus, and Fallopian tubes. Although there is often a sense of dull pressure during this part of the exam, it is not usually painful.

Not all health-care professionals are equally adept or sensitive to women's feelings when it comes to pelvic exams. It's important for a woman to find a doctor or nurse with whom she feels comfortable and is able to communicate. If a woman is tense and anxious before her pelvic exam, it can cause tenseness in her pelvic muscles so that it is more likely that the examination will be uncomfortable. A good health-care professional can help in this situation by teaching the woman several relaxation techniques and by using an unhurried approach. In addition, many women find that if each part of the exam is explained to them in advance and they are told at each step what is being done, they are less apprehensive. Finally, many women appreciate the opportunity to watch the exam in a hand-held mirror.

We strongly suggest that all women who are sexually active have a pelvic exam and Pap

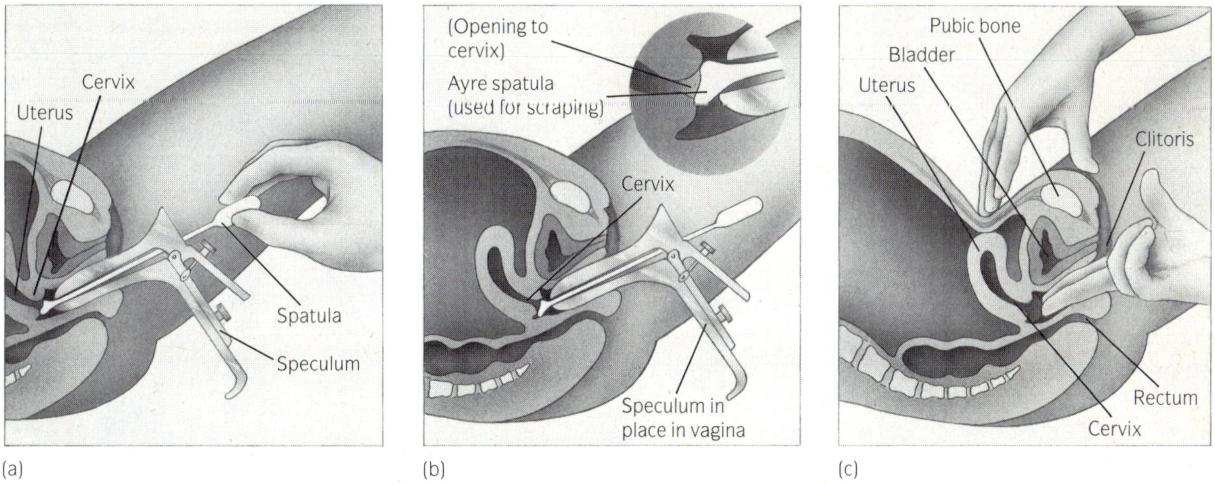

The pelvic exam. (a) The speculum in place for a pelvic exam. (b) The Ayre spatula is used to get a sample of cells for the Pap smear. (c) The bimanual pelvic exam.

smear once a year. Women who are using birth control pills or who have a history of genital herpes should have a Pap smear twice a year. The most recent recommendations of the American Cancer Society are that (1) all women age 20 and over should have a Pap smear annually for two negative exams and then at least every three years until age 65; (2) pelvic exams should be done as part of a general physical exam every three years from age 20 to 40 and annually thereafter; (3) any of the following factors suggest the need for more frequent tests: early age at first intercourse, multiple sex partners, infertility, abnormal uterine bleeding, history of genital herpes or genital warts, obesity, or use of estrogens.

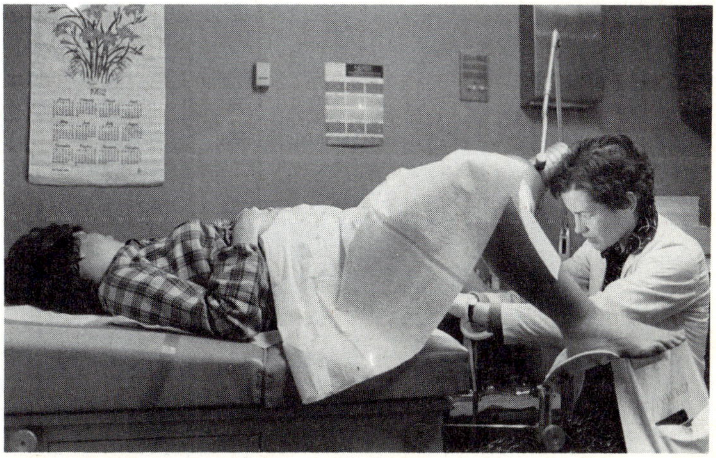

ful to try to find out the dosage of the DES-type drug received, when in the pregnancy it was first administered, and for how long, such information is not always available. Nevertheless, a medical examination is in order if you (or your child) had such an exposure or think you may have.

DES daughters should undergo a pelvic examination including a Pap smear and should have a test using an iodine solution to stain the lining of the vagina temporarily. The physician may also use a special magnifying instrument called a colposcope for this examination, and if there are areas of the vagina that appear abnormal, a biopsy (removal and examination of tissue specimens) may be taken. Usually this type of biopsy causes relatively little discomfort, although a slight amount of bleeding (less than during menstrual flow) may occur for 12 to 24 hours after the procedure is done.

The situation for DES sons is not yet completely understood, but we suggest that until more information is available, they undergo a medical examination on an annual basis.

Generally, treatment is *not* required for DES-related abnormalities, and over 98 percent of exposed individuals will be found to be cancer-free. Nevertheless, follow-up examinations (advisable at least every six months if abnormalities are found, or once a year if not) are important because the success of treating the types of cancer that can develop is partly dependent on detecting it in its earliest stages.

Needless to say, knowledge of DES exposure can lead to anger, guilt, fear of cancer, and concerns about fertility and sex. One 24-year-old nurse summarizes her reactions:

> When I first learned that my mother had used DES while she was pregnant with me, I didn't fully comprehend what it meant. Now that I realize that the risk of cancer is remote, I'm less afraid, but I'd be dishonest if I didn't say that I consider myself abnormal and I constantly worry about what will happen. Statistics mean very little when you're on the line yourself.
> *(Authors' files)*

Other DES daughters voice dismay at being advised not to use birth control pills (it is possible that the pill might aggravate the DES-induced changes, although whether or not this actually happens is not currently clear) or worry about their future childbearing risks. Fortunately, there are several groups available to help them deal with such concerns, including DES Action (Long Island Jewish Hospital, New Hyde Park, NY 11040), National Women's Health Network (2025 I Street, N.W., Suite 105, Washington, DC 20006), and the National Cancer Institute (Department DES, Office of Cancer Communications, Bethesda, MD 20205).

Alcoholism

The alcoholic man or woman has a high chance of having sexual problems. Not all these problems result from the alcoholism, however: in more than a few cases preexisting sexual difficulties may have played an important role in starting a person on a path toward heavy drinking. Here, the use of alcohol may help people cope with feelings of sexual inadequacy by making them less interested in sex or less critical of their own performance. Given the popular notion that drinking is "manly" and that liquor can be used to seduce a woman by lowering her resistance, it is easy to see how drinking seems to be "beneficial" from a man's sexual viewpoint. Women who feel guilty or inhibited about sex may find that drinking loosens these restraints and lets them feel more comfortable.

We have found that about 40 percent of alcoholic men have problems with erections and 5 to 10 percent have retarded ejaculation. Thirty to 40 percent of alcoholic women have difficulties in sexual arousal, and 15 percent have problems being orgasmic (Kolodny, Masters, and Johnson, 1979; Murphy et al., 1980). Sexual desire is also apt to be low in alcoholics (Schiavi, 1990).

There are several reasons behind these problems. Alcoholism directly affects hormone production and lowers testosterone in men (Van Thiel, 1976; Lindholm et al., 1978) and estrogen in women (Ryback, 1977). Shrunken testes and breast enlargement are common in alcoholic men. Other medical complications of alcoholism include liver damage, nerve damage, lowered resistance to infection, and poor nutrition, all of which may provide a biological basis for sexual impairment. Relevant psychosocial factors include fears of performance and spectatoring, marital conflicts, low self-esteem, guilt, and depression.

Even when an alcoholic has stopped drinking completely, there is no guarantee that his or her sexual difficulties will disappear. About half of the time these problems continue, requiring professional counseling to be resolved.

Penile Implants

When injury or illness causes complete inability to have erections, sexual functioning can be restored to a significant degree by the use of various types of mechanical devices that can be implanted in the penis with surgery. Although these devices can provide firm enough erections for intercourse to take place, they cannot restore sensation to the penis or normal ejaculation if these have been lost due to organic causes.

There are two basic types of penile implants. The simplest is a pair of fixed, semirigid rods that are placed inside the shaft of the penis. The earliest version of these rods produced a permanent state of partial erection that was embarrassing to some men. Now there are several additional types of rods that have either a bendable silver wire core or a hinge to allow the partly erect penis to be bent down against the inner thigh when the man is dressed, and embarrassment doesn't seem to be much of a problem.

More complicated and expensive, but more realistic in appearance and function, is an inflatable device (Figure 10–1) that also requires surgical placement. Two tapered inflatable cylinders are inserted into the penis and are connected by a tubing system to a fluid storage reservoir implanted in the lower abdomen. By pinching a simple pump and valve in the scrotum, fluid moves into the cylinders, causing a natural-looking erection. Releasing the valve moves the fluid out of the cylinders back to the reservoir (returning the penis to the flaccid state).

Either device may seem somewhat artificial to the man or his partner: in some cases this feeling is so problematic after surgery, the man only uses his implant a few times (Renshaw, 1979). For many men facing a "hopeless" situation, however, penile implants can restore a sense of manhood and improve self-esteem considerably. Thus, penile implants are currently used to treat men with erectile dysfunction resulting from spinal cord injuries, diabetes, multiple sclerosis and other neurological disease, and men with impotence resulting from severe vascular problems that are not correctable by surgery.

Unfortunately, penile implant surgery is not without its technical problems. In three reports, complications with the inflatable device—including infection and mechanical failure—were noted to occur in more than 40 percent of patients, often requiring removal of the device or at least one repeat operation to correct the problem (Apte, Gregory, and Purcell, 1984; Fallon, Rosenberg, and Culp, 1984; Joseph, Bruskewitz, and Benson, 1984). While the rate of complications with noninflatable rods is much lower, it is plain that this type of surgery is not the simple solution most men imagine it should be.

FIGURE 10–1

The Inflatable Penile Implant

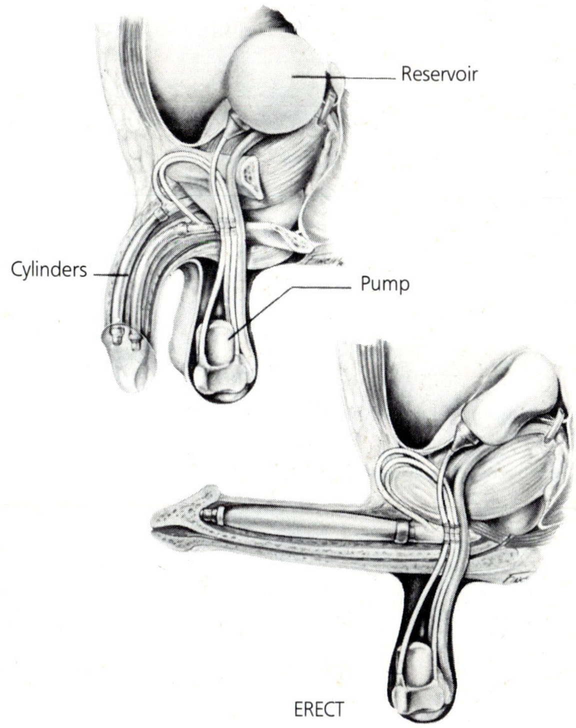

SEXUAL ASPECTS OF PSYCHIATRIC ILLNESSES

Mood Disorders

The mood disorders, also known as affective disorders, are marked by a prolonged disturbance of emotion that affects a person's whole life. These disturbances generally take the form of either depressed moods, elevated moods (euphoria or mania), or alterations of depressed and elevated moods (American Psychiatric Association, 1987). The latter condition has traditionally been called manic–depressive illness but is now also called bipolar disorder. Depression that occurs without accompanying bouts of mania is considered a unipolar disorder.

The features of depression are depressed mood (sometimes described as feelings of sadness, hopelessness, or despondency) and/or loss of interest in or pleasure from all or almost all of a person's ordinary activities (American Psychiatric Association, 1987). The most typical symptoms are loss of appetite, weight loss, difficulty sleeping, decreased energy, feelings of worthlessness or excessive or inappropriate guilt, difficulty thinking or concentrating, and recurrent thoughts of death or suicide (American Psychiatric Association, 1987; Goodwin and Guze, 1989).

The core features of mania are inappropriate, sustained euphoria; hyperactivity; and "flight of ideas"—the rapid, often chaotic, jumping from one idea to another. In unbridled mania, a person's speech generally changes from its natural style to a fast, rushing delivery; it may also be filled with puns, rhymes, and jokes, as well as highly dramatic pronouncements. There is usually a decreased need for sleep and a great sense of restlessness: manic people have a very tough time sitting still or listening, uninterruptingly, to anyone else. The person typically feels sublimely self-confident and advises others about matters in which he or she has no special knowledge—like how to attain world peace or how to run a world-class hotel. At the same time, the manic person often starts, and then abandons, ambitious projects for which he or she has little or no background, one minute announcing that they've started a novel, then calling friends to say that they've devised a new system for beating the stock market, then claiming that they've been hired to promote a U2 concert. The hallmark of such actions is their grandiosity, their impulsivity, and their disorganization; these features carry over into other behavior, as well, in which rash acts such as going on a major buying spree, driving recklessly, or resigning abruptly from a job occur.

Mood disorders are among the most common psychiatric conditions, with most studies reporting that more females are affected than males. The proportion of the adult population in the United States that currently has a mood disorder is thought to be approximately 5 percent (Myers, Weissman, and Tischler, 1984; Fishman, 1990). The lifetime risk of ever having a mood disorder has been estimated by Wing and Bebbington (1985) as 12 percent for men and 20 percent for women. Mania occurs far less often than depression, but both conditions tend to recur. About 70 percent of people with a major depressive episode will have at least one additional bout of depression in their lifetime, and about 12 percent will have subsequent bouts of mania (U.S. Public Health Service, 1986).

The sexual effects of the mood disorders are varied. The majority of depressed persons experience a marked reduction in their sex drives, but overt sexual dysfunction such as erectile dysfunction or anorgasmia occurs in less than one-third of these cases (Tamburello and Seppecher, 1977; Kolodny, Masters, and Johnson, 1979). In chronic depression, inhibited sexual desire is common (Kaplan, 1983), and the capacity for enjoying sexual fantasies is often lost (Woods, 1981). As we have noted elsewhere (Kolodny, Masters, and Johnson, 1979, p. 301):

> It is common to find that the depressed patient has few sexual fantasies or thoughts about sex; it is also common to find a significant decrease in initiatory sexual behavior, although the sexual receptivity of depressed persons is somewhat less affected. Mechanisms of sexual arousal (erectile function in the male and vaginal lubrication in the female) are more likely to be intact than to be impaired, but often the perception of sexual arousal is negatively affected.

When a true sexual dysfunction occurs as a result of depression, it is sometimes masked by other problems. In one case, a married 42-year-old man suffering from depression withdrew from virtually all social interaction with his wife, even insisting on eating his meals alone; months later, it turned out that this self-imposed social isolation was in part his response to guilt over erectile difficulties that first appeared as part of the depressive symptoms (Authors' files). Similarly, because depression in one partner obviously has some impact on many aspects of a couple's intimacy, it is no surprise that it may interfere with their sex relations.

Infrequently, depression may trigger unusual forms of sexual behavior, such as incest, pedophilia, or exhibitionism. And in some cases, depressed persons may start an affair to stimulate both their mood and their sexual performance.

Mania affects sexual behavior in a number of different ways, but its main effect is to make sexual behavior very impulsive. During a bout of mania (which typically lasts for weeks or months), hypersexuality is common (Tsuang, 1975). Ordinary social and sexual inhibitions may be loosened or shattered, with both male and female manics suddenly (and uncharacteristically) having sex with numerous partners, including partners who are total strangers, as the following case summaries show:

> *Case 1:* A 28-year-old married female accountant who had a past history of psychiatric hospitalization for both manic and depressive episodes occurring sporadically since her early twenties called her husband from work one day to announce that she had taken all the money from their joint checking account and was off to the West Coast to see some friends. After flying from Boston to Los Angeles, she suddenly boarded another plane for Las Vegas. In four days there, she picked up seven different men at her hotel bar and had sex with them; the last two men agreed to a sexual threesome at her insistence.

> *Case 2:* A 37-year-old sociology professor was taken to a psychiatrist after she suddenly disrobed at a faculty meeting and began masturbating. The psychiatrist discovered that she had cancelled all her office hours for the past several weeks and had squandered $25,000 from a research grant she had received earlier that semester. The diagnosis of mania was easily established.

Hospitalized manic patients often disrupt the psychiatric ward by similar displays of overt, inappropriate sexuality or by attempts to have sex with fellow patients or hospital staff members. In addition, some manic persons show their hypersexuality by a frantic search for sexual partners or constant seductive behavior (Woods, 1981), or by participation in forms of sexual activity that they never tried previously, including bisexuality, homosexuality, or group sex.

Mania is often treated with a drug called lithium carbonate. Although this is usually effective in controlling the manic episode and in preventing recurrences, lithium occasionally causes sexual difficulties in males, including erectile problems and decreased sexual desire (Blay, Ferraz, and Calil, 1982). One of the reasons for this effect may be that lithium decreases testosterone levels in the blood (Sanchez et al., 1976). There are no reports of lithium producing negative sexual effects in females.

A number of different medications are used to treat depression, often in combination with a program of cognitive psychotherapy (Goodwin and Guze, 1989). Virtually all the antidepressant drugs can affect sexual functioning adversely in both males and females, although this problem occurs in only a small minority of patients (Kolodny, Masters, and Johnson, 1979; Segraves et al., 1985; Jani and Wise, 1988; Segraves, 1988). (In males, the most common sexual difficulty is inhibited ejaculation, while in females inhibited orgasm is the most frequent problem.) As a practical matter, however, the sexual effects of antidepressant drugs are generally beneficial because they bring about an improvement in the mood disorder: they usually boost a person's sexual interest back to its pre-illness level. In addition, if sexual dysfunction occurred as a result of the depression, as the depression lifts, the dysfunction often disappears.

Anorexia Nervosa and Bulimia

Anorexia nervosa, the self-starvation disorder, and **bulimia,** the binge–purge eating disorder, are related conditions marked by disturbances in body image and obsessive–compulsive concerns focusing on food and eating. Both disorders characteristically start in adolescence or young adulthood and affect females much more frequently than males (American Psychiatric Association, 1987). There is mounting evidence that anorexia and bulimia have increased in frequency in the general population in the past two decades; the problem of bulimia appears to be especially acute on college campuses throughout the nation, where some studies have estimated that more than 10 percent of college females engage in bulimic behavior, which they learn from other females in what has been termed a "copy cat" manner (Thompson and Schwartz, 1981; Pope et al., 1984; Johnson and Connors, 1987). The increased occurrence of both eating disorders may partly reflect the emphasis our culture puts on thinness as a way of providing attractiveness and personal self-worth (N. Kolodny, 1987).

The essential features of anorexia nervosa are: (1) progressive weight loss, to a point more than 15 percent below minimal normal weight for age and height (or failure to gain weight in a period of body growth); (2) disgust with food (often accompanied by a preoccupation with thoughts about food); (3) intense fear of gaining weight or becoming fat, even when the victim is so thin that she or he looks like a skeleton; (4) distorted body image so that the person "feels fat" even when emaciated; and (5) loss of menstrual

anorexia nervosa an eating disorder marked by self-starvation. Anorexia nervosa usually occurs in females in their teens or early twenties.

bulimia an eating disorder marked by frequent episodes of binge eating (consuming large quantities of food) followed immediately by purging the food just eaten by self-induced vomiting or use of laxatives.

periods in females (American Psychiatric Association, 1987; Goodwin and Guze, 1989). The disorder, while treatable, is sometimes fatal and often requires hospitalization.

Although the cause of anorexia is not known, one frequently expressed view is that it is a form of rejection of developing adult sexuality (Goodwin and Guze, 1989). Other theories have held that, through starvation, anorectic females reject a wish to be pregnant (Halmi, 1985) or that the anorexic's avoidance of food results from sexual and social tensions generated by the physical changes that occur with puberty (Crisp, 1967).

The anorectic female actually makes her body regress sexually by severely restricting her food intake. She can postpone the onset of menarche (if she hasn't yet started to have menstrual periods) or make her menstrual periods stop by losing a lot of weight; this effect occurs by suppression of luteinizing hormone and follicle stimulating hormone production (Copeland, 1985). By disrupting her ovarian functioning (estrogen production is kept at basically prepubertal levels in anorexia), the anorexic also can often postpone her breast development or cause her breasts to shrink back to a less threateningly sexual degree of flatness. Similarly, testosterone levels are low in male anorexics, and the development of secondary sex characteristics such as facial hair and lowering of the voice is delayed.

Anorectic females typically show little or no interest in sex; in fact, they often appear frightened of sex. Most anorectic females avoid dating, do not masturbate, and have no desire to give up their much-coveted virginity. Adolescents with anorexia nervosa are often shy and withdrawn and appear childlike in their social interactions. In some cases, a history of sexual abuse or assault precedes the development of anorexia (Goldfarb, 1987; Schecter, Schwartz, and Greenfeld, 1987). Even among married adult anorexics, avoidance of sex is common and sexual dysfunctions such as primary anorgasmia or vaginismus are frequently seen (Renshaw, 1990).

Bulimia is characterized by binge eating—the consumption of large amounts of food in a relatively short time period (generally less than two hours)—usually followed by self-induced vomiting or abuse of laxatives or diuretics. The binges, which are usually planned, typically involve rapidly eating food with a high calorie content and a lot of sugar—such as ice cream, donuts, cookies, or chocolates—and are usually carried out in private, gobbling down the food with little chewing (American Psychiatric Association, 1987). The bulimic feels out of control during a binge and worries that she won't be able to stop eating. Immediately after the binge, the bulimic is often depressed and guilty over her lack of control. Sometimes, but not always, there is an anorectic eating pattern between binges; more commonly, the bulimic is preoccupied with her weight and pursues various diet plans and stringent daily exercising as a way of staying thin.

In contrast to anorexics, bulimics tend to be socially outgoing and sexually active at an early age (Hazard, 1985; Johnson and Connors, 1987; Haimes and Katz, 1988). However, as Renshaw (1990) points out, bulimics have a relatively high rate of sexual dysfunction as well as inhibited sexual desire. Renshaw also notes that many bulimics feel guilty about masturbation, which she observes is "strikingly similar to their binge–guilt–purge eating cycle." On the other hand, some bulimic females lead very satisfying sex lives, so it is incorrect to assume that anyone with bulimia is automatically sexually dysfunctional.

DRUGS AND SEX

For many centuries, there has been an avid search for **aphrodisiacs**—substances that could increase a person's sexual powers or desire. The long list of substances that have been claimed to have such an effect include oysters, ginseng root, powdered rhinoceros horn, animal testicles, and turtles' eggs, but there is no evidence that an actual aphrodisiac response occurs. "Spanish fly," the most famous supposed aphrodisiac, is made from beetles found in southern Europe. The beetles are ground into a powder and, when taken internally, the substance irritates the bladder and urethra and can also cause ulcers, diarrhea, and even death. The burning sensation in the penis due to irritation of the urethra has been interpreted by some men as a sign of lust.

Aphrodisiacs aside, both prescription drugs and drugs used recreationally (or illicitly, depending on your viewpoint) have some specific effects on sexuality.

Prescription Drugs

Many of the medications used to treat high blood pressure cause sexual difficulties for men and women. For example, Aldomet (alphamethyldopa), one of the drugs most commonly used to treat this condition, causes erectile dysfunction in 10 to 15 percent of men at low doses and in up to half of men in high doses (Kolodny, 1978a). Decreased libido and impaired sexual arousal is found in similar proportions of women using this drug. A different type of problem is found with Ismelin (guanethidine), which inhibits ejaculation in more than half of the men using it. Usually these difficulties disappear within a week or two after stopping the medication, but in some cases the sexual dysfunction may persist because of anxiety. Fortunately, there are many medications available to treat high blood pressure. Some have low rates of sexual side effects, and it is almost always possible to find a combination that will leave sexual function intact while simultaneously controlling high blood pressure (Croog et al., 1988).

Tranquilizers such as Librium (chlordiazepoxide) and Valium (diazepam) can sometimes cause erectile dysfunction, anorgasmia, or decreased sexual desire but in other instances may be beneficial by reducing sexual anxiety. Barbiturates and related drugs such as Quaalude (methaqualone) have also been reported to cause a variety of sexual problems (Gay et al., 1975; Bush, 1980), although Quaalude has developed a street reputation as an aphrodisiac. Our research has shown that some people using Quaalude temporarily lose some of their sexual inhibitions, which they translate as a sexual "stimulant" effect. The problem, as a number of experienced drug users confirm, is that Quaalude also depresses the function of the nervous system and can actually impair sexual performance (Gay et al., 1975).

Antihistamines, used in allergy pills and sinus medications, can affect sexuality in two ways. Drowsiness is a prime side effect and one not likely to improve the quality of sex. In women, these drugs often cause a reduction in vaginal lubrication so they may sometimes cause painful intercourse.

The effects of hormones on sexual function were discussed in Chapter 3. A more detailed discussion of the sexual effects of prescription drugs is given in the several references listed at the end of this chapter.

Nonprescription Drugs

ALCOHOL

The effects of alcohol on sexuality have fascinated people throughout history. In *Macbeth*, Shakespeare reported that "it provokes the desire but it takes away the performance" (Act 2, scene 3, line 34), and modern research has shown that this view is fairly accurate. In one study, college men were given alcohol in three different doses while watching erotic movies (Farkas and Rosen, 1976). Amounts of alcohol well below the legal levels of intoxication suppressed erections. Similar studies in women showed that alcohol had a negative impact on physiologic signs of sexual arousal (Wilson and Lawson, 1976, 1978). Alcohol

FOCUS IN BRIEF

Sex and Alcohol: Physiological Effects

1. Acute actions
   Male: Very low blood concentrations of alcohol seem to have a mildly enhancing effect on erections in men, but at blood concentrations corresponding to two to three shots of liquor, erections are mildly suppressed and ejaculation is delayed. At higher blood alcohol concentrations, many males are unable to ejaculate and have marked difficulty obtaining or maintaining erections.
   Female: Very low blood alcohol concentrations seem to have minimal effects on sexual responsivity, but moderate concentrations cause a reduction in vaginal blood flow, a delayed time to reach orgasm, and less orgasmic intensity. High blood alcohol concentrations can block orgasmic responsivity and can interfere with vaginal lubrication.
2. Chronic actions
   Male: Chronic alcohol abuse commonly causes low sex desire and erectile dysfunction possibly due to the depression of testosterone production.
   Female: Chronic alcohol abuse causes low sexual interest, difficulties becoming sexually aroused, and problems with orgasmic response. The cause of these problems is unclear.

aphrodisiac (af' rō dēz' ē ak) a substance that increases or is believed to increase a person's sexual powers or desire.

has also been shown to weaken male masturbatory effectiveness and to decrease the pleasure and intensity of male orgasm (Malatesta, 1979), and alcohol, even in moderate amounts, makes it more difficult for women to reach orgasm (Malatesta et al., 1982).

Despite the *physical* inhibition of even two or three drinks of an alcoholic beverage (due to a depressant effect on the nervous system), most people believe that alcohol *increases* their sexual responsiveness. This is partly because alcohol has a "disinhibiting" effect: it lowers the sexual inhibitions a person may ordinarily have, thus making it possible for sexual desire to emerge (Crowe and George, 1989). The belief that alcohol enhances sex also stems from advertising and cultural myths.

NARCOTICS

Addictive drugs such as heroin and morphine produce many sexual problems (Cushman, 1973; Mintz et al., 1974; Cicero et al., 1975). One large survey found that in 162 male addicts, erectile dysfunction occurred in 48 percent, retarded ejaculation in 59 percent, and low sexual interest in 66 percent; in 85 female addicts, 27 percent had orgasmic dysfunction and 57 percent had low sexual interest (Kolodny, 1983a). This is a complex area to evaluate, however, because drug addiction may be a means of trying to escape from preexisting sexual difficulties or may be a substitute for sex. Factors such as hormone problems (Azizi et al., 1973; Santen et al., 1975; Mirin et al., 1980), infections, and poor nutrition, which occur as a result of addiction, also play a role in causing sexual difficulties.

Narcotic addicts are also likely to have other problems that complicate their sex lives. Rosenbaum (1981) has noted that (1) female addicts usually have partners who are also addicted; (2) many addicts find that the "hit" of mainlining heroin is far more pleasurable, intense, and easy to get than an orgasm (in fact, many ex-addicts say the feeling is like dozens of orgasms rolled up into one); and (3) the sensuality and sharing that accompany narcotic use become a replacement for the sharing and sensuality of sex. Furthermore, since most female addicts must turn to prostitution to raise money for their habit, it is not surprising that sex becomes less appealing to them.

AMPHETAMINES AND COCAINE

Amphetamines ("speed," "uppers," "pep pills") reportedly increase sexual responsiveness when used in low doses but have the opposite effect in high doses or when used on a long-term basis.

Cocaine ("coke," "snow") has a street reputation as a strong sexual stimulant, but there are also reports of sexual dysfunction with its use (Gay et al., 1975; Bush, 1980; Cocores, Dackis, and Gold, 1986). Kolodny (1983) found that 17 percent of 168 male cocaine users had episodes of erectile failure when they used this drug, and 4 percent had experienced priapism (painful, persistent erections) at least once during or immediately after the use of cocaine. Similarly, Wesson (1982) found evidence of male erectile difficulties during the use of cocaine, and Siegel (1982) reported that the dangerous practice of "free-basing" cocaine consistently leads to sexual disinterest and situational impotence (20 of 23 men were affected in his study). In addition, the recent appearance of a highly potent form of cocaine called "crack" has led to addiction occurring very quickly. One study of 60 male crack users found that more than two-thirds of this group were sexually dysfunctional, while 23 of 30 female crack users reported decreased sexual interest and responsivity (Kolodny, 1987). A more recent report noted:

> At some point, nearly all chronic high-dose cocaine users become sexually dysfunctional (i.e., impotent and nonorgasmic). But despite their inability to perform physically, many chronic users find that their sexual feelings and fantasies are still heightened by cocaine, and their sexual acting-out behavior continues. At this point, however, sexual arousal and stimulation are often reduced to a purely mental (psychological) experience for the chronic user. *(Washton, 1989, p. 34)*

Because crack use is often combined with the practice of bartering sexual services in exchange for the drug, females who become addicted to crack commonly have sex with a number of partners each day in order to feed their habit (Macdonald et al., 1988; Fullilove and Fullilove, 1989). Partly because of this, crack use has been tied to soaring rates of STDs in the past few years (Goldsmith, 1988; Chaisson et al., 1989; Fullilove et al., 1990). In addition, Washton (1989) claims that many people who become addicted to crack are also driven to compulsive sexuality (see the Case Study on page 297).

Cocaine use as a purported sexual stimulant is interesting for several other reasons. For one thing, many users believe that rubbing cocaine on the tip of the clitoris increases female sexual sensitivity and arousal, but how this could occur is difficult to understand since cocaine is used medically as a topical anesthetic, that is, to deaden nerve endings. The continued use of this practice may indicate how powerful expectations are in interpreting our experiences.

CASE STUDY

Twin Peaks

Jeff was a 36-year-old stockbroker who had an unhappy marriage, two young children, and a five-year dual addiction to cocaine and compulsive sexuality. His two addictions fed each other in a seemingly unending circle: whenever he used cocaine, it triggered his uncontrollable sexual appetite for prostitutes and pornographic movies, and whenever he paid a visit to a prostitute, it triggered an intense urge to get high on cocaine.

Jeff's sexual history was relatively unremarkable before he tried cocaine for the first time. As his cocaine use escalated—and particularly after he switched from snorting to smoking cocaine freebase—he developed a severe sexual compulsion. His sexual compulsion involved repeated, marathon encounters with prostitutes and/or incidents of prolonged masturbation while he watched hard-core porn movies. Typically, he would disappear for two or three days at a time for his cocaine and sex binges. With the huge expenditures he had to pay for his cocaine habit and for his desperately needed nonstop partying with prostitutes, he gradually drove his family close to the verge of bankruptcy.

As the realization of his monetary plight set in, Jeff's self-esteem reached an all-time low. He felt ashamed of himself, guilty about his infidelities and his financial irresponsibility, and profoundly depressed over being so totally out of control. In addition, he was horrified when he first realized that he had undoubtedly exposed himself and his wife to infection with the AIDS virus, especially since he knew that some of his favorite prostitutes were hooked on IV drugs.

At the end of his proverbial rope, Jeff agreed to get treatment only after his wife threatened him with divorce and his employer threatened to fire him. During his admission interview, Jeff kept quiet about his cocaine-related sexual behavior. He was too ashamed of it and too afraid of being seen as a "pervert" by the interviewer to raise the issue. Because this issue was overlooked, he continued to have relapses with some frequency. Following more recent therapy, in which the sexual compulsion was identified and dealt with simultaneously with the drug abuse problem, Jeff has now been drug-free for more than two years and has been able to discard his compulsive sexual behavior.

Comment: There are several elements in Jeff's case that are of interest. First, many cocaine abusers get caught in a pattern of escalating sexual behavior that is associated with their drug abuse. They may or may not have a true sexual compulsion, but they simply find that the expectation and the opportunity for sex is there, so they take it. (Male crack users who frequent "crack houses" almost always find women hanging around the premises who are willing to trade sex for drugs.) Second, Jeff became amenable to treatment only when he had almost reached the end of the line. This pattern is particularly true for cocaine abusers—indeed, most drug abusers—who are somehow always able to convince themselves that they're in control, that they can stop whenever they want to, right up until the curtain drops on them (e.g., coming to the brink of bankruptcy, or having a brush with death). Finally, Jeff had a number of relapses during treatment, which is characteristic of dealing with persons with dual addictions. In fact, there are no certainties at all that treatment will be successful, since so much of the outcome depends on the participant's degree of motivation.

Source: Case Study/Twin Peaks, adapted from Arnold Washton, MEDICAL ASPECTS OF HUMAN SEXUALITY 23 (12): 32–39, December 1989. Reprinted by permission of the author.

A second interesting point is that cocaine clearly acts as a sexual facilitator in a social sense. When a man offers cocaine to a woman (or vice versa) there is usually a sexual invitation implied. As Kolodny (1985) notes:

> Widely available at singles bars and in the economically advantaged "just-got-a-divorce" crowd, cocaine literally opens the doors of sexual access for many males and provides a convenient excuse for many females who otherwise might pass on having "instant sex" with a partner they hardly know.

MARIJUANA

Marijuana ("pot," "dope," "grass") is generally reported to enhance sexual feelings. In our own research with more than 1000 men and women aged 18 to 35 who had used this drug as an accompaniment to sex, 83 percent of the men and 81 percent of the women said that marijuana improved their sexual experience (Kolodny, Masters, and Johnson, 1979). Most users, however, denied that marijuana led to more sexual desire, quicker sexual arousal, or more intense orgasms. Instead, they indicated that marijuana gave them an increased awareness of touch all over their bodies, led to greater relaxation (both mentally and physically), and put them more in tune with their partners. These are highly subjective judgments which cannot be verified fully in experimental research. However, generally similar findings have been reported by others; for example, Halikas, Weller, and Morse (1982) described self-reports of enhanced touch awareness and physical closeness in a majority of both male and female users.

In nonsexual situations, it has been shown that instead of *increasing* touch sensitivity, marijuana actually produces no change or *lessens* touch perception (Reese, 1977). There is also considerable documentation that marijuana use slows reflex reactions (Klonoff, 1974; Manno et al., 1974; Jones, 1976; Jaffe, 1980). The fact that marijuana users say that if *they* are "high" but their partner is not, the sexual experience is unpleasant (disjointed?) also indicates that there is a strongly subjective element to the reported effects.

Some other research findings also bear examination. Erectile dysfunction has been found to affect about 20 percent of men using marijuana daily, although no association between marijuana use and sexual dysfunction in women has been noted (Kolodny, 1981). However, some women who use marijuana report that it causes temporary vaginal dryness, which can sometimes cause painful intercourse. Furthermore, heavy marijuana use has been reported to lower testosterone production in animals and men (Collu et al., 1975; Harmon et al., 1976; Smith et al., 1976; Kolodny et al., 1974, 1976, 1979) and to disturb sperm production as well (Kolodny et al., 1974; Hembree, Zeidenberg, and Nahas, 1976).[1] Although these effects are reversible once the drug is stopped, they may sometimes contribute to sexual problems. One study of chronic, frequent marijuana use in women showed menstrual cycle abnormalities and hormone changes but no negative sexual effects (Bauman et al., 1979).

ANABOLIC STEROIDS

Anabolic steroids are synthetic forms of testosterone that were developed in order to minimize the masculinizing effects of testosterone while amplifying its growth-promoting (anabolic) properties. While this class of hormones has authentic medical uses as a prescription drug (e.g., in the treatment of osteoporosis, endometriosis, breast cancer, and some anemias), they have become notorious because of their widespread illicit use by athletes. Because the anabolic properties of the drug increase the body's conversion of nitrogen from protein food sources into muscle, the drugs are commonly used by athletes in sports such as football, wrestling, weight lifting, bodybuilding, and track and field in which increased muscle size is beneficial. Whether anabolic steroids actually increase strength or speed or otherwise improve athletic performance is unclear at present (Wilson, 1988).

Although use of anabolic steroids has long been "athletes' darkest and best-kept secret" (Hallagan, Hallagan, and Snyder, 1989), the world's attention was focused on this issue with the disqualification of Canadian sprinter Ben Johnson, winner of the 1988 Olympic 100-meter dash, after he acknowledged that he had used anabolic steroids during training (*Washington Post*, June 13, 1989, p. E1). But it is hardly just elite, world-class athletes who use anabolic ste-

[1] One carefully designed research study found that three weeks of daily marijuana smoking under controlled conditions did *not* lower testosterone in men (Mendelson et al., 1974). However, a similar study, using the same carefully controlled conditions but administering marijuana daily over a three-*month* period found that the testosterone-lowering effect did not show up for five to six weeks (Kolodny, Masters, and Johnson, 1979, Figure 13–2).

roids: one recent survey found that 6.6 percent of 12th grade male students ($N = 3403$) drawn from 46 public and private high schools across the country had used anabolic steroids, with two-thirds of this group starting at age 16 or younger (Buckley et al., 1988). Another survey documented that high school females, as well as males, sometimes use anabolic steroids; 1 percent of the female high school seniors in this study reported that they had used these drugs during their athletic careers (Newman, 1986). Among college athletes, usage is both far more common and far riskier because of higher doses and the frequent practice of "stacking"—using two or more anabolic drugs at the same time.

There are a number of undesirable or harmful side effects associated with the use of anabolic steroids. In most cases, the frequency and severity of these effects increase with the dose of the drug(s) used (Gilman, Goodman, and Gilman, 1988). Since it is not unusual for athletes who get anabolic steroids on the black market to use them in doses 10 to 50 times higher than the amounts used for medical purposes, the rates of harmful side effects are much higher than they are when used for strictly medical purposes. In both sexes, there is a significant risk of liver abnormalities (including chemically induced hepatitis, jaundice, and tumors), high blood pressure, and endocrine and reproductive effects. In women, the most visible effects are masculinizing ones: growth of facial and body hair, male pattern baldness, and enlargement of the clitoris. Women also are apt to have menstrual irregularities and blocked or inhibited ovulation as a result of using anabolic steroids. In males, these drugs typically cause a sharp drop in circulating testosterone (because their weak androgenic action is enough to keep the hypothalamus from triggering the hormonal signals for more testosterone production) and shrinkage of the testes. Sperm production is seriously impaired with prolonged use, and the resulting sterility is not always reversed after the anabolic steroids are discontinued (Lamb, 1984; Wilson, 1988). Gynecomastia (enlargement of the male breasts) is another common finding.

Many males using high doses of anabolic steroids develop low levels of sexual desire and erectile dysfunction—presumably as a result of their lowered testosterone production—but they are apt to attribute their lack of sexual interest to "being in training," rather than to hormonal changes of which they are unaware. Because they are not particularly interested in sex, they may not discover that they are having difficulties with erection until many months after the problem first begins.

There are also potential psychological effects from use of high doses of anabolic steroids. The most prominent is a form of increased aggressiveness known colloquially as "'roid rage." Rapid mood swings are also frequently noted, and one report found that 12 percent of users had psychotic symptoms (Pope and Katz, 1988). It has been theorized that the rapid mood swings and aggressiveness of steroid abuse may sometimes contribute to sexual assault committed by male athletes (Kolodny, 1990), although this is a complex issue in which blame should not be put entirely on the drugs.

Finally, when the anabolic steroids are injected (rather than taken in pill form), there is an increased risk of infections associated with sharing needles, including hepatitis and HIV (Sklarek et al., 1984).

INFECTIONS

Certain types of infections that affect the sex organs are not usually transmitted through sexual intercourse, unlike the sexually transmitted diseases that we have previously discussed. These infections, which *can* be sexually transmitted, can produce troublesome symptoms that interfere with sexual pleasure or cause considerable emotional turmoil. Fortunately, the most common of these infections are easily treatable and have no major health risks. We discuss them here to avoid the implication that they are always or usually of sexual origin.

Cystitis

Cystitis, or infection of the bladder, is closely related to sexual activity in women. Sexual intercourse leads to an increase in bacteria in the urine (Buckley, McGuckin, and MacGregor, 1978) presumably because of inward pressure on the urethra during coital thrusting. Because the female urethra is short (about 2.5 cm, or 1 inch) compared to the male urethra (usually more than 15 cm, or 6 inches), cystitis is far

anabolic steroids synthetic hormones that promote the build-up of muscle mass. Commonly used by athletes in an attempt to increse their size and strength.

cystitis (sis tī′ tis) infection or inflammation of the bladder.

more common in women than men (the bacteria have a shorter distance to travel).

The symptoms of cystitis include burning during urination, frequent urination, cloudy or bloody urine, and pain in the lower abdomen. The diagnosis can be made by examining a urine sample under the microscope and by taking a culture to identify the specific bacteria involved. Broad-spectrum antibiotics such as tetracycline or ampicillin are often prescribed.

One special variety of this infection is the so-called honeymoon cystitis that can occur either when a woman first becomes coitally active (not always on her honeymoon) or when coital activity is resumed after a prolonged period of inactivity.

Toxic Shock Syndrome

Toxic shock syndrome (TSS) first came to public attention in 1980 when it was widely reported as a serious, sometimes fatal illness suddenly striking healthy menstruating women who used tampons. Although TSS was named in 1978 by Todd and coworkers, who reported on a small number of cases appearing in children, it now is clear that it is actually a rare form of scarlet fever that was initially described in 1927 (Stevens, 1927; Reingold, 1983).

TSS is marked by high fever, vomiting, diarrhea, muscle pain, and a skin rash that resembles a severe sunburn. Fainting spells, low blood pressure, and dizziness are other common symptoms. TSS is caused by a toxin, or poison, produced by a bacteria called *Staphylococcus aureus*, and it occurs primarily in menstruating women who use tampons. Most of the cases encountered in 1980 were associated with the use of Rely tampons, which were subsequently found to have a relative risk of developing TSS 11 times greater than Playtex tampons, 28 times higher than OB tampons, 38 times higher than Kotex tampons, and 77 times higher than Tampax (Schlech et al., 1982). However, both the absorbency and the chemical composition of tampons are thought to play a role, with low-absorbency tampons being much less risky (Berkley et al., 1987). After Rely tampons were withdrawn from the market, the number of cases of TSS linked

FIGURE 10–2

Reported Cases of Toxic-Shock Syndrome, by Quarter, United States, January 1, 1979–March 31, 1990*

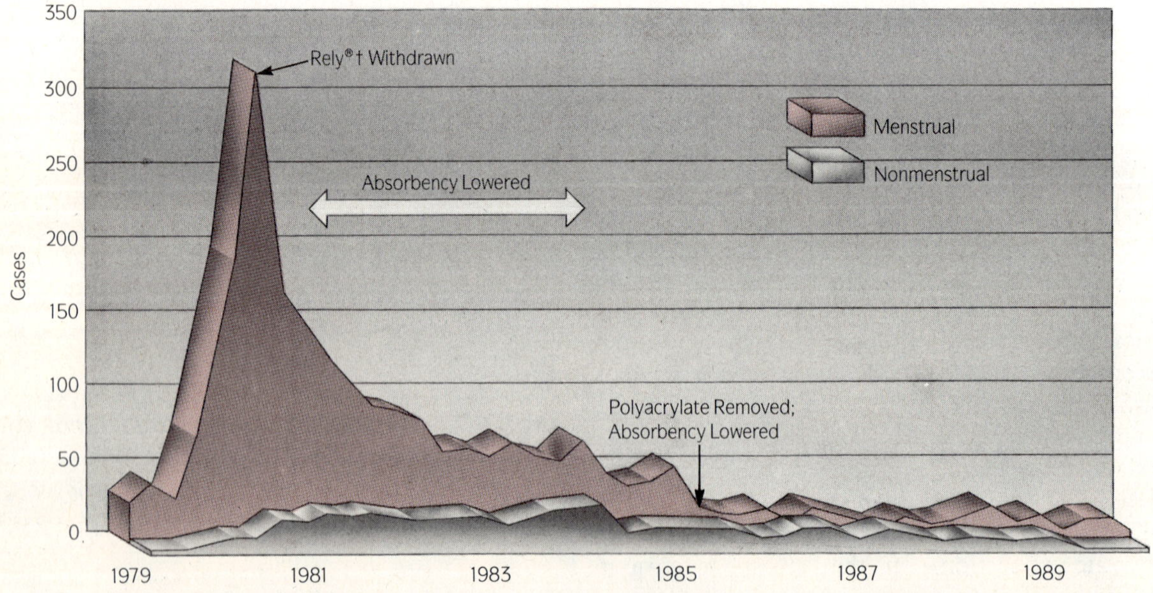

* Includes only cases meeting the CDC case definition.
† Use of trade names is for identification only and does not imply endorsement by the Public Health Service or the U.S. Department of Health and Human Services.

Source: MMWR 39:25, 1990.

with tampon use dropped (Reingold et al., 1982), and by 1983, approximately 15 percent of the cases being reported were unrelated to menstruation (Reingold, 1983) (see Figure 10–2). It is now clear that TSS can affect men as well as women and all age groups—including infants and the elderly—but the group at highest risk still seems to be tampon-using white females aged 15 to 25.

While women using tampons have the greatest risk of TSS and a few cases have been linked to use of the contraceptive sponge as well as to use of a diaphragm, the chances of developing this illness are very low. Preventive measures that can be taken to reduce this risk still further include (1) switching to sanitary napkins or minipads entirely; (2) alternating the use of tampons and minipads or sanitary napkins several times each day; or (3) changing tampons three or four times daily. If you develop symptoms suggestive of TSS while you are menstruating, you should immediately see a physician since TSS is a rapidly progressive illness that is fatal in about 4 percent of cases. Fortunately, with proper medical management—including hospitalization, treatment of shock, and aggressive antibiotic therapy—it is now clear that TSS is not as frightening as it first seemed to be.

Prostatitis

Prostatitis, or inflammation of the prostate, can be either acute (sudden) or chronic (long-lasting). The infecting organism is usually *E. coli*, a normal inhabitant of the intestines. Acute prostatitis is marked by fever, chills, perineal or rectal pain, painful urination, and urinary frequency and is likely to interfere with sexual function (painful ejaculation is common). Chronic prostatitis may involve no symptoms at all, or low back pain or perineal discomfort may be present. Chronic prostatitis has sometimes been thought to cause premature or bloody ejaculation (Davis and Mininberg, 1976). Antibiotic treatment usually clears up acute prostatitis but may be ineffective in curing the chronic form of this disease.

SUMMARY

1. A number of myths exist about the sexuality of disabled people that present obstacles to their freedom of sexual expression. In recent years, these myths have been countered by a better understanding of the fact that being disabled does not prevent a person from having sexual feelings and needs and by recognition that a broad range of sexual expression is possible even if a disability partially interferes with sexual functioning.
2. Although spinal cord injury (SCI) commonly causes a variety of sexual problems (including erectile difficulties and disruption of ejaculation in men and impairment of vaginal lubrication and anorgasmia in women), as well as loss of sensations in the genitals, many SCI persons are able to be sexually active. In addition to noncoital options for intimacy and sexual sharing (such as oral–genital sex, massage, and cuddling), some SCI men can have intercourse using a "stuffing" technique and others choose to have a penile implant.
3. People who have been blind or deaf since birth are often hampered in learning about sex. While these conditions do not impair the physical reflexes of sexual response, they may at times create interpersonal problems that make sexual relationships difficult.
4. Many mildly or moderately mentally retarded persons are able to learn the basic facts necessary for responsible sexual behavior if this information is presented to them in a manner geared to their learning level.
5. A number of medical conditions can interfere physiologically with sexual function. For example, neurologic problems such as multiple sclerosis commonly cause erectile dysfunction and female anorgasmia. Erectile dysfunction occurs in 50 percent of diabetic men and 40 percent of male alcoholics; anorgasmia is found in about one-third of diabetic women and 15 percent of female alcoholics. Other illnesses may be closely associated with anxiety about sex that limits sexual enjoyment. Heart attacks, breast cancer, and conditions that require hysterectomy are examples of such health problems.
6. Psychiatric illnesses frequently cause changes in sexual behavior. Loss of interest in sex is very common in depression, whereas hypersexual behavior is more typically seen with mania. Persons with anorexia nervosa are likely to be quite sexually withdrawn and childlike, whereas bulimia (the binge–purge eating disorder) has a far less noticeable impact on sexuality.

toxic shock syndrome (TSS) an illness of rapid onset caused by infection with *Staphylococcus aureus* bacteria; symptoms include fever, vomiting, muscle pain, and a sunburn-like skin rash. Most, but not all, cases have occurred in menstruating women, and the syndrome is thought to be related to the use of high-absorbency vaginal tampons.

prostatitis inflammation of the prostate, caused by infection.

7. DES (diethylstilbestrol), which was widely used over three decades to treat problem pregnancies, is known to cause a variety of problems in the children of women who took this drug while pregnant. Although cancer of the vagina or cervix is infrequent in DES-exposed daughters, noncancerous abnormalities are common and should be followed closely by a physician. DES-exposed sons have an increased rate of reproductive abnormalities and may also have a heightened risk of cancer of the testis (although this has not been proved yet).
8. No true aphrodisiac has ever been found, although many people claim that alcohol, marijuana, cocaine, or amphetamines enhance their sexual experiences. Others report that these same substances lower their sexual desire or impair their sexual responses.
9. Prescription medications that can cause sexual problems include drugs used to treat high blood pressure, tranquilizers, barbiturates, and antihistamines.
10. Toxic shock syndrome (TSS) is a serious disorder caused by a toxin produced by the *Staphylococcus aureus* bacteria. Marked by an abrupt onset of fever, vomiting, muscle pain, skin rash, and low blood pressure, about 85 percent of TSS occurs in menstruating women. Although the TSS outbreak has slowed now compared to what it was in 1979–1980, it is advisable for women to change their tampons three or four times daily while they are menstruating or to switch to the use of sanitary napkins or minipads to minimize the risk of this illness.
11. Cystitis is inflammation of the bladder that can occur in either sex, while prostatitis is inflammation caused by infection of the prostate. Either condition may cause pain or burning with urination and can make sexual functioning uncomfortable.

Thought Questions

1. How have your friends and acquaintances responded to mastectomy or hysterectomy? Do you know of cases where orgasmic experience appeared to decline following hysterectomy? How do you think most men would respond to their wife or lover if she had to have a mastectomy? Is losing a breast different from losing an arm or leg from a sexual point of view?
2. Why is it that there are so many more operations done in this country to remove ovaries than to remove testes?
3. Imagine a friend of yours who is in a wheelchair who has lost a partner and is now ready to develop a new relationship. What should he or she do to get back into the mainstream again? What encouragement or advice would you give?
4. Researchers have shown that alcohol and marijuana have (if anything) deleterious effects on sexual functioning. But most users believe that they enhance sex. Why? What do you think about it?
5. Students and other young people often make fun of penile implants. Why? If you or your male partner lost the ability to get erect, would you want one of these implants? Why or why not?

Suggested Readings

Bullard, David, and Knight, Susan, eds. *Sexuality and Physical Disability*. St. Louis: C. V. Mosby, 1981. The first half of this book provides an extraordinary collection of personal reflections on the sexual needs and experiences of the disabled. The second half of the book, which is less engaging, consists of a number of papers of uneven quality discussing professional issues in this field.

Bush, Patricia. *Drugs, Alcohol and Sex*. New York: Richard Marek Publishers, 1980. Broad coverage of the physical and psychological effects of drugs and alcohol on sex, conveyed with a sense of humor.

Gregg, Charles. "Toxic Shock." In *A Virus of Love and Other Tales of Medical Detection*, by Charles Gregg, pp. 93–112. New York: Charles Scribner's Sons, 1983. A superb recounting of the whole toxic shock syndrome story including a scientific viewpoint and a revealing look at the commercial side of the issues involving Procter & Gamble, the makers of Rely tampons.

Kolodny, Robert; Masters, William; and Johnson, Virginia. *Textbook of Sexual Medicine*. Boston: Little Brown, 1979. A comprehensive but sometimes technical discussion of the impact of illness, drugs, and surgery on sexuality.

Meyers, Robert. *D.E.S.: The Bitter Pill*. New York: Putnam, 1983. The story of DES and its effects on millions is told with accuracy, insight, and compassion. Nontechnical but scientifically sound, this book is must reading for those who have been exposed to DES.

Monat, Rosalyn. *Sexuality and the Mentally Retarded.* San Diego: College-Hill Press, 1982. A thoughtful overview of a much-neglected topic.

Rabin, Barry. *The Sensuous Wheeler: Sexual Adjustment for the Spinal Cord Injured.* San Francisco: Multi Media Resource Center, 1980. A thoughtful, creative approach to a difficult subject, written in an informal tone. Deserves an award for its title!

Schover, L. R., and Jensen, S. B. *Sexuality and Chronic Illness.* New York: Guilford Press, 1988. A concise yet comprehensive discussion of sexual aspects of many medical conditions.

Appendix Resource Guide

MAJOR ORGANIZATIONS IN THE FIELD OF SEXUALITY

AASECT (American Association of Sex Educators, Counselors, and Therapists)
435 North Michigan Avenue, Suite 1717
Chicago, IL 60611
312-644-0828

AASECT publishes the quarterly *Journal of Sex Education & Therapy* as well as a monthly newsletter, *Contemporary Sexuality*. It will provide a list of certified sex therapists in your locale if you need it.

SIECUS (Sex Information and Education Council of the U.S.)
130 West 42nd Street, Suite 2500
New York, NY 10036
212-819-9770

SIECUS publishes the bimonthly *SIECUS Report* and maintains an extensive sexuality library at New York University. It provides pre-printed comprehensive bibliographies on many sexual topics and will arrange to do computer searches of its data base on a very reasonable fee-for-service basis.

SOCIETY FOR THE SCIENTIFIC STUDY OF SEX
Box 208
Mount Vernon, IA 52314

SSSS publishes the bimonthly *Journal of Sex Research*.

INSTITUTIONS IN THE FIELD OF SEXOLOGY

KINSEY INSTITUTE FOR RESEARCH IN SEX, GENDER, AND REPRODUCTION
Morrison Hall
Indiana University
Blooming, IN 47405
812-855-7686

The Kinsey Institute has the most extensive library collection of materials related to sexuality in the United States.

MASTERS & JOHNSON INSTITUTE
24 South Kingshighway
St. Louis, MO 63108
314-361-2377

While the MJI does not maintain a research library or other materials to assist students conducting research, it does have an active sex therapy program that accepts couples from around the world.

ORGANIZATIONS PROVIDING AIDS INFORMATION

AIDS ACTION COUNCIL
729 8th Street SE, Suite 200
Washington, DC 20003
202-547-3101

AIDS INFORMATION
U.S. Public Health Service
Office of Public Affairs, Room 721-H
200 Independence Avenue SW
Washington, DC 20201
202-245-6867

AIDS-RELATED DISCRIMINATION UNIT
American Civil Liberties Union
132 West 43rd Street
New York, NY 10036
212-944-9800, Ext. 545

AMERICANS FOR A SOUND AIDS POLICY (ASAP)
P. O. Box 17433
Washington, DC 20041
703-471-7350

AMERICAN FOUNDATION FOR AIDS RESEARCH (AMFAR)
1515 Broadway, Suite 3601
New York, NY 10036
212-719-0033

GAY MEN'S HEALTH CRISIS
P. O. Box 274
129 West 20th Street
New York, NY 10011
212-807-6655

NATIONAL AIDS NETWORK
2033 M Street, Suite 800
Washington, DC 20036
202-293-2437

NATIONAL ASSOCIATION OF PEOPLE WITH AIDS
P. O. Box 65472
Washington, DC 20335
202-483-7979

HIV/AIDS HOTLINES

NATIONAL AIDS HOTLINE: 800-342-AIDS
NATIONAL AIDS INFORMATION CLEARINGHOUSE: 800-458-5231

This service, provided by the Centers for Disease Control, distributes up-to-date information related to HIV/AIDS statistics and services. Its data base contains descriptions of more than 12,000 organizations working in the field and more than 6,000 AIDS-related educational materials, as well as information about funding opportunities for community-based HIV/AIDS service organizations. All of the Clearinghouse's services (including its publications) are free.

NATIONAL GAY TASK FORCE: 800-221-7044

Note: Additional listings of national and community-based AIDS organizations can be found in *AIDS Information Sourcebook: Second Edition, 1989–90* (H. R. Malinowsky and G. Perry, eds.), published by Oryx Press, Phoenix, Arizona (800-457-6799).

ORGANIZATIONS PROVIDING RESEARCH ON CONTRACEPTION

ALAN GUTTMACHER INSTITUTE
111 Fifth Avenue
New York, NY 10003
212-254-5656

One of the most prolific sources of new research in contraception, the AGI publishes two outstanding journals, *Family Planning Perspectives* and *International Family Planning Perspectives,* as well as several useful newsletters such as the biweekly "Washington Memo," which summarizes political actions and legal decisions that affect family planning issues, including the fast-changing area of abortion law.

PLANNED PARENTHOOD FEDERATION OF AMERICA
810 Seventh Avenue
New York, NY 10019
212-541-7800

Planned Parenthood has local clinics in cities throughout the country. (You can usually locate them through your local telephone directory; if not, you can contact the national office.) This organization offers a broad range of information on virtually every aspect of family planning and sex education through a series of pamphlets and classes, as well as providing clinical services such as contraceptive counseling, pregnancy testing, voluntary sterilization, preventive health-care exams (including Pap smears and breast exams), and early abortion services. (In some locations, Planned Parenthood also offers confidential testing for HIV.)

POPULATION INFORMATION PROGRAM
Johns Hopkins University
527 St. Paul Place
Baltimore, MD 21202

This program publishes the highly readable but thoroughly documented *Population Reports* about various family planning issues on a five times a year basis; back issues are available for many issues. They also run POPLINE, a computerized collection of more than 200,000 citations with abstracts, and will perform searches of this data base for a nominal fee.

ORGANIZATIONS PROVIDING INFORMATION AND SERVICES RELATED TO HOMOSEXUALITY

INSTITUTE FOR THE PROTECTION OF GAY AND LESBIAN YOUTH
110 East 23rd Street
New York, NY 10010
212-473-1113

LAMBDA LEGAL DEFENSE AND EDUCATION FUND
132 West 43rd Street
New York, NY 10036
212-944-9488

NATIONAL GAY AND LESBIAN TASK FORCE
1517 U Street NW
Washington, DC 20009
202-332-6483

NATIONAL LESBIAN AND GAY HEALTH FOUNDATION
P. O. Box 65472
Washington, DC 20035
202-797-3708

ORGANIZATIONS HELPING INCEST VICTIMS OR SURVIVORS

ADULTS MOLESTED AS CHILDREN UNITED
P. O. Box 592
San Jose, CA 95108
408-280-5055

INCEST SURVIVORS ANONYMOUS
P. O. Box 5613
Long Beach, CA 90805
213-428-5599

INCEST RECOVERY ASSOCIATION
6200 North Central Expressway, Suite 209
Dallas, TX 75206
214-373-6607

LOOKING UP (for adult incest survivors)
P. O. Box K
Augusta, ME 04330
207-626-3402

NATIONAL CENTER ON CHILD ABUSE AND NEGLECT
P. O. Box 1182
Washington, DC 20013
202-245-2858

NATIONAL RESOURCE CENTER ON CHILD SEXUAL ABUSE
106 Lincoln Street
Huntsville, AL 35801
800-543-7006

VOICES in Action, Inc. (VOICES is an acronym for Victims of Incest Can Emerge Survivors.)
P. O. Box 148309
Chicago, IL 60614
312-327-1500

CHILD ABUSE/INCEST HOTLINES

National Child Abuse Hotline (Referral Service): 800-422-4453

ORGANIZATIONS PROVIDING INFERTILITY SERVICES

AMERICAN FERTILITY SOCIETY
2140 Eleventh Avenue, Suite 200
Birmingham, AL 35205

Provides a large number of informational brochures on topics such as endometriosis, the medical evaluation of infertility, and IVF. Also makes referrals to medical specialists in your locale.

NATIONAL SOCIETY OF GENETIC COUNSELORS
233 Canterbury Drive
Wallingford, PA 19086
215-872-7608

Provides information and referrals on genetic counseling services.

RESOLVE, INC.
5 Water Street
Arlington, MA 02174
617-643-2424

A valuable, national self-help group for infertile couples that provides physician and IVF referrals, many informational brochures, a monthly newsletter, and telephone counseling. It has support groups throughout the nation. If you are having problems with infertility and are thinking about obtaining treatment, we strongly recommend that you join this group, both for the information it will provide and the numerous ways in which it can help you deal with the emotional ups and downs of this odyssey.

ORGANIZATIONS PROVIDING PREGNANCY-RELATED SERVICES

AMERICAN COLLEGE OF NURSE MIDWIVES
1522 K Street NW
Washington, DC 20005

Provides information on midwife-assisted childbirth.

AMERICAN COLLEGE OF OBSTETRICIANS AND GYNECOLOGISTS
409 12th Street SW
Washington, DC 20024
202-638-5577

This national organization has a resource center that provides a number of educational pamphlets as well as lists of ob-gyns in various locations.

AMERICAN SOCIETY FOR PSYCHOPROPHYLAXIS IN OBSTETRICS/LAMAZE
1840 Wilson Boulevard, Suite 204
Arlington, VA 22201

Despite its intimidating name, this organization provides useful brochures about the Lamaze method and offers a referral service to certified Lamaze instructors in your area. It also publishes a magazine on pregnancy, childbirth, and early childhood.

INTERNATIONAL CHILDBIRTH EDUCATION ASSOCIATION
P. O. Box 20048
Minneapolis, MN 55420

Dedicated to family-centered maternity care and freedom of choice in childbirth, this organization publishes a number of informative brochures and periodicals and will refer you to the Childbirth Education Association in your area.

LaLECHE LEAGUE INTERNATIONAL
9616 Minneapolis Avenue
Franklin Park, IL 60131

A nationwide organization that offers practical advice about breast-feeding. Organizes local monthly meetings in many cities and provides a variety of useful publications.

STD INFORMATION

HEPATITIS HOTLINE: 404-332-4555

This service provided by the C.D.C. gives information on modes of transmission, prevention, and statistics related to all forms of viral hepatitis.

HERPES RESOURCE CENTER: 415-328-7710

STD NATIONAL HOTLINE: 800-227-8922

A service provided by the American Social Health Association, this hotline deals with questions on any STDs.

MAJOR JOURNALS

Archives of Sexual Behavior
Plenum Publishing Company
233 Spring Street
New York, NY 10013

Family Planning Perspectives
Alan Guttmacher Institute
111 Fifth Avenue
New York, NY 10003

Journal of Homosexuality
The Haworth Press
10 Alice Street
Binghamton, NY 13904

Journal of Psychology & Human Sexuality
Haworth Press
10 Alice Street
Binghamton, NY 13904

Journal of Sex Education & Therapy
435 North Michigan Avenue, Suite 1717
Chicago, IL 60611

Journal of Sex & Marital Therapy
Brunner/Mazel, Inc.
19 Union Square West
New York, NY 10003

Journal of Sex Research
P. O. Box 208
Mount Vernon, IA 52314

Medical Aspects of Human Sexuality
Cahners Publishing
249 West 17th Street
New York, NY 10011

Sex Roles
Plenum Publishing Company
233 Spring Street
New York, NY 10013

Sexuality and Disability
Human Sciences Press
233 Spring Street
New York, NY 10013

Siecus Report
130 West 42nd Street, Suite 2500
New York, NY 10036

MISCELLANEOUS

AMERICAN CANCER SOCIETY (National Office)
90 Park Avenue
New York, NY 10016

With more than 3,000 local units, which you can find by consulting your local telephone directory, this organization provides many informational and educational services related to cancer. The "Reach to Recovery" program for women who have had mastectomies is particularly noteworthy.

NATIONAL ABORTION RIGHTS ACTION LEAGUE
1101 14th Street NW
Washington, DC 20005
202-371-0779

This is the leading pro-choice abortion group in America; it maintains a high political profile and is frequently in the news. NARAL produces a number of educational materials, such as videotapes and brochures, advocating women's right to abortion.

NATIONAL CANCER INSTITUTE CANCER INFORMATION SERVICE: 800-4-CANCER

Provides a wide range of brochures, reprints, and bibliographies at no charge, as well as answering all cancer-related questions.

NATIONAL CENTER FOR THE PREVENTION AND CONTROL OF RAPE
National Institutes of Mental Health
5600 Fisher's Lane
Rockville, MD 20857
301-433-1910

NATIONAL COALITION AGAINST SEXUAL ASSAULT
8787 State Street
East St. Louis, IL 62203
618-398-7764

NATIONAL RIGHT TO LIFE COMMITTEE
419 7th Street NW
Washington, DC 20004
202-626-8800

This is one of the leading anti-abortion groups. Like others in this field, it is primarily a political organization.

NATIONAL SELF-HELP CLEARINGHOUSE
33 West 42nd Street
New York, NY 10036
212-840-1259

If you need help in finding a self-help organization that we haven't listed here, this national clearinghouse will help you find it.

SEX ADDICTS ANONYMOUS
P. O. Box 3038
Minneapolis, MN 55403
612-871-1520

Glossary

abortion Termination of a pregnancy before the fetus can survive outside the uterus. *Spontaneous* abortions occur naturally due to medical problems; *induced* abortions are done intentionally.

abstention (abstinence) The act of voluntarily not engaging in some act, such as sexual intercourse. A highly effective method of birth control if practiced consistently.

acquired immune deficiency syndrome See *AIDS*.

acrosome (ak′ ro sōm) Chemical reservoir in the head of the spermatozoon.

actual effectiveness The observed effectiveness of a contraceptive method in real life, including user failures and method failures.

adolescent growth spurt A period of fast bone growth usually occurring in the early or middle teens caused by the rising sex hormone levels of puberty.

adrenogenital syndrome (a drē′ nō jen′ i tul) An inherited disorder involving an enzyme block in the adrenal glands. Females born with this condition frequently have masculinized genitals because of excess androgen exposure prenatally. In males, genital appearance is usually unaffected.

ageism An attitude of prejudice against the elderly.

AIDS (acquired immune deficiency syndrome) A condition of increased susceptibility to unusual forms of cancer and infection due to disturbances of the body's immune defenses; a majority of cases have occurred in male homosexuals.

AIDS-related complex (ARC) A constellation of signs and symptoms of infection with HIV, including such features as swollen lymph nodes and fevers or night-sweats, that falls short of a full-blown case of AIDS. A substantial number of cases of ARC eventually progress to AIDS.

Alzheimer's disease A progressive form of degenerative brain disease that causes dementia (deterioration of mental abilities).

amniocentesis (am′ nē ō sen tē′ sis) Procedure used to obtain a sample of amniotic fluid from the uterus of a pregnant woman to be analyzed for a variety of genetic disorders and biochemical abnormalities in the fetus.

amnion (am′ nē on) The inner of the thin sacs of tissue (fetal membranes) that enclose the developing fetus.

amniotic fluid (am′ nē ot′ ik) The liquid in which the developing fetus is suspended. It keeps the temperature constant and cushions shock.

anabolic steroids Synthetic hormones that promote the build-up of muscle mass. Commonly used by athletes in an attempt to increase their size and strength.

androgens (an′ dro jinz) Hormones such as testosterone that develop and maintain secondary sex characteristics in males and, if in large quantities, promote masculinization in females.

anorexia nervosa An eating disorder marked by self-starvation. Anorexia nervosa usually occurs in females in their teens or early twenties.

anorgasmia (an′ or gaz′ mē uh) The inability of a woman to reach orgasm. Can be classified as primary (always existing), secondary (having been orgasmic in the past), situational (existing only in certain situations), coital (existing only during coitus), or random (existing on a frequent basis during different types of sexual activity).

aphrodisiac (af′ rō dēz′ ē ak) A substance that increases or is believed to increase a person's sexual powers or desire.

areola (a rē′ o luh) The circular area of dark skin around the nipple.

asymptomatic carrier state The phase of HIV infection in which a person is symptom-free (although able to infect others); this period may last for years.

azidothymidine (AZT) (or zidovudine) A medication that has been shown to prolong life in HIV-infected persons and to slow the progression to symptomatic AIDS.

bacterial vaginosis A bacterial infection of the vagina marked by a malodorous grayish-white discharge and symptoms of burning or itching; this condition is caused by an overgrowth of various bacteria, including *Garduerella vaginalis*.

Bartholin's glands (bahr′ tō linz) Small glands adjacent to the vaginal opening. Although they produce minimal amounts of lubrication, their function is unknown.

basal body temperature (BBT) Temperature taken immediately after awakening and used to predict ovu-

---

Long vowels are marked. Short vowels are left alone or changed to show the sound they make. Major (′) and minor (′) accents are marked.

lation for the rhythm method of birth control. *See temperature method of birth control.*

bisexual (bī sek′ shoo ul) A person sexually attracted to both males and females.

blastocyst (blas′ tō sist) A spherical mass of cells with a hollow inner portion containing fluid produced by the cleavage of the fertilized egg.

bonding (parent-child) The emotional link partly created by cuddling, cooing, and physical and eye contact by the parent early in an infant's life.

brain tumors Abnormal growths in the brain, which can either be malignant (cancerous) or nonmalignant.

Braxton-Hicks contractions Painless short episodes of muscle tightening sometimes mistaken for the onset of labor.

breech presentation The childbirth presentation in which the buttocks or feet are the first part of the baby to pass through the opening of the vagina.

bulbocavernosus (bul′ bō kav ur nō′ sus) A muscle encircling and supporting the entrance to the vagina.

bulimia An eating disorder marked by frequent episodes of binge eating (consuming large quantities of food) followed immediately by purging the food just eaten by self-induced vomiting or use of laxatives.

calendar method of birth control A technique of determining the days in the menstrual cycle when the risk of pregnancy is low; a form of the rhythm method.

capacitation (kuh pas′ i tā′ shun) The process by which sperm become capable of penetrating an egg.

castration anxiety (kas trā′ shun) According to Freud, the unconscious fear in boys about the possible loss of their penis as a terrible form of punishment.

cephalic presentation (se fal′ ik) The childbirth presentation in which the head is the first part of the baby's body to pass through the birth canal.

cervical cap (ser′ vi kul kap) A small plastic or rubber contraceptive device worn on the cervix to provide a barrier to sperm.

cervical os (ser′ vi kul oss′) The mouth or opening of the cervix.

cervix (ser′ viks) The cylindrical part of the uterus that protrudes into the vagina. The point where sperm cells enter the uterus and menstrual flow exits is called the *cervical os.*

cesarean section (seez air′ ee uhn) A surgical method of childbirth in which delivery occurs through an incision in the abdomen and uterus.

chancre (shan′ ker) A painless sore that appears in the primary stage of syphilis.

chloasma (klō as′ muh) Brown pigmented spots, usually on the face, caused either by birth control pills or hormones produced naturally during pregnancy.

chorion (kor ee on′) The outer sac of tissue that encloses the developing fetus inside the uterus.

chorionic villi sampling (CVS) A method for diagnosing defects in the developing fetus; done by inserting a catheter through the vagina and cervix to take a small piece of tissue from the edge of the chorion, the membrane surrounding the fetus.

chromosomes (krō′ muh sōmz) The genetic material in the nucleus of every cell in the body. Sperm and eggs each have 23 chromosomes; all other cells normally have 46.

cilia (sil′ ē uh) The hairlike filaments in the inside of the Fallopian tubes that propel the egg along to the uterus.

circumcision (sur′ kum sizh′ un) Surgical removal of the foreskin of the penis.

climacteric (klī mak′ tur ik) Syndrome experienced by about 5 percent of men over 60, marked by weakness, fatigue, poor appetite, decreased sexual drive, reduction or loss of potency, irritability, and impaired ability to concentrate. Also see *menopause*, which is sometimes called the female climacteric.

clitoral glans (klit′ o rul) The tip or head and the only visible part of the clitoris, resembling a small button.

clitoral hood The fold of skin covering the clitoral shaft. Sometimes referred to as the female foreskin.

clitoral shaft Part of the external female genitals; two small erectile bodies enclosed in a fibrous membrane and ending in a glans. Corresponds to the *corpus cavernosa* in the penis.

clitoris (klit′ o ris) Part of the external genitals of the female, situated at the anterior meeting of the labia minora and made up of two small erectile bodies, a glans and a hood. Its only known function is to focus and accumulate sexual sensations and erotic pleasure.

coitus interruptus (kō′ i tus in tur rup′ tus) The removal of the penis from the vagina before ejaculation occurs.

colostrum (kohl ah′ strum) A thin, watery fluid secreted by the breasts late in pregnancy as a precursor to breast milk.

combination pill A birth control pill containing both estrogen and progesterone.

congenital syphilis Syphilis contracted by the fetus from an infected mother, causing various abnormalities in the unborn child.

coronal ridge (kor′ ō nul) The rim of tissue that separates the glans from the shaft of the penis.

corpora cavernosa (kor′ por ruh kav ur nō′ suh) The two parallel cylindrical bodies of erectile tissue that make up the larger part of the shaft of the penis and the clitoris. Also called cavernous bodies.

corpus luteum (kor′ pus lew′ tē um) The part of the capsule of the ovarian follicle left in the ovary after an egg is expelled. It secretes hormones and, if pregnancy does not occur, degenerates.

corpus spongiosum (kor′ pus spon′ jē ō′ sum) The cylinder of erectile tissue along the underside of the penis containing the urethra. The distal portion expands to form the *glans.* Also called spongy body.

couvade syndrome (koo vahd′) A condition in which a male experiences symptoms mimicking pregnancy and/or childbirth.

Cowper's glands (kow′ perz) Two pea-sized structures connected to the urethra just below the prostate gland. They produce fluid before ejaculation but otherwise have no known function.

crowning In childbirth, the appearance of the baby's head at the opening of the vagina.

crura (kroo′ ruh) The internal branches of the clitoral shaft and the corpus cavernosa attached to the bony pelvis.

cryptorchid (krip tor′ kid) Undescended testes.

cystitis (sis tī′ tis) Inflammation of the bladder.

diabetes A chronic disorder of how the body handles sugar because of an insulin deficiency. Complications of this disease include circulatory and neurological problems.

diaphragm (dī′ uh fram) A dome-shaped rubber contraceptive device that is positioned inside the vagina so that it blocks the cervix; it must be used with a spermicide to be effective.

dihydrotestosterone (dī hī′ drō tes tos′ ter ōn) A hormone similar to testosterone that stimulates development of the penis, scrotum, and prostate gland in the embryo.

dilatation (dil′ uh tā′ shun) Opening of the mouth of the cervix in preparation for birth.

dilatation and curettage (D&C) (kyur e tazh′) Process involving dilating the cervix and then gently scraping the lining of the uterus with a metal instrument. Sometimes used as a form of abortion.

dilatation and evacuation (D&E) A method for abortion involving widening the mouth of the cervix, followed by removing the products of conception by a combination of suction and scraping.

douching (dūsh′ ing) Using a liquid to flush the vagina.

Down's syndrome A chromosome disorder that causes mental retardation and defects of the heart, kidneys, and intestines. Also known as trisomy 21 or mongolism.

dysfunctional (dis funk′ shun ul) Abnormally impaired.

dysmenorrhea (dis men′ or ē′ uh) Painful menstruation, usually including backache, headache, cramps, and a bloated feeling.

dyspareunia (dis′ puh roo′ nē uh) Painful intercourse.

eclampsia (e klamp′ sē uh) A condition occurring during the latter half of pregnancy marked by high blood pressure, edema, protein in the urine, and convulsions, sometimes resulting in coma or death. Also known as toxemia of pregnancy.

ectopic pregnancy (ek top′ ik) A misplaced pregnancy. The implantation of the blastocyst occurs outside the uterus, for example in the tubes or abdomen.

edema (e dē′ muh) Swelling due to fluid retention.

effacement (e fāce′ munt) The thinning or flattening of the cervix during labor.

effleurage (ef′ lu razh′) The circular stroking movement used in massage of the abdomen during labor in the Lamaze method.

egg donors Women who volunteer to provide their eggs for the purposes of treating anovulatory infertility or avoiding the transmittal of a genetic disorder in another woman.

ejaculatory ducts (ē jak′ you luh tō′ rē) Paired tubelike structures that carry sperm from the vas deferens and fluid from the seminal vesicles into the prostatic urethra.

ejaculatory incompetence The inability to ejaculate within the vagina. Can be classified as primary (always existing) or secondary (having been able to ejaculate in the past).

ejaculatory inevitability The first stage of orgasm in men, a feeling of having passed the point where ejaculation can be controlled as the vas deferens, seminal vesicles, and prostate start contracting.

embryo (em′ brē ō) The unborn child during the first eight weeks after fertilization.

embryo freezing A technique of freezing pre-embryo (usually zygotes or blastocysts) for use in subsequent menstrual cycles so as to reduce the risk of multiple gestations and reduce the cost of treating infertility.

embryo transplant A method of treating female infertility that involves artificially inseminating a donor female, then removing the pre-implantation pre-embryo and transplanting it to the infertile woman's uterus.

encephalitis A viral infection of the brain that is among the most serious opportunistic infections persons with AIDS face.

endocervical canal (en′ dō ser′ vi kul) The tubelike connection between the mouth of the cervix and the uterine cavity containing numerous secretory glands that produce mucus.

endometriosis The occurrence of endometrial tissue in locations other than the uterus; a frequent cause of female infertility.

endometrium (en′ dō mē′ trē um) The inner lining of the uterus in which the egg implants and which is partially shed during menstruation.

engagement The settling of the fetal head into position against the pelvic bones for birth. It usually occurs during the last few weeks of pregnancy in women having their first child and during labor with subsequent pregnancies. Also called dropping or lightening.

enzyme-linked immunoabsorbent assay (ELISA) The screening test used to detect HIV antibodies in blood samples; positive ELISA results must always be confirmed with a second, more specific, test, such as the Western blot.

epididymis (ep′ i did′ i mis) The tightly coiled tubing network folded against the back surface of each testis in which sperm cells spend several weeks maturing.

epilepsy A disease of unknown origin marked by the periodic occurrence of seizures (convulsions)

episiotomy (e piz′ ē ot′ uh mē) During a vaginal delivery, the incision in the mother's perineum that gives the baby's head more room to emerge.

erectile dysfunction The inability to have or maintain an erection firm enough for coitus. Can be classified as primary (always existing) or secondary (having functioned in the past). See *impotence*.

estrogens (es′ tro jinz) Hormones present in both sexes, but primarily considered female. Produced in the ovaries and adrenal glands in the female, they maintain the lining of the vagina and produce breast growth. Also important in controlling the menstrual cycle.

excitement phase First phase of the human sexual response cycle caused by physical and/or psychological stimulation. It is characterized by increasing levels of myotonia and by vasocongestion.

extra nipples More than two paired nipples; about one person in 1000 has this condition.

Fallopian tubes (fuh lō′ pē un) The tubes that transport eggs from the ovaries to the uterus. Also called oviducts.

false labor Irregular contractions that do not become regular. They are felt mainly in the lower abdomen and groin in contrast to true labor, which is felt in the back and abdomen.

fellatio (fe lā′ shē ō) Stimulation of the male genitals by oral contact.

fetal alcohol syndrome The effects on the unborn child of heavy use of alcohol by the pregnant woman, including growth deficiencies, nervous system damage, and facial abnormalities.

fetal membranes Two thin sacs of tissue, the inner amnion and the outer chorion, that enclose the developing baby.

fetal monitor Electronic equipment used during labor to check the progress of the baby, especially its heartbeat, and the duration, frequency, and intensity of uterine contractions.

fimbria (fim′ brē uh) Long, fingerlike extensions at the entrance to the Fallopian tubes.

first stage of labor The early portion of labor in which cervical effacement and dilatation occurs.

follicle (fol′ i kul) A thin capsule of tissue surrounding immature eggs.

follicle stimulating hormone (FSH) A substance produced in the pituitary gland that prepares the ovary for ovulation and stimulates the production of sperm cells in the testes.

follicular phase (fol ik′ ū lar) The first phase of the menstrual cycle, in which ovarian follicles begin to mature as a result of stimulation by FSH. See also *follicle stimulating hormone*.

foreskin (for′ skin) The freely movable skin that covers the penis. Also the hood of the clitoris.

frenulum (fren′ ū lum) A small, triangular fold of skin on the underside of the penis connecting the glans with the foreskin.

frigidity (fri jid′ i tē) An outdated term formerly used to describe female sexual difficulties.

FSH See *follicle stimulating hormone*.

gamete intrafallopian transfer (GIFT) The direct placement of a mixture of sperm and eggs into the Fallopian tube as a treatment for infertility.

gender identity The inner sense a person has of being male or female.

gender role Behavior that conveys to others that an individual is either male or female.

genital herpes (jen′ i tul her pēz) Painful blisters of the genitals caused by infection with the herpes virus; outbreaks typically are recurrent and are highly contagious.

genital warts Dry, painless warts on or near the genitals or anus that are caused by a sexually transmitted virus. Sometimes referred to as venereal warts.

genitals (jen′ i tulz) Sex organs in the pelvic region. Customarily refers to the penis, the testes, and scrotum in the male and the vulva and vagina in the female.

glans (glanz) The tip or head of the penis or clitoris.

gonad Ovary or testicle.

gonadotropin releasing hormone (GnRH) (gō nad′ ō trō′ pin) A substance produced by the hypothalamus that controls the production and release of LH and FSH by the pituitary.

gonorrhea A sexually transmitted disease caused by the bacterium *Neisseria gonorrheae*. First symptoms in men include a puslike discharge from the tip of the penis and frequent urination, but many affected women are symptomless. Untreated, gonorrhea can cause serious complications, especially infertility in women.

granulosa cells (gran′ ū lō′ suh) The cells lining the ovarian follicle that enlarge and form the corpus luteum.

G spot (Gräfenberg spot) A proposed region of the front wall of the vagina claimed by some researchers to have a high degree of erotic sensitivity.

gynecomastia (jīn′ e kō mas′ tē uh) Enlargement of one or both male breasts.

hepatitis (hep ah tie′ tis) An infection or inflammation of the liver.

hermaphrodite (hur maf′ rō dīt) A person with both testicular and ovarian tissue.

heterosexual (het′ ur ō sek′ shoo ul) A person with sexual preference for partners of the opposite sex.

homosexual (hō′ mō sek′ shoo ul) A person with sexual preference for partners of his or her own sex.

hormone Chemical substance secreted by the endocrine system into the bloodstream to be carried directly to the tissue on which it acts.

hot flash Sudden sensations of warmth, blushing, and sweating, sometimes with dizziness, that occur commonly in menopausal women.

human immunodeficiency virus (HIV) The retrovirus that causes AIDS; prior to 1986, this virus was generally called HTLV-III.

hymen (hī′ mun) A thin tissue membrane covering the opening of the vagina.

hypothalamus (hī′ pō thal′ uh mus) The portion of the brain that has primary control over most endocrine pathways. It reacts to the level of hormones in the blood supply which regulate many sexual responses and direct their production.

hysterectomy (his′ tur ek′ tuh mē) Partial or total removal of the uterus.

hysterotomy (his tur ot′ uh mē) Incision of the uterus. Infrequently used for abortion during the second trimester.

implantation The attachment of the blastocyst to the lining of the uterus.

impotence (im′ puh tence) The inability to have or maintain an erection firm enough for coitus. See *erectile dysfunction*.

induced labor Labor started artificially, usually by infusing oxytocin into a vein.

infertility The inability of a couple to achieve pregnancy, usually defined after a year or more of sexual intercourse without pregnancy.

inhibited sexual desire (ISD) A condition marked by very low interest in sexual behavior.

inner lips See *labia minora*.

intrauterine device (IUD) (in truh ū′ ter in) A small object, either plastic or metal, placed inside the uterus for birth control.

introitus The opening of the vagina.

inverted nipples Congenital condition in which the nipples are not protuberant.

***in vitro* fertilization** A procedure involving removing eggs from a woman's body and fertilizing them with sperm in a laboratory. After successful fertilization, the embryo is surgically implanted in the woman's uterus.

Kaposi's sarcoma A previously rare form of cancer of the small blood vessels, causing purplish spots on the skin or in the mouth; a common sign of AIDS in homosexual men.

Klinefelter's syndrome A sex chromosome abnormality marked by an extra X chromosome in a genetic male, giving a 47, XXY pattern. Most of these men tend to be tall with poor muscular development and small testes. Sexual desire is often low and impotence common.

labia majora (la′ bē uh muh jor′ uh) The two outer folds of skin on either side of the inner lips, the clitoris, and the urethral and vaginal openings.

labia minora (la′ bē uh mī nor′ uh) The two inner folds of skin enclosing the urethral and vaginal openings.

labor The processes involved in giving birth, especially uterine contractions.

lactation (lak tā′ shun) The production of milk by the breasts, usually beginning a few days after birth.

laparoscopy An exploratory visualization of the pelvic and abdominal organs using a tube-like instrument.

laparotomy (lap uh rot′ uh mē) Any operation involving an incision through the abdominal wall. Now used for sterilization only if other surgery is required in the abdomen.

larynx The voice box.

latency stage In Freudian theory, the period from about six years to puberty when sexual impulses are quiescent and are sublimated into nonsexual behaviors and interests.

latent stage (syphilis) Period in the course of syphilis when symptoms disappear and the disease is no longer contagious. During this stage infecting organisms burrow into most organs of the body.

Leydig cells (lī′ dig) The cells in the testes where hormone production occurs.

luteal phase (lū′ tē ul) The third phase of the menstrual cycle, after ovulation. The corpus luteum produces large amounts of progesterone and estrogen, which prepare the uterus to receive the fertilized egg.

luteinizing hormone (LH) (lū′ tē in īz′ ing) Produced by the pituitary gland, LH triggers ovulation and stimulates the Leydig cells to manufacture testosterone.

lymphokines Messenger proteins secreted by macrophages that activate the immune response.

macromastia (mak′ rō mas′ tē uh) Abnormally large breasts.

mammary hyperplasia or macromastia Abnormally large breasts.

mastectomy (mas tek′ tuh mē) Surgical removal of the breast.

meiosis (mī ō′ sis) The process by which each immature egg divides into four cells, only one of which is a mature egg.

menarche (me nar′ kē) The onset of menses.

menopause (men′ ō paws) The period during which menstruation gradually stops, usually occurring in the late forties. Sometimes called female climacteric.

menstruation (men stroo′ ā′ shun) A flow of blood from the lining of the uterus occurring about once a month in females from puberty until the late forties or early fifties.

minipill A contraceptive pill containing only progesterone in low dosage.

molluscum contagiosum A skin disease caused by a pox virus; the skin breaks out in small, bumpy lesions with a pearly top.

mongolism See *Down's syndrome.*

monilial vaginitis (mon il′ ee all vaj in eye′ tis) Infection of the vagina caused by a fungus; usually accompanied by a thick, cheesy discharge with intense itching.

mons veneris (mōnz ven′ e ris) The area over the pubic bone of the female, which consists of a cushion of fatty tissue covered by skin and pubic hair. Also called mons pubis or mound of Venus.

morula (more′ u lah) A spherical mass of cells resulting from cleavage of the fertilized egg.

mucosa (mew kō′ suh) Mucous membrane. The membrane lining of the body openings, especially of the vagina, kept moist by the secretions of various types of glands.

Müllerian duct (mew ler′ ē un) One of two pairs of embryonic genital ducts. In females, this duct system develops into the Fallopian tubes, uterus, and inner part of the vagina. In males, a substance secreted by the embryonic testes causes the Müllerian duct system to shrink and practically disappear.

multiorgasmic (mul′ tē or gaz′ mik) The potential ability of women to have a series of identifiable orgasmic responses without dropping below the plateau level of arousal. Men do not share this capacity.

multiple sclerosis (MS) A chronic neurological disorder affecting both motor and sensory function in an episodic but progressive fashion.

myometrium (mī′ ō mē′ trē um) The muscular component of the uterus, important in labor and delivery.

myotonia (mī′ ō tō nē uh) Involuntary contraction of muscle.

neuromuscular tension (new′ rō mus′ kew lur) Buildup of energy in the nerves and muscles sometimes caused by sexual arousal.

neurosis A psychological disorder usually characterized by anxiety and/or tension. In contrast to more severe forms of psychological problems, called psychoses, with a neurosis a person's sense of reality is not greatly altered.

nipple Protuberance located at the tip of the breast consisting principally of smooth muscle fibers and a network of nerve endings and containing in the female the outlets of the milk ducts.

nocturnal emissions Involuntary male orgasm and ejaculation during sleep (sometimes called wet dreams).

occiput presentation The childbirth presentation in which the back part of the baby's head is the first part to pass through the birth canal.

Oedipus complex (ed′ i pus) In Freudian theory, the sexual attraction of a young boy toward his mother, accompanied by a mixture of fear and rivalry toward his father. See also *Electra complex.*

orgasm (or′ gas um) The third and shortest phase of the human sexual response cycle. A total body response involving the sudden discharge of accumulated sexual tension.

orgasmic dysfunction (or gaz′ mik) The inability of a female to reach orgasm. See also *anorgasmia.*

orgasmic platform The narrowing of the vagina during sexual excitement due to vasocongestion.

os penis Pelvis bone present in some species but not in humans or other primates.

osteoporosis (ah stee oh porh oh′ sis) A condition in which the bones become thin and brittle due to mineral loss; a common occurrence in postmenopausal women.

outer lips See *labia majora.*

ovariectomy (ō vuh′ rē ek′ tuh mē) Surgical removal of the ovaries.

ovaries (ō′ vur ēz) Paired structures located on each side of the uterus that contain and release eggs and secrete hormones such as estrogen and progesterone. The female gonads.

ovulation (ōv you lā′ shun) The second phase of the menstrual cycle; the release of the egg from the ovary.

ovulation method of birth control A method that depends on changes in the cervical mucus thought to indicate the time of ovulation. The mucus changes from cloudy, white, and tacky to clear and stretchy at the time of ovulation. Intercourse is thought to be safe four days after the ovulatory mucus begins and when the mucus has returned to a cloudy, tacky consistency. Failure rate is high.

ovum (ō′ vum) A mature egg cell that is capable, after maturation and fertilization, of becoming another member of the same species.

oxytocin (ahk′ sē to′ sin) A hormone made in the posterior pituitary thought to play a role in uterine contractions and lactation stimulation.

paraplegia Paralysis of both lower extremities.

parent-child bonding The process of attachment and identification that usually occurs during early infancy.

penis (pē′ nis) The male organ of copulation. It consists primarily of three cylinders of spongy tissue, interspersed with many small, thin-walled blood vessels and bound in a thick membrane sheath.

penis envy In Freudian theory, the girl's unconscious sense of inadequacy and jealousy at not having a penis.

pentamidine A medication used to prevent *Pneumocystis carinii* pneumonia.

perimenopausal years (perry men oh paws′ uhl) The years immediately before and after menopause.

perineum (per i nē′ um) The hairless area of skin between the vagina and anus in the female and between the scrotum and anus in the male.

phagocytes White blood cells that engulf invading microorganisms.

pituitary (pi tew′ i ter′ ē) An acorn-sized gland at the base of the brain which, at the direction of the hypothalamus, secretes several hormones important to sexual development and function. Once believed to control most of the endocrine system, it is now known to act only as a relay station.

placenta (pluh sen′ tuh) The organ attached to the wall of the uterus that performs the functions of nutrition, respiration, and excretion for the unborn child. It is also an endocrine organ secreting large amounts of several hormones.

plateau phase The phase of human sexual response following excitement, in which a leveling off of sexual tensions occurs. This phase can be short or long prior to reaching levels required to trigger orgasm.

Pneumocystis carinii A microorganism that causes life-threatening pneumonia in persons with AIDS; one of the leading causes of death in AIDS patients.

polar bodies Cells that arise in the development of the ovum during meiosis.

polio An infection caused by a virus that can, in severe forms, cause paralysis.

postmenopausal years The period of a woman's life after menstruation ceases.

postpartum depression The letdown many women experience after giving birth. They are tearful and depressed and may have frightening dreams. Also called baby blues.

precocious puberty (pree koh′ shus pew′ burr tee) Physical changes of puberty occurring before age 8 in girls or age 10 in boys.

preeclampsia (prē′ e klamp′ sē uh) A condition occurring during the latter half of pregnancy characterized by high blood pressure, edema, and protein in the urine. May progress to *eclampsia*.

pre-embryo stage The interval from the completion of fertilization until the appearance of a single primitive streak.

premature ejaculation Unintentional ejaculation during noncoital play, while the male is trying to enter his partner, or soon after intercourse begins.

premenstrual syndrome (PMS) Fatigue, irritability, depression, and bloated feeling some women experience a few days before menstruation. Physical, psychological, and social causes are debated.

prenatal care The combined efforts of doctor, nurse, and mother to see that the pregnant women stays healthy and the unborn child has everything needed to grow and develop.

prenatal period The time from conception to birth.

primitive streak An embryonic structure that appears on about the fourteenth day of development, eventually degenerating and disappearing.

procreational sex (pro′ krē ā′ shun ul) Sexual intercourse solely for reproduction. Sometimes advocated by some churches and groups as the only acceptable reason for sex.

progesterone (prō jes′ tur ōn) A hormone present in both sexes, but primarily known as a female hormone. Present in high levels during pregnancy.

prolapsed cord Condition whereby the umbilical cord is compressed to the point where the blood supply to the baby is cut off.

prostaglandin-induced abortion Evacuation of the contents of the pregnant uterus produced by infusion of prostaglandins.

prostatectomy (pros′ tuh tek′ tuh mē) Surgical removal of the prostate gland.

prostate gland (pros′ tāt) Gland located directly below the bladder, surrounding the urethra as it exits the bladder. It secretes part of the seminal fluid and is a major site of the synthesis of prostaglandins.

prostatitis (pros tuh tī′ tis) Inflammation of the prostate, caused by infection.

pseudohermaphrodite (sue′ dō hur mat′ rō dīt) An individual born with gonads matching the sex chromosomes but a genital appearance that resembles the opposite sex.

pubic lice Parasites that invade the pubic region, often transmitted during sexual intercourse.

pubococcygeus (pew bō kock sij′ ē us) A muscle encircling and supporting the vagina.

quadriplegia (kwahd ruh pleej′ ee ah) Paralysis of all limbs.

quickening The time during pregnancy when a woman can first feel the fetus moving.

rapid orgasm The female counterpart of premature ejaculation, marked by characteristically having orgasm so quickly in a sexual encounter that it is distressful. This is a very rare complaint.

recreational sex Sexual activity primarily for pleasure. Emotional involvement and intimacy are purposefully limited.

rectum (rek′ tum) The lower part of the large intestine.

refractory period In the male, the period immediately following ejaculation during which further orgasm is physiologically impossible. This period is not present in the female response cycle.

relational sex Sexual activity in the context of emotional involvement and intimacy in a relationship.

resolution phase Last phase of human sexual response following orgasm or maximum excitement in which the body returns to an unaroused state.

retarded ejaculation Condition in which ejaculation in the vagina occurs only after a lengthy time period and strenuous efforts.

retrograde ejaculation Condition in which the semen spurts backward into the bladder during orgasm because the bladder neck does not close off properly. It occurs in men with multiple sclerosis and diabetes and following some types of prostate surgery.

Rh incompatibility Condition in which antibodies from the mother's bloodstream destroy red blood cells in the fetus, causing anemia, mental retardation, or fetal death.

rhythm method Any form of birth control based on periodic abstinence. Although most rhythm methods seek to identify the most fertile portion of the menstrual cycle, they are generally of poor reliability. Rhythm methods are acceptable to the Catholic church, which views them as "natural" forms of birth control.

rubella (roo bel′ uh) German measles. If the virus crosses the placental barrier to the fetus, it can cause serious malformations including deafness, eye problems, and mental retardation.

Rubin's test A procedure to check for obstructed Fallopian tubes. Carbon dioxide is inserted into the uterus to see if it passes into the abdomen.

saline-induced abortion Evacuation of the contents of the pregnant uterus produced by infusion of a salt solution into the amniotic fluid.

scrotum (skrō′ tum) The thin, loose sac of skin that contains the testes and has a layer of muscle fibers that contract involuntarily.

second stage of labor The portion of labor from full cervical dilatation to delivery of the baby.

seminal fluid (sem′ uh nul) The thick white, yellow, or gray liquid portion of the male ejaculate.

seminal vesicles (sem′ uh nul ves′ e kulz) In the male, paired pouchlike bodies that empty into the ejaculatory ducts and provide the major part of fluid in the ejaculate.

seminiferous tubules (sem′ i nif′ ur us tū′ bewls) Microscopic tube-shaped structures in the testes where sperm is produced.

sensate focus Graduated touching experiences (not necessarily sexual) assigned to couples in therapy to reduce anxiety and teach nonverbal communication skills.

sex flush A temporary reddish, spotty, rashlike color change sometimes developing during sexual excitement. Usually on the abdomen and breasts, it can spread to any areas of the body.

sexual aversion A severe phobia (irrational fear) of sexual activity or the thought of sexual activity, which generally leads to avoidance of sexual situations.

sexual differentiation The process that begins at the moment of conception to create a normal male or female.

sexual dysfunction Conditions in which the ordinary physical responses of sexual excitement or orgasm are impaired. Can be classified as psychosocial (caused by psychological, interpersonal, environmental, and cultural factors) or organic (caused by physical or medical factors such as illness, injury, or drugs).

sexuality A broadly encompassing term used to refer to all aspects of being and feeling sexual.

sexually transmitted disease (STD) Infection spread mainly by sexual contact.

shingles A painful, blistering skin rash caused by the herpes zoster virus.

smegma (smeg′ muh) Glandular secretions, dead cells, dirt particles, and bacteria that accumulate under the foreskin of the penis or the hood of the clitoris.

spongy body See *corpus spongiosum.*

squeeze technique Method for reducing the tendency for rapid ejaculation.

sterilization Surgical procedure performed on men (vasectomy) or women (tubal ligation; hysterectomy) to prevent union of sperm and egg.

syphilis (sif′ uh lis) A sexually transmitted disease caused by *Treponema pallidum.* Its stages consist of primary (characterized by chancres), secondary (characterized by rash, fever, aches and pains, weight loss, and hair loss), and tertiary (characterized by serious heart problems and brain or spinal cord damage).

temperature method of birth control A technique of determining the part of the menstrual cycle when pregnancy is likely to occur so that intercourse can be avoided then. Involves daily recording of basal body temperature to pinpoint ovulation. Intercourse is not allowed from the day menstrual flow stops until two to four days after a temperature rise. Failure rate is high.

teratogen (teh rat′ ō jin) A substance, such as a drug or chemical, that causes birth defects.

testes (tes′ tēz) The paired male reproductive glands contained in the scrotum. The male gonads.

testicular feminization syndrome An inherited condition in which tissues are insensitive to the effects of testosterone. The individual is born with a 46, XY chromosome pattern (male) but with female genitals.

testosterone (tes tos′ tur ōn) The most important hormone in sexual function, present in both sexes. Often called the male hormone, it is secreted by the testes and adrenals in the male and the ovaries and adrenals in the female.

theoretical effectiveness The ideal effectiveness of a contraceptive method when used correctly and consistently.

third stage of labor The period immediately following delivery of the baby, concluding with separation and expulsion of the placenta.

thrush An infection of the mouth and throat caused by monilia; this type of infection is more bothersome than life-threatening.

toxemia A complication of pregnancy marked by sudden increase in blood pressure, edema, and protein in the urine.

toxic shock syndrome (TSS) An illness of rapid onset caused by infection with *Staphylococcus aureus* bacteria; symptoms include fever, vomiting, muscle pain, and a sunburn-like skin rash. Most, but not all, cases have occurred in menstruating women, and the syndrome is thought to be related to the use of high-absorbency vaginal tampons.

transudation (trans′ ū dā′ shun) The passing of a fluid through a membrane, especially the lubrication in the vagina during sexual arousal.

transverse position The childbirth presentation in which the baby lies across the uterus and a shoulder or arm is first to be seen at the opening of the vagina. A cesarean section is often necessary if the baby cannot be turned.

trichomonas vaginitis (trick o mōn′ ess) An infection of the vagina caused by bacteria called trichomonas vaginalis. Accompanied by a frothy, thin, greenish or yellowish gray, foul-smelling discharge and burning and itching.

trimester A three-month period; generally used to describe the progression of pregnancy in three such periods.

trisomy 21 (trī′ sō mē) See *Down's syndrome*.

tubal ligation (tū′ bull lī gā′ shun) Literally, tying the tubes—cutting, cauterizing, and blocking the Fallopian tubes to prevent conception.

Turner's syndrome A sex chromosome abnormality caused by a missing chromosome. The individual has a 45, X chromosome pattern and may appear fairly normal until puberty, when nonfunctioning gonads prevent development of the secondary sex characteristics and the adolescent growth spurt. May also be accompanied by webbing of the neck, increased carrying angle of the elbow, heart defects, and other abnormalities.

umbilical cord The cylindrical structure connecting the fetus to the placenta. It contains two arteries and a vein.

urethra (u rē′ thruh) A tube beginning at the bladder and ending at the urethral meatus, carrying urine in the female and urine or semen in the male.

urethral meatus (u re′ thral mē a′ tus) The urinary opening.

urinary stress incontinence A condition in which urine leaks from the urethra during coughing, laughing, and/or sexual arousal.

uterus (ū′ tur us) A hollow, pear-shaped muscular organ, part of the female internal genitals, in which the fertilized egg becomes embedded and the embryo and the fetus are nourished. Sometimes called the womb.

vacuum aspiration The method usually chosen for abortion during the first trimester. The cervix is dilated and the contents of the uterus are removed through a plastic tube connected to a pump.

vagina (va jī′ nuh) The canal in the female that receives the penis in copulation, existing as a potential space capable of contraction and expansion. The opening is called the vaginal introitus.

vaginismus (vaj in iz′ mus) Involuntary spasms of the muscles around the vagina in response to attempts at penetration.

vaginitis (vaj in ī′ tis) Vaginal inflammation from infection or chemical irritation.

vas deferens (vas def′ ur enz) One of two long, tube-like structures that convey spermatozoa from the testes.

vasectomy (vas ek′ tuh mē) Surgical procedure for sterilization of the male consisting of cutting and tying each vas deferens. The operation does not stop sperm production but blocks its passage from the testes.

vasocongestion (vas′ o kun jes′ chun) An increased amount of blood concentrated in body tissues, especially in the genitals and female breasts during sexual arousal. In the male it causes erection and in the female an increase in the size of the clitoris and transudation of fluid in the vagina.

venereal warts Dry, usually painless, sexually transmitted nodules that grow on or near the genitals and are caused by a virus.

vertex presentation (vur′ teks) The childbirth presentation in which the crown of the baby's head is first to be seen at the opening of the vagina.

viral hepatitis Infection of the liver by a virus causing a debilitating acute illness and sometimes a chronic condition.

vulva (vul′ vuh) The external sex organs of the female: the mons, labia, clitoris, and vaginal orifice.

Western blot test A confirmatory test used to supplement ELISA testing. Western blot tests are more accurate than ELISA tests, but their complexity and expense precludes their use as the primary screening method in testing for HIV.

wet dreams See *nocturnal emissions*.

withdrawal The removal of the penis from the vagina before ejaculation occurs. When used as a birth control method, failure rate is high. See *coitus interruptus*.

Wolffian duct (wool′ fē un) One of two primitive duct systems in the embryo. Develops in the male to form the epididymis, vas deferens, seminal vesicles, and prostate; it shrinks in the female to nonfunctioning remnants.

zona pellucida (zō′ nuh pe lew′ sē duh) The jellylike material surrounding the mature egg.

zygote (zī′ gōt) The single cell created by the penetration of an egg by the sperm. An organism produced by the union of two gametes.

zygote intrafallopian transfer (ZIFT) A technique of assisted reproductive technology in which the woman's eggs are fertilized *in vitro*, after which the zygote is placed in the Fallopian tube.

References

Aarskog, D. "Maternal Progestins as a Possible Cause of Hypospadias." *New England Journal of Medicine* 300:75–78, 1979.

Abel, G. G., et al. "Women's Vaginal Responses During REM Sleep." *Journal of Sex and Marital Therapy* 5:5–14, 1979.

Abitbol, M. M., and Davenport, J. H. "Sexual Dysfunction After Therapy for Cervical Carcinoma." *American Journal of Obstetrics and Gynecology* 119:181–189, 1974.

Adams, D. B.; Gold, A. R.; and Burt, A. D. "Rise in Female-Initiated Sexual Activity at Ovulation and Its Suppression by Oral Contraceptives." *New England Journal of Medicine* 299:1145–1150, 1978.

Addiego, F., et al. "Female Ejaculation: A Case Study." *Journal of Sex Research* 17(1):13–21, 1981.

Adler, N. E., et al. "Psychological Responses After Abortion." *Science* 248:41–44, 1990.

Alderman, P. M. "The Lurking Sperm." *Journal of the American Medical Association* 259:3142–3144, 1988.

Alexander, L. "Treatment of Impotency and Anorgasmia by Psychotherapy Aided by Hypnosis." *American Journal of Clinical Hyponosis* 17:33–43, 1974.

Alington-MacKinnon, D., and Troll, L. E. "The Adaptive Function of the Menopause: A Devil's Advocate Position." *Journal of the American Geriatrics Society* 29:349–353, 1981.

Allen, J. A. "Premenstrual Frenzy." *New York Magazine,* pp. 37–42, November 1, 1982.

Alter, M., et al. "Hepatitis B Virus Transmission Between Heterosexuals." *Journal of the American Medical Association* 256:1307–1310, 1986.

Alter, M. J., and Sampliner, R. E. "Hepatitis C: And Miles to Go Before We Sleep." *New England Journal of Medicine* 321:1538–1540, 1989.

Alter, M. J., et al. "The Importance of Heterosexual Activity and Intravenous Drug Use in the Transmission of Hepatitis B and Non-A, Non-B Hepatitis." *Journal of the American Medical Association* 262:1201–1205, 1989.

———. "The Changing Epidemiology of Hepatitis B in the United States." *Journal of the American Medical Association* 263:1218–1222, 1990.

Altman, L. K., "Some Optimism Amid Grim Predictions as 87-Nation AIDS Meeting Opens." *The New York Times,* June 5, 1989, p. B4 (1989a).

———. "Who's Stricken and How: AIDS Pattern Is Shifting." *The New York Times,* Section 1, pp. 1 & 28, February 5, 1989.

Alvarez, F., et al. "New Insights on the Mode of Action of Intrauterine Contraceptive Devices in Women." *Fertility and Sterility* 49:768–773, 1988.

Alzate, H., and Hoch, Z. "The 'G Spot' and 'Female Ejaculation': A Current Appraisal." *Journal of Sex & Marital Therapy* 12:211–220, 1986.

Alzate, H., and Londono, M. L. "Vaginal Erotic Sensitivity." *Journal of Sex & Marital Therapy* 10:49–56, 1984.

American Cancer Society. "Guidelines for the Cancer-Related Checkup." *Ca-A Cancer Journal for Clinicians* 30:194–240, 1980.

American Psychiatric Association. *Diagnostic and Statistical Manual of Mental Disorders,* 3rd ed. rev. Washington, DC: American Psychiatric Association, 1987.

American Psychiatric Association. *Diagnostic and Statistical Manual of Mental Disorders,* 3rd ed. (DSM-III). Washington, DC: American Psychiatric Association, 1980.

Anderson, B. G. *The Aging Game: Success, Sanity and Sex After 60.* New York: McGraw-Hill, 1979.

Andrews, M. C., et al. "An Analysis of the Obstetric Outcome of 125 Consecutive Pregnancies Conceived *in vitro* and Resulting in 100 Deliveries." *American Journal of Obstetrics and Gynecology* 154:848–854, 1986.

Annon, J. S. *The Behavioral Treatment of Sexual Problems: Brief Therapy.* New York: Harper & Row, 1976.

Antunes, C. M., et al. "Endometrial Cancer and Estrogen Use: Report of a Large Case–Control Study." *New England Journal of Medicine* 300:9–13, 1979.

Apfelbaum, B. (ed.). *Expanding the Boundaries of Sex Therapy,* 2nd ed. Berkeley, CA: Berkeley Sex Therapy Group, 1983.

Apte, S. M.; Gregory J.; and Purcell, M. "The Inflatable Penile Prosthesis: Reoperation and Patient Satisfaction." *Journal of Urology* 131:894–895, 1984.

Arentewicz, G., and Schmidt, G. (eds.). *The Treatment of Sexual Disorders.* New York: Basic Books, 1983.

Arms, S. *Immaculate Deception.* Boston: Houghton Mifflin, 1975.

Arno, P. S., et al. "Economic and Policy Implications of Early Intervention in HIV Disease." *Journal of the American Medical Association* 262:1493–1498, 1989.

Arvin, A. M., et al. "Failure of Antepartum Maternal Cultures to Predict the Infant's Risk of Exposure to Herpes Simplex Virus at Delivery." *New England Journal of Medicine* 315:796–800, 1986.

Ashford, J. *The Whole Birth Catalog.* Trumansburg, NY: The Crossing Press, 1983.

Ayalah, D., and Weinstock, I. J. *Breasts.* New York: Summit Books, 1979.

Azizi, F., et al. "Decreased Serum Testosterone Concentration in Male Heroin and Methadone Addicts." *Steroids* 22:467–472, 1973.

Bachetti, P., and Moss, A. R. "Incubation Period of AIDS in San Francisco." *Nature* 338:251–253, 1989.

Bakwin, H. "Erotic Feelings in Infants and Young Children." *Medical Aspects of Human Sexuality* 8(10):200–215, 1974.

Baldwin, J. D., and Baldwin, J. I. "Factors Affecting AIDS-Related Risk-Taking Behavior Among College Students." *Journal of Sex Research* 25:181–196, 1988.

Ballinger, C. B. "The Menopause and Its Syndromes." In Howells, J. G. (ed.), *Modern Perspectives in the Psychiatry of Middle Age,* pp. 279–303. New York: Brunner/Mazel, 1981.

Bancroft, J. "The Behavioral Approach to Treatment." In Money, J., and Musaph, H. (eds.), *Handbook of Sexology,* pp. 1197–1225. Amsterdam: Elsevier/North-Holland, 1977.

———. "The Relationship Between Hormones and Sexual Behavior in Humans." In Hutchison, J. B. (ed.), *Biological Determinants of Sexual Behavior,* pp. 493–519. New York: Wiley, 1978.

———. "Hormones and Human Sexual Behavior." *Journal of Sex & Marital Therapy* 10:3–21, 1984.

Bancroft, J., et al. "Mood, Sexuality, Hormones and the Menstrual Cycle: III. Sexuality and the Role of Androgens." *Psychosomatic Medicine* 45:509–524, 1983.

Barbach, L. G. *For Yourself: The Fulfillment of Female Sexuality.* New York: Doubleday, 1975.

———. *Women Discover Orgasm.* New York: Free Press, 1980.

———. *For Each Other: Sharing Sexual Intimacy.* Garden City, NY: Anchor Press, 1982.

Barbach, L. G., and Levine, L. *Shared Intimacies.* Garden City, NY: Anchor Press/Doubleday, 1980.

Barlow, D. *Sexually Transmitted Diseases: The Facts.* New York: Oxford University Press, 1979.

Barocas, R., and Karoly, P. "Effects of Physical Appearance on Social Responsiveness." *Psychology Review* 31:495–500, 1972.

Barrett-Connor, E. "Post-Menopausal Estrogen Replacement and Breast Cancer." *New England Journal of Medicine* 321:319–320, 1989.

Bart, P. B., and Grossman, M. "Menopause." In Notman, M. T., and Nadelson, C. C. (eds.), *The Woman Patient,* pp. 337–354. New York: Plenum Press, 1978.

Bates, G. "On the Nature of the Hot Flash." *Clinical Obstetrics and Gynecology* 24(1):231–241, 1981.

Battaglia, F. C. "Reducing the Cesarean-Section Rate Safely." *New England Journal of Medicine* 319:1540–1541, 1988.

Baulieu, E. "Contragestion and Other Clinical Applications of RU 486, an Antiprogesterone at the Receptor." *Science* 245:1351–1357, 1989.

———. "RU-486 as an Antiprogesterone Steroid." *Journal of the American Medical Association* 262:1808–1814, 1989a.

Bauman, J. E. "Basal Body Temperature: Unreliable Method of Ovulation Detection." *Fertility and Sterility* 36:729, 1981.

Bauman, J. E., et al. "Effectos Endocrinos Del Uso Cronico De La Marijuana in Mujeres." *Cuadernos Cientificos Cemesam* 10:85–97, July 1979.

Bayer, R.; Levine, C.; and Wolf, S. "HIV Antibody Screening." *Journal of the American Medical Association* 256:1768–1774, 1986.

Becker, E. F. *Female Sexuality Following Spinal Cord Injury.* Bloomington, IN: Accent Special Publication, Cheever Publishing, 1978.

Becker, M. H., and Joseph, J. G. "AIDS and Behavioral Change to Reduce Risk: A Review." *American Journal of Public Health* 78:394–410, 1988.

Beerthuizen, R. J., et al. "IUD and Salpingitis." *European Journal of Obstetrics, Gynecology, and Reproductive Biology* 13(1):31–41, 1982.

Belliveau, F., and Richter, L. *Understanding Human Sexual Inadequacy.* New York: Bantam, 1970.

Belzer, E. "Orgasmic Expulsions of Women: A Review and Heuristic Inquiry." *Journal of Sex Research* 17:1–12, 1981.

Benigni, A., et al. "Effect of Low-Dose Aspirin on Fetal and Maternal Generation of Thromboxane by Platelets in Women at Risk for Pregnancy-Induced Hypertension." *New England Journal of Medicine* 321:357–362, 1989.

Bennett, C. J., et al. "Sexual Dysfunction and Electroejaculation in Men with Spinal Cord Injury." *Journal of Urology* 139:453–457, 1988.

Benson, R. C. *Current Obstetric & Gynecologic Diagnosis & Treatment.* Los Altos, CA: Lange Medical Publications, 1978.

Beral, V., et al. "Epidemiology of Kaposi's Sarcoma in AIDS Patients: United States." Fifth International Conference on AIDS, Montreal, June 4–9, 1989. (Abstract # M.A.O.30, p. 50)

Berger, G.; Goldstein, M.; and Fuerst, M. *The Couple's Guide to Fertility.* New York: Doubleday, 1989.

Berger, R. M. *Gay and Gray: The Older Homosexual Male.* Urbana: University of Illinois Press, 1982.

Bergkvist, L., et al. "The Risk of Breast Cancer After Estrogen and Estrogen-Progestin Replacement." *New England Journal of Medicine* 321:293–297, 1989.

Berkley, S. F., et al. "The Relationship of Tampon Characteristics to Menstrual Toxic Shock Syndrome." *Journal of the American Medical Association* 258:917–920, 1987.

Berne, E. *Sex in Human Loving.* New York: Pocket Books, 1971.

Bernstein, G., et al. "Results of a Comparative Study of the Diaphragm and Cervical Cap." Paper presented at the annual meeting of the American Public Health Association, Las Vegas, September 29–October 2, 1986.

Binkin, N. J., and Alexander, E. R. "Neonatal Herpes: How Can It Be Prevented?" *Journal of the American Medical Association* 250:3094–3095, 1983.

Blay, S. L.; Ferraz, M. P. T.; and Calil, H. M. "Lithium-Induced Male Sexual Impairment." *Journal of Clinical Psychiatry* 43:497–498, 1982.

Blume, E. "Methodological Difficulties Plague PMS Research." *Journal of the American Medical Association* 249:2866, 1983.

Boehm, D. "The Cervical Cap: Effectiveness as a Contraceptive." *Journal of Nurse-Midwifery* 28(1):3–6, 1983.

Bohlen, J. G. " 'Female Ejaculation' and Urinary Stress Incontinence." *Journal of Sex Research* 18:360–363, 1982.

Bohlen, J. G., et al. "Development of a Woman's Multiple Orgasm Pattern: A Research Case Report." *Journal of Sex Research* 18:130–145, 1982.

Booth, A. W. "AIDS and Insects." *Science* 237:355–356, 1987.

Boston Women's Health Book Collective. *Our Bodies, Ourselves,* 2nd ed. New York: Simon & Schuster, 1976.

Boston Women's Health Book Collective. *The New Our Bodies, Ourselves.* New York: Simon & Schuster, 1984.

Bracken, M. B. "Spermicidal Contraceptives and Poor Reproductive Outcomes: The Epidemiologic Evidence Against an Association." *American Journal of Obstetrics and Gynecology* 151:552–556, 1985.

Bragonier, J. R. "Influence of Oral Contraception on Sexual Response." *Medical Aspects of Human Sexuality* 10(10):130–143, October 1976.

Brandt, E. N., Jr. "Physicians and Sexually Transmitted Disease: A Call to Action." *Journal of the American Medical Association* 248:2032, 1982.

Brecher, E. *The Sex Researchers.* Boston: Little, Brown, 1969.

Brecher, E. M. "History of Human Sexual Research and Study." In Freedman, A. M.; Kaplan, H. I.; and Sadock, B. J. (eds.), *Comprehensive Textbook of Psychiatry/II,* pp. 1327–1357. Baltimore: Williams & Wilkins, 1975.

Brecher, R., and Brecher, E. *An Analysis of Human Sexual Response.* New York: New American Library, 1966.

Breen, J. L. "A 21-Year Survey of 654 Ectopic Pregnancies." *American Journal of Obstetrics and Gynecology* 106:1004–1019, 1970.

Breo, D. "AMA AIDS Expert's Grim Message." *American Medical News,* pp. 3 & 32, December 5, 1986.

Brindley, G. S., and Gillan, P. "Men and Women Who Do Not Have Orgasms." *British Journal of Psychiatry* 45:351–356, 1982.

Brock, B. V., et al. "Frequency of Asymptomatic Shedding of Herpes Simplex Virus in Women with Genital Herpes." *Journal of the American Association* 263:418–420, 1990.

Brody, Jane E. "Study Finds Women in 40's Benefit from Mammograms." *The New York Times,* p. B5, September 21, 1988.

Brown, J. *Nutrition for Your Pregnancy.* Minneapolis: University of Minnesota Press, 1983.

Brown, J. M., and Chaves, J. F. "Hypnosis in the Treatment of Sexual Dysfunction." *Journal of Sex & Marital Therapy* 6(1):63–74, 1980.

Brownmiller, S. *Against Our Will.* New York: Simon & Schuster, 1975.

Bryson, Y. J., et al. "Treatment of First Episodes of Genital Herpes Simplex Virus Infection with Oral Acycolvir." *New England Journal of Medicine* 308:916–921, 1983.

Buchanan, R. "Breast-feeding: Aid to Infant Health and Fertility Control." *Population Reports,* Series J(4): July 1975.

Buckley, R. M., Jr.; McGuckin, M.; and MacGregor, R. R. "Urine Bacterial Counts After Sexual Intercourse." *New England Journal of Medicine* 298:321–324, 1978.

Buckley, W. E., et al. "Estimated Prevalence of Anabolic Steroid Use Among Male High School Seniors." *Journal of the American Medical Association* 260:3441–3445, 1988.

Bullard, D. G., and Knight, S. E. (eds.). *Sexuality and Physical Disability.* St. Louis, MO: C. V. Mosby, 1981.

Bullough, V. L. *Sexual Variance in Society and History.* New York: Wiley, 1976.

Bullough, V., and Bullough, B. *Sin, Sickness, and Sanity.* New York: New American Library, 1977.

Burgess, A. W., and Holmstrom, L. L. *Rape: Victims of Crisis.* Bowie, MD: Robert J. Brady, 1974.

Burke, D. S., et al. "Measurement of the False Positive Rate in a Screening Program for Human Immunodeficiency Virus Infections." *New England Journal of Medicine* 319:961–964, 1988.

———. "Human Immunodeficiency Virus Infections in Teenagers." *Journal of the American Medical Association* 263:2074–2077, 1990.

Bush, P. *Drugs, Alcohol and Sex.* New York: Richard Marek Publishers, 1980.

Butler, R. M., and Lewis, M. I. *Sex After Sixty.* New York: Harper & Row, 1976.

Cadden, V. "The Psychiatrists Versus Masters and Johnson." In LoPiccolo, J., and LoPiccolo, L. (eds.), *Handbook of Sex Therapy,* pp. 485–490. New York: Plenum Press, 1978.

Cagen, R. "The Cervical Cap as a Barrier Contraceptive." *Contraception* 33:496, 1986.

Caird, W., and Wincze, J. P. *Sex Therapy: A Behavioral Approach.* New York: Harper & Row, 1977.

Cannon, R. O., et al. "Association of Herpes Simplex Virus Type 2 with HIV Infection in Heterosexual Patients Attending Sexual Transmitted Disease Clinics." Presented at the Fourth International Conference on AIDS, Stockholm, June 12–16, 1988. (Abstract Book 2, p. 201)

Caron, S. L., and McMullen, T. "AIDS and the College Student: The Need for Sex Education." *SIECUS Report* 15(6):6–7, July/August 1987.

Carroll, James. "Change Starts with Our Own Attitudes." In Alyson, S. (ed.), *You Can Do Something About AIDS,* 2nd ed., pp. 19–21. Boston: The Stop AIDS Project, 1990.

Carson, S. A. "Sex Selection: The Ultimate in Family Planning." *Fertility & Sterility* 50:16–18, 1988.

Carter, C. S., and Greenough, W. T. "Sending the Right Sex Messages." *Psychology Today,* p. 112, September 1979.

Casper, R. F.; Yen, S. S. C.; and Wilkes, M. M. "Menopausal Flushes; A Neuroendocrine Link with Pulsatile Luteinizing Hormone Secretion." *Science* 205:823–825, 1979.

Castleman, M. *Sexual Solutions.* New York: Touchstone, 1989.

Catania, J. A., and White, C. B. "Sexuality in an Aged Sample: Cognitive Determinants of Masturbation." *Archives of Sexual Behavior* 11:237–245, 1982.

Cates, W., Jr.; Weisner, P. J.; and Curran, J. W. "Sex and Spermicides: Preventing Unintended Pregnancy and Infection." *Journal of the American Medical Association* 248:1636–1637, 1982.

Catterall, R. D. *A Short Textbook of Venereology.* Philadelphia: Lippincott, 1974.

Cavero, C. "Modern Midwifery: Complicated Rebirth of an Ancient Art." *Family and Community Health* 2(3):29–39, November 1979.

Cefalu, E., et al. "Successful Gamete Intrafallopian Transfer Following Failed Artificial Insemination by Donor: Evidence for a Defect in Gamete Transfer?" *Fertility & Sterility* 50:279–282, 1988.

Centers for Disease Control. "Oral Contraceptive Use and the Risk of Ovarian Cancer." *Journal of American Medical Association* 249:1596–1599, 1983.

———. "Oral Contraceptive Use and the Risk of Endometrial Cancer." *Journal of the American Medical Association* 249:1600–1604, 1983a.

———. *"Chalamydia Trachomatis* Infections: Policy Guidelines for Prevention and Control." *MMWR* 34(Suppl.):53S—74S, 1985.

———. "1989 Sexually Transmitted Diseases Treatment Guidelines." *Morbidity and Mortality Weekly Report* 38(S-8), 1989.

———. "Ectopic Pregnancy—United States, 1986." *Morbidity and Mortality Weekly Report* 38:481–484, 1989a.

Chaisson, R. E., et al. "Cocaine Use and HIV Infection in Intravenous Drug Users in San Francisco." *Journal of the American Medical Association* 261:561–565, 1989.

Chasnoff, I. J., et al. "Temporal Patterns of Cocaine Use in Pregnancy." *Journal of the American Medical Association* 261:1741–1744, 1989.

Chasnoff, I. J.; Landress, H. J.; and Barrett, M. E. "The Prevalence of Illicit-Drug or Alcohol Use During Pregnancy and Discrepancies in Mandatory Reporting in Pinellas County, Florida." *New England Journal of Medicine* 322:1202–1206, 1990.

Cherfas, J. "The Pill of Choice?" *Science* 245:1319–1324, 1989.

Cherfas, J., and Palca, J. "Hormone Antagonist with Broad Potential." *Science* 245:1322, 1989.

Chesler, P. *Sacred Bond: The Legacy of Baby M.* New York: Times Books, 1988.

Chesser, E. *The Sexual Marital and Family Relationships of the English Woman.* London: Hutchinson's Medical Publications, 1956.

Chiasson, M. A.; Stoneburner, R. L.; and Joseph, S. C. "Human Immunodeficiency Virus Transmission Through Artificial Insemination." *Journal of AIDS* 3:69–72, 1990.

Chipouras, S., et al. *Who Cares? A Handbook on Sex Education and Counseling Services for Disabled People.* Washington, DC: George Washington University, 1979.

Cicero, T. J., et al. "Function of the Male Sex Organs in Heroin and Methadone Users." *New England Journal of Medicine* 292:882–887, 1975.

Clark, L. "Is There a Difference Between a Clitoral and a Vaginal Orgasm?" *Journal of Sex Research* 6:25–28, 1970.

Clarke, D. H. "Erectile Dysfunction in Diabetes." *Clinical Diabetes* 6:103–105, 1988.

Clarkson, T. B., and Alexander, N. J. "Long-Term Vasectomy: Effects on the Occurrence and Extent of Atherosclerosis in Rhesus Monkeys." *Journal of Clinical Investigation* 65(1):15–25, 1980.

Clarren, S. K., and Smith, D. W. "The Fetal Alcohol Syndrome." *New England Journal of Medicine* 298:1063–1067, 1978.

Cochran, S. D., and Mays, V. M. "Sex, Lies, and HIV." *New England Journal of Medicine* 322:774–775, 1990.

Cocores, J.; Dackis, C.; and Gold, M. "Sexual Dysfunction Secondary to Cocaine Abuse." *Journal of Clinical Psychiatry* 47:384–385, 1986.

Cohen, H.; Rosen, R. C.; and Goldstein, L. "Electroencephalographic Laterality Changes During Human Sexual Orgasm." *Archives of Sexual Behavior* 5:189–199, 1976.

Cohen, P. T.; Sande, M. A.; and Volberding, P. A. (eds.). *The AIDS Knowledge Base.* Waltham, MA: The Medical Publishing Group, 1990.

Colditz, G. A., et al. "Menopause and the Risk of Coronary Heart Disease in Women." *New England Journal of Medicine* 316:1105–1110, 1987.

Cole, H. M. "Intrauterine Devices." *Journal of the American Medical Association* 261:2127–1230, 1989.

Coleman, S., and Piotrow, P. "Spermicides: Simplicity and Safety Are Major Assets." *Population Reports.* Series H(5): September 1979.

Coleman, S.; Piotrow, P. T.; and Rinehart, W. "Tobacco: Hazards to Health and Human Reproduction." *Population Reports,* Series L(1): March 1979.

Collier, A. C., et al. "A Pilot Study of Low-Dose Zidovudine in Human Immunodeficiency Virus Infection." *New England Journal of Medicine* 323:1015–1021, 1990.

Collins, E., and Turner, C. "Maternal Effects of Regular Salicylate Ingestion in Pregnancy." *Lancet* 2:335–339, 1975.

Collins, J. A., et al. "Treatment-Independent Pregnancy Among Infertile Couples." *New England Journal of Medicine* 309:1201–1206, 1983.

Collu, R., et al. "Endocrine Effects of Chronic Administration of Psychoactive Drugs to Prepubertal Male Rats. I: Δ^9-Tetrahydrocannabinol." *Life Sciences* 16:533–542, 1975.

Comfort, A. *The Joy of Sex.* New York: Crown, 1972.

Committee on Contraceptive Development, *Developing New Contraceptives: Obstacles and Opportunities,* Washington, DC: National Academy Press, 1990.

Conant, M., et al. "Condoms Prevent Transmission of AIDS-associated Retrovirus." *Journal of the American Medical Association* 255:1706, 1986.

Consensus Conference. "The Impact of Routine HTLV-III Antibody Testing of Blood and Plasma Donors on Public Health." *Journal of the American Medical Association* 256:1778–1783, 1986.

Conway, G. A., et al. "Underreporting of AIDS Cases in South Carolina, 1986 and 1987." *Journal of the American Medical Association* 262:2859–2863, 1989.

Coolfont Report. "A PHS Plan for Prevention and Control of AIDS and the AIDS Virus." *Public Health Reports* 101:341–348, 1986.

Cooper, D. A., et al. "Acute AIDS Retrovirus Infection: Definition of a Clinical Illness Associated with Seroconversion." *Lancet* 1:537–546, 1985.

Copeland, P. M. "Neuroendocrine Aspects of Eating Disorders." In Emmett, S. W. (ed.), *Theory and Treatment of Anorexia Nervosa and Bulimia,* pp. 51–72. New York: Brunner/Mazel, 1985.

Corbitt, G.; Bailey, A. S.; and Williams, G. "HIV Infection in Manchester, 1959." *Lancet* 336:51, 1990.

Corey, L., and Holmes, K. K. "Sexual Transmission of Hepatitis A in Homosexual Men: Incidence and Mechanism." *New England Journal of Medicine* 302:435–438, 1980.

———. "Genital Herpes Simplex Virus Infections: Current Concepts in Diagnosis, Therapy, and Prevention." *Annals of Internal Medicine* 98:973–983, 1983.

Corey, L., et al. "Double-blind Controlled Trial of Topical Acyclovir in Genital Herpes Simplex Virus Infections." *American Journal of Medicine* 73:326–334, 1982.

———. "Genital Herpes Simplex Virus Infections: Clinical Manifestations, Course, and Complications." *Annals of Internal Medicine* 98:958–972, 1983.

Corsan, G. H.; Ghazi, D.; and Kemmann, E. "Home Urinary Luteinizing Hormone Imunoassays: Clinical Applications," *Fertility & Sterility* 53:591–601, 1990.

Costello, John. *Virtue Under Fire.* Boston: Little, Brown, 1985.

Cotten-Huston, A. L., and Wheeler, K. A. "Preorgasmic Group

Treatment: Assertiveness, Marital Adjustment and Sexual Function in Women." *Journal of Sex & Marital Therapy* 9:296–302, 1983.

Council on Scientific Affairs. "Estrogen Replacement in the Menopause." *Journal of the American Medical Association* 249:359–361, 1983.

———. "Mammographic Screening in Asymptomatic Women Aged 40 Years and Older." *Journal of the American Medical Association* 261:2535–2542, 1989.

Couzinet, B., et al. "Termination of Early Pregnancy by the Progesterone Antagonist RU 486." *New England Journal of Medicine* 315:1565–1569, 1986.

Covington, T. R., and McClendon, J. R. *Sex Care: The Complete Guide to Safe and Healthy Sex.* New York: Pocket Books, 1987.

Cramer, D. W., et al. "The Relationship of Tubal Infertility to Barrier Method and Oral Contraceptive Use." *Journal of the American Medical Association* 257:2446–2450, 1987.

———. "The Sexual Aversion Syndrome." *Journal of Sex & Marital Therapy* 11:285–292, 1985.

Crisp, A. H. "The Possible Significance of Some Behavioral Correlates of Weight and Carbohydrate Intake." *Journal of Psychosomatic Research* 11:117–131, 1967.

Croog, S. H., et al. "Sexual Symptoms in Hypertensive Patients." *Archives of Internal Medicine* 148:788–794, 1988.

Crowe, L. C., and George, W. H. "Alcohol and Human Sexuality: Review and Integration." *Psychological Bulletin* 105:374–386, 1989.

Cunningham, F. G., and Gant, N. F. "Prevention of Preeclampsia—A Reality?" *New England Journal of Medicine* 321:606–607, 1989.

Cunningham, F. G.; MacDonald, P. C.; and Gant, N. F. (eds.). *Williams Obstetrics.* East Norwalk, CT: Appleton and Lange, 1989.

Curran, J. W. "AIDS: Two Years Later." *New England Journal of Medicine* 309:609–611, 1983.

Cushman, P., Jr. "Plasma Testosterone in Narcotic Addiction." *American Journal of Medicine* 55:452–458, 1973.

Dalton, H. L., Burris, S. and the Yale AIDS Law Project. *AIDS and the Law.* New Haven, CT: Yale University Press, 1987.

Dalton, K. "Menstruation and Acute Psychiatric Illness." *British Medical Journal,* pp. 148–149, January 17, 1959.

———. "Menstruation and Accidents." *British Medical Journal* 2:1425–1426, 1960.

———. *The Premenstrual Syndrome.* Springfield, IL: Charles C. Thomas, 1964.

———. "The Influence of Mother's Menstruation on Her Child." *Proceedings of the Royal Society of Medicine* 59:1014–1016, 1966.

———. "Menstruation and Examinations." *Lancet* 2:1386–1388, 1968.

———. "Children's Hospital Admissions and Mother's Menstruation." *British Medical Journal* 2:27–28, 1970.

———. "Cyclical Criminal Acts in Premenstrual Syndrome." *Lancet* 2:1070–1071, 1980.

Dan, A. J. "Behavioral Variability and the Menstrual Cycle." Presented at the American Psychological Association Annual Convention, Washington, DC, 1976.

Dan, B. D. "Sex and the Singles' Whirl: The Quantum Dynamics of Hepatitis B." *Journal of the American Medical Association* 256:1344, 1986.

Danforth, D. N. "Cesarean Section." *Journal of the American Medical Association* 253:811–818, 1985.

Darling, C. A.; Davidson, J. K.; and Conway-Welch, C. "Female Ejaculation: Perceived Origins, The Grafenburg Spot/Area, and Sexual Responsiveness." *Archives of Sexual Behavior* 19:29–47, 1990.

David, H. P. "Abortion: A Continuing Debate." *Family Planning Perspectives* 10:313–316, 1978.

Davis, G. L., et al. "Treatment of Chronic Hepatitis C with Recombinant Interferon Alfa." *New England Journal of Medicine* 321:1501–1506, 1989.

Davis, J. E., and Mininberg, D. T. "Prostatitis and Sexual Function." *Medical Aspects of Human Sexuality* 10(8):32–40, 1976.

Davis, K. B. *Factors in the Sex Life of Twenty-Two Hundred Women.* New York: Harper, 1929.

DeBuono, B. A., et al. "Sexual Behavior of College Women in 1975, 1986, and 1989." *New England Journal of Medicine* 322:821–825, 1990.

DeCasper, A. J., and Fifer, W. P. "Of Human Bonding: Newborns Prefer Their Mothers' Voices." *Science* 208:1174–1176, 1980.

DeGowin, E. L., and DeGowin, R. L. *Bedside Diagnostic Examination,* 3rd ed. New York: Macmillan, 1976.

Delaney, J.; Lupton, M. J.; and Toth, E. *The Curse: A Cultural History of Menstruation.* New York: New American Library, 1977.

del Rosario, N. C.; Blair, E.; and Rickman, L. "A Herpetic Hickey." *New England Journal of Medicine* 317:54–55, 1987.

D'Emilio, J., and Freedman, E. B. *Intimate Matters: A History of Sexuality in America.* New York: Harper & Row, 1988.

Dennerstein, L., and Burrows, G. D. "Hormone Replacement Therapy and Sexuality in Women." *Clinics in Endocrinology and Metabolism* 11(3):661–679, November 1982.

Dennerstein, L.; Wood, C.; and Burrows, G. D. "Sexual Response Following Hysterectomy and Oophorectomy." *Obstetrics and Gynecology* 49:92–96, 1977.

Derogatis, L. R., and Kourlesis, S. M. "An Approach to Evaluation of Sexual Problems in the Cancer Patient." *Ca-A Cancer Journal for Clinicians* 31:46–50, 1981.

Diagram Group. *Man's Body: An Owner's Manual.* New York: Paddington Press, 1976.

Diamond, M. "Sexual Identity, Monozygotic Twins Reared in Discordant Sex Roles and a BBC Follow-up." *Archives of Sexual Behavior* 11:181–186, 1982.

Di Bisceglie, A. M., et al. "Recombinant Interferon Alfa Therapy for Chronic Hepatitis C." *New England Journal of Medicine* 321:1506–1510, 1989.

Dick-Read, G. *Childbirth Without Fear.* New York: Harper & Row, 1932.

Diokno, A. C.; Brown, M. B.; and Herzog, A. R. "Sexual Function in the Elderly." *Archives of Internal Medicine* 150:197–200, 1990.

Djerassi, C. *The Politics of Contraception.* New York: Norton, 1979.

Dodson, B. *Liberating Masturbation*. New York: Bodysex Designs, 1974.

Doel, et al. "Persistence of High Risk Sexual Behavior in Homosexual/Bisexual Men: A Multicenter Study." Presented at the Fifth International Conference on AIDS, Montreal, June 1989. (Abstract # M.D.P. 23, p. 714)

Dornblaser, C., and Landry, U. *The Abortion Guide: A Handbook for Women and Men*. New York: Berkley, 1982.

Dorris, Michael. *The Broken Cord*. New York: Harper & Row, 1989.

Douglas, J., et al. "A Double-blind Study of Oral Acyclovir for Suppression of Recurrences of Genital Herpes Simplex Virus Infection." *New England Journal of Medicine* 310:1551–1556, 1984.

Drill, V. A. "Oral Contraceptives: Relation to Mammary Cancer, Benign Breast Lesions, and Cervical Cancer." *Annual Review of Pharmacology* 15:367–385, 1975.

Dunn, H. G., et al. "Maternal Cigarette Smoking During Pregnancy and the Child's Subsequent Development, II: Neurological and Intellectual Maturation to the Age of 6½ Years." *Canadian Journal of Public Health* 68:43–50, 1977.

Dunn, M. E., and Trost, J. E. "Male Multiple Orgasms: A Descriptive Study." *Archives of Sexual Behavior* 18:377–388, 1989.

Eckholm, E., and Tierney, J. "AIDS in Africa: A Killer Rages On." *The New York Times*, pp. 1, 15–16, September 16, 1990.

Eddy, D. M. *Screening for Cancer: Theory, Analysis and Design*. Englewood Cliffs, NJ: Prentice-Hall, 1980.

Eddy, D. M., et al. "The Value of Mammography Screening in Women under Age 50." *Journal of the American Medical Association* 259:1512–1519, 1988.

Edmiston, Susan. "Hers." *The New York Times*, p. Y20, July 22, 1982.

Ehrhardt, A., and Meyer-Bahlburg, H. "Effects of Prenatal Sex Hormones on Gender-Related Behavior." *Science* 211(4488):1312–1318, 1981.

Ehrhardt, A. A.; Evers, K.; and Money, J. "Influence of Androgen and Some Aspects of Sexual Dimorphic Behavior in Women with the Late-Treated Adrenogenital Syndrome." *Johns Hopkins Medical Journal* 123:115–122, 1968.

Ehrhardt, A. A.; Grisanti, G. C.; and Meyer-Bahlburg, H. F. "Prenatal Exposure to Medroxyprogesterone Acetate (MPA) in Girls." *Psychoneuroendocrinology* 2:391–398, 1977.

Ekstrand, M. L., et al. "Risky Sex Relapse, The Next Challenge for AIDS Prevention Programs." Fifth International Conference on AIDS, Montreal, June 4–9 1989. (Abstract # T.D.O.8, p. 699)

Eliasson, R., and Lindholmer, C. "Functions of Male Accessory Genital Organs." In Hafez, E. S. (ed.), *Human Semen and Fertility Regulation in Men*. St. Louis, MO: Mosby, 1976.

Ellis, A. *The American Sexual Tragedy*. New York: Twayne Publishers, 1959.

———. "Treatment of Erectile Dysfunction." In Leiblum, S. R., and Pervin, L. A. (eds.), *Principles and Practice of Sex Therapy*, pp. 235–262. New York: Guilford Press, 1980.

Erlich, K. S., et al. "Acyclovir-Resistant Herpes Simplex Virus Infections in Patients with the Acquired Immunodeficiency Syndrome." *New England Journal of Medicine* 320:293–296, 1989.

Erlik, Y., et al. "Association of Waking Episodes with Menopausal Hot Flushes." *Journal of the American Medical Association* 245:1741–1744, 1981.

Ernst, M. L., and Loth, D. *American Sexual Behavior and the Kinsey Report*. New York: Greystone Press, 1948.

Essex, M., and Kanki, P. "The Origins of the AIDS Virus." *Scientific American*, pp. 64–71, October 1988.

Ettinger, B., et al. "Long-Term Estrogen Replacement Prevents Bone Loss and Fractures." *Annals of Internal Medicine* 102:319–329, 1985.

European Collaborative Study. "Mother-to-Child Transmission of HIV Infection." *Lancet* 2:1039–1043, 1988.

Fabbri, R., Jr. "Hypnosis and Behavioral Therapy: A Coordinated Approach to the Treatment of Sexual Disorders." *American Journal of Clinical Hypnosis* 19:4–8, 1976.

Fahey, B. J., and Henderson, D. K. "Minimizing Risks for Occupational Blood-borne Infections." *Journal of the American Medical Association* 264:1189–1190, 1990.

Faich, G., et al. "Toxic Shock Syndrome and the Vaginal Contraceptive Sponge." *Journal of the American Medical Association* 255:216–218, 1986.

Falicov, C. J. "Sexual Adjustment During First Pregnancy and Post-Partum." *American Journal of Obstetrics and Gynecology* 117:991–1000, 1973.

Fallon, B.; Rosenberg, S.; and Culp, D. "Long-Term Follow-up in Patients with an Inflatable Penile Prothesis." *Journal of Urology* 132:270–271, 1984.

Family Planning Perspectives. "Depo-Provera May Be Linked to Uterine Cancer, Preliminary Data Imply." *Family Planning Perspectives*, 11:47, 1979.

Farkas, G. M., and Rosen, R. C. "Effect of Alcohol on Elicited Male Sexual Response." *Journal of Studies on Alcohol* 37:265–272, 1976.

Farzadegan, H. "Loss of Human Immunodeficiency Virus Type 1 (HIV-1) Antibodies with Evidence of Viral Infection in Asymptomatic Homosexual Men." *Annals of Internal Medicine* 108:785–790, 1988.

Fausto-Sterling, A. *Myths of Gender*. New York: Basic Books, 1985.

Fawaz, K. A., and Matloff, D. S. "Viral Hepatitis in Homosexual Men." *Gastroenterology* 81:537–538, 1981.

Federation of Feminist Women's Health Center. *A New View of a Woman's Body*. New York: Simon & Schuster, 1981.

Feldblum, P. J.; Bernardik, E.; and Rosenberg, M. J. "Spermicide Use and Sexually Transmitted Disease." *Journal of the American Medical Association* 259:2851, 1988.

Fielding, J. E. "Adolescent Pregnancy Revisited." *New England Journal of Medicine* 299:893–896, 1978.

Fiscella, K. "Relationships of Weight Change to Required Size of Vaginal Diaphragm." *Nurse Practitioner* 7(7):21, 25, July–August 1982.

Fischl, M., et al. "Evaluation of Heterosexual Partners, Children, and Household Contacts of Adults with AIDS." *Journal of the American Medical Association* 257:640–644, 1987.

Fischl, M. A., et al. "The Efficacy of Azidothymidine (AZT) in the Treatment of Patients with AIDS and AIDS Related Complex." *New England Journal of Medicine* 317:192–197, 1987a.

Fischl, M. A., et al. "Seroprevalence of HIV Antibody in a Sexually Active Heterosexual Population." Presented at the Fourth International AIDS Conference, Stockholm, June 1988. (Abstract #4067, 1988a)

Fischl, M. A., et al. "A Randomized Controlled Trial of a Reduced Daily Dose of Zidovudine in Patients with Acquired Immunodeficiency Syndrome." *New England Journal of Medicine* 323:1009–1014, 1990.

Fisher, Bernard, et al. "Eight Year Results of a Randomized Clinical Trial Comparing Total Mastectomy and Lumpectomy With or Without Irradiation in the Treatment of Breast Cancer." *New England Journal of Medicine* 320:822–828, 1989.

Fisher, S. *The Female Orgasm.* New York: Basic Books, 1973.

Fisher, W. A.; Branscombe, N. R.; and Lemery, C. R. "The Bigger the Better? Arousal and Attributional Responses to Erotic Stimuli That Depict Different Size Penises." *Journal of Sex Research* 19:337–396, 1983.

Fishman, H. "Clinical Issues in Treatment-Resistant Depression." *The Psychiatric Times* Supplement, October 1990.

FitzGerald, M., and FitzGerald, D. "Deaf People Are Sexual Too!" *SIECUS Report* 6(2):1, 13–15, 1977.

Ford, C. S., and Beach, F. A. *Patterns of Sexual Behavior.* New York: Harper & Brothers, 1951.

Forrest, J. D., and Fordyce, R. R. "U.S. Women's Contraceptive Attitudes and Practice: How Have They Changed in the 1980s?" *Family Planning Perspectives* 20:112–118, 1988.

Forrest, J. D., and Henshaw, S. K. "What U.S. Women Think and Do About Contraception." *Family Planning Perspectives* 15:157–166, 1983.

Forrest, J. D., and Singh, S. "Public-Sector Savings Resulting from Expenditures for Contraceptive Services." *Family Planning Perspectives* 22:6–15, 1990.

Forrest, K. A., et al. "Vaginal Douching as a Risk Factor for Pelvic Inflammatory Disease." *Journal of the National Medical Association* 81:159–165, 1989.

Foster, R. S., Jr., et al. "Breast Self-Exam Practices and Breast-Cancer Stage." *New England Journal of Medicine* 299:265–270, 1978.

Fox, C. A., and Fox, B. "Blood Pressure and Respiratory Patterns During Human Coitus." *Journal of Reproduction and Fertility* 19:405–415, 1969.

Francis, D., and Chin, J. "The Prevention of Acquired Immunodeficiency Syndrome in the United States." *Journal of the American Medical Association* 257:1357–1366, 1987.

Francis, D. P., et al. "Targeting AIDS Prevention and Treatment Toward HIV-1-Infected Persons: The Concept of Early Intervention." *Journal of the American Medical Association* 262:2572–2576, 1989.

Frank, D., et al. "Mastectomy and Sexual Behavior: A Pilot Study." *Sexuality and Disability* 1:16–26, 1978

Frank, R. "The Hormonal Causes of Premenstrual Tension." *Archives of Neurology and Psychiatry* 26:1053–1057, 1931.

Franklin, E. W., and Zeiderman, A. M. "Tubal Ectopic Pregnancy: Etiology and Obstetric and Gynaecologic Sequelae." *American Journal of Obstetrics and Gynecology* 117:220–225, 1973.

Freud, S. *A General Introduction to Psychoanalysis*. Garden City, NY: Garden City Publishing, 1943.

Fried, P. A. "Postnatal Consequences of Maternal Marijuana Use in Humans." *Annals of the New York Academy of Sciences* 562:123–132, 1989.

Friedland, G., et al. "Lack of Transmission of HTLV-III/LAV Infection to Household Contacts of Patients with AIDS or AIDS-Related Complex with Oral Candidiasis." *New England Journal of Medicine* 314:344–349, 1986.

Friedland, G. H. "Early Treatment for HIV." *New England Journal of Medicine* 322:1000–1002, 1990.

Frieze, I. H., et al. *Women and Sex Roles: A Social Psychological Perspective*. New York: Norton, 1978.

Frisch, R. E., and McArthur, J. W. "Menstrual Cycles: Fatness as a Determinant of Minimum Weight for Height Necessary for Their Maintenance or Onset." *Science* 185:949–951, 1974.

Frisch, R. E.; Wyshak, G.; and Vincent, L. "Delayed Menarche and Amenorrhea in Ballet Dancers." *New England Journal of Medicine* 303:17–19, 1980.

Froland, S. S., et al. "HIV-1 Infection in a Norwegian Family Before 1970." *Lancet* 1:1344–1345, 1988.

Fuchs, K., et al. "Vaginismus: The Hypno-Therapeutic Approach." *Journal of Sex Research* 11:39–45, 1975.

Fugger, E. F. "Clinical Status of Human Embryo Cryopreservation in the United States of America," *Fertility & Sterility* 52:986–990, 1989.

Fullilove, M. T., and Fullilove, R. E. "Intersecting Epidemics: Black Teen Crack Use and Sexually Transmitted Disease." *Journal of the American Medical Women's Association* 44:146–153, 1989.

Fullilove, R. E., et al. "Risk of Sexually Transmitted Disease Among Black Adolescent Crack Users in Oakland and San Francisco, Calif." *Journal of the American Medical Association* 263:851–855, 1990.

Furstenberg, F. F., Jr. "The Social Consequences of Teenage Parenthood." *Family Planning Perspectives* 8:148–164, 1976.

Gabuzda, D. H., and Hirsch, M. H. "Neurologic Manifestations of Infection with Human Immunodeficiency Virus," *Annals of Internal Medicine* 107:383–391, 1987.

Gadpaille, W. J. *The Cycles of Sex*. New York: Scribner, 1975.

Gail, M. H., et al. "Projecting Individualized Probabilities of Developing Breast Cancer for White Females Who Are Being Examined Annually." *Journal of the National Cancer Institute* 81:1879–1886, 1989.

Gambrell, R. D., et al. "Changes in Sexual Drives of Patients on Oral Contraceptives." *Journal of Reproductive Medicine* 17(3):165–171, September 1976.

Gambrell, R. D., Jr. "The Menopause: Benefits and Risks of Estrogen–Progestogen Replacement Therapy." *Fertility & Sterility* 37:457–464, 1982.

Gambrell, R. D., Jr., et al. "Reduced Incidence of Endometrial Cancer Among Postmenopausal Women Treated with Progestogens." *Journal of the American Geriatrics Society* 27:389–398, 1979.

Garry, R. F., et al. "Documentation of an AIDS Virus Infection in the United States in 1968." *Journal of the American Medical Association* 260:2085–2087, 1988.

Gay, G. R., et al. "Drug–Sex Practice in the Haight-Ashbury or 'The Sensuous Hippie.' " In Sandler, M., and Gessa, G. L. (eds.), *Sexual Behavior: Pharmacology and Biochemistry,* pp. 63–79. New York: Raven Press, 1975.

Gay, P. *The Bourgeois Experience: Victoria to Freud,* Vol. 1: *Education of the Senese.* New York: Oxford Press, 1983.

George, L. K., and Weiler, S. J. "Sexuality in Middle and Later Life." *Archives of General Psychiatry* 38:919–923, 1981.

Gibbs, C. J., et al. "HIV Immunization and Challenge of HIV Seropositive and Seronegative Chimpanzees." Fifth International Conference on AIDS, Montreal, June 4–9, 1989. (Abstract #C.Th.C.O. 46, p. 541)

Gilbaugh, J. H., Jr., and Fuchs, P. C. "The Gonococcus and the Toilet Seat." *New England Journal of Medicine* 301:91–93, 1979.

Gill, W. B.; Schumacher, G. F. B.; and Bibbo, M. "Pathological Semen and Anatomical Abnormalities of the Genital Tract in Human Male Subjects Exposed to Diethylstilbestrol in Utero." *Journal of Urology* 117:477–480, 1977.

Gillespie, O. *Herpes: What to Do When You Have It.* New York: Grosset & Dunlap, 1982.

Gilman, A. G.; Goodman, L. S.; and Gilman, A. (eds.). *The Pharmacological Basis of Therapeutics.* New York: Macmillan, 1988.

Gilman, L. *The Adoption Resource Book,* New York: Harper & Row, 1987.

Gissmann, L., and Schwarz, E. "Persistence and Expression of Human Papillomavirus DNA in Genital Cancer." In Everd, D., and Clark, S. (eds.), *Papillomaviruses,* pp. 190–197. Chicester, England: Wiley, 1986.

Glaser, J. B.; Strange, T. J.; and Rosati, D. "Heterosexual Human Immunodeficiency Virus Transmission Among the Middle Class." *Archives of Internal Medicine* 149:645–649, 1989.

Glass, R., and Ericsson, R. *Getting Pregnant in the 1980s.* Berkeley: University of California Press, 1982.

Goedert, J. J. "A Prospective Study of Human Immunodeficiency Virus Type 1 Infection and the Development of AIDS in Subjects with Hemophilia." *New England Journal of Medicine* 321:1141–1148, 1989.

Goedert, J., et al. "Three Year Incidence of AIDS in Five Cohorts of HTLV-III Infected Risk Groups." *Science* 231:992–995, 1986.

Goldberg, D. C., et al. "The Grafenberg Spot and Female Ejaculation: A Review of Initial Hypotheses." *Journal of Sex and Marital Therapy* 9:27–37, 1983.

Goldfarb, L. A. "Sexual Abuse Antecedent to Anorexia Nervosa, Bulimia, and Compulsive Overeating: Three Case Reports." *International Journal of Eating Disorders,* 6:675–680, 1987.

Goldman, B. D. "Developmental Influences of Hormones on Neuroendocrine Mechanisms of Sexual Behavior: Comparisons with Other Sexually Dimorphic Behaviors." In Hutchison, J. B. (ed.), *Biological Determinants of Sexual Behavior,* pp. 127–152. New York: Wiley, 1978.

Goldsmith, M. "Sexually Transmitted Diseases May Reverse the 'Revolution.' " *Journal of the American Medical Association* 255:1665–1672, 1986.

Goldsmith, M. F. "Sex in the Age of AIDS Calls for Common Sense and Condom Sense." *Journal of the American Medical Association* 257:2261–2266, 1987.

———. "Sex Tied to Drugs = STD Spread." *Journal of the American Medical Association* 260:2009, 1988.

———. " 'Silent Epidemic' of 'Social Disease' Makes STD Experts Raise Their Voices." *Journal of the American Medical Association* 261:3509–3510, 1989.

Golub, S. "The Effect of Premenstrual Anxiety and Depression on Cognitive Function." *Journal of Personality and Social Psychology* 34:99–104, 1976.

———. (ed.) *Menarche: The Transition from Girl to Woman.* Lexington, MA: Lexington Books, D. C. Heath, 1983.

González, E. R. "Premenstrual Syndrome: An Ancient Woe Deserving of Modern Scrutiny." *Journal of the American Medical Association* 245(14):1393–1396, 1981.

Goodwin, D. W., and Guze, S. B., *Psychiatric Diagnosis.* New York: Oxford University Press, 1989.

Goodwin, F. K. "Which Kids Use Condoms—Or Don't." *Journal of the American Medical Association* 264:1389, 1990.

Gordis, R. "Designated Discussion." In Masters, W. H.; Johnson, V. E.; and Kolodny, R. C. (eds.), *Ethical Issues in Sex Therapy and Research,* pp. 32–38. Boston: Little, Brown, 1977.

Gordon, S. Speech at the Annual Meeting of the American Association for Sex Educators, Counselors, and Therapists, New York, March 13, 1982. (Printed in *Impact 1982/83,* Institute for Family Research and Education, Syracuse University.)

Gostin, L. O. "Public Health Strategies for Confronting AIDS." *Journal of the American Medical Association* 261:1621–1630, 1989.

Gould, J. B., et al. "Socioeconomic Differences in Rates of Cesarean Sections." *New England Journal of Medicine* 321:233–239, 1989.

Gould, S. J. "The Terrifying Normalcy of AIDS." *The New York Times Magazine,* pp. 32–33, April 19, 1987.

Goyert, G. L., et al. "The Physician Factor in Cesarean Birth Rates." *New England Journal of Medicine* 320:706–709, 1989.

Graber, B. (ed.). *Circumvaginal Musculature and Sexual Function.* New York: Karger, 1982.

Graber, B., and Kline-Graber, G. "Clitoral Foreskin Adhesions and Female Sexual Function." *Journal of Sex Research* 15:205–212, 1979.

Grad, R., et al. *The Father Book: Pregnancy and Beyond.* Washington, DC: Acropolis Books, 1981.

Grafenberg, E. "The Role of the Urethra in Female Orgasm." *International Journal of Sexology* 3:145–148, 1950.

Graham, S. "Alcohol and Breast Cancer." *New England Journal of Medicine* 316:1211–1213, 1987.

Graham, S., et al. "Sex Patterns and Herpes Simplex Virus Type 2 in the Epidemiology of Cancer of the Cervix." *American Journal of Epidemiology* 115:729–735, 1982.

Green, A. W. "Sexual Activity and the Postmyocardial Infarction Patient." *American Heart Journal* 89:246–252, 1975.

Green, C. P., and Potteiger, K. "Teenage Pregnancy: A Major Problem for Minors." Washington, DC: Zero Population Growth, 1977.

Greenblatt, R., et al. "Update on the Male and Female Climacteric." *American Geriatrics Society* 27(11):481–490, 1979.

Greenblatt, R. B., and Stoddard, L. D. "The Estrogen–Cancer Controversy." *Journal of the American Geriatrics Society* 26:1–8, 1978.

Greenhouse, S. "A Fierce Battle." *The New York Times Magazine* pp. 23–26, February 12, 1989.

Greer, D. M., et al. "A Technique for Foreskin Reconstruction and Some Preliminary Results." *Journal of Sex Research* 18:324–330, 1982.

Gregg, Charles. "Toxic Shock." In Gregg, C. (ed.), *A Virus of Love and Other Tales of Medical Detection,* pp. 93–112. New York: Charles Scribner's Sons, 1983.

Grimes, D. "Reversible Contraception for the 1980s." *Journal of the American Medical Association* 255:69–75, 1986.

Grimes, D. A., and Cates, W., Jr. "Abortions: Methods and Complications." In Hafez, E. S. (ed.), *Human Reproduction: Conception and Contraception,* pp. 796–813. New York: Harper & Row, 1980.

Grossman, F.; Eichler, L.; and Winickoff, S. *Pregnancy, Birth and Parenthood.* San Francisco: Jossey-Bass, 1980.

———. "The Neuroendocrinology of Puberty." *Hospital Practice,* pp. 51–60, March 1980.

Hadler, S., et al. "Long-Term Immunogenicity and Efficacy of Hepatitis B Vaccine in Homosexual Men." *New England Journal of Medicine* 315:209–214, 1986.

Hahn, R. A., et al. "Prevalence of HIV Infection Among Intravenous Drug Users in the United States." *Journal of the American Medical Association* 261:2677–2684, 1989.

Hahn, S. R., and Paige, K. E. "American Birth Practices: A Critical Review." In Parsons, J. E. (ed.), *The Psychobiology of Sex Differences and Sex Roles,* pp. 145–175. New York: McGraw-Hill/Hemisphere, 1980.

Haimes, A. L., and Katz, J. L., "Sexual and Social Maturity Versus Social Conformity in Restricting Anorectic, Bulimic, and Borderline Women." *International Journal of Eating Disorders* 7:331–341, 1988.

Halbreich, U.; Endicott, J.; and Nee, J. "Premenstrual Depressive Changes." *Archives of General Psychiatry* 40:535–542, 1983.

Halikas, J.; Weller, R.; and Morse, C. "Effects of Regular Marihuana Use on Sexual Performance." *Journal of Psychoactive Drugs* 14:59–70, 1982.

Hallagan, J. B.; Hallagan, L. F.; and Snyder, M. B., "Anabolic–Androgenic Steroid Use by Athletes." *New England Journal of Medicine* 321:1042–1045, 1989.

Haller, J. S., and Haller, R. M. *The Physician and Sexuality in Victorian America.* New York: Norton, 1977.

Hallstrom, T. "Sexuality of Women in Middle Age: The Goteborg Study." *Journal of Biosocial Sciences (Suppl.)* 6:165–175, 1979.

Halmi, K. A. "Anorexia Nervosa." In Kaplan, H. I., and Sadock, B. J. (eds.), *Comprehensive Textbook of Psychiatry,* 4th ed., pp. 1143–1148, Baltimore: Williams & Wilkins, 1985.

Handsfield, H. "Gonorrhea and Uncomplicated Gonococcal Infection." In Holmes, K. K., et al. (eds.), *Sexually Transmitted Diseases,* pp. 205–220. New York: McGraw-Hill, 1984.

Handsfield, H., et al. "Criteria for Selective Screening for *Chlamydia trachomatis* Infection in Women Attending Family Planning Clinics." *Journal of the American Medical Association* 255:1730–1734, 1986.

Handsfield, H. H., et al. "Localized Outbreak of Penicillinase-Producing *Neisseria gonorrhoeae.*" *Journal of the American Medical Association* 261:2357–2361, 1989.

Harbison, R. D., and Mantilla-Plata, B. "Prenatal Toxicity, Maternal Distribution and Placental Transfer of Tetrahydrocannabinol." *Journal of Pharmacology and Experimental Therapy* 180:446–453, 1972.

Harlap, S. "Gender of Infants Conceived on Different Days of the Menstrual Cycle." *New England Journal of Medicine* 300:1445–1448, 1979.

Harlap, S., et al. "A Prospective Study of Spontaneous Fetal Losses After Induced Abortions." *New England Journal of Medicine* 301:677–681, 1979.

Harmon, J. W., et al. "Interference with Testicular Development with Δ^9-tetrahydrocannabinol." *Surgical Forum* 27:350–352, 1976.

Harrison, F. *The Dark Angel: Aspects of Victorian Sexuality.* New York: University Books, 1977.

Harrison, H., and Alexander, E. "*Chlamydia trachomatis* Infections of the Infant." In Holmes, K. K., et al. (eds.), *Sexually Transmitted Diseases,* pp. 270–280. New York: McGraw-Hill, 1984.

Haseltine, W. A., and Wong-Staal, F. "The Molecular Biology of the AIDS Virus." *Scientific American* 259(4):52–62, October, 1988.

Haskett, R. F., et al. "Severe Premenstrual Tension: Delineation of the Syndrome." *Biological Psychiatry* 15:121–139, 1980.

Hass, A. *Teenage Sexuality.* New York: Macmillan, 1979.

Hatcher, R. A., et al. *Contraceptive Technology* 1982–1983. New York: Irvington Publishers, 1982.

Haverkos, H. W., and Edelman, R. "The Epidemiology of Acquired Immunodeficiency Syndrome Among Heterosexuals." *Journal of the American Medical Association* 260:1922–1929, 1988.

Hazard, C. *Feminine Self-Concept in Bulimic Women.* Unpublished manuscript, Texas A&M University, 1985; cited in Johnson and Connors, 1987.

Heiman, J.; LoPiccolo, L.; and LoPiccolo, J. *Becoming Orgasmic: A Sexual Growth Program for Women.* Englewood Cliffs, NJ: Prentice-Hall, 1976.

Heiman, J. R., and LoPiccolo, J. *Becoming Orgasmic: A Sexual and Personal Growth Program for Women,* rev. ed. Englewood Cliffs, NJ: Prentice-Hall, 1988.

Heinonin, O. P., et al. "Cardiovascular Birth Defects and Antenatal Exposure to Female Sex Hormones." *New England Journal of Medicine* 296:67–70, 1977.

Helmrich, S. P., et al. "Risk Factors for Breast Cancer." *American Journal of Epidemiology* 117:35–45, 1983.

Helsinga, K. *Not Made of Stone: The Sexual Problems of Handicapped People.* Springfield, IL: Charles C. Thomas, 1974.

Hembree, W. C.; Zeidenberg, P.; and Nahas, G. G. "Marihuana Effects upon Human Gonadal Function." In Nahas, G. G. (ed.), *Marihuana: Chemistry, Biochemistry and Cellular Effects.* New York: Springer-Verlag, 1976.

Henshaw, S. K., and O'Reilly, K. "Characteristics of Abortion Patients in the United States, 1979 and 1980." *Family Planning Perspectives* 15(1):5–15, 1983.

Henshaw, S. K., and Silverman, J. "The Characteristics and Prior Contraceptive Use of U.S. Abortion Patients." *Family Planning Perspectives* 20:158–168, 1988.

Henshaw, S. K., and Van Vort, J. *Abortion Services in the United States.* New York: Alan Guttmacher Institute, 1988.

Herbst, A. L.; Ulfelder, H.; and Poskanzer, D. C. "Adenocarcinoma of the Vagina: Association of Maternal Stilbestrol Therapy with Tumor Appearance in Young Women." *New England Journal of Medicine* 284:878–881, 1971.

Herman, R. C. "Risk of HIV Exposure to Medical Students and

Health Care Personnel." *Journal of the American Medical Association* 264:1187, 1990.

Herzberg, B. N., et al. "Oral Contraceptives, Depression, and Libido." *British Medical Journal* 3:495–500, 1971.

Herzog, L. W. "Urinary Tract Infections and Circumcision: A Case–Control Study," *American Journal of Diseases of Children* 143:348–350, 1989.

Heywood, W. L., and Curran, J. W. "The Epidemiology of AIDS in the U.S." *Scientific American* 259(4):72–81, 1988.

Hicks, D. R., et al. "Inactivation of HTLV-III-Infected Cultures of Normal Human Lymphocytes by Nonoxynol-9 in Vitro." *Lancet* II:1422–1423, 1985.

Hicks, J. M., and Iosefsohn, M. "Reliability of Home Pregnancy-Test Kits in the Hands of Laypersons." *New England Journal of Medicine* 320:320–321, 1989.

Hill, L. M.; Breckle, R.; and Gehrking, W. C. "The Prenatal Detection of Congenital Malformations by Ultrasonography." *Mayo Clinic Proceedings* 58:805–826, 1983.

Hilts, P. J. "World AIDS Epidemic Draws New Warnings." *The New York Times,* p. D19, December 1, 1989.

Hirsch, M. S., and Schooley, R. T. "Drug Therapy: Treatment of Herpesvirus Infections (second of two parts)." *New England Journal of Medicine* 309:1034–1039, 1983.

Hirsch, M. S., and Schooley, R. T. "Resistance to Antiviral Drugs: The End of Innocence." *New England Journal of Medicine* 320:313–314, 1989.

Hite, S. *The Hite Report.* New York: Dell, 1977.

———. *The Hite Report on Male Sexuality.* New York: Alfred A. Knopf, 1981.

Ho, D. D., et al. "The Acquired Immunodeficiency Syndrome (AIDS) Dementia Complex." *Annals of Internal Medicine* 111:400–410, 1989.

Hogan, D. R. "The Effectiveness of Sex Therapy: A Review of the Literature." In LoPiccolo, J., and LoPiccolo, L. (eds.), *Handbook of Sex Therapy,* pp. 57–84. New York: Plenum Press, 1978.

Hogge, W.; Schonberg, S.; and Golbus, M. "Chorionic Villus Sampling: Experience of the First 1,000 Cases." *American Journal of Obstetrics and Gynecology* 154:1249–1252, 1986.

Holden, C. "Koop Finds Abortion Evidence 'Inconclusive'." *Science* 243:730–731, 1989.

Holmberg, S. D., et al. "Prior Herpes Simplex Virus Type 2 Infection as a Risk Factor for HIV Infection." *Journal of the American Medical Association* 259:1048–1050, 1988.

Holmes, K. K. "Syphilis." In Isselbacher, K. J., et al. (eds.), *Harrison's Principles of Internal Medicine,* 9th ed., pp. 716–726. New York: McGraw-Hill, 1980.

———. "The *Chlamydia* Epidemic." *Journal of American Medical Association* 245:1718–1723, 1981.

Holmes, K. K., and Stamm, W. E. "Chlamydial Genital Infections: A Growing Problem." *Hospital Practice,* pp. 105–117, October 1979.

Holmes, K. K., et al. "Etiology of Nongonococcal Urethritis." *New England Journal of Medicine* 292:1199–1205, 1975.

Holmes, K. K., et al. (eds.), *Sexually Transmitted Diseases,* 2nd ed. New York: McGraw-Hill, 1989.

Hoofnagle, J. H. "Toward Universal Vaccination Against Hepatitis B Virus." *New England Journal of Medicine* 321:1333–1334, 1989a.

———. "Type D (Delta) Hepatitis." *Journal of the American Medical Association* 261:1321–1325, 1989.

Hoover, R. N.; Gray, L. A.; and Fraumeni, J. D., Jr. "Stilbestrol (Diethylstilbestrol) and the Risk of Ovarian Cancer." *Lancet* 2:533–534, 1977.

Hopkins, K. R., and Johnston, W. B. *The Incidence of HIV Infection in the United States,* Indianapolis: Hudson Institute, 1988.

Horsman, A., et al. "Effect of Estrogen Dose on Postmenopausal Bone Loss." *New England Journal of Medicine* 309:1405–1407, 1983.

Howard, L., et al. "Evaluation of Chlamydiazyme for the Detection of Genital Infection Caused by *Chlamydia trachomatis.*" *Journal of Clinical Microbiology* 23:329–332, 1986.

Hunt, M. *Sexual Behavior in the 1970s.* New York: Dell, 1975.

Hutchison, J. B. (ed.). *Biological Determinants of Sexual Behavior.* New York: Wiley, 1978.

Illa, R. V. "Possible Salivary Transmission of AIDS: Case Report." First International Symposium on Oral AIDS, Montreal, June 1–3, 1989, Abstract #3.6.

Imagawa, D. T., et al. "Human Immunodeficiency Virus Type 1 Infection in Homosexual Men Who Remain Seropositive for Prolonged Periods." *New England Journal of Medicine* 320:1458–1462, 1989.

Imperato-McGinley, J., and Peterson, R. "Male Pseudohermaphroditism: The Complexities of Male Phenotypic Development." *American Journal of Medicine* 61:251–272, 1976.

Imperato-McGinley, J., et al. "Androgens and the Evolution of Male-Gender Identity Among Male Pseudohermaphrodites with 5α-Reductase Deficiency." *New England Journal of Medicine* 300(22): 1233–1237, 1979.

Institute of Medicine/National Academy of Sciences. *Confronting AIDS: Directions for Public Health, Health Care, and Research.* Washington, DC: National Academy Press, 1986.

———. *Confronting AIDS: Update 1988.* Washington, DC: National Academy Press, 1988.

Jacobs, L. S., et al. "Primary Microsurgery for Postinflammatory Tubal Infertility." *Fertility & Sterility* 50:855–859, 1988.

Jaffe, J. H. "Drug Addiction and Drug Abuse." In Gilman, A. S.; Goodman, L. S.; and Gilman, A. (eds.), *The Pharmacological Basis of Therapeutics,* pp. 535–583. New York: Macmillan, 1980.

James, Robin. "HIV Testing and Counseling: Crisis and Coping for Adolescents and Adults." In Anderson, G., (ed.), *Courage to Care,* pp. 271–283. Washington, DC: Child Welfare League of America, 1990.

James, W. H. "Coital Rates and the Pill." *Nature* 234:555–556, 1971.

Jamison, P. L., and Gebhard, P. G., "Penis Size Increase Between Flaccid and Erect States: An Analysis of the Kinsey Data." *Journal of Sex Research* 24:177–183, 1988.

Janerich, D. T.; Piper, J. M.; and Glebatis, D. M. "Oral Contraceptives and Congenital Limb-Reduction Defects." *New England Journal of Medicine* 291:697–700, 1974.

Jani, N. N., and Wise, T. N. "Antidepressants and Inhibited Female Orgasm: A Literature Review." *Journal of Sex & Marital Therapy* 14:279–284, 1988.

Jason, J. M., et al. "HTLV-III/LAV Antibody and Immune Status of Household Contacts and Sexual Partners of Persons with Hemophilia." *Journal of the American Medical Association* 255:212–215, 1986.

Jelliffe, D. B. "Community and Sociopolitical Considerations of Breast-Feeding." In Ciba Foundation Symposium 45 (new series), *Breast-Feeding and the Mother,* pp. 231–245. New York: Elsevier/North-Holland, 1976.

Jensen, P., et al. "Sexual Dysfunction in Male and Female Patients with Epilepsy: A Study of 86 Outpatients." *Archives of Sexual Behavior* 19:1–14, 1990.

Jensen, S. "Sexual Dysfunction in Insulin-Treated Diabetics." *Archives of Sexual Behavior* 15:271–283, 1986.

Jick, H., et al. "Myocardial Infarction and Other Vascular Diseases in Young Women: Role of Estrogens and Other Factors." *Journal of the American Medical Association* 240:2548–2552, 1978.

———. "Vaginal Spermicides and Gonorrhea." *Journal of the American Medical Association* 248:1619–1621, 1982.

Johnson, C., and Connors, M. E. *The Etiology and Treatment of Bulimia Nervosa.* New York: Basic Books, 1987.

Johnson, J. H. "Weighing the Evidence on the Pill and Breast Cancer." *Family Planning Perspectives* 21:89–92, 1989.

Johnson, R. E., et al. "A Seroepidemiologic Survey of the Prevalence of Herpes Simplex Virus Type 2 Infection in the United States." *New England Journal of Medicine* 321:7–12, 1989.

Johnson, V. E., and Masters, W. H. "Intravaginal Contraceptive Study, Phase I: Anatomy." *Western Journal of Surgery, Obstetrics, and Gynecology* 70:202–207, 1962.

Jonas, H. S., and Dooley, S. L. "The Search for a Lower Cesarean Rate Goes On." *Journal of the American Medical Association* 262:1512–1513, 1989.

Jones, E. F., and Forrest, J. D. "Contraceptive Failure in the United States: Revised Estimates from the 1982 National Survey of Family Growth." *Family Planning Perspectives* 21:103–109, 1989.

Jones, H. W., Jr., and Schrader, C. "And Just What Is A Pre-Embryo?" *Fertility & Sterility* 52:189–191, 1989.

Jones, K. L., et al. "Pattern of Malformations in the Children of Women Treated with Carbamazepine During Pregnancy." *New England Journal of Medicine* 320:1661–1666, 1989.

Jones, R. B., et al. "Recovery of *Chlamydia trachomatis* from the Endometrium of Women at Risk for Chlamydial Infection." *American Journal of Obstetrics and Gynecology* 155:35–39, 1986.

Jones, R. T. "Human Effects." In Petersen, R. C. (ed.), *Marihuana Research Findings: 1976,* pp. 128–178. NIDA Dept. of HEW (ADM) 78-501. Washington, DC: U.S. Government Printing Office, 1976.

Joseph, D.; Bruskewitz, R.; and Benson, R. "Long-Term Evaluation of the Inflatable Penile Prosthesis." *Journal of Urology* 131:670–673, 1984.

Joseph, J. G., et al. "Magnitude and Determinants of Behavioral Risk Reduction: Longitudinal Analysis of a Cohort at Risk for AIDS." *Psychological Health* 1:73–96, 1987.

Jost, A. "Problems of Fetal Endocrinology: The Gonadal and Hypophyseal Hormones." *Recent Progress in Hormone Research* 8:379–418, 1953.

———. "A New Look at Mechanisms Controlling Sex Differentiation in Mammals." *Johns Hopkins Medical Journal* 130:38–53, 1972.

Judson, F. "Fear of AIDS and Gonorrhea Rates in Homosexual Men." *Lancet* II:159–160, 1983.

Kaeser, L. "Reconsidering Age Limits on Pill Use." *Family Planning Perspectives* 21:273–274, 1989.

Kaiser, F. E., et al. "Impotence and Aging: Clinical and Hormonal Factors." *Journal of the American Geriatric Society* 36:511–519, 1988.

Kalter, H., and Warkany, J. "Congenital Malformations." *New England Journal of Medicine* 308:491–497, 1983.

Kanki, P., et al. "New Human T-Lymphotropic Retrovirus Related to Simian T-Lymphotropic Virus Type III (STLV III)." *Science* 232:238–243, 1986.

Kant, S. "The Transmission of HTLV-III." *Journal of the American Medical Association* 253:1901, 1985.

Kaplan, H. *The Evaluation of Sexual Disorders.* New York: Brunner/Mazel, 1983.

Kaplan, H. S. *The New Sex Therapy.* New York: Brunner/Mazel, 1974.

———. *The Illustrated Manual of Sex Therapy.* New York: Quadrangle/New York Times, 1975.

———. *Disorders of Sexual Desire.* New York: Brunner/Mazel, 1979.

Kaplan, Helen S. *How to Overcome Premature Ejaculation.* New York: Brunner/Mazel, 1989.

———. "Homosexuality in History." In Marmor, J. (ed.), *Homosexual Behavior,* pp. 75–99. New York: Basic Books, 1980.

Karmel, M. *Thank You, Dr. Lamaze.* Philadelphia: Lippincott, 1959.

Kasan, P. N., and Andrews, J. "Oral Contraception and Congenital Anomalies." *British Journal of Obstetrics and Gynaecology* 87:548–551, 1980.

Kassel, V. "Sex in Nursing Homes." *Medical Aspects of Human Sexuality* 10(3):129–131, March 1976.

Katchadourian, H. *The Biology of Adolescence.* San Francisco: W. H. Freeman, 1977.

Kaufman, D. W., et al. "Decreased Risk of Endometrial Cancer Among Oral Contraceptive Users." *New England Journal of Medicine* 303:1045–1047, 1980.

Kay, C. R., and Hannaford, P. C. "Breast Cancer and the Pill." *British Journal of Cancer* 58:675–680, 1988.

Kegel, A. "Sexual Functions of the Pubococcygeus Muscle." *Western Journal of Surgery, Obstetrics, and Gynecology* 60:521–524, 1952.

Kelley, D. B., and Pfaff, D. W. "Generalizations from Comparative Studies on Neuroanatomical and Endocrine Mechanisms of Sexual Behavior." In Hutchison, J. B. (ed.), *Biolo... terminants of Sexual Behavior,* pp. 225–254. New ... 1978.

Kelsey, J. L., et al. "Exogenous Estrogens and O... the Epidemiology of Breast Cancer." *Journal ... Cancer Institute* 67:327–333, 1981.

Kemeny, M. E., et al. "Psychological and Im... tors of Genital Herpes Recurrence." *Psyc...* 51:195–208, 1989.

Kempton, W. "Sex Education for the Mentally Handicapped." *Sex and Disability* 1(2):137–146, 1978.

Kennard, E. A. D., et al. "A Program for Matched, Anonymous Oocyte Donation." *Fertility & Sterility* 51:655–660, 1989.

Kennedy, L. "Human Papillomavirus: A Study of Male Sexual Partners." *Medical Journal of Australia* 149:309–311, 1988.

Kennedy, S., and Over, R. "Psychophysiological Assessment of Male Sexual Arousal Following Spinal Cord Injury." *Archives of Sexual Behavior* 19:15–28, 1990.

Kern, S. "Freud and the Discovery of Child Sexuality." *History of Childhood Quarterly* 1:117–141, 1973.

Kessler, I. I. "On the Etiology and Prevention of Cervical Cancer: A Status Report." *Obstetrics and Gynecological Survey* 34:790–794, 1979.

Keye, W. R. "Update: Premenstrual Syndrome." *Endocrine & Fertility Forum* 6(4):1–3, Fall 1983.

Kilmann, P. R. "The Treatment of Primary and Secondary Orgasmic Dysfunction: A Methodological Review of the Literature Since 1970." *Journal of Sex & Marital Therapy* 4:155–176, 1978.

Kilmann, P. R., and Auerbach, R. "Treatment of Premature Ejaculation and Psychogenic Impotence: A Critical Review of the Literature." *Archives of Sexual Behavior* 8:81–100, 1979.

King, S. "Not Everyone Agrees with New Mammographic Screening Guidelines Designed to End Confusion." *Journal of the American Medical Association* 262:1154–1155, 1989.

Kingsley, L.A., et al. "Sexual Transmission Efficiency of Hepatitis B Virus and Human Immunodeficiency Virus Among Homosexual Men." *Journal of the American Medical Association* 264:230–234, 1990.

Kinsey, A. C., et al. *Sexual Behavior in the Human Female*. Philadelphia: Saunders, 1953.

Kinsey, A. C.; Pomeroy, W. B.; and Martin, C. E. *Sexual Behavior in the Human Male*. Philadelphia: Saunders, 1948.

Kish, L. S., et al. "An Ancient Method and a Modern Scourge: The Condom as a Barrier Against Herpes." *Journal of the American Academy of Dermatology* 9:769–770, 1983.

Klaus, M. H., et al. "Maternal Attachment: Importance of the First Post-Partum Days." *New England Journal of Medicine* 286:460–463, 1972.

Kline-Graber, G., and Graber, B. "Diagnosis and Treatment Procedures of Pubococcygeal Deficiencies in Women." In LoPiccolo, J., and LoPiccolo, L. (eds.), *Handbook of Sex Therapy*, pp. 227–239. New York: Plenum Press, 1978.

Klitsch, M. "FDA Approval Ends Cervical Cap's Marathon." *Family Planning Perspectives* 20:137–138, 1988.

Klonoff, H. "Marijuana and Driving in Real-Life Situations." *Science* 186:317–324, 1974.

Klonoff-Cohen, H. S., et al. "An Epidemiologic Study of Contraception and Preeclampsia." *Journal of the American Medical Association* 262:3143–3147, 1989.

Koeske, R. "Lifting the Curse of Menstruation: Toward a Feminist Perspective on the Menstrual Cycle." *Women and Health* 8:1–16, 1983.

Koeske, R. K. "Premenstrual Emotionality: Is Biology Destiny?" *Women and Health* 1:11–14, 1976.

[illegible]ke, R. K., and Koeske, G. F. "An Attributional Approach to [illegible]ods and the Menstrual Cycle." *Journal of Personality and [illegible] Psychology* 31:474–478, 1975.

Kolata, G. "AIDS Is Spreading in Teen-Agers, A New Trend Alarming to Experts." *The New York Times*, Section 1, pp. 1 & 30, October 8, 1989.

———. "NIH Panel Urges Fewer Cesarean Births." *Science* 210:176–177, 1980a.

Kolodny, N. *When Food's a Foe*. Boston: Little, Brown, 1987.

Kolodny, R., and Kolodny, N. "Current Trends in Sexual Behavior and the Impact of AIDS Anxiety." Presented at the Third Annual Symposium of the Behavioral Medicine Institute, New York, April 25, 1987.

Kolodny, R. C. "Sexual Dysfunction in Diabetic Females." *Diabetes* 20(8):557–559, 1971.

———. "Effects of Alpha-Methyldopa on Male Sexual Function." *Sexuality and Disability* 1:223–228, 1978.

———. "Ethical Issues in the Prevention of Sexual Problems." In Qualls, C. B.; Wincze, J. P.; and Barlow, D. H. (eds.), *The Prevention of Sexual Disorders*, pp. 183–196. New York: Plenum Press, 1978a.

———. "Effects of Marihuana on Sexual Behavior and Function." Paper presented at the Midwestern Conference on Drug Use, St. Louis, February 16, 1981.

———. "Drugs and Sex: "New Findings and Old Problems." Presented at the Second Annual Symposium on Psychopharmacology and Human Behavior, Cambridge, MA, September 10, 1987.

———. "Evaluating Sex Therapy: Process and Outcome at the Masters & Johnson Institute." *Journal of Sex Research* 17:301–318, 1981a.

———. Unpublished observations, 1981b.

———. "Sexual Issues in Mid-Adulthood." Presented at the Las Vegas Psychiatric Symposium, Las Vegas, NV, January 23, 1983.

———. Unpublished research, 1983a.

———. "The Clinical Management of Sexual Problems in Substance Abusers." In Bratter, T. E., and Forrest, G. (eds.), *Current Management of Alcoholism and Substance Abuse*. New York: Free Press, 1985.

———. "Anabolic Steroids and Sexual Assault." Presented at the First Annual Florida Sex Therapy Association Training Program, March 16, 1990, Miami.

Kolodny, R. C., and Bauman, J. E. "Female Sexual Activity at Ovulation" (letter). *New England Journal of Medicine* 300:626, 1979.

Kolodny, R. C., and Kolodny, N. J. "Dynamics of the HIV/AIDS Epidemic as a Reflection of Sexual Behavior Patterns in the Early 1990s." Presented at the Behavioral Medicine Institute Symposium on Sexuality, New York, June 1, 1990.

Kolodny, R. C., et al. "Depression of Plasma Testosterone Levels After Chronic Intensive Marijuana Use." *New England Journal of Medicine* 290:872–874, 1974.

———. "Sexual Dysfunction in Diabetic Men." *Diabetes* 23:306–309, 1974a.

———. "Depression of Plasma Testosterone with Acute Marihuana Administration." In Braude, M. C., and Szara, S. (eds.), *The Pharmacology of Marihuana*, pp. 217–225. New York: Raven Press, 1976.

———. "Endocrine Status of Men During Chronic Marihuana Use." Paper presented at Washington University Medical Center Research Seminar. St. Louis, April 1979.

———. "Endocrine Effects of Chronic Marihuana Use by Women." Paper presented at the University of Rochester Medical School Endocrine Grand Rounds, Rochester, NY, February 1980.

Kolodny, R. C.; Masters, W. H.; and Johnson, V. E. *Textbook of Sexual Medicine*. Boston: Little, Brown, 1979.

Kols, A., et al. "Oral Contraceptives in the 1980s." *Population Reports,* Series A, No. 6, May–June, 1982.

Komaroff, A. L., et al. "Chlamydial Pharyngitis." *Annals of Internal Medicine* 111:537–538, 1989.

Konner, Melvin. "The Gender Option." *The Sciences* 27(6):2–4, November–December 1987.

Koonin, L. M., et al. "Maternal Mortality Surveillance, United States, 1980–1985," *Morbidity and Mortality Weekly Report* 37 (Suppl. No. SS-5), pp. 19–29, December 1988.

Koop, C. E. "The U.S. Surgeon General on the Health Effects of Abortion." *Population and Development Review* 15:172–175, 1989.

Koralnik, I. J., et al. "A Controlled Study of Early Neurologic Abnormalities in Men with Asymptomatic Human Immunodeficiency Virus Infection." *New England Journal of Medicine* 323:864–870, 1990.

Kramer, Larry. "A 'Manhattan Project' for AIDS." *The New York Times,* p. A15, July 16, 1990.

Krane, R. J., and Siroky, M. B. "Neurophysiology of Erection." *Urologic Clinics of North America* 8:91–102, 1981.

Kuo, G., et al. "An Assay for Circulating Antibodies to a Major Etiologic Virus of Non-A, Non-B Hepatitis." *Science* 244:362–364, 1989.

Kurinij, N.; Shiono, P.; and Rhodes, G. "Breast-Feeding Incidence and Duration in Black and White Women." *Pediatrics* 81:365–371, 1988.

Ladas, A. K.; Whipple, B.; and Perry, J. D. *The G Spot and Other Recent Discoveries About Human Sexuality.* New York: Holt, Rinehart & Winston, 1982.

Lafferty, W. E., et al. "Recurrences After Oral and Genital Herpes Simplex Virus Infection." *New England Journal of Medicine* 316:1444–1449, 1987.

Lake, A. "Childbirth in America." *McCall's,* p. 128, January 1976.

Lamaze, F. *Painless Childbirth*. Chicago: Regnery, 1970.

Lamb, D. R. "Anabolic Steroids in Athletes: How Well Do They Work and How Dangerous Are They?" *American Journal of Sports Medicine* 12:31–38, 1984.

Lamb, E. J., and Leurgans, S. "Does Adoption Affect Subsequent Fertility?" *American Journal of Obstetrics and Gynecology* 134:138–144, 1979.

Lambert, B. "10 Years Later, Hepatitis Study Still Yields Critical Data on AIDS." *The New York Times,* p. C3, July 17, 1990.

Lamberti, J. "Sexual Adjustment After Radiation Therapy for Cervical Carcinoma." *Medical Aspects of Human Sexuality* 13(3):87–88, 1979.

Lammer, E., et al. "Retinoic Acid Embryopathy." *New England Journal of Medicine* 313:837–841, 1985.

Lane, H. C., et al. "Abnormalities of B-Cell Activation and Immunoregulation in Patients with the Acquired Immunodeficiency Syndrome." *New England Journal of Medicine* 309:453–458, 1983.

Langenberg, A., et al. "Development of Clinically Recognizable Genital Lesions Among Women Previously Identified as Having 'Asymptomatic' Herpes Simplex Virus Type 2 Infection." *Annals of Internal Medicine* 110:882–887, 1989.

Langone, John. *AIDS: The Facts.* Boston: Little, Brown, 1988.

Langston, Deborah. *Living with Herpes*. Garden City, NY: Doubleday, 1983.

Larder, B. A.; Draby, G.; and Richman, D. D. "HIV with Reduced Sensitivity to Zidovudine (AZT) Isolated During Prolonged Therapy." *Science* 243:1731–1734, 1989.

Larsen, B., and Galask, R. P. "Vaginal Microbial Flora: Composition and Influences of Host Physiology." *Annals of Internal Medicine* 96 (Part 2):926–930, 1982.

Larson, T., and Bryson, Y. "Fomites and Herpes Simplex Virus: The Toilet Seat Revisited (abstract)." *Pediatric Research* 16:244, 1982.

Lattimer, J. K., et al. "The Optimum Time to Operate for Cryptorchidism." *Pediatrics* 53:96–99, 1974.

Laumann, E. O., et al. "Monitoring the AIDS Epidemic in the United States: A Network Approach." *Science* 244:1186–1189, 1989.

LaVecchia, C., et al. "General Epidemiology of Breast Cancer in Northern Italy." *International Journal of Epidemiology* 16:347–355, 1987.

Lawson, Carol. "Surrogate Mothers Grow in Numbers Despite Questions." *The New York Times,* pp. C1 & C18, October 1, 1986.

Layde, P. M. "Smoking and Cervical Cancer: Cause or Coincidence?" *Journal of the American Medical Association* 261:1631–1633, 1989.

Lazarus, A. A. "Psychological Treatment of Dyspareunia." In Leiblum, S. R., and Pervin, L. A. (eds.), *Principles and Practice of Sex Therapy,* pp. 147–166. New York: Guilford Press, 1980.

Leary, W. E. "Sharp Rise in Rare Sex-Related Diseases." *The New York Times,* p. B6, July 14, 1988.

Leary, W. E. "Why Fewer Blacks Choose to Breast-Feed Than Do Whites." *The New York Times,* p. B7, April 7, 1988a.

LeBolt, S. A.; Grimes, D. A.; and Cates, W., Jr. "Mortality from Abortion and Childbirth." *Journal of the American Medical Association* 248:188–191, 1982.

Lee, N. C., et al. "Type of Intrauterine Contraceptive Device and the Risk of Pelvic Inflammatory Disease." *Obstetrics and Gynecology* 62:1–7, 1983.

Lee, N. C.; Rubin, G. L.; and Borucki, R. "The Intrauterine Device and Pelvic Inflammatory Disease Revisited: New Results from the Women's Health Study." *Obstetrics and Gynecology* 72:1–6, 1988.

Lee, P. A. "The Relationship of Concentrations of Serum Hormones to Pubertal Gynecomastia." *Journal of Pediatrics* 86:212–215, 1975.

Leiblum, S., and Rosen, R. (eds.). *Sexual Desire Disorders.* New York: Guilford Press, 1988.

———. *Principles and Practice of Sex Therapy: Update for the 1990s,* 2nd ed. New York: Guilford Press, 1989.

Leiblum, S., et al. "Vaginal Atrophy in the Postmenopausal Woman: The Importance of Sexual Activity and Hormones."

Journal of the American Medical Association 249:2195–2198, 1983.

Leiblum, S. R., and Pervin, L. A. *Principles and Practice of Sex Therapy.* New York: Guilford Press, 1980.

Lenton, E. A.; Weston, G. A.; and Cooke, I. D. "Problems in Using Basal Body Temperature Recordings in an Infertility Clinic." *British Medical Journal* 1:803–805, 1977.

Levin, A. A., et al. "Association of Induced Abortion with Subsequent Pregnancy Loss." *Journal of the American Medical Association* 243:2495–2499, 1980.

Levin, R. J., and Levin, A. "Sexual Pleasure: The Surprising Preferences of 100,000 Women." *Redbook,* pp. 51–58, September 1975.

Levine, A., et al. "Immunization with Inactivated, Envelope-Depleted HIV Immunogen in HIV Infected Men with ARC." Fifth International Conference on AIDS, Montreal, June 4–9, 1989. (Abstract #Th.B.O.44, p. 219)

Levine, S. B. "Marital Sexual Dysfunction: Introduction Concepts." *Annals of Internal Medicine* 84:448–453, 1976.

Levy, J. A. "Human Immunodeficiency Viruses and the Pathogenesis of AIDS." *Journal of the American Medical Association* 261:2997–3006, 1989.

Liang, A. P., et al. "Risk of Breast, Uterine Corpus and Ovarian Cancer in Women Receiving Medroxyprogesterone Injections." *Journal of the American Medical Association* 249:2909–2912, 1983.

Lief, H. I. "Inhibited Sexual Desire." *Medical Aspects of Human Sexuality* 11(7):94–95, 1977.

Lilius, H. G.; Valtonen, E. J.; and Wikström, J. "Sexual Problems in Patients Suffering from Multiple Sclerosis." *Journal of Chronic Diseases* 29:643–647, 1976.

Lindholm, F. B., et al. "Pituitary-Testicular Function in Patients with Chronic Alcoholism." *European Journal of Clinical Investigation* 8:269–272, 1978.

Linn, L. S., et al. "Recent Sexual Behaviors Among Homosexual Men Seeking Primary Care." *Archives of Internal Medicine* 149:2685–2690, 1989.

Lipkin, M., Jr., and Lamb, G. S. "The Couvade Syndrome: An Epidemiologic Study." *Annals of Internal Medicine* 96:509–511, 1982.

Lipnick, R. J., et al. "Oral Contraceptives and Breast Cancer." *Journal of the American Medical Association* 255:58–61, 1986.

Lipsett, M. B. "Estrogen Use and Cancer Risk." *Journal of the American Medical Association* 237:1112–1115, 1977.

Liskin, L., and Blackburn, R. "AIDS: A Public Health Crisis." *Population Reports,* Ser. L. no. 6, July–August 1986.

Liskin, L.; Pile, J. M.; and Quillin, W. F. "Vasectomy: Safe and Simple." *Population Reports,* Series D, no. 4, November–December 1983.

Lo, B., et al. "Voluntary Screening for Human Immunodeficiency Virus (HIV) Infection." *Annals of Internal Medicine* 110:727–733, 1989.

Loche, M., and Mach, B. "Identification of HIV-infected Seronegative Individuals by a Direct Diagnostic Test Based on Hybridization to Amplified Viral DNA." *Lancet* 2:418–421, 1988.

Long Laws, J. *The Second X.* New York: Elsevier, 1979.

LoPiccolo, J. "Direct Treatment of Sexual Dysfunction in the Couple." In Money, J., and Musaph, H. (eds.), *Handbook of Sexology,* pp. 1227–1244. Amsterdam: Elsevier/North Holland, 1977.

LoPiccolo, J., and Heiman, J. "The Role of Cultural Values in the Prevention and Treatment of Sexual Problems." In Qualls, C. B.; Wincze, J. P.; and Barlow, D. H. (eds.), *The Prevention of Sexual Disorders,* pp. 43–71. New York: Plenum Press, 1978.

LoPiccolo, J., and Lobitz, W. C. "The Role of Masturbation in the Treatment of Orgasmic Dysfunction." *Archives of Sexual Behavior* 2:163–171, 1972.

LoPiccolo, J., and LoPiccolo, L. (eds.), *Handbook of Sex Therapy.* New York: Plenum Press, 1978.

LoPiccolo, J., et al. "Effectiveness of Single Therapists Versus Cotherapy Teams in Sex Therapy." *Journal of Consulting & Clinical Psychology* 53:287–294, 1985.

LoPiccolo, L. "Low Sexual Desire." In Leiblum, S. R., and Pervin, L. A. (eds.), *Principles and Practice of Sex Therapy,* pp. 29–64. New York: Guilford Press, 1980.

Louik, C., et al. "Maternal Exposure to Spermicides in Relation to Certain Birth Defects." *New England Journal of Medicine* 317:474–476, 1987.

Lui, K.-J.; Darrow, W. W.; and Rutherford, G. W., III. "A Model-Based Estimate of the Mean Incubation Period for AIDS in Homosexual Men." *Science* 240:1333–1335, 1988.

Lund, D. S. "Survey: Many Women Found Breast Cancer 'Accidentally'." *American Medical News,* p. 35, June 17, 1988.

Lundberg, P. O. "Sexual Dysfunction in Patients with Neurological Disorders." In Gemme, R., and Wheeler, C. C. (eds.), *Progress in Sexology,* pp. 129–139. New York: Plenum Press, 1977.

Lundberg, P. O., and Wide, L. "Sexual Function in Males with Pituitary Tumors." *Fertility and Sterility* 29:175–179, 1978.

Lycke, E., et al. "The Risk of Transmission of Genital *Chlamydia trachomatis* Infection Is Less Than That of Genital *Neisseria gonorrhea* Infection." *Sexually Transmitted Diseases* 7:6, 1980.

McBride, G. "Putting a Better Cap on the Cervix." *Journal of the American Medical Association* 243(16):1617–1618, 1980.

MacDonald, K. L., et al. "Performance Characteristics of Serologic Tests for Human Immunodeficiency Virus Type 1 (HIV-1) Among Minnesota Blood Donors." *Annals of Internal Medicine* 110:617–621, 1989.

MacDonald, N. E., et al. "High-Risk STD/HIV Behavior Among College Students." *Journal of the American Medical Association* 263:3155–3159, 1990.

Macdonald, P. T., et al. "Heavy Cocaine Use and Sexual Behavior." *Journal of Drug Issues* 18:437–455, 1988.

McDougall, J. K., et al. "Cervical Carcinoma: Detection of Herpes Simplex Virus RNA in Cells Undergoing Neoplastic Change." *International Journal of Cancer* 25:1–8, 1980.

McEwen, B. "Neural Gonadal Steroid Actions." *Science* 211(4488):1303–1311, 1981.

McKinley, H., and Drew, B. "The Nursing Home: Death of Sexual Expression." *Health and Social Work* 2(3):180–187, August 1977.

McKusick, L., and Hoff, C. C. "Relationship Betwen HIV Awareness, Partner Selection Criteria, and Early Relationship Formation in Two Groups of San Francisco Bar Patrons."

Presented at the Fifth International Conference on AIDS, Montreal, June 1989. (Abstract No. W.D.O. 2, p. 704)

McLane, M.; Krop, H.; and Mehta, J. "Psychosexual Adjustment and Counseling After Myocardial Infarction." *Annals of Internal Medicine* 92:514–519, 1980.

MacLusky, N., and Naftolin, F. "Sexual Differentiation of the Central Nervous System." *Science* 211(4488):1294–1303, 1981.

Madore, C., et al. "A Study on the Effects of Induced Abortion on Subsequent Pregnancy Outcome." *American Journal of Obstetrics and Gynecology* 139(5):516–521, 1981.

Maine, D. "Depo: The Debate Continues." *Family Planning Perspectives* 10:342, 1978.

Malatesta, V. J. "Alcohol Effects on the Orgasmic-Ejaculatory Response in Human Males." *Journal of Sex Research* 15:101–107, 1979.

Malatesta, V. J., et al. "Acute Alcohol Intoxication and Female Orgasmic Response." *Journal of Sex Research* 18:1–17, 1982.

Malinowski, B. *The Sexual Life of Savages*. New York: Harcourt, Brace & World, 1929.

Mann, J. I., and Inman, W. H. "Oral Contraceptives and Death from Myocardial Infarction." *British Medical Journal* 2:245–248, 1975.

Mann, D., et al. "Myocardial Infarction and Angina Pectoris in Young Women." *Journal of Epidemiology and Community Health* 41:215–219, 1987.

Manno, J. E., et al. "Motor and Mental Performance with Marijuana: Relationship to Administered Dose of Δ^9-tetrahydrocannabinol and Its Interaction with Alcohol." In Miller, L. L. (ed.), *Marihuana: Effects on Human Behavior,* pp. 45–72. New York: Academic Press, 1974.

March, C. "Update: Home Tests for Ovulation and Pregnancy." *Endocrine & Fertility Forum* 8(4):2–6, 1985.

Marchbanks, P. A., et al. "Risk Factors for Ectopic Pregnancy." *Journal of the American Medical Association* 259:1823–1827, 1988.

Marcus, S. *The Other Victorians*. New York: Bantam Books, 1967.

Marmor, J. "Clinical Aspects of Male Homosexuality." In Marmor, J. (ed.), *Homosexual Behavior,* pp. 267–279. New York: Basic Books, 1980a.

Marshall, W. A. "Growth and Sexual Maturation in Normal Puberty." *Clinics in Endocrinology and Metabolism* 4:3–25, 1975.

———. *Human Growth and Its Disorders*. New York: Academic Press, 1977.

Marshall, W. A., and Tanner, J. M. "Variation in the Pattern of Pubertal Changes in Girls." *Archives of Disease in Childhood* 44:291–303, 1969.

———. "Variation in the Pattern of Pubertal Changes in Boys." *Archives of Disease in Childhood* 45:13–23, 1970.

Martin, C. E. "Sexual Activity in the Aging Male." In Money, J., and Musaph, H. (eds.), *Handbook of Sexology,* pp. 813–824. New York: Elsevier/North Holland Biomedical Press, 1977.

Martin, J. L. "Psychological, Social and Serological Correlates of Sexual Behavior Changes Among Gay Men." Paper presented at the International Academy of Sex Research 12th Annual Meeting, Amsterdam, the Netherlands, September 19, 1986.

Martinez, G. A., and Dodd, D. A. "Milk Feeding Patterns in the U.S. During the First 12 Months of Life." *Pediatrics* 68:863–868, 1982.

Marx, J. L. "Circumcision May Protect Against the AIDS Virus." *Science* 245:470–471, 1989.

———. "How DNA Viruses May Cause Cancer." *Science* 243:1012–1013, 1989a.

Massey, F. J., et al. "Vasectomy and Health." *Journal of the American Medical Association* 252:1023–1029, 1984.

Masters, W. H. "Update on Sexual Physiology." Paper presented at the Masters & Johnson Institute's Postgraduate Workshop on Human Sexual Function and Dysfunction, St. Louis, October 20, 1980.

———. "Update on Sexual Physiology." Presented at the Masters & Johnson Institute's Advanced Workshop on Human Sexuality, St. Louis, June 12, 1982.

Masters, W. H., et al. *Ethical Issues in Sex Therapy and Research,* vol. 2. Boston: Little, Brown, 1980.

———. "Outcome Studies at the Masters & Johnson Institute." Presented at the Sixth World Congress of Sexology, Washington, DC, May 26, 1983.

Masters, W. H., and Johnson, V. E. *Human Sexual Response*. Boston: Little, Brown, 1966.

———. "Human Sexual Inadequacy. Boston: Little, Brown, 1970.

———. *The Pleasure Bond*. New York: Bantam Books, 1976.

———. *Homosexuality in Perspective*. Boston: Little, Brown, 1979.

———. "Facts and Fallacies in Sexual Physiology." Paper presented at the Fifth National Meeting of the American Association of Sex Educators, Counselors, and Therapists, San Francisco, April 4, 1981.

Masters, W. H.; Johnson, V. E.; and Kolodny, R. C. Unpublished observations, 1980.

———. *Crisis: Heterosexual Behavior in the Age of AIDS*. New York: Grove Press, 1988.

Masterson, A., et al. "Marked Underreporting of CDC Defined AIDS Due to Poor Utilization of the HIV Antibody Test." Fifth International Conference on AIDS, Montreal, June 4–9, 1989. (Abstract T.A.O. 5, p. 55)

Mastroianni, L., Jr.; Donaldson, P. J.; and Kane, T. T. "Development of Contraceptives—Obstacles and Opportunities." *New England Journal of Medicine* 322:482–484, 1990.

Masur, F. T. "Resumption of Sexual Activity Following Myocardial Infarction." *Sexuality and Disability* 2:98–114, 1979.

May, R. "Mood Shifts and the Menstrual Cycle." *Journal of Psychosomatic Research* 20:125–130, 1976.

Medical Research International and Society for Assisted Reproductive Technology. "In Vitro Fertilization–Embryo Transfer in the United States: 1988 Results from the IVF–ET Registry." *Fertility & Sterility* 53:13–20, 1990.

Mehta, J., and Krop, H. "The Effect of Myocardial Infarction on Sexual Functioning." *Sexuality and Disability* 2:115–121, 1979.

Mendelson, J. H., et al. "Plasma Testosterone Levels Before, During, and After Chronic Marihuana Smoking." *New England Journal of Medicine* 291:1051–1055, 1974.

Mertz, G. J., et al. "Double-Blind Placebo-Controlled Trial of Oral Acyclovir in First-Episode Genital Herpes Simplex Virus Infection." *Journal of the American Medical Association* 254:1147–1151, 1984.

Mertz, G. J., et al. "Long-Term Acyclovir Suppression of Frequently Recurring Genital Herpes Simplex Virus Infection." *Journal of the American Medical Association* 260:201–206, 1988a.

Mertz, G. J., et al. "Transmission of Genital Herpes in Couples with One Symptomatic and One Asymptomatic Partner: A Prospective Study." *Journal of Infectious Disease* 157:1169–1177, 1988.

Merz, B. "Greater IUD Perforation Risk, Lactation Linked." *Journal of the American Medical Association* 249:3152, 1983.

Messenger, M. *The Breastfeeding Book.* New York: Van Nostrand Reinhold, 1982.

Metzger, D. "It Is Always the Woman Who Is Raped." *American Journal of Psychiatry* 133:405–408, 1976.

Meyer, H. "Prostitutes, Politics Heighten Thailand's AIDS Dilemma." *American Medical News,* pp. 3 & 26–28, July 27, 1990.

Meyer-Bahlburg, H. F. "Behavioral Effects of Estrogen Treatment in Human Males." *Pediatrics* 62(Suppl.):1171–1177, 1978.

Meyer-Bahlburg, H., et al. "HIV-Positive Gay Men: Sexual Dysfunction." Fifth International Conference on AIDS, Montreal, 1989. (Abstract # T.D.O. 22, p. 701)

Meyers, Robert. *D.E.S.: The Bitter Pill.* New York: Seaview/Putnam, 1983.

Miller, D. B. "Sexual Practices and Administrative Policies in Long Term Care Institutions." In Solnick, R. L. (ed.), *Sexuality and Aging,* rev. ed., pp. 163–175. Los Angeles: University of Southern California Press, 1978.

Miller, D. R., et al. "Breast Cancer Before Age 45 and Oral Contraceptive Use: New Findings." *American Journal of Epidemiology* 129:269–277. 1989.

Miller, H. *Tropic of Cancer.* New York: Grove Press, 1961.

Miller, H. G., Turner, C. F., and Moses, L. E. *AIDS—The Second Decade.* Washington, DC: National Academy Press, 1990.

Miller, L., Downer, A., and Krueger, L. "Reported Sexual Behavior Differences Between Heterosexual and Gay/Bisexual Populations." Presented at the IV International Conference on AIDS, Stockholm, June 12–16, 1988.

Mills, J. L., et al. "Maternal Alcohol Consumption and Birth Weight." *Journal of the American Medical Association* 252:1875–1879, 1984.

Mindel, A., et al. "Prophylactic Oral Acyclovir in Recurrent Genital Herpes." *Lancet* 2:57–59, 1984.

Minkoff, H. L., et al. "Routinely Offered Prenatal HIV Testing." *New England Journal of Medicine* 319:1018, 1988.

Mintz, J., et al. "Sexual Problems of Heroin Addicts." *Archives of General Psychiatry* 31:700–703, 1974.

Minuk, G. Y.; Bohme, C. E.; and Bower, T. J. "Condoms and Hepatitis B Virus Infection." *Annals of Internal Medicine* 104:584, 1986.

Mirin, S., et al. "Opiate Use and Sexual Function." *American Journal of Psychiatry* 173:909–915, 1980.

Mishell, D. R., Jr. "Contraception." *New England Journal of Medicine* 320:777–787, 1989.

———. "Current Status of Intrauterine Devices." *New England Journal of Medicine* 312:984–985, 1985.

Mishell, D. R., Jr. "Intrauterine Devices." *Journal of the American Medical Association* 263:235–236, 1990.

Mishell, D. R., Jr., et al. "The Intrauterine Device: A Bacteriologic Study of the Endometrial Cavity." *American Journal of Obstetrics and Gynecology* 96:119, 1966.

MMWR. "Rubella and Congenital Rubella: United States, 1983." *Journal of the American Medical Association* 251:2774–2775, 1984.

Moghissi, K. S. "Accuracy of Basal Body Temperature for Ovulation Detection." *Fertility and Sterility* 27:1415–1421, 1976.

Mohr, J. C. *Abortion in America: The Origins and Evolution of National Policy, 1800–1900.* New York: Oxford University Press, 1978.

Mohr, J. W.; Turner, R. E.; and Jerry, M. B. *Pedophilia and Exhibitionism.* Toronto: University of Toronto Press, 1964.

Monat, R. K. *Sexuality and the Mentally Retarded.* San Diego: College-Hill Press, 1982.

Money, J. "Ablatio Penis: Normal Male Infant Sex-Reassigned as a Girl." *Archives of Sexual Behavior* 4:65–72, 1975.

———. *Love and Love Sickness.* Baltimore: Johns Hopkins University Press, 1980.

Money, J., and Ehrhardt, A. E. *Man & Woman, Boy & Girl.* Baltimore: Johns Hopkins University Press, 1972.

Money, J., and Schwartz, M. "Dating, Romantic and Nonromantic Friendships, and Sexuality in 17 Early-Treated Adrenogenital Females, Aged 16–25." In Lee, P. A., et al. (eds.), *Congenital Adrenal Hyperplasia.* Baltimore: University Park Press, 1977.

Mooney, T. O.; Cole, T. M.; and Chilgren, R. A. *Sexual Options for Paraplegics and Quadraplegics.* Boston: Little, Brown, 1975.

Moore, D. E., et al. "Transmission of Genital Herpes by Donor Insemination." *Journal of the American Medical Association* 261:3441–3443, 1989.

Moos, R. H. "Typology of Menstrual Cycle Symptoms." *American Journal of Obstetrics and Gynecology* 103:390–402, 1969.

Morin, N. C., et al. "Congenital Malformations and Psychosocial Development in Children Conceived by In Vitro Fertilization." *Journal of Pediatrics* 115:222–227, 1989.

Moss, A. R., et al. "Seropositivity for HIV and the Development of AIDS or AIDS Related Condition." *British Medical Journal* 296:745–750, 1988.

Mulligan, T., and Katz, P. G. "Erectile Failure in the Aged: Evaluation and Treatment." *Journal of the American Geriatrics Society* 36:54–62, 1988.

Mulligan, T., et al. "The Role of Aging and Chronic Disease in Sexual Dysfunction." *Journal of the American Geriatrics Society* 36:520–524, 1988.

Munjack, D. J., and Kanno, P. H. "Retarded Ejaculation: A Review." *Archives of Sexual Behavior* 8:139–150, 1979.

Munjack, D. J., and Oziel, L. J. *Sexual Medicine and Counseling in Office Practice.* Boston: Little, Brown, 1980.

Murphy, W. D., et al. "Sexual Dysfunction and Treatment in Alcoholic Women." *Sexuality and Disability* 3:240–255, 1980.

Murphy-Corb, M., et al. "A Formalin-Inactivated Whole SIV Vaccine Confers Protection in Macaques." *Science* 246:1293–1297, 1989.

Murray, P. P., et al. "Oral Contraceptive Use in Women with a Family History of Breast Cancer." *Obstetrics and Gynecology* 73:977–983, 1989.

Myers, J. K.; Weissman, M. M.; and Tischler, G.C. "Six-month Prevalence of Psychiatric Disorders in Three Communities." *Archives of General Psychiatry* 41:959–967, 1984.

Myers, S. A., and Gleicher, N. "A Successful Program to Lower Cesarean-Section Rates." *New England Journal of Medicine* 319:1511–1516, 1988.

Nadelson, C. C. "The Emotional Impact of Abortion." In Notman, M. T., and Nadelson, C. C. (eds.), *The Woman Patient,* Vol. 1, pp. 173–179. New York: Plenum Press, 1978.

Nadelson, C. C., et al. "A Follow-up Study of Rape Victims." *American Journal of Psychiatry* 139:1266–1270, 1982.

Nahmias, A. J., et al. "Perinatal Risk Associated with Maternal Genital Herpes Simplex Virus Infection." *American Journal of Obstetrics and Gynecology* 110:825–832, 1971.

———. "Evidence for Human Infection with an HTLV-III/LAV-like Virus in Central Africa, 1959. *Lancet* 1:1279–1280, 1986.

National Coordinating Group for Male Contraceptives, Shanghai. "Gossypol: A New Male Contraceptive." *Chinese Medical Journal* 58:455–458, 1978.

Nerurkar, L. S., et al. "Survival of Herpes Simplex Virus in Water Specimens Collected from Hot Tubs in Spa Facilities and on Plastic Surfaces." *Journal of the American Medical Association* 250:3081–3083, 1983.

Newhouse, M. L., et al. "A Case–Control Study of Carcinoma of the Ovary." *British Journal of Preventive and Social Medicine* 31(3):148–153, September 1977.

Newman, G., and Nichols, C. R. "Sexual Activities and Attitudes in Older Persons." *Journal of the American Medical Association* 173:117–119, 1960.

Newman, M. *Michigan Consortium of Schools Student Survey.* Minneapolis: Hazelden Research Services, 1986.

Nichols, S. E. "Psychosocial Reactions of Persons with the Acquired Immunodeficiency Syndrome." *Annals of Internal Medicine* 103:765–767, 1985.

Niswander, K. R.; Singer, J.; and Singer M. "Psychological Reaction to Therapeutic Abortion, II: Objective Response." *American Journal of Obstetrics and Gynecology* 114:29–33, 1972.

Nora, A. H., and Nora, J. J. "Maternal Exposure to Exogenous Progestogen/Estrogen as a Potential Cause of Birth Defects." *Advances in Planned Parenthood* 12(3):156–169, 1978.

Nora, J. J., and Nora, A. H. "Birth Defects and Oral Contraceptives." *Lancet* 1:941–942, 1973.

Norman, C. "Politics and Science Clash on African AIDS." *Science* 230:1140–1141, 1986.

Norris, R. V., and Sullivan, C. *PMS: Premenstrual Syndrome.* New York: Rawson Wade, 1983.

North, B. B., and Vorhauer, B. W. "Use of the Today Contraceptive Sponge in the United States." *International Journal of Fertility* 30:81–84, 1985.

Notman, M. T. "A Psychological Consideration of Mastectomy." In Notman, M. T., and Nadelson, C. C. (eds.), *The Woman Patient,* Vol. 1, pp. 247–255. New York: Plenum Press, 1978.

Notzon, F. C.; Placek, P. J.; and Taffel, S. M. "Comparisons of National Cesarean-Section Rates." *New England Journal of Medicine* 316:386–389, 1987.

Olweus, D., et al. "Testosterone, Aggression, Physical and Personality Dimensions in Normal Adolescent Males." *Psychosomatic Medicine* 42:253–270, 1980.

Oriel, J. D., et al. "Genital Yeast Infections." *British Medical Journal* 4:761–764, 1972.

Ory, H. W.; Rosenfeld, A.; and Landman, L. C. "The Pill at 20: An Assessment." *Family Planning Perspectives* 12:278–283, 1980.

Ory, S. J. "Ectopic Pregnancy: Current Evaluation and Treatment." *Mayo Clinic Proceedings* 64:874–877, 1989.

Osborne, N. G.; Grubin, L.; and Pratson, L. "Vaginitis in Sexually Active Women: Relationship to Nine Sexually Transmitted Organisms." *Obstetrics and Gynecology* 142:962–967, 1982.

Osofsky, J. D., et al. "Psychologic Effects of Legal Abortion." *Clinical Obstetrics and Gynecology* 14(1):215–234, 1971.

Ouellette, E. M., et al. "Adverse Effects on Offspring of Maternal Alcohol Abuse During Pregnancy." *New England Journal of Medicine* 297:528–530, 1977.

Padwick, M. L., et al. "Efficacy, Acceptability, and Metabolic Effects of Transdermal Estradiol in the Management of Postmenopausal Women." *American Journal of Obstetrics and Gynecology* 152:1085–1091, 1985.

Paige, K. E. "Women Learn to Sing the Menstrual Blues." *Psychology Today,* pp. 41–46, April 1973.

Paige, K. "The Declining Taboo Against Menstrual Sex." *Psychology Today* 12(7):50–51, 1978.

Palmore, E. "Published Reactions to the Kinsey Report." *Social Forces* 31:165–170, December 1952.

Parlee, M. B. "The Premenstrual Syndrome." *Psychological Bulletin* 80:454–465, 1973.

Parsons, J. E. "Psychosexual Neutrality: Is Anatomy Destiny?" In Parsons, J. E. (ed.), *The Psychobiology of Sex Differences and Sex Roles,* pp. 3–29. New York: Hemisphere Publishing, 1980.

Payne, S. F., et al. "Effect of Multiple Disease Manifestations on Length of Survival for AIDS Patients in San Francisco." Fifth International Conference on AIDS, Montreal, June 4–9, 1989. (Abstract # W.A.P. 80, p. 133)

Pekkanen, J. "Are We Closing in on AIDS?" *Reader's Digest,* pp. 79–85, December 1989.

Percival-Smith, R. K., and Abercrombie, B. "Postcoital Contraception with DL-Norgestrel/Ethinyl Estradiol Combination: Six Years Experience in a Student Medical Clinic." *Contraception* 36:287–292, 1987.

Perelman, M. A. "Treatment of Premature Ejaculation." In Leiblum, S. R., and Pervin, L. A. (eds.), *Principles and Practice of Sex Therapy,* pp. 199–233. New York: Guilford Press, 1980.

Perkins, R. P. "Sexual Behavior and Response in Relation to Complications of Pregnancy." *American Journal of Obstetrics and Gynecology* 134:498–505, 1979.

Perlmutter, J. F. "A Gynecological Approach to Menopause." In Notman, M. T., and Nadelson, C. C. (eds.), *The Woman Patient,* pp. 323–335. New York: Plenum Press, 1978.

Pernoll, M. L., and Benson, R. C. *Current Obstetric and Gynecologic Diagnosis & Treatment.* Norwalk, CT: Appleton & Lange, 1987.

Perrin, E. B., et al. "Long-Term Effect of Vasectomy on Coronary Heart Disease." *American Journal of Public Health* 74:128–132, 1984.

Perrone, J. "Controversial Abortion Approach." *American Medical News,* pp. 9 & 18–22. January 12, 1990.

Perry, J. D., and Whipple, B. "Pelvic Muscle Strength of Female Ejaculators: Evidence in Support of a New Theory of Orgasm." *Journal of Sex Research* 17(1):22–39, 1981.

Perry, S.; Jacobsberg, L.; and Fogel, K. "Orogenital Transmission of Human Immunodeficiency Virus (HIV)." *Annals of Internal Medicine* 11:951–952, 1989.

Persky, H. "Reproductive Hormones, Moods and the Menstrual Cycle." In Friedman, R. C.; Richard, R. M.; and Vande Wiele, R. L. (eds.), *Sex Differences in Behavior,* pp. 455–466. New York: Wiley, 1974.

Persky, H., et al. "Plasma Testosterone Level and Sexual Behavior of Couples." *Archives of Sexual Behavior* 7:157–173, 1978.

Peter, J. B.; Bryson, Y.; and Lovett, M. A. "Genital Herpes: Urgent Questions, Elusive Answers." *Diagnostic Medicine,* pp. 71–74, 76–88, *March/April* 1982.

Peterman, T. A., and Curran, J. W. "Sexual Transmission of Human Immunodeficiency Virus." *Journal of the American Medical Association* 256:2222–2226, 1986.

Peterman, T. A., et al. "Risk of HIV Transmission from Heterosexual Adults with Transfusion-Associated Infections." *Journal of the American Medical Association* 259:55–58, 1988.

Petravage, J. B. "Outcomes of Three Birthing Rooms." *Journal of Family Practice* 16:929, 1983.

Pfeiffer, E., and Davis, G. C. "Determinants of Sexual Behavior in Middle and Old Age." *Journal of the American Geriatrics Society* 20:151–158, 1972.

Pfeiffer, E.; Verwoerdt, A.; and Davis, G. C. "Sexual Behavior in Middle Life." *American Journal of Psychiatry* 128:1262–1267, 1972.

Pfeffer, M. A. "Diabetic Sexual Dysfunction," *Clinical Diabetes* 6:97–100, 118, 1988.

Piazza, M., et al. "Passionate Kissing and Microlesions of the Oral Mucosa: Possible Role in AIDS Transmission." *Journal of the American Medical Association* 261:244–245, 1989.

Piotrow, P. T.; Rinehart, W.; and Schmidt, J. C. "IUDs: An Update on Safety, Effectiveness, and Research." *Population Reports,* Series B(3), May 1979.

Pivar, D. J. *Purity Crusade, Sexual Morality, and Social Control, 1868–1900.* Westport, CT: Greenwood Press, 1973.

Placek, P.; Taffel, S.; and Liss, T. "The Cesarean Future." *American Demography* 9:46–47, 1987.

Plapinger, L., and McEwen, B. S. "Gonadal Steroid–Brain Interactions in Sexual Differentiation." In Hutchison, J. B. (ed.), *Biological Determinants of Sexual Behavior,* pp. 153–218. New York: Wiley, 1978.

Platt, R.; Rice, P. A.; and McCormack, W. M. "Risk of Acquiring Gonorrhea and Prevalence of Abnormal Adnexal Findings Among Women Recently Exposed to Gonorrhea." *Journal of the American Medical Association* 250:3205–3209, 1983.

Platzker, A. C.; Lew, C. D.; and Stewart D. "Drug 'Administration' Via Breast Milk." *Hospital Practice,* pp. 111–122, September 1980.

Podolsky, S. "Erectile Impotence in the Diabetes Patient." *Practical Gastroenterology* 7(1):40–43, January/February 1983.

Pokrovsky, V. V., and Eramova, E. U. "Nosocomial Outbreak of HIV Infection in Elista, USSR." Fifth International Conference on AIDS, Montreal, June 4–9, 1989. (Abstract # W.A.O.5, p. 63)

Poland, R. L. "The Question of Routine Neonatal Circumcision." *New England Journal of Medicine* 322:1312–1315, 1990.

Pomeroy, W. B. "The Masters–Johnson Report and the Kinsey Tradition." In Brecher, R., and Brecher, E. (eds.), *An Analysis of Human Sexual Response,* pp. 111–123. New York: Signet Books, 1966.

———. *Your Child and Sex: A Guide for Parents.* New York: Delacorte, 1976.

Pope, H. G., and Katz, D. L. "Affective and Psychotic Symptoms Associated with Anabolic Steroid Use." *American Journal of Psychiatry* 145:487–490, 1988.

Pope, H. G., et al. "Prevalence of Anorexia Nervosa and Bulimia in Three Student Populations." *International Journal of Eating Disorders* 3:45–51, 1984.

Population Reports. Published five times per year by Population Information Program of the Johns Hopkins University, 624 N. Broadway, Baltimore, MD 21205.

Potts, M. "Birth Control Methods in the United States." *Family Planning Perspectives* 20:288–297, 1988.

Powell, M. G., et al. "Contraception with the Cervical Cap: Effectiveness, Safety, Continuity of Use, and User Satisfaction." *Contraception* 33:215–232, 1986.

Powledge, T. M. "Unnatural Selection." In Holmes, H. B.; Hoskins, B. B.; and Gross, M. (eds.), *The Custom-Made Child? Women Centered Perspectives.* Clifton, NJ: Humana Press, 1981.

Prather, R. C. "Sexual Dysfunction in the Diabetic Female: A Review." *Archives of Sexual Behavior* 17:277–284, 1988.

Presidential Commission on the Human Immunodeficiency Virus Epidemic. *Report of the Presidential Commission on the Human Immunodeficiency Virus Epidemic.* Washington, DC: U.S. Government Printing Office, 1988.

Presser, H. B. "Guessing and Misinformation About Pregnancy Risk Among Urban Mothers." *Family Planning Perspectives* 9:111–115, 1977.

Pritchard, J. A., and MacDonald, P. C. *William's Obstetrics,* 16th ed. New York: Appleton-Century-Crofts, 1980.

Prober, C. G., et al. "Low Risk of Herpes Simplex Virus Infections in Neonates Exposed to the Virus at the Time of Vaginal Delivery to Mothers with Recurrent Genital Herpes Simplex Infections." *New England Journal of Medicine* 316:240–244, 1987.

Prober, C. G., et al. "Use of Routine Viral Cultures at Delivery to Identify Neonates Exposed to Herpes Simplex Virus." *New England Journal of Medicine* 318:887–891, 1988.

Proctor, F.; Wagner, N.; and Butler, J. "The Differentiation of Male and Female Orgasm: An Experimental Study." In Wagner, N. (ed.), *Perspectives on Human Sexuality.* New York: Behavioral Publications, 1974.

Pugh, B. "An Evaluation of the Effects of Various Lubricants on Latex Condoms." Presented at the Fifth International Conference on AIDS, Montreal, June 4–9, 1989. (Abstract # W.A.P. 95, p. 135)

Quadagno, D. M., et al. "Postpartum Moods in Men and Women." *American Journal of Obstetrics and Gynecology* 154:1018–1023, 1986.

Queenan, J. T. "The C-Section Crisis: Why We Must Solve It Ourselves." *Contemporary Obstetrics and Gynecology* 31(2):9–10, 1988.

Quinn, T. C., et al. "Human Immunodeficiency Virus Infection Among Patients Attending Clinics for Sexually Transmitted Diseases." *New England Journal of Medicine* 318:197–203, 1988.

Rabin, B. *The Sensuous Wheeler: Sexual Adjustment for the Spinal Cord Injured*. San Francisco: Multi-Focus Resource Center, 1980.

Rachman, S. J., and Wilson, G. T. *The Effects of Psychological Therapy,* 2nd ed. New York: Pergamon Press, 1980.

Raisz, L. G. "Local and Systemic Factors in the Pathogenesis of Osteoporosis." *New England Journal of Medicine* 318:818–828, 1988.

Ramcharan, S. *The Walnut Creek Contraceptive Drug Study: A Prospective Study of the Side Effects of Oral Contraceptives*. Bethesda, MD: U.S. Department of Health and Human Services, National Institutes of Health (publication NIH 81-564), 1981.

Ramcharan, S., et al. "The Walnut Creek Contraceptive Study." *Journal of Reproductive Medicine* 25(Suppl.) 346–376, 1980.

Rando, R. F. "Human Papillomavirus: Implications for Clinical Medicine." *Annals of Internal Medicine* 108:628–630, 1988.

Ranki, A., et al. "Long Latency Precedes Overt Seroconversion in Sexually Transmitted Human Immunodeficiency Virus Infections." *Lancet* 2:589–593, 1987.

———. "In Vitro Fertilization Enters Stormy Adolescence as Experts Debate the Odds." *Journal of the American Medical Association* 259:464–469, 1988.

———. "New Use for Old Method of Inducing Ejaculation May Give Hope of Fatherhood to Some Spinal Cord-Injured Men." *Journal of the American Medical Association* 258:743–744, 1987.

Redfield, R. R., and Burke, D. S. "HIV Infection: The Clinical Picture." *Scientific American* 259(4):90–98, October 1988.

Reese, C. R. "Neurophysiological Studies of Cannabis in Human Subjects." *Journal of Substance Use and Abuse* 4:118–127, 1977.

Reeves, W. C., et al. "Human Papillomavirus Infection and Cervical Cancer in Latin America." *New England Journal of Medicine* 320:1437–1441, 1989.

Reichman, R. C., et al. "Treatment of Recurrent Genital Herpes Simplex Infections with Oral Acyclovir." *Journal of the American Medical Association* 251:2103–2107, 1984.

Reid, R., et al. "Genital Warts and Cervical Cancer." *Cancer* 53:943–953, 1984.

Reiner, N. E., et al. "Asymptomatic Rectal Mucosal Lesions and Hepatitis B Surface Antigen at Sites of Sexual Contact in Homosexual Men with Persistent Hepatitis B Virus Infection." *Annals of Internal Medicine* 96:170–173, 1982.

Reingold , A. L. "Nonmenstrual Toxic Shock Syndrome: The Growing Picture." *Journal of the American Medical Association* 249:932, 1983.

———. "Toxic Shock Syndrome and the Contraceptive Sponge." *Journal of the American Medical Association* 255:242–243, 1986.

Reingold, A. L., et al. "Toxic Shock Syndrome Surveillance in the United States, 1980 to 1981." *Annals of Internal Medicine* 96(Part 2):875–880, 1982.

Reinisch, J. M. "Fetal Hormones, the Brain, and Human Sex Differences: A Heuristic, Integrative Review of the Recent Literature." *Archives of Sexual Behavior* 3:51–90, 1974.

———. "Prenatal Exposure to Synthetic Progestins Increases Potential for Aggression in Humans." *Science* 211:1171–1173, 1981.

Reinisch, June. *The Kinsey Institute New Report on Sex*. New York: St. Martin's Press, 1990.

Renshaw, D. "Inflatable Penile Prosthesis." *Journal of the American Medical Association* 241:2637–2638, 1979.

———. "Sex and Eating Disorders." *Medical Aspects of Human Sexuality* 24(4):68–77, 1990.

Rhoads, G. G., et al. "The Safety and Efficacy of Chorionic Villus Sampling for Early Prenatal Diagnosis of Cytogenetic Abnormalities." *New England Journal of Medicine* 320:609–617, 1989.

Richart, R. M., and Barron, B. A. "Screening Strategies for Cervical Cancer and Cervical Intraepitheleal Neoplasia." Presented at the American Cancer Society National Conference on Cancer Prevention and Detection, Chicago, April 17–19, 1980.

Richwald, G. A., et al. "Are Condom Instructions Readable? Results of a Readability Study." *Public Health Reports* 103:355–358, 1988.

———. "Sexual Activities in Bathhouses in Los Angeles County: Implications for AIDS Prevention Education." *Journal of Sex Research* 25:169–180, 1988.

Riesenberg, D. E. "AIDS-Prompted Behavior Changes Reported." *Journal of the American Medical Association* 255:171, 176, 1986.

Rietmeijer, C. A. M., et al. "Condoms as Physical and Chemical Barriers Against Human Immunodeficiency Virus." *Journal of the American Medical Association* 259:1851–1853, 1988.

Riis, B.; Thomsen, K.; and Christiansen, C. "Does Calcium Supplementation Prevent Postmenopausal Bone Loss?" *New England Journal of Medicine* 316:173–177, 1987.

Rinehart, W. "Postcoital Contraception: An Appraisal." *Population Reports,* Series J(9):January 1976.

Rinehart, W., and Piotrow, P. T. "OCs: Update on Usage, Safety, and Side Effects." *Population Reports,* Series A(5):January 1979.

Robbins, M., and Jensen, G. D. "Multiple Orgasm in Males." *Journal of Sex Research* 14:21–26, 1978.

Robboy, S. J., et al. *Prenatal Diethylstilbestrol (DES) Exposure: Recommendations of the Diethylstilbestrol Adenosis (DESAD) Project for the Identification and Management of Exposed Individuals*. Washington, DC: U.S. Department of Health and Human Services, NIH Publication No. 81–2049, 1981.

Robertson, D. H.; McMillan, A.; and Young, H. *Clinical Practice in Sexually Transmissible Diseases*. Kent, England: Pitman Medical, 1980.

Robinson, J. E., and Short, R. V. "Changes in Breast Sensitivity at Puberty, During the Menstrual Cycle, and at Parturition." *British Medical Journal* 1:1188–1191, 1977.

Rodgers, D. A., and Ziegler, F. J. "Psychological Reactions to Surgical Contraception." In Fawcett, J. T. (ed.), *Psychological Perspectives on Population,* pp. 306–326. New York: Basic Books, 1973.

Roeske, N. C. "Hysterectomy and Other Gynecological Surgeries: A Psychological View." In Notman, M. T., and Nadelson, C. C. (eds.), *The Woman Patient,* Vol. 1, pp. 217–232. New York: Plenum Press, 1978.

Romieu, I., et al. "Prospective Study of Oral Contraceptive Use and Risk of Breast Cancer in Women." *Journal of the National Cancer Institute* 81:1313–1321, 1989.

Ronald, A. R., and Albritton, W. L. "Chancroid and *Haemophilus ducreyi.*" In Holmes, K. K., et al. (eds.), *Sexually Transmitted Diseases,* pp. 385–393. New York: McGraw-Hill, 1984.

Rooks, J. P., et al. "Outcomes of Care in Birth Centers." *New England Journal of Medicine* 321:1804–1811, 1989.

Rooney, J. F., et al. "Acquisition of Genital Herpes from an Asymptomatic Sexual Partner." *New England Journal of Medicine* 314:1561–1564, 1986.

Rosen, M. G., and Thomas, L. *The Cesarean Myth.* New York: Viking Penguin, 1989.

Rosenbaum, M. "When Drugs Come into the Picture, Love Flies Out the Window: Women Addicts' Love Relationships." *International Journal of the Addictions* 16:1197–1206, 1981.

Rosenberg, L., et al. "Oral Contraceptive Use in Relation to Nonfatal Myocardial Infarction." *American Journal of Epidemiology* 111:59–66, 1980.

Rosenberg, M. J., et al. "Effect of the Contraceptive Sponge on Chlamydia Infection, Gonorrhea, and Candidiasis." *Journal of the American Medical Association* 257:2308–2312, 1987.

Rosenblatt, R. "The Baby in the Factory." *Time,* p. 90, February 14, 1983.

Rosenfield, A., et al. "The Food and Drug Administration and Medroxyprogesterone Acetate: What Are the Issues? *Journal of the American Medical Association* 249:2922–2928, 1983.

Ross, C., and Piotrow, P. T. "Birth Control Without Contraceptives." *Population Reports,* Series I(1):June 1974.

Ross, J. A. "Contraception: Short-Term vs. Long-Term Failure Rates." *Family Planning Perspectives* 21:275–277, 1989.

Rossi, A. S., and Rossi, P. E. "Body Time and Social Time: Mood Patterns by Menstrual Cycle and Day of Week." *Social Science Research* 6:273–308, 1977.

Rousseau, S., et al. "The Expectancy of Pregnancy for 'Normal' Infertile Couples." *Fertility & Sterility* 40:768–772, 1983.

Rowland, D. L., et al. "Penile and Finger Sensory Thresholds in Young, Aging, and Diabetic Males." *Archives of Sexual Behavior* 18:1–12, 1989.

Royal College of General Practitioners' Oral Contraception Study. "Mortality Among Oral-Contraceptive Users." *Lancet* 2:727–731, October 8, 1977.

Royal College of General Practitioners. *Oral Contraception and Health: An Interim Report from the Oral Contraception Study.* New York: Pitman, 1974.

Rozenbaum, W., et al. "HIV Transmission by Oral Sex." *Lancet* 2:1395, 1988.

Rubin, R.; Reinisch, J.; and Haskett, R. "Postnatal Gonadal Steroid Effects on Human Behavior." *Science* 211(4488):1318–1324, 1981.

———. *Liking and Loving: An Introduction to Social Psychology.* New York: Holt, Rinehart and Winston, 1973.

Ruble, D. N.; Brooks-Gunn, J.; and Clarke, A. "Research on Menstrual-Related Psychological Changes: Alternative Perspectives." In Parsons, J. E. (ed.), *The Psychobiology of Sex Differences and Sex Roles,* pp. 227–243. New York: McGraw-Hill/Hemisphere, 1980.

Rush, D., and Callahan, K. R. "Exposure to Passive Cigarette Smoking and Child Development: A Critical Review." *Annals of the New York Academy of Sciences* 562:74–100, 1989.

Ryback, R. S. "Chronic Alcohol Consumption and Menstruation" (letter). *Journal of the American Medical Association* 238:2143, 1977.

Ryder, N. B. "Contraceptive Failure in the United States." *Family Planning Perspectives* 5(3):133–142, 1973.

Sairam, M. R., et al. "Isolation, Structure, and Synthesis of a Human Seminal Plasma Peptide with Inhibin-like Activity." *Science* 223:1199–1201, 1984.

Sanchez, R. S., et al. "Pituitary–Testicular Axis in Patients on Lithium Therapy." *Fertility & Sterility* 27:667–669, 1976.

Sandberg, E. C. "Psychological Aspects of Contraception." In Sadock, B. J.; Kaplan, H. I.; and Freedman, A. M. (eds.), *The Sexual Experience,* pp. 335–349. Baltimore: Williams & Wilkins, 1976.

Sanders, L. L., Jr., et al. "Treatment of Sexually Transmitted Chlamydial Infections." *Journal of the American Medical Association* 255:1750–1756, 1986.

Santen, R. J., et al. "Mechanism of Action of Narcotics in the Production of Menstrual Dysfunction in Women." *Fertility and Sterility* 26:538–548, 1975.

Schacter, J. "Chlamydial Infections." *New England Journal of Medicine* 298:428–435, 1978.

Schacter, J., et al. "Prospective Study of Perinatal Transmission of *Chlamydia trachomatis.*" *Journal of the American Medical Association* 255:3374–3377, 1986.

Schacter, J.; Stone, E.; and Moncada, J. "Screening for Chlamydial Infections in Women Attending Family Planning Clinics." *Western Journal of Medicine* 138:375–379, 1983.

Schatten, G., and Schatten, H. "The Energetic Egg." *The Sciences* 23(5):28–34, 1983.

Schatzkin, A., et al. "Alcohol Consumption and Breast Cancer in the Epidemiologic Follow-up Study of the First National Health and Nutrition Examination Survey." *New England Journal of Medicine* 316:1169–1173, 1987.

Schecter, J. O.; Schwartz, H. P.; and Greenfeld, D. G. "Sexual Assault and Anorexia Nervosa." *International Journal of Eating Disorders* 6:313–316, 1987.

Schiavi, R. "Chronic Alcoholism and Male Sexual Dysfunction." *Journal of Sex & Marital Therapy* 16:23–33, 1990.

Schiff, E., et al. "The Use of Aspirin to Prevent Pregnancy-Induced Hypertension and Lower the Ratio of Thromboxane A2 to Prostacyclin in Relatively High Risk Pregnancies." *New England Journal of Medicine* 321:351–356, 1989.

Schiller, P. *The Sex Profession.* Washington, DC: Shilmark House, 1981.

Schlech, W. F., III, et al. "Risk Factors for Development of Toxic Shock Syndrome." *Journal of the American Medical Association* 248:835–839, 1982.

Schmid, G. P., et al. "Chancroid in the United States." *Journal of the American Medical Association* 258:3265–3268, 1987.

Schmidt, C. W., and Lucas, J. "The Short-Term, Intermittent, Conjoint Treatment of Sexual Disorders." In Meyer, J. K.

(ed.), *Clinical Management of Sexual Disorders*. Baltimore: Williams & Wilkins, 1976.

Schneider, E. L. (ed.). *The Aging Reproductive System*. New York: Raven Press, 1978.

Schoen, E. J. "The Status of Circumcision of Newborns." *New England Journal of Medicine* 322:1308–1312, 1990.

Schofield, C. B. *Sexually Transmitted Diseases*. New York: Churchill Livingstone, 1979.

Scholl, T. O., et al. "Effects of Vaginal Spermicides on Pregnancy Outcome." *Family Planning Perspectives* 15:244–250, 1983.

Schover, L. R., and LoPiccolo, J. "Treatment Effectiveness for Dysfunctions of Sexual Desire." *Journal of Sex & Marital Therapy* 8:179–197, 1982.

Schover, L. R., et al. "The Multi-axial Problem-Oriented Diagnostic System for the Sexual Dysfunctions: An Alternative to DSM-III." *Archives of General Psychiatry* 39:614–619, 1982.

Schover, Leslie R., et al. "Orgasm Phase Dysfunction in Multiple Sclerosis." *Jouranl of Sex Research* 25:548–554, 1988.

Schover, Leslie R., and Jensen, S. B. *Sexuality and Chronic Illness: A Comprehensive Approach*. New York: Guilford Press, 1988.

Schreeded, M. T., et al. "Hepatitis B in Homosexual Men: Prevalence of Infection and Factors Related to Transmission." *Journal of Infectious Diseases* 146:7–15, 1982.

Schreiner-Engel, P., and Schiavi, R. "Sexual Arousability in Women." Paper presented at the Sixth Annual Meeting of the Society for Sex Therapy and Research, Cambridge, MA, May 31, 1980.

Schreiner-Engel, P., et al. "Sexual Arousability and the Menstrual Cycle." *Psychosomatic Medicine* 43:199–214, 1981.

Schulman, A. "Organs and Orgasms." In Gornick, V., and Moran, B. K. (eds.), *Women in Sexist Society*. New York: Basic Books, 1971.

Schultz, S., et al. "Declining Rates of Rectal and Pharyngeal Gonorrhea Among Men: New York City." *Journal of the American Medical Association* 252:327–331, 1984.

———. "Female-to-Male Transmission of HTLV-III." *Journal of the American Medical Association* 255:1703, 1986.

Schultz, W. C. M., et al. "Vaginal Sensitivity to Electric Stimuli: Theoretical and Practical Implications." *Archives of Sexual Behavior* 18:87–95, 1989.

Schumacher, S. "Effectiveness of Sex Therapy." In Gemme, R., and Wheeler, C. C., *Progress in Sexology*, pp. 141–151. New York: Plenum Press, 1977.

Schwartz, D. "Female Fecundity as a Function of Age." *New England Journal of Medicine* 306:404–406, 1982.

Schwartz, M. F., and Bauman, J. E. "Hyperprolactinemia and Sexual Dysfunction in Men." Presented at the Seventh Annual Meeting of the Society for Sex Therapy and Research, New York, March 1981.

Schwartz, P., et al. "Type II Herpes Simplex Virus and Vulvar Carcinoma in Situ." *New England Journal of Medicine* 305:517–518, 1981.

Segal, S. J. "Methods of Fertility Regulation in Clinical Trial." In *Contraception: Science, Technology, and Application*, pp. 135–146. Washington, DC: National Academy of Sciences, 1979.

Segraves, R. T. "Psychiatric Drugs and Inhibited Female Orgasm." *Jouranl of Sex and Marital Therapy* 14:202–207, 1988.

Segraves, R. T., et al. "Erectile Dysfunction Association with Pharmacologic Agents." In Segraves, R. T., and Schoenberg, H. W. (eds.), *Diagnosis and Treatment of Erectile Disturbances*. New York: Plenum Press, 1985.

———. "Spontaneous Remission in Erectile Dysfunction: A Partial Replication." *Behavioral Research and Therapy* 23(2):203–204, 1985.

Seibel, M. "A New Era in Reproductive Technology." *New England Journal of Medicine* 318:828–834, 1988.

Seibel, M.; Ranoux, C.; and Kearnan, M. "In Vitro Fertilization: How Much Is Enough?" *New England Journal of Medicine* 321:1052–1053, 1989.

Seibel, M. M.; Freeman, M.; and Graves, W. "Carcinoma of the Cervix and Sexual Function." *Obstetrics and Gynecology* 55:484–487, 1980.

Semmens, J. P., and Wagner, G. "Estrogen Deprivation and Vaginal Function in Postmenopausal Women." *Journal of the American Medical Association* 248:445–448, 1982.

Sevely, J., and Bennett, J. "Concerning Female Ejaculation and the Female Prostate." *Journal of Sex Research* 14:1–20, 1978.

Shafer, M. A., et al. "Urinary Leukocyte Esterase Screening Test for Asymptomatic Chlamydial and Gonococcal Infections in Males." *Journal of the American Medical Association* 262:2562–2566, 1989.

Shainess, N. "How 'Sex Experts' Debase Sex." *World* 2(1):21–25, 1973.

Shane, J. M.; Schiff, I.; and Wilson, E. A. The Infertile Couple: Evaluation and Treatment. *Clinical Symposia* 28(5), 1976.

Shapira, J., and Cummings, J. L. "Alzheimer's Disease: Changes in Sexual Behavior." *Medical Aspects of Human Sexuality* 23(No.6):32–36, June 1989.

Shapiro, H. I. *The New Birth-Control Book: A Complete Guide for Women and Men*. Englewood Cliffs, NJ: Prentice-Hall, 1988.

Shapiro, S., et al. "Birth Defects and Vaginal Spermicides." *Journal of the American Medical Association* 247:2381–2384, 1982.

Sherfey, M. J. *The Nature and Evolution of Female Sexuality*. New York: Random House, 1972.

Sherif, C. W. "A Social Psychological Perspective on the Menstrual Cycle." In Parsons, J. E. (ed.), *The Psychobiology of Sex Differences and Sex Roles*, pp. 245–268. New York: McGraw-Hill/Hemisphere, 1980.

Sherris, J. D.; Lewison, D.; and Fox, G. "Update on Condoms: Products, Protection, Promotion." *Population Reports*, Series H, No. 6, 1982.

Sherris, J. D.; Moore, S. H.; and Fox, G. "New Developments in Vaginal Contraception." *Population Reports*, Series H, No. 7, January/February 1984.

Shettles, L., and Rorvik, D. *Your Baby's Sex: Now You Can Choose*. New York: Dodd, Mead, 1970.

Shilts, R. *And the Band Played On: Politics, People, and the AIDS Epidemic*. New York: St. Martin's Press, 1987.

Shiono, P. H.; Klebanoff, M. A.; and Rhoads, G. G. "Smoking and Drinking During Pregnancy." *Journal of the American Medical Association* 255:82–84, 1986.

Shostak, A.; McLouth, G.; and Seng, L. *Men and Abortions: Lessons, Losses, and Love*. New York: Praeger, 1984.

Shuckit, M. A., et al. "Premenstrual Symptoms and Depression in a University Population." *Diseases of the Nervous System* 36:516–517, 1975.

Sidi, A. A., et al. "Recent Advances in the Diagnosis and Management of Impotence. *Urology Clinics of North America* 13(3):489–500, August 1986.

Siegel, K., et al. "Patterns of Change in Sexual Behavior Among Gay Men in New York City." *Archives of Sexual Behavior* 17:481–497, 1988.

Siegel, O. "Personality Development in Adolescence." In Wolman, B. B., et al. (eds.), *Handbook of Development Psychology,* pp. 537–548. Englewood Cliffs, NJ: Prentice-Hall, 1982.

Siegel, R. K. "Cocaine and Sexual Dysfunction." *Journal of Psychoactive Drugs* 14:71–74, 1982.

Silver, H. "Autologous Blood Donation." *Transfusion Medicine Topic Update* 2(1):1–4, January 1989.

Silverberg, E. "Cancer Statistics, 1981." *Ca-A Cancer Journal for Clinicians* 31(1):13–28, 1981.

Silverman, S. "Scope, Specifics of Maternal Drug Use, Effects on Fetus Are Beginning to Emerge from Studies." *Journal of the American Medical Association* 261:1688–1689, 1989.

Singer, J., and Singer, I. "Types of Female Orgasm." *Journal of Sex Research* 8:255–267, 1972.

Singh, J., et al. "Sex Life and Psychiatric Problems After Myocardial Infarction." *Journal of the Association of Physicians of India* 18:503–507, 1970.

Sklarek, H. M., et al. "AIDS in a Bodybuilder Using Anabolic Steroids." *New England Journal of Medicine* 311:1701, 1984.

Slattery, M. L. "Cigarette Smoking and Exposure to Passive Smoke Are Risk Factors for Cervical Cancer." *Journal of the American Medical Association* 261:1593–1598, 1989.

Sloan, L. A. "Abortion Attitude Scale." *Health Education* 14(3):41–42, 1983.

Smith, C. G., et al. "Effect of Delta-9-tetrahydrocannabinol (THC) on Secretion of Male Sex-Hormone in Rhesus Monkey." *Pharmacologist* 18:248, 1976.

Smith, D. W. "The Fetal Alcohol Syndrome." *Hospital Practice,* pp. 121–128, October 1979.

Smith, Diana G. "Thailand: AIDS Crisis Looms." *Lancet* 335:781–782, 1990.

Smith, P. C. "Saving Lives with a Testicular Self-Examination." *Sexual Medicine Today* 4(6):11–12, 1980.

Smith, T. F., et al. "The Phylogenetic History of Immunodeficiency Viruses." *Nature* 333:573–575, 1988.

Sobel, J. D. "Bacterial Vaginosis—An Ecologic Mystery." *Annals of Internal Medicine* 111:551–551, 1989.

Sorokin, P. A. *The American Sex Revolution.* Boston: Porter Sargent, 1956.

Soules, M. R., and Bremmer, W. J. "The Menopause and Climacteric: Endocrinologic Basis and Associated Symptomatology." *Journal of the American Geriatrics Society* 30:547–561, 1982.

Spear, L. P.; Kirstein, C. L.; and Frambes, N. A. "Cocaine Effects on the Developing Central Nervous System: Behavioral, Psychopharmacological, and Neurochemical Studies." *Annals of The New York Academy of Sciences* 562:290–307, 1989.

Speroff, L.; Glass, R. H.; and Kase, N. G. *Clinical Gynecologic Endocrinology and Infertility,* 3rd ed. Baltimore: Williams & Wilkins, 1983.

Spitzer, P. G., and Weiner, N. J. "Transmission of HIV Infection from a Woman to a Man by Oral Sex." *New England Journal of Medicine* 320:251, 1989.

Spring-Mills, E., and Hafez, E. S. "Male Accessory Sexual Organs." In Hafez, E. S. (ed.), *Human Reproduction,* pp. 60–90. New York: Harper & Row, 1980.

Stall, R., et al. "Alcohol and Drug Use During Sexual Activity and Compliance with Safe Sex Guidelines for AIDS." *Health Education Quarterly* 13:359–371, 1986.

Stamm, W. E. "Diagnosis of *Chlamydia trachomatis* Genitourinary Infections." *Annals of Internal Medicine* 108:710–717, 1988.

Stamm, W. E., et al. "Causes of the Acute Urethral Syndrome in Women." *New England Journal of Medicine* 303:409–415, 1980.

———. "Effect of Treatment Regimens for *Neisseria gonorrhoeae* on Simultaneous Infection with *Chlamydia trachomatis.*" *New England Journal of Medicine* 310:545–549, 1984.

———. "CDC Update: *Chlamydia trachomatis Infections.*" *Urban Health* 14:10–29, July/August 1985.

Stamm, W. E., et al. "The Association Between Genital Ulcer Disease and Acquisition of HIV Infection in Homosexual Men." *Journal of the American Medical Association* 260:1429–1433, 1988.

Starr, B. D., and Weiner, M. B. *The Starr–Weiner Report on Sex and Sexuality in the Mature Years.* New York: Stein & Day, 1981.

Staver, S. "Women Found Contracting HIV via Unprotected Sex." *American Medical News,* p. 4, June 1, 1990.

Stearns, P. "Interpreting the Medical Literature on Aging." Presented at the Family and Community History Colloquia: The Physican and Social History, Chicago, October 30, 1975 (cited in Bart and Grossman, 1978).

Stempel, R. R., and Moss, A. R. "Changes in Sexual Behavior by Gay Men in Response to AIDS." Fourth International Conference on AIDS, Stockholm, June 12–16, 1988. (Abstract #6538)

Stevens, C. E., et al. "Epidemiology of Hepatitis C. Virus." *Journal of the American Medical Association* 263:49–53, 1990.

Stevens, F. A. "The Occurrence of *Staphylococcus aureus* Infection with a Scarlatiniform Rash." *Journal of the American Medical Association* 88:1957–1958, 1927.

Stevens, W. K. "Fear of AIDS Brings Explicit Advice to Campus, Caution to Singles Bars." *The New York Times,* p. 9, February 17, 1987.

Stewart, F., et al. *My Body, My Health: The Concerned Woman's Guide to Gynecology.* New York: Wiley, 1979.

Stibbe, J. "Heterosexual Infectivity of LAV/HTLV-III as Judged by Antibody Testing in Spouses of Seropositive Hemophiliacs," p. 122. Presented at the Second International Conference on AIDS, Paris, June 23–25, 1986.

Stomper, P. C., et al. "Is Mammography Painful?" *Archives of Internal Medicine* 148:521–524, 1988.

Stout, A. L., et al. "Premenstrual Symptoms in Black and White Community Samples." *American Journal of Psychiatry* 143:1436–1439, 1986.

Stovall, T. G.; Ling, F. W.; and Buster, J. E. "Outpatient Chemotherapy of Unruptured Ectopic Pregnancy." *Fertility & Sterility* 51:435–438, 1989.

Straus, S. E., et al. "Suppression of Frequently Recurring Genital Herpes: A Placebo-Controlled Double-Blind Trial of Oral

Acyclovir." *New England Journal of Medicine* 310:1545–1550, 1984.

———. "Herpes Simplex Virus Infections: Biology, Treatment, and Prevention." *Annals of Internal Medicine* 103:404–419, 1985.

———. "Acyclovir Suppression of Frequently Recurring Genital Herpes." *Journal of the American Medical Association* 260:2227–2230, 1988.

Streissguth, A. P.; Sampson, P.; and Barr, H. M. "Neurobehavioral Dose–Response Effects of Prenatal Alcohol Exposure in Humans from Infancy to Adulthood." *Annals of the New York Academy of Sciences* 562:145–158, 1989.

Stryker, J. "IV Drug Use and AIDS: Public Policy and Dirty Needles." *Journal of Health Politics, Policy and Law* 14:719–740, 1989.

Sullivan, J. M., et al. "Postmenopausal Estrogen Use and Coronary Atherosclerosis." *Annals of Internal Medicine* 108:358–363, 1988.

Sullivan-Bolyai, J., et al. "Neonatal Herpes Simplex Virus Infection in King County, Washington." *Journal of the American Medical Association* 250:3059–3062, 1983.

Sulloway, F. J. *Freud: Biologist of the Mind.* New York: Basic Books, 1979.

Sultan, F. E., and Chambles, D. L. "Pubococcygeal Function and Orgasm in a Normal Population." In Graber, B. (ed.), *Circumvaginal Musculature and Sexual Function,* pp. 74–87. New York: Karger, 1982.

Surgeon General, U.S. Public Health Service. *Surgeon General's Report on Acquired Immune Deficiency Syndrome.* Washington, DC: U.S. Government Printing Office, 1986.

Sussman, N. "Sex and Sexuality in History." In Sadock, B. J.; Kaplan, H. I.; and Freedman, A. M. (eds.), *The Sexual Experience,* pp. 7–70. Baltimore: Williams & Wilkins, 1976.

Szasz, G., and Carpenter, C. "Clinical Observations in Vibratory Stimulation of the Penis of Men with Spinal Cord Injury." *Archives of Sexual Behavior* 18:461–474, 1989.

Szasz, T. *Sex by Prescription.* New York: Anchor Press/Doubleday, 1980.

Tabar, L., et al. "Reduction in Mortality from Breast Cancer After Mass Screening with Mammography." *Lancet* 1:829–832, 1985.

Tam, M. R. "Culture-Independent Diagnosis of *Chlamydia trachomatis* Using Monoclonal Antibodies." *New England Journal of Medicine* 310:1146–1150, 1984.

Tamburello, A., and Seppecher, M. F. "The Effects of Depression on Sexual Behavior: Preliminary Results of Research." In Gemme, R., and Wheeler, C. C. (eds.), *Progress in Sexology,* pp. 107–128. New York: Plenum Press, 1977.

Tannahill, R. *Sex in History.* New York: Stein & Day. 1980.

Tanne, J. H. "The Last Word on Avoiding AIDS." *New York,* pp. 28–34, October 7, 1985.

Tanner, J. M. "Sequence and Tempo in the Somatic Changes in Puberty." In Grumbach, M. M.; Grave, G. D.; and Mayer, F. E. (eds.), *Control of the Onset of Puberty.* New York: Wiley, 1974.

Taylor, G. R. *Sex in History.* New York: Vanguard, 1954.

Tejada, I. S. D., et al. "Impaired Neurogenic and Endothelium-Mediated Relaxation of Penile Smooth Muscle from Diabetic Men with Impotence." *New England Journal of Medicine* 320:1025–1030, 1989.

Thin, R. N.; Leighton, M.; and Dixon, M. J. "How Often Is Genital Yeast Infection Sexually Transmitted?" *British Medical Journal* 2:93–94, 1977.

Thompson, M., and Schwartz, D. "Life Adjustment of Women with Anorexia Nervosa and Anorexia-like Behavior." *International Journal of Eating Disorders* 2:47–60, 1981.

Thompson, S. E., and Washington, A. E. "Epidemiology of Sexually Transmitted *Chlamydia trachomatis* Infections." *Epidemiology Review* 5:96–123, 1983.

Thornton, C. E. "Sexuality Counseling of Women with Spinal Cord Injuries." *Sexuality and Disability* 2:267–277, 1979.

Tietze, C. "Induced Abortion." In Money, J., and Musaph, H. (eds.), *Handbook of Sexology,* pp. 605–620. New York: Elsevier/North-Holland, 1977.

Tietze, C., and Lewit, S. "Legal Abortion." *Scientific American* 236:16, 21–27, 1977.

Todd, J., et al. "Toxic-Shock Syndrome Associated with Phage-Group-I Staphylococci." *Lancet* 2:1116–1118, 1978.

Todd, W. D., and Tapley, D. F. *The Columbia University College of Physicians and Surgeons Complete Guide to Pregnancy.* New York: Crown Publishers, 1988.

Tolor, A., and DiGrazia, P. V. "Sexual Attitudes and Behavior Patterns During and Following Pregnancy." *Archives of Sexual Behavior* 5:539–551, 1976.

Tong, S. M.; Zhou, X. H.; and Zhou, Y. X. "Human Antifertility Effect on Gossypol: Cytologic Observation of Semen." *Chinese Medical Journal* 95(5):355–362, May 1982.

Trause, M. A.; Kennell, J.; and Klaus, M. "Parental Attachment Behavior." In Money, J., and Musaph, H. (eds.), *Handbook of Sexology,* pp. 789–799. New York: Elsevier/North-Holland, 1977.

Treiman, K., and Liskin, L. "IUDS—A New Look." *Population Reports,* Series B, No. 5, March 1988.

Trudel, G., and Saint Laurent, S. "A Comparison Between the Effects of Kegel's Exercises and a Combination of Sexual Awareness Relaxation and Breathing on Situational Orgasmic Dysfunction in Women." *Journal of Sex & Marital Therapy* 9:204–209, 1983.

Trussell, J., and Grummer-Strawn, L. "Contraceptive Failure of the Ovulation Method of Periodic Abstinence." *Family Planning Perspectives* 22:65–75, 1990.

Trussell, J., and Westoff, C. F. "Contraceptive Practice and Trends in Coital Frequency." *Family Planning Perspectives* 12:246–249, 1980.

Tsuang, M. T. "Hypersexuality in Man Patients." *Medical Aspects of Human Sexuality* 9(11):83–89, 1975.

Tucker, J., et al. "HTLV-III Infection Associated with Glandular-Fever-like Illness in a Hemophiliac." *Lancet* 1:585, 1985.

Turner, B. F., and Adams, C. G. "Reported Change in Preferred Adult Sexual Activity Over the Adult Years." *Journal of Sex Research* 25:289–303, 1988.

Turner, C. F.; Miller, H. G.; and Moses, L. E., eds. *AIDS: Sexual Behavior and Intravenous Drug Use.* Washington, DC: National Academy Press, 1989.

Udry, J. R., and Cliquet, R. L. "A Cross-Cultural Examination of the Relationship Between Ages at Menarche, Marriage, and First Birth." *Demography* 19:53–63, 1982.

Udry, J. R., and Morris, N. "Distribution of Coitus in the Menstrual Cycle." *Nature* 220:593–596, 1968.

———. "Effect of Contraceptive Pills on the Distribution of Sexuality Activity in the Menstrual Cycle." *Nature* 227:502–503, 1970.

Unger, R. K. "Toward a Redefinition of Sex and Gender." *American Psychologist* 34(11):1085–1094, 1979.

U.S. Department of Health, Education, and Welfare. *Age at Menarche in the United States.* DHEW Publication No. (HRA)74:1615, p. 3, 1973.

U.S. Public Health Service. *Mood Disorders: Pharmacologic Prevention of Recurrence.* Washington, DC: Department of Health and Human Services, Public Health Service Monograph Vol. 5, No. 4, 1986.

———. "Public Health Service Plan for the Prevention and Control of AIDS and the AIDS Virus." Report of the Coolfont Planning Conference, June 4–6, 1986.

Upton, G. V. "Lipids, Cardiovascular Disease, and Oral Contraceptives: A Practice Perspective." *Fertility & Sterility* 53:1–12, 1990.

Utian, W. H. "Effect of Hysterectomy, Oophorectomy and Estrogen Therapy on Libido." *International Journal of Obstetrics and Gynaecology* 13:97–100, 1975.

Utian, W. H., et al. "Successful Pregnancy After in Vitro Fertilization and Embryo Transfer from an Infertile Woman to a Surrogate." *New England Journal of Medicine* 313:1351–1352, 1985.

van Griesven, G. J. P., et al. "Effect of Human Immunodeficiency Virus (HIV) Antibody Knowledge on High-Risk Sexual Behavior with Steady and Nonsteady Sexual Partners Among Homosexual Men." *American Journal of Epidemiology* 129:596–603, 1989.

Van Thiel, D. H. "Testicular Atrophy and Other Endocrine Changes in Alcoholic Men." *Medical Aspects of Human Sexuality* 10(6):153–154, 1976.

Vermund, S. H., et al. "Acquired Immunodeficiency Syndrome Among Adolescents." *American Journal of Diseases of Children* 143:1220–1225, 1989.

Vessey, M., and Wiggins, P. "Use-Effectiveness of the Diaphragm in a Selected Family Planning Clinic Population in the United Kingdom." *Contraception* 9:15–21, 1974.

Vessey, M., et al. "Outcome of Pregnancy in Women Using Intrauterine Device." *Lancet* 1:495–498, 1974.

———. "Fertility After Stopping Different Methods of Contraception." *British Medical Journal* 1:265–267, 1978.

Vessey, M.; Lawless, M.; and Yeates, D. "Efficacy of Different Contraceptive Methods." *Lancet* 1(8276):841–842, 1982.

Vessey, M. P. "Oral Contraceptives and Breast Cancer." *International Planned Parenthood Federation Medical Bulletin* 21(6):1–2, 1987.

Vessey, M. P., et al. "Pelvic Inflammatory Disease and the Intrauterine Device." *British Medical Journal* 282(6267):855–857, 1981.

Vittecoq, D., et al. "Acute HIV Infection After Acupuncture Treatment." *New England Journal of Medicine* 320:250–251, 1989.

Voeller, B. "Persistent Condom Breakage." Presented at the Fifth International Conference on AIDS, Montreal, June 4–9, 1989. (Abstract W.A.P. 99, p. 136)

Voeller, Bruce. Personal communication, November 1986.

Voger, F. T. "Sex Life of American Indians." In Ellis, A., and Abarbanel, A. (eds.), *The Encyclopedia of Sexual Behavior,* pp. 90–109. New York: Hawthorn Books, 1961.

Volberding, P. A. "The Clinical Spectrum of Acquired Immunodeficiency Syndrome: Implications for Comprehensive Patient Care." *Annals of Internal Medicine* 103:729–733, 1985.

Volberding, P. A., et al. "Zidovudine in Asymptomatic Human Immunodeficiency Virus Infection." *New England Journal of Medicine* 322:941–949, 1990.

Vollman, R. F. *The Menstrual Cycle.* Philadelphia: Saunders, 1977.

Vontver, L. A., et al. "Recurrent Genital Herpes Simplex Virus Infection in Pregnancy: Infant Outcome and Frequency of Asymptomatic Recurrences." *American Journal of Obstetrics and Gynecology* 143:75–81, 1982.

Wallace, J. I.; Mann, J.; and Beatrice, S. "HIV-1 Exposure Among Clients of Prostitutes." Fifth International Conference on AIDS, Stockholm, June 12–16, 1988.

Walsh, R. N., et al. "The Menstrual Cycle, Sex and Academic Performance." *Archives of General Psychiatry* 38:219–221, 1981.

Ward, J. W., et al. "Transmission of Human Immunodeficiency Virus (HIV) by Blood Transfusions Screened as Negative for HIV Antibody." *New England Journal of Medicine* 318:473–478, 1988.

Washton, A. M. "Cocaine Abuse and Compulsive Sexuality." *Medical Aspects of Human Sexuality* 23(12):32–39, December 1989.

Wasow, M., and Loeb, M. "Sexuality in Nursing Homes." *Journal of the American Geriatrics Society* 27:73–79, 1979.

Waterman, C. K., and Chiauzzi, E. J. "The Role of Orgasm in Male and Female Sexual Enjoyment." *Journal of Sex Research* 18:146–159, 1982.

Watkins, R. N. "Vaginal Spermicides and Congenital Disorders: The Validity of a Study." *Journal of the American Medical Association* 256:3095, 1986.

Webster, S. K.; Bauman, J. E.; and Kolodny, R. C. "The Biochemistry of Dysmenorrhea: Failure to Validate the Distinction Between Spasmodic and Congestive Dysmenorrhea." Presented at the First Dysmenorrhea Symposium, St. Louis University, St. Louis, MO, 1978.

Weideger, P. *Menstruation and Menopause,* rev. ed. New York: Delta Books, 1977.

Weiss, H. D. "The Physiology of Human Penile Erection." *Annals of Internal Medicine* 76:793–799, 1972.

Weiss, N. S., and Sayvetz, T. A. "Incidence of Endometrial Cancer in Relation to the Use of Oral Contraceptives." *New England Journal of Medicine* 302:551–554, 1980.

Weiss, S. H. "Links Between Cocaine and Retroviral Infection." *Journal of American Medical Association* 261:607–609, 1989.

Weitz, C. M. "Vaginal Birth After Cesarean Section." *Postgraduate Obstetrics and Gynecology* 5(11):1–4, 1985.

Wellisch, D. K.; Jamison, K. R.; and Pasnau, R. O. "Psychosocial Aspects of Mastectomy, II: The Man's Perspective." *American Journal of Psychiatry* 135:543–546, 1978.

Wertz, R. W., and Wertz, D. C. *Lying-in: A History of Childbirth in America*. New York: Free Press, 1977.

Wesson, D. R. "Cocaine Use by Masseuses." *Journal of Psychoactive Drugs* 14:75–76, 1982.

Westoff, C. F., and McCarthy, J. "Sterilization in the United States." *Family Planning Perspectives* 11:147–152, 1979.

Wharton, C., and Blackburn, R. "Lower-Dose Pills." *Population Reports,* Series A, No. 7, November, 1988.

Wickware, F. S. "Report on the Kinsey Report." *Life* 25:86–90, August 2, 1948.

Wilcox, A. J., et al. "Incidence of Early Loss of Pregnancy." *New England Journal of Medicine* 319:189–194, 1988.

Wilcox, D., and Hager, R. "Toward Realistic Expectation for Orgasmic Response in Women." *Journal of Sex Research* 16:162–179, 1980.

Wilson, G. T., and Lawson, D. M. "Effects of Alcohol on Sexual Arousal in Women." *Journal of Abnormal Psychology* 85:489–497, 1976.

———. "Effects of Alcohol on Sexual Arousal in Male Alcoholics." *Journal of Abnormal Psychology* 87:609–616, 1978.

Wilson, J.; George, F.; and Griffin, J. "The Hormonal Control of Sexual Development." *Science* 211(4488):1278–1284, 1981.

Wilson, J. D. "Androgen Abuse by Athletes." *Endocrine Reviews* 9:181–199, 1988.

Wilson, J. G. "Embryotoxicity of Drugs in Man." In Wilson, J. G., and Fraser, F. C. (eds.), *Handbook Teratology,* Vol. 1: *General Principles and Etiology,* pp. 209–255. New York: Plenum Press, 1977.

Winder, A., and Winder, B. "Patient Counseling: Clarifying a Woman's Choice for Breast Reconstruction." *Patient Education and Counseling* 7:65–75, 1985.

Wing, J. K., and Bebbington, P. "Epidemiology of Depression." In Beckham, E. E., and Leber, W. R. (eds.), *Handbook of Depression,* pp. 765–794. Homewood, IL: Dorsey Press, 1985.

Winkelstein, W., Jr., et al. "Selected Sexual Practices of San Francisco Heterosexual Men and Risk of Infection by the Human Immunodeficiency Virus." *Journal of the American Medical Association* 257:1470–1471, 1987.

Winkenwerder, W., Kessler, A. R., and Stolec, R. M. "Federal Spending for Illness Caused by the Human Immunodeficiency Virus." *New England Journal of Medicine* 320:1598–1603, 1989.

Wissell, T. E., et al. "Declining Frequency of Circumcision: Implications for Changes in the Absolute Incidence and Male to Female Sex Ratio of Urinary Tract Infections in Early Infancy." *Pediatrics* 79:338–342, 1987.

Witkin, M. H. "Sex Therapy and Mastectomy." *Journal of Sex & Marital Therapy* 1:290–304, 1975.

Wofsy, C. B., et al. "Isolation of AIDS-Associated Retrovirus from Genital Secretions of Women with Antibodies to the Virus." *Lancet* 1:527–529, 1986.

Wolner-Hanssen, P., et al. "Association Between Vaginal Douching and Acute Pelvic Inflammatory Disease." *Journal of the American Medical Association* 263:1936–1941, 1990.

Wolpe, J. *Psychotherapy by Reciprocal Inhibition.* Stanford, CA: Stanford University Press, 1958.

———. *The Practice of Behavior Therapy.* Oxford: Pergamon, 1969.

Woods, S. M. "Sexuality and Mental Disorders." In Lief, H. L. (ed.), *Sexual Problems in Medical Practice,* pp. 199–209. Chicago: American Medical Association, 1981.

Working Group on the Very Low Birth Weight Infant. "European Community Collaborative Study of Pregnancy Between 22 and 28 Weeks' Gestation." *Lancet* 336:782–784, 1990.

World Health Organization. *Special Programme of Research, Development and Research Training: Seventh Annual Report.* Geneva: WHO, November 1978.

———. "A Prospective Multicentre Trial of the Ovulation Method of Natural Family Planning II: The Effectiveness Phase." *Fertility & Sterility* 36:591–598, 1981.

Wortman, J. "Vasectomy: What Are the Problems?" *Population Reports,* Series D(2), January 1975.

Wortman, J., and Piotrow, P. T. "Laparoscopic Sterilization, II: What Are the Problems?" *Population Reports,* Series C(2), March 1973.

Wright, N. H., et al. "Neoplasia and Dysplasia of the Cervix Uteri and Contraception: A Possible Protective Effect of the Diaphragm." *British Journal of Cancer* 38(2):273–279, August 1978.

Wyngaarden, J. B. "Identifying Factors That Reactivate Herpes Simplex Virus." *Journal of the American Medical Association* 259:1922, 1988.

Yalom, I. D.; Green, R.; and Fisk, N. "Prenatal Exposure to Female Hormones." *Archives of General Psychiatry* 28:554–561, 1973.

Zacharias, L., and Wurtman, R. J. "Age at Menarche: Genetic and Environmental Influences." *New England Journal of Medicine* 280:868–875, 1969.

Zarutskie, P. W., et al. "The Clinical Relevance of Sex Selection Techniques." *Fertility & Sterility* 52:891–905, 1989.

Zeiss, A. M. "Expectation for the Effects of Aging on Sexuality in Parents and Average Married Couples." *Journal of Sex Research* 18:47–57, 1982.

Zelnick, M., and Kantner, J. F. "Reasons for Nonuse of Contraception by Sexually Active Women Aged 15–19." *Family Planning Perspectives* 11:289–296, 1979.

Ziegler, J. B., et al. "Postnatal Transmission of AIDS-associated Retrovirus from Mother to Infant." *Lancet* 1:896–898, 1985.

Zilbergeld, B. *Male Sexuality: A Guide to Sexual Fulfillment.* Boston: Little, Brown, 1978.

———. "Alternatives to Couples Counseling for Sex Problems: Group and Individual Therapy." *Journal of Sex & Marital Therapy* 6(1):3–18, 1980.

Zilbergeld, B., and Evans, M. "The Inadequacy of Masters and Johnson." *Psychology Today* 14:29–43, 1980.

Ziporyn, T. "Search for Male Contraceptive Complicated by Adverse Effects." *Journal of the American Medical Association* 252:1101–1103, 1984.

Zorgniotti, A. W., et al. "Auto-injection of the Corpus Cavernosum with a Vasoactive Drug Combination for Vasculogenic Impotence." *Journal of Urology* 133:39–41, 1985.

Zuckerman, A. J. "Viral Hepatitis." *Practical Gastroenterology* 6(6):16, 21–27, November/December 1982.

Zuckerman, B., et al. "Effects of Maternal Marijuana and Cocaine Use on Fetal Growth." *New England Journal of Medicine* 320:762–768, 1989.

Zussman, J. U.; Zussman, P. P.; and Dalton, K. K. "Postpubertal Effect of Prenatal Administration of Progesterone." Paper presented at the Society for Research in Child Development, Denver, April 1975.

———. Abstract, Third Annual Meeting of the International Academy of Sex Research, Bloomington, IN, 1977.

Zussman, L., et al. "Sexual Response After Hysterectomyoophorectomy: Recent Studies and Reconsideration of Psychogenesis. *American Journal of Obstetrics and Gynecology* 140:725–729, 1981.

Zwerner, J. "Sexual Issues of Women with Spinal Cord Injury." *Sexuality and Disability* 5:158–171, 1982.

Photo Credits

Chapter 1 p. 3 (top left), Jerry Howard/Positive Images; (top right), Eli Reed/ Magnum Photos; (center), Jim Whitmer; (bottom left), Michael O'Brien; (bottom right), Joel Gordon Photography. p. 9 (top left), Art Resource, NY; (top right), The Bettmann Archive; (bottom), Art Resource, NY. p. 10, The Bettmann Archive. p. 13, The Bettmann Archive. p. 14, The Bettmann Archive.

Chapter 3 p. 61, Norman Hurst/Stock Boston. p. 70, 1990 Gail Machlis.

Chapter 4 p. 76, Dr. Landrum B. Shettles. p. 79, Photri, Inc. p. 80, Photri, Inc. p. 82, Photri, Inc. p. 84, Custom Medical Stock Photo. All Rights Reserved. p. 91, Susan Lapides/Design Conceptions. p. 94, S.I.U./Peter Arnold, Inc. p. 98, Jerry Howard/Stock Boston.

Chapter 5 p. 124, Frank Siteman. p. 127, Scott, Foresman. p. 128, Frank Siteman. p. 132, Population Reports, Population Information Program. p. 134, Frank Siteman. p. 137, Scott, Foresman. p. 139, Scott, Foresman.

Chapter 6 p. 163, Courtesy, Clifford C. Synder, M.D. p. 167, Donald Dietz/Stock Boston, p. 174, Mary Ellen Mark/Archive Pictures Inc. p. 198, Ken Green/Visuals Unlimited.

Chapter 7 p. 192, From Herbert Blough, "Successful Treatment of Human Genital Herpes Infections," JOURNAL OF THE AMERICAN MEDICAL ASSOCIATION 241:279–281, 1979, p. 279, figure 2, copyright 1979 American Medical Association. p. 196 (all), Lippincott, From *Sexually Transmitted Diseases,* by David Barlow, photographed by Tom Treasure, Published by Oxford University Press. © 1979 David Barlow.

Chapter 8 p. 218 (left), Michael J. Okoniewski/The Image Works; (right), Courtesy, The Center for Attitudinal Healing, Tiburon, CA. p. 219, Bob Daemmrich/The Image Works. p. 224, Bob Mahoney/Picture Group, p. 227, G. Schachmes/Sygma. p. 233, James D. Wilson/Woodfin Camp & Associates. p. 242 (top left), Liane Enkelis/Stock Boston; (bottom left), Shahn Kerami/Gamma-Liaison; (right), Courtesy, San Francisco AIDS Foundation & Haight-Ashbury Free Clinics, Inc., with the generous financial support of the Herman Goldman Foundation. Photography by Warwick May.

Chapter 9 p. 263 (all), Scott F. Johnson. p. 264, Frank Siteman.

Chapter 10 p. 277 (top left), Abraham Menaske/Photo Researchers; (top right), Even Johnson/Jeroboam Inc.; (bottom), Joel Gordon Photography. p. 228, Betty Medsger. p. 281, Ellis Herwig/The Picture Cube. p. 285, Courtesy, American Cancer Society. p. 289. Lincoln Russell/ Stock Boston.

Color Insert: Human Conception and Development

Plate 1, Photo 1 M. Abbey/Photo Researchers, Inc.

Plate 1, Photo 2 Dr. G. Schatten/Photo Researchers, Inc.

Plate 1, Photo 3 Dr. Sue Sundstrom/Gamma-Liaison

Plate 1, Photo 4 Dr. Sue Sundstrom/Gamma-Liaison

Plate 2, Photo 5 © Petit Format-Nestle/Science Source/ Photo Researchers, Inc.

Plate 2, Photo 6 © Lennart Nilsson, from *A Child Is Born* (New York: Dell, 1977, p. 41), Courtesy Bonnier Fakta.

Plate 2, Photo 7 © Lennart Nilsonn, from *A Child is Born* (New York: Dell, 1977, p. 81), Courtesy Bonnier Fakta.

Plate 3, Photo 8 © Lennart Nilsson, from *A Child Is Born* (New York: Dell, 1977, p. 96), Courtesy Bonnier Fakta.

Plate 3, Photo 9 © Lennart Nilsson, from *A Child Is Born* (New York: Dell, 1977, p. 96), Courtesy Bonnier Fakta.

Plate 3, Photo 10 © Petit Format-Nestle/Science Source/ Photo Researchers, Inc.

Plate 4, Photo 11 Courtesy Dr. Landrum B. Shettles.

Plate 4, Photo 12 © Lennart Nilsson, from *A Child Is Born* (New York: Dell, 1977, p. 117), Courtesy Bonnier Fakta.

Plate 4, Photo 13 © Petit Format-Nestle/Science Source/ Photo Researchers, Inc.

Color Insert: Sexually Transmitted Diseases

Plate 5, Photo 1 Centers for Disease Control, Atlanta.
Plate 5, Photo 2 Massachusetts Department of Public Health.
Plate 6, Photo 3 National Institutes of Health.
Plate 6, Photo 4 Centers for Disease Control, Atlanta.
Plate 6, Photo 5 Centers for Disease Control, Atlanta.
Plate 6, Photo 6 Peter Arnold, Inc.
Plate 7, Photo 7 Zeva Delbaum/Peter Arnold, Inc.
Plate 7, Photo 8 Centers for Disease Control, Atlanta.
Plate 8, Photo 10 Centers for Disease Control, Atlanta.

Color Insert: HIV and AIDS

Plate 9, Photo 1 From *AIDS IN 1988,* by Robert C. Gallo. © 1988 Scientific American, Inc. All rights reserved. October 1988, Vol. 259, No. 4, page 43, illustrations by George V. Kelvin/Science Graphics.
Plate 10, Photo 2 Adapted from drawing by Ina Worpole, from *HIV INFECTION: THE CLINICAL PICTURES,* by Robert R. Redfield and Donald S. Burke, October 1988. Copyright © 1988 by Scientific American, Inc. All rights reserved.
Plate 11, Photo 3 Adapted from drawing by Hank Iken from *AIDS THERAPIES,* by Robert Yarchoan, Hiroaki Mitsuya, and Samuel Broader, October 1988. Copyright © 1988 by Scientific American, Inc. All rights reserved.
Plate 11, Photo 4 Lennart Nilsson/Boehringer Ingelheim International GmbH.
Plate 12, Photo 5 Laurie Burnham.
Plate 12, Photo 6 Alon Reininger/Contact Press Images/ Woodfin Camp & Associates.
Plate 12, Photo 7 David Burnett/Contact Press Images/ Woodfin Camp & Associates.

Index

Note: Page numbers followed by *n* indicate material in notes.